25. Colloquium der Gesellschaft für Biologische Chemie

25. Colloquium
der Gesellschaft für Biologische Chemie,
25.—27. April 1974 in Mosbach / Baden

Biochemistry
of Sensory Functions

Edited by L. Jaenicke

With 288 Figures

Springer-Verlag New York Heidelberg Berlin 1974

Professor Dr. L. JAENICKE, Institut für Biochemie der Universität Köln, D-5000 Köln, An der Bottmühle 2/Federal Republic of Germany

ISBN 0-387-07038-9 Springer-Verlag New York · Heidelberg · Berlin
ISBN 3-540-07038-9 Springer-Verlag Berlin · Heidelberg · New York

Library of Congress Cataloging in Publication Data. Gesellschaft für Biologische Chemie. Biochemistry of sensory functions. English or German. Includes index. 1. Senses and sensation—Congresses. 2. Biological chemistry—Congresses. I. Jaenicke, Lothar, 1923-ed. II. Title. [DNLM: 1. Neurochemistry—Congresses. 2. Sense organs—Physiology—Congresses. WL700 M894b 1974]. QP431. G5 1974. 591.1'82. 74-23671.

Typesetting, Printing and Binding: Brühlsche Universitätsdruckerei, Gießen

Preface

This volume contains the Proceedings of the 25th Mosbach Colloquium, the general theme of which is the *Biochemistry of Sensory Functions*. It was intended, continuing the silver-tradition of these Colloquia, to provide the uninitiated biochemist with an insight into the current status of a line of research in Molecular Biology which, more than many other fields in Biochemistry, has maintained its contacts with and respect for Physiology.

The speakers were asked to attempt to outline their topic sufficiently to define the fundamentals and to build up upon this basis the more sophisticated details of their own studies. It is for the reader to evaluate how well both organizer and participants have attained this end[1]. These Proceedings not only mirror the hubs around which several groups of scientists wheel but may also serve as a source of literature references and for the advanced student as an introduction to this highly up-to-date branch of Biochemistry, although no index is provided as the table of contents is considered sufficient to locate most of the sought-for information.

Kind words were spoken on occasion of this symposium — much to the pleasure of the receiving end. They have nevertheless been left unrecorded to save space for the additional hard facts that were chiseled out during the discussions. However, I do not want to forget to thank here everyone who helped to make this 25th Mosbach Colloquium an event worthy of praise.

Unfortunately, in spite of great efforts on the part of the editor, Dr. WALD failed to submit the manuscript of his excellent review.

---

[1] English speaking readers may find themselves irritated now and then or even harassed by occasional idiomatic peculiarities. At such times some German may help.

This omission, of course, detracts from the intended value of the work. However, I had to consider that if reports had appeared at a later date their expected usefulness would have been lessened. I had therefore to compromise — it is hoped to the satisfaction of the readers of this book!

Köln, October 1974   L. JAENICKE

Contents

Photoreception

Chemoreception

Energy Transfer and Signal Conversion

Neurotransmission

Biochemistry of Learning Processes

Prologue: Opening Remarks on Occasion of the 25th Mosbach Colloquium

This is the 25th Mosbach Colloquium sponsored by the Gesellschaft für Biologische Chemie. Anniversaries usually commemorate important landmarks in the history of science. This is not the case here; but nevertheless a few words seem appropriate on this occasion. The first Mosbach Colloquium was held in 1950. It signified, like the foundation of our society about a year earlier, a new beginning in a democratic German society. The preceding catastrophe had destroyed millions of human lives and irreparably damaged our scientific tradition and reputation. Among the scientific disciplines the relatively new fields of biochemistry and biochemical genetics had suffered most under political repression and racial persecution, which led to Germany's virtually complete isolation from the world scientific community. It was therefore indeed a memorable event when some of the leading German biochemists, among them OTTO WARBURG, assembled here in Mosbach together with their students for the first time, 25 years ago. But the man who deserves most of the credit for bringing the Mosbach Colloquia into existence was the late KURT FELIX, Professor of Physiological Chemistry at the University of Frankfurt. Uppermost in the mind of the Founding Fathers was the hope to reestablish international connections in order to gain information on developments in biochemical research, which were either unknown in Germany or only known by hearsay. This was understandable because in the intervening years some most important concepts and techniques had been developed, and these had revolutionized biochemistry. During the time when darkness fell upon Germany, the center of gravity in biochemical research had shifted to the United States: AVERY, MacLEOD and McCARTHY did their transformation experiments, establishing DNA rather than protein as the principal component of the gene. BEADLE and TATUM formulated the one gene-one enzyme hypothesis. FRITZ LIPMANN created the idea of phosphoryl group transfer potentials and discovered CoA. The CORIS described, for the first time, the synthesis of a macromolecule, glycogen, *in vitro*, and HERMAN KALCKAR and others quantitized oxidative phosphorylation. The first antibiotics had been discovered and changed medicine, liberating mankind from the scourge of bacterial infections. Isotopic tracers facilitated the study of intermediary metabolism. These, to name only a few, were among the biochemical news of that time. We, who had just begun to study biochemistry, heard of these and other developments overseas for the first time here in Mosbach. For us, the young adepts, the early Mosbach Colloquia were certainly among the most formative influences.

The special character of these early Mosbach Colloquia has survived to this day. This has never been a symposium or a workshop for a select few. It is still a meeting with a remarkably heterogeneous audience, to which biochemists of very different creeds come to get first-hand information from the best experts on recent developments in very divergent fields. Another remarkable feature, which also has survived despite the exponential growth of population, technology and industry with its mostly undesirable consequences for the natural environment, is the peaceful and quaint character of the medieval city of Mosbach and the unspoiled beauty of its countryside, which casts its spell on every visitor, letting us forget for a few days the hectic aspects of life in our times. Therefore I wish to express our gratitude to the *Bürgermeister* and the *Rat der Stadt Mosbach* for their hospitality and for the special consideration which they have always given to the wishes of our society and to the needs of the Mosbach Colloquia. Thanks to the cooperation of Springer-Verlag, and to Dr. MAYER-KAUPP, who until his recent retirement supervised as, editor in chief for the last 25 years the publication of the Mosbach Colloquia, but especially thanks to the efforts of his successor, Dr. HARALD WIEBKING, I can present to the library of the city of Mosbach a complete collection of all the Mosbach Colloquia, some of which are out of print and which will soon include the 25th. With this gift on the occasion of the 25th anniversary of the Mosbach Colloquia we wish to show our appreciation for the decision of the *Stadtrat* of Mosbach to spend a considerable sum of money on remodelling and modernizing the *Markthalle* fitting it out for future Mosbach Colloquia.

But certainly the focal point in commemorating the 25th anniversary of the Mosbach Colloquia is the Meeting itself, which was held in Mosbach from 24th to 27th April 1974. Thanks to the unusual commitment, the enthusiasm and the hard work which our colleague LOTHAR JAENICKE has devoted to the organization of the "Jubilee" Colloquium, and thanks to the contributions of very distinguished guests from the United States and Europe, the Anniversary Colloquium fits the occasion. It is a representative report on some of the most significant developments in one of the most exciting fields of biology. This meeting more than anything else sets an example of the spirit of the Mosbach Colloquia which is worth remembering. This we owe to the speakers and the discussants, and to Dr. LOTHAR JAENICKE who made it all possible.

Ernst J.M. HELMREICH
Chairman
Gesellschaft für Biologische Chemie

Photoreception

Biochemistry of Visual Pigments in Relation to Visual Excitation

S. L. Bonting and F. J. M. Daemen

Dept. of Biochemistry, University of Nijmegen, Nijmegen, The Netherlands

With 12 Figures

Introduction

The visual mechanism in the vertebrate rod photoreceptor cell involves one key substance, the visual pigment rhodopsin, and two key structures, the photoreceptor membrane and the outer membrane of the rod cell. Figure 1 is a schematic drawing of a vertebrate rod, showing from top to bottom: the outer segment with numerous rod sacs, the narrow cilium leading to the inner segment with mitochondria, endoplasmatic reticulum, nucleus and the synapse with the bipolar cells.

The visual mechanism begins with the absorption of a photon by a molecule of rhodopsin, located in the rod sac membrane or photoreceptor membrane, which eventually leads to the excitation of the synapse and the generation of a nerve impulse which travels to the brain. Between light absorption and synaptic stimulation a series of chemical and physical processes takes place, lasting about 100 msec.

The crucial questions to be answered are: what happens to the visual pigment, and what happens in the photoreceptor and outer membranes? This paper will be restricted entirely to the visual mechanism of the vertebrate rod, while Hubbard and Stieve will deal with invertebrate systems, and Oesterhelt will discuss comparative aspects of light-sensitive retinaldehyde-protein complexes in vertebrates, invertebrates and bacteria.

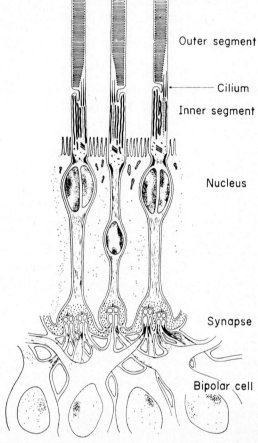

Outer segment

Cilium

Inner segment

Nucleus

Synapse

Bipolar cell

Fig. 1. Structure of vertebrate rod photoreceptor cell

Properties of Rhodopsin

Rhodopsin consists of a protein (opsin) and a chromophoric group (retinaldehyde). It has two characteristic properties: 1. its typical absorption spectrum, 2. its photosensitivity.

Before illumination the absorption spectrum has three absorption peaks, the α-peak at 500 nm, the β-peak around 340 nm and the high γ-peak at 278 nm (Fig. 2, solid line). The α- and β-peaks

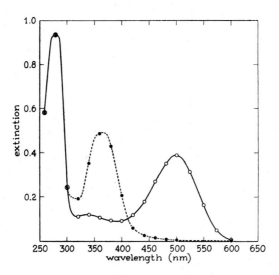

Fig. 2. Absorption spectrum of rhodopsin

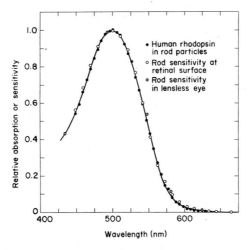

Fig. 3. Agreement between the difference spectrum of human rhodopsin and human scotopic visibility curve at the retinal surface or in the lensless eye. [From WALD and BROWN (1958)]

are due to the chromophore, the γ-peak to the opsin. Upon illumination the α-peak disappears, and one at 380 nm (or 360 nm in the presence of NH_2OH) appears, leading to the absorption spectrum indicated by the dotted line in Fig. 2. This drastic change in absorption spectrum upon illumination causes a color change from red purple to pale yellow ("bleaching"). The accompanying drop in 500 nm absorbance is used to determine the amount of rhodopsin present, its molar absorbance at this wavelength being 40 300 (DAEMEN et al., 1970; ROTMANS et al., 1972; DAEMEN et al., 1972).

Proof that rhodopsin is the key substance of rod vision was obtained by WALD (WALD, 1938; WALD and BROWN, 1958) from the close agreement between the human rhodopsin absorption spectrum and the human scotopic visibility curve (Fig. 3).

Structure of the Rod Cell

The rod outer segment develops from a primitive cilium to an organelle containing 500—2000 regularly stacked sacs or disks (DE ROBERTIS, 1960). Simultaneously with the formation of the sacs, the visual pigment rhodopsin appears (BONTING et al., 1961). All sacs appear to be separate from each other and all but the bottom few are closed and separate from the outer membrane. Autoradiographic studies have shown that the sacs are formed continuously at the bottom through invagination of the outer membrane and then move up to the top in about 10 days in warm-blooded vertebrates (YOUNG, 1867, 1971). Then they are shed in groups of 8—30 and removed through phagocytic action of the overlying pigment epithelium.

The inner segment contains the metabolic machinery of the cell for biosynthesis and energy metabolism. Here the major building blocks of the photoreceptor membrane, opsin and phospholipids are prefabricated and sent through the cilium to the base of the outer segment, where they are incorporated into the membrane of the newly formed sacs.

The regular stacking of the sacs in the mature rod outer segment permits X-ray diffraction studies of the photoreceptor membrane. Results of such studies (*e.g.* BLASIE, 1972) indicate a structure as shown in Fig. 4 for this membrane. Confirmation of this basic structure has been obtained from chemical analysis and from freeze-cleavage electronmicroscopy (*e.g.* OLIVE and BENEDETTI, 1974). Immunofluorescent and tracer studies have shown that rhodopsin is located in the photoreceptor membrane (DEWEY et al., 1966; HALL et al., 1969). It appears to be embedded on one side of the membrane, most likely the outer side.

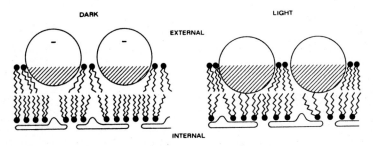

Fig. 4. Structure of rod sac membrane as derived from chemical and X-ray diffraction studies. Large circles represent rhodopsin molecules, immersed for $\frac{1}{3}$ before and for $\frac{1}{2}$ after illumination in the phospholipid layer, as suggested by BLASIE (1972)

Isolation and Composition of Photoreceptor Membranes

Mild homogenization of the retina breaks off the rod outer segments at the cilium. Centrifugation of the suspension in a sucrose density gradient (1 hr, $27\,000 \times g$, $10°$ C) yields a heavy sediment and two layers. The upper, purple layer contains the rod outer segments. In the case of cattle eyes obtained from the slaughter house an appreciable part of the pigment is in the bleached state, particularly in the summer season (Fig. 5, open bars). Treatment of the purple layer with excess 11-*cis*-retinaldehyde regenerates the bleached pigment, leading to a maximal and reproducible rhodopsin yield (8.3 ± 0.1 nmol per mg dry membrane preparation; shaded bars, Fig. 5) throughout the year (DE GRIP et al., 1972). Aqueous suspensions of such enriched photoreceptor membranes offer several advantages over detergent-solubilized rhodopsin preparations for the study of visual pigment properties (BONTING et al., 1974).

The chemical composition of the photoreceptor membranes is presented in Table 1. Lipid extraction with chloroform-methanol,

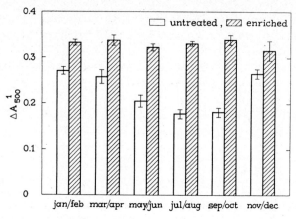

Fig. 5. Seasonal effects and effects of enrichment on rhodopsin content

followed by quantitative thin layer chromatography yields the phospholipid pattern, while fatty acids are determined by gas chromatography (BORGGREVEN et al.,1970). Protein and cholesterol are determined colorimetrically.

Striking features are the high phospholipid content, the low cholesterol content and the high content of unsaturated fatty acids

Table 1. Chemical composition of lyophilized photoreceptor membrane

Protein		38%
rhodopsin protein	85%	
Lipids		50%[a]
phosphatidyl ethanolamine	34%	
phosphatidyl choline	30%	
phosphatidyl serine	11%	
other phospholipids	15%	
cholesterol	6%	
other lipids	4%	
Carbohydrates		2%
Water		6%
Unknown		4%
		100%

[a] Fatty acids: unsaturated 52%, incl. 34% C22 : 6.

(esp. C22 : 6). This indicates a highly fluid lipid bilayer, which is in agreement with the calculation by CONE (1972) that its viscosity is equal to that of olive oil.

Of the total membrane protein 85% is rhodopsin (DAEMEN et al., 1972), in agreement with which sodium dodecylsulfate gel electrophoresis yields only one major band. The molecular weight, derived from gel electrophoresis and from amino acid analysis of detergent-extracted rhodopsin, is 39000 (DAEMEN et al., 1972). These studies also prove that one chromophoric group is present per rhodopsin molecule.

Rhodopsin and the Lipid Bilayer

Treatment of an aqueous suspension of photoreceptor membranes with the phospholipid splitting enzymes phospholipase C and A removes over 95% of the phospholipids with little effect on the rhodopsin content and its spectral properties (BORGGREVEN et al., 1971, 1972). The regeneration capacity of the rhodopsin in the delipidated preparation remains for 70% intact under suitable conditions.

This relatively easy and complete removal of phospholipids from the membrane fits with the membrane structure shown in Fig. 4. Since the residual contents of the amino group containing phospholipids phosphatidylethanolamine and phosphatidylserine are only 0.1 mole per mole chromophore (Fig. 6), these compounds cannot be the binding site for the chromophore in native rhodopsin (see also: DAEMEN et al., 1971).

These findings indicate that there is little association between rhodopsin and the phospholipids in the membrane. This is confirmed by the finding that the rhodopsin molecules rotate freely and rapidly (rotation time 20 µsec) in the plane of the membrane (BROWN, 1972; CONE, 1972), and that they also diffuse in this plane with a molecular velocity of 0.3 µm/sec (LIEBMAN and ENTINE, 1974). There appears to be no energy transfer between rhodopsin molecules (HAGINS and JENNINGS, 1959; LIEBMAN, 1962; EBREY, 1971), which is not surprising for rhodopsin spheres rotating and diffusing freely in a lipid layer. This is a strong argument against a solid-state process in visual excitation (BONTING, 1969, p. 393).

The chromophore is always oriented in the plane of the photoreceptor membrane, since the rod shows steady linear dichroism only in the axial plane, but not in the membrane plane (SCHMIDT, 1938; DENTON, 1954). This represents the most favorable condition for light absorption *in vivo*.

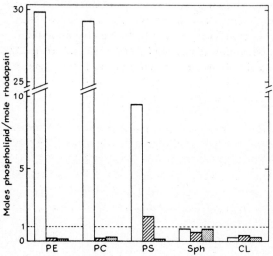

Fig. 6. Phospholipid composition of rod sac membrane before and after treatment with phospholipases

Chromophore Conformation and Binding Site

The identity of the chromophoric group with retinaldehyde has long been established (BALL et al., 1948). Evidence that in native rhodopsin it is present as the 11-*cis* isomer has been reported by WALD and HUBBARD (HUBBARD and WALD, 1952; WALD and BROWN, 1956; HUBBARD, 1958). More direct evidence for this fact has recently been obtained by thin layer chromatography of the chromophore, extracted with organic solvent from rhodopsin in darkness at room temperature, followed by spectral identification through iodine-catalyzed isomerization (ROTMANS et al., 1972). During illumination the chromophore is isomerized to the all-*trans* form.

Retinaldehyde is linked through its aldehyde groups to an amino group of opsin. This link is a protonated aldimine bond $-\overset{H}{C}=\overset{H}{\underset{+}{N}}-$

(MORTON and PITT, 1957; RIMAI et al., 1970), which is not stable against acid hydrolysis. This excludes identification of the binding site through hydrolysis of rhodopsin. Prior reduction with $NaBH_4$ stabilizes such a bond, but $NaBH_4$ does not react with rhodopsin in darkness. Illumination in the presence of $NaBH_4$ does give reduction, and subsequent hydrolysis has permitted to identify the chromophore-carrying amino group as the ε-amino group of lysine (BOWNDS and WALD, 1965; AKHTAR et al., 1965). This is then the binding site in bleached rhodopsin (Metarhodopsin II), but not necessarily that in native rhodopsin, since there is a distinct possibility of transiminization during bleaching.

Table 2. Dansylated groups from rhodopsin after 0 and 97% amidination, dansylation, hydrolysis and thin layer chromatography

	Molar ratio	
	0%	97%
Lysine	16.4 ± 0.8	1.4 ± 0.2
Ethanolamine	27.9 ± 1.0	0.4 ± 0.2
Serine	8.2 ± 0.6	0.2 ± 0.2

This problem has now been solved by a different approach. All free amino groups in photoreceptor membranes are blocked by amidination with methylacetimidate (MAI), which does not attack the chromophoric bond (DE GRIP et al., 1973 a and b). This preparation is then treated with Dansyl chloride, which displaces the chromophore and forms a hydrolysis-resistant link with the chromophore bearing group. Hydrolysis followed by quantitative thin-layer chromatography permits identification of this group. The results in Table 2 prove that it is again the ε-amino group of lysine, bearing in mind that (phosphatidyl) ethanolamine has already been excluded as a binding site by the phospholipid removal experiments (BORGGREVEN et al., 1971, 1972). So retinaldehyde is bound to lysine, both in native and in bleached rhodopsin (Metarhodopsin II).

Chromophore Migration During Photolysis

Since there are 14—16 lysine residues present per rhodopsin molecule and the protonated aldimine bond readily reacts with unprotonated amino groups, there still remains a possibility of migration of the chromophoric group during photolysis.

Photolysis of rhosopsin consists of a series of chemical changes, beginning with the isomerization of 11-*cis*-retinaldehyde to its all-*trans* isomer, and ending *in vivo* with the release of retinol. The intermediates have been spectrally identified:

Rhodopsin (500 nm) → prelumirhodopsin (543 nm) → lumirhodopsin (497 nm) → metarhodopsin I (480 nm) → metarhodopsin II (380 nm) → metarhodopsin III (465 nm) → all-*trans*-retinol (330 nm) + opsin.

(In parentheses the wavelength of maximal absorbance; see Bonting, 1969, pp. 369—377.) The only light-requiring step is the first one, involving chromophore isomerization and formation of pre-lumirhodopsin. At physiological temperature the conversion of rhodopsin to metarhodopsin I takes place in microseconds, the conversion of metarhodopsin I → II in milliseconds, and the decay of the latter substance requires several minutes. This indicates that visual excitation takes place at the latest during the conversion of metarhodopsin I → II. Hence, the possibility of chromophore migration during this conversion is of interest for our understanding of the excitation process.

We have studied this possibility by adding $NaBH_4$ during or after illumination, and then probing the chromophore binding site by treatment with 11-*cis*-retinaldehyde and determining whether light-sensitive pigment is formed (Bonting et al., 1973; Rotmans et al., 1974). Figure 7 explains how migration of the chromophore would lead to the formation of a new photopigment under these conditions. If reduction is complete within 5 sec after illumination,

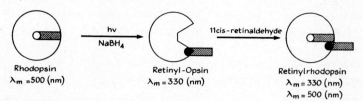

Rhodopsin
$\lambda_m = 500$ (nm)

Retinyl-Opsin
$\lambda_m = 330$ (nm)

Retinylrhodopsin
$\lambda_m = 330$ (nm)
$\lambda_m = 500$ (nm)

Fig. 7. Formation of retinylrhodopsin upon incubation of illuminated and reduced rhodopsin with 11-*cis* retinaldehyde (○ aldimine bond at original binding site, ● reduced aldimine bond). This reaction can only occur if the chromophore migrates to a new binding site prior to reduction

we find no pigment formation. If, however, the time interval between reduction and illumination is lengthened, an increasing amount of photopigment is formed (Fig. 8, solid line). These experiments indicate that in metarhodopsin II the chromophore is still bound to the same lysine residue as in rhodopsin, but that during

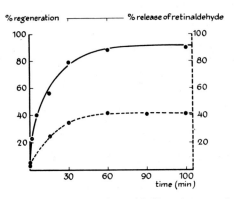

Fig. 8. Percentage of the chromophoric binding sites vacated (———) and retinaldehyde release from rhodopsin (- - -) as a function of the time elapsing after illumination

the decay of this intermediate the chromophore begins to migrate. Determination of the liberation of the chromophore (retinaldehyde rather than retinol, since NADPH is absent in these experiments) shows that liberation is slower and less complete (Fig. 8, dotted line) than migration. About 60% of the chromophore remains bound to sites other than the original binding site, mostly to protein amino groups, minor amounts to phospholipid amino groups.

Involvement of Retinoldehydrogenase in Chromophore Migration

In the presence of NADPH enzymatic reduction of free and aldimine-linked retinaldehyde to retinol by means of the retinoldehydrogenase present in the photoreceptor membrane takes place (DE PONT et al., 1970). Hence, one of the sites to which the chromophore migrates could be the active site of this enzyme. Evidence for an intermediary linking of retinaldehyde to an amino group in this active site has been obtained by measuring the retinoldehydrogenase activity as a function of the time elapsing between illumination of $NaBH_4$ (Fig. 9). Presence of retinaldehyde on the active site during $NaBH_4$ addition will yield a stable single bond, thus inactivating the enzyme. The minimum activity about 15 min after

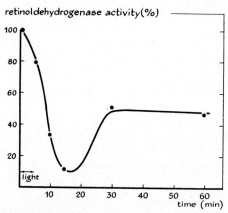

Fig. 9. Retinoldehydrogenase activity as a function of the time interval between illumination and addition of $NaBH_4$

illumination suggests that at that time (and in the absence of NADPH) the active site of retinoldehydrogenase is maximally occupied by migrated chromophore molecules. Supporting evidence comes from the amidination experiments (Table 3). After four consecutive treatments with MAI in darkness 40% of the retinoldehydrogenase activity is left. A fifth treatment with MAI completes amidination, leaving 15% retinoldehydrogenase activity if carried

Table 3. Effect of NH_2-blocking on retinoldehydrogenase activity

Treatment	NH_2 blocked (%)	Rhodopsin left (%)	Regenern. capacity (%)	Retinol DH activity (%)
MAI, 4 × in dark	92	80	75	40
MAI, 5th time, light	97	2	0	15
MAI, 5th time, dark	97	70	70	0

out in the light and no activity if carried out in the dark. In the former case retinaldehyde can migrate to the enzyme protecting the active site from amidination, while in the latter case no chromophore migration occurs and the active site remains unprotected.

The possibility that metarhodopsin III could represent the enzyme-substrate complex has occurred to us. However, in 80% amidinated preparations we find virtually no metarhodopsin III ($\sim$ 10%) formed upon illumination, while retinoldehydrogenase activity is largely intact (> 80%). This makes it very unlikely that metarhodopsin III represents the enzyme-substrate complex of retinoldehydrogenase.

Sulfhydryl Groups in Visual Excitation

Various investigators have reported that illumination of detergent-solubilized rhodopsin unmasks two SH-groups in addition to the two available before illumination (WALD and BROWN, 1951; OSTROY et al., 1966; ZORN and FUTTERMAN, 1971). This has led to the suggestion that in addition to an amino group a SH-group might be involved in the binding of the chromophore (HELLER, 1968).

The availability of detergent-free photoreceptor membrane preparations has prompted a reinvestigation of this matter (DE GRIP et al., 1973c). The membrane preparations are treated with 5,5'-dithio-bis-(2-nitro-benzoic acid) (DTNB) under optimal reaction conditions and oxidation of SH-groups is prevented by working under nitrogen. Table 4 shows that 2 SH-groups, both before and after illumination, are modified without effect on the 500 nm absorbance (before illumination) and the regeneration capacity (before and after illumination). Reaction with N-ethylmaleimide (NEM) gives identical results. In detergent solutions the earlier findings are confirmed, and the regeneration capacity is sharply decreased, even in the case of the mild detergent digitonin.

These results indicate that the appearance of SH-groups during photolysis is an artifact due to denaturation effects of the detergents. They also rule out the covalent participation of an SH-group in the binding of the chromophore.

With p-chloromercuribenzoate (pCMB) two SH-groups of the membrane suspension react fast, and an additional two SH-groups react slowly in the dark, but then the regeneration capacity of

Table 4. Number of reactive SH-groups per mole of rhodopsin as determined
by reaction with DTNB

	Number of SH-groups	
	Dark	Light
Membrane suspension:	1.8 ± 0.1	1.8 ± 0.2 (5)
ΔA_{500}	100%	—
Regeneration capacity	95%	98%
Detergent solution:		
Digitonin	2.0 ± 0.1	3.9 ± 0.2 (4)
Triton-X-100	3.0 ± 0.1	6.0 ± 0.2 (5)
CTAB	3.6 ± 0.3	5.8 ± 0.3 (2)
Sodium dodecylsulfate	5.9 ± 0.2	5.9 ± 0.2 (5)

In parentheses the number of samples determined.

rhodopsin is lost. After illumination the remaining two SH-groups
become available for reaction with pCMB. This indicates the presence of three differently located pairs of SH-groups in the rhodopsin molecule (Fig. 10): one pair on the surface of the molecule
(reacting with DTNB and NEM in darkness and light, and fast
reacting with pCMB), one pair inside the molecule, but not close to
the chromophore (reacting slowly with pCMB), and one pair near
the chromophore (reacting with DTNB and NEM in the light in the
presence of detergent (reacting with pCMB in the light).

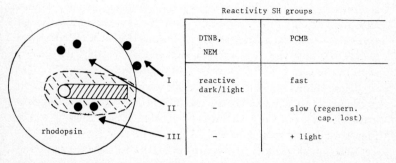

Fig. 10. Schematic presentation of the localization of the six sulfhydryl groups
(●) of rhodopsin. The cross-hatched bar represents the chromophoric group

Events in the Outer Membrane during Visual Excitation

Electrophysiological studies have greatly elucidated the events taking place in the outer membrane of the rod cell after illumination, and which lead to stimulation of the synapse with the bipolar cells. TOMITA (1970) has been able to record membrane potential and

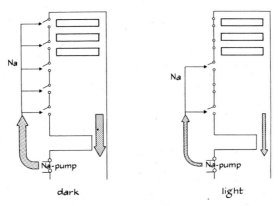

Fig. 11. Schematic presentation of the sodium current in the vertebrate rod. In darkness all sodium channels are open, and the current is large. Upon illumination sodium channels close and the current is reduced

resistance by means of a microelectrode placed inside an individual rod cell. He observes in the dark a small membrane potential (10—20 mV, inside negative), which upon illumination hyperpolarizes by 13—15 mV. This hyperpolarization is accompanied and apparently caused by an increase in membrane resistance, which represents a decrease in sodium permeability. HAGINS (1972) concludes from measurements with multiple, extracellularly placed microelectrodes the existence of a dark current consisting of a flow of sodium ions from the inner segment along the rod to the outer segment, where the outer membrane is highly permeable to sodium ions. This dark current is sensitive to cyanide and ouabain, which means that it is energy-dependent and driven by a Na^+-K^+-activated ATPase pump (see: BONTING, 1970). Light reduces this dark current by the decrease in sodium permeability of the outer segment membrane.

These findings are represented schematically in Fig. 11. In darkness there is a large sodium current, because the sodium channels in the outer segment membrane are open. Upon illumination part of the sodium channels close, leading to a decrease in the sodium current. Supporting evidence has been obtained by observing the effect of light on the rate of swelling and shrinking of freshly isolated rod outer segments in hyper- and hypotonic salt solutions (Korenbrot and Cone, 1972; Korenbrot, 1973). There are an estimated 1000 sodium channels per frog rod, passing a total of 2×10^9 ions/sec. Per photon the dark current decreases by about 1%, which would mean closing of about 10 sodium channels. Hagins has calculated that this small decrease in dark current should just be "noticeable" at the synapse above the random fluctuations. This explains the fact that absorption of a single photon can excite a rod cell, provided we may assume that the bleaching of a single rhodopsin molecule will close some 10 sodium channels.

Calcium as a Transmitter between Photoreceptor and Outer Membrane

This brings us to our final point: how is the signal of the photolysis of a rhodopsin molecule in the photoreceptor membrane transmitted to the outer membrane, which is separated by a 75—400 Å space from the nearest photoreceptor membrane ?

Yoshikami and Hagins (1973) have observed that raising the external calcium ion concentration from 1.4 to 20 mM rapidly and reversibly abolishes the dark current and the effect of light on it. Lowering the external calcium concentration to 10^{-7} M by means of EGTA has more or less the opposite effect: the dark current and the effect of light on it are initially multiplied severalfold. This leads these authors to the hypothesis that calcium ions act as a transmitter between the two membranes (Fig. 12). The rod sacs would act as calcium stores, while the cytoplasmic calcium concentration would be very low in the resting state, as is the case in resting muscle where the sarcoplasmic reticulum is the calcium store. Bleaching of rhodopsin would release calcium ions to the cytoplasm, which then diffuse to the outer membrane where they block the sodium channels.

Evidence for such a mechanism has recently been obtained in our laboratory (HENDRIKS et al., 1974). In freshly isolated frog rod outer segments the calcium content, determined by atomic absorption spectrophotometry, is very high: 11—13 mol/mol rhodopsin or 30 mmol/l outer segment volume. when isolation takes place in the

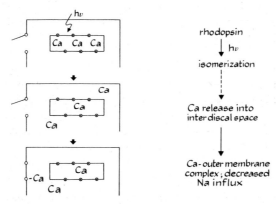

Fig. 12. Schematic presentation of the calcium transmitter hypothesis. Calcium ions, released from the rod sacs upon photolysis of rhodopsin, diffuse to the outer membrane and close sodium channels

presence of ATP (Table 5). This calcium concentration is even higher than that in squid axon mitochondria (20 mM). In the absence of ATP the calcium content is significantly lower, suggesting the presence of an ATP-dependent accumulation process. Illumination of untreated outer segments causes no significant change in the calcium content. However, illumination, followed by rapid lysis through addition of 4 vol. H_2O, causes a 16% loss of

Table 5. Calcium content of isolated frog rod outer segments

Medium	mol Ca^{2+}/mol rhodopsin	Nr. of experiments
Ringer, 3 mM ATP	11.0 ± 1.2	21
Ringer, 3 mM ATP, 10 mM EDTA	12.8 ± 1.6	4
Ringer, no ATP, no EDTA	7.8 ± 0.6	10

Table 6. Light-induced calcium loss from frog rod outer segment preparations

Treatment of outer segments	% loss of sedimentable Ca^{2+}	Nr. of experiments	
Untreated, light	0	10	
Light, lysis	16	4	P = 0.01
Lysis, light	6	2	
Lysis, restoration to isotonicity, light	24	5	P < 0.01

calcium from the sedimentable fraction (Table 6). Reversal of the order (lysis, followed immediately by a light flash) gives a small loss of 6%, but when the lysed rods are first restored to the normal isotonic medium, illumination gives a large (24%) and significant loss of calcium from the sedimentable fraction. The latter loss remains constant, when the percentage photolysis is decreased down to 15% (Table 7).

Table 7. Light-induced calcium loss from lysed frog rod outer segment preparations

% Rhodopsin photolyzed	% loss of sedimentable Ca^{2+}	Nr. of experiments
85	24 ± 1	5
40	20	1
15	27 ± 4	5

The most likely interpretation of these experiments is that the rod sacs store large amounts of calcium by an ATP-requiring process, thus keeping the cytoplasmic calcium concentration very low. Accumulation may either be by transport into the sac interior space or by adsorption on the sac membrane. Photolysis of rhodopsin leads to a release of calcium from the sacs. Diffusion of the released calcium ions to the outer membrane, which could occur in a few milliseconds (fast enough for excitation), would lead to a closing of sodium channels. At 15% photolysis 20 calcium ions are released per rhodopsin molecule bleached, which is probably a lower limit to the number that can be released by single photon absorption. It is, therefore, quite conceivable that this process could close about 10 sodium channels per photon, as required for the observed decrease in the dark current and for the explanation of the fact that a single photon can excite a rod cell.

Summary

The rod sac membrane consists of a highly fluid lipid bilayer, in which rhodopsin molecules float and spin (probably in the outer face).
Absorption of a photon leads to photolysis of rhodopsin, consisting of chromophore isomerization, followed by a number of thermal conversions. The chromophore remains bound to the same ε-amino group of lysine until Metarhodopsin II begins to decay. Then it migrates to other binding sites, incl. retinoldehydrogenase, which in the presence of NADPH reduces it to retinol.
The rod sacs have a high calcium content through accumulation by an ATP-dependent process. Photolysis of rhodopsin leads to release of part of the calcium ions, which diffuse to the outer membrane and close part of the sodium channels in this membrane. This reduces the dark current of sodium ions, extruded by an Na^+-K^+ ATPase pump from the inner segment and passively entering the outer segment. The reduction of the dark current stimulates the synapse with the bipolar cells.

References

AKHTAR, M., BLOSSE, P. T., DEWHURST, P. B.: Life Sci. **4**, 1221 (1965).
BALL, S., GOODWIN, T. W., MORTON, R. A.: Biochem. J. **42**, 516 (1948).
BLASIE, J. K.: Biophys. J. **12**, 191, 205 (1972).
BONTING, S. L.: Curr. Topics Bioenergetics **3**, 351 (1969).
BONTING, S. L.: In: BITTAR, E. E. (Ed.): Membranes and ion transport, Vol. I, p. 257. London: Wiley 1970.
BONTING, S. L., CARAVAGGIO, L. L., GOURAS, P.: Exp. Eye Res. **1**, 14 (1961).
BONTING, S. L., ROTMANS, J. P., DAEMEN, F. J. M.: In: LANGER, H. (Ed.): Biochemistry and physiology of visual pigments, p. 39. Berlin: Springer 1973.
BONTING, S. L., DE GRIP, W. L., ROTMANS, J. P., DAEMEN, F. J. M.: Exp. Eye Res. **18**, 77 (1974).
BORGGREVEN, J. M. P. M., DAEMEN, F. J. M., BONTING, S. L.: Biochim. biophys. Acta (Amst.) **202**, 374 (1970).
BORGGREVEN, J. M. P. M., ROTMANS, J. P., BONTING, S. L., DAEMEN, F. J. M.: Arch. Biochem. Biophys. **145**, 290 (1971).

Borggreven, J.M.P.M., Daemen, F.J.M., Bonting, S.L.: Arch. Biochem. Biophys. **151**, 1 (1972).

Bownds, D., Wald, G.: Nature (Lond.) **205**, 254 (1965).

Brown, P.K.: Nature (Lond.) New Biol. **236**, 35 (1972).

Cone, R.A.: Nature (Lond.) New Biol. **236**, 39 (1972).

Daemen, F.J.M., Borggreven, J.M.P.M., Bonting, S.L.: Nature (Lond.) **227**, 1260 (1970).

Daemen, F.J.M., Jansen, P.A.A., Bonting, S.L.: Arch. Biochem. Biophys. **145**, 300 (1971).

Daemen, F.J.M., de Grip, W.J., Jansen, P.A.A.: Biochim. biophys. Acta (Amst.) **271**, 419 (1972).

Denton, E.J.: J. Physiol. **124**, 17 (1954).

Dewey, M.M., Davies, P., Blasie, J.K.: J. Histochem. Cytochem. **14**, 789 (1966).

Ebrey, T.G.: Proc. nat. Acad. Sci. (Wash.) **68**, 713 (1971).

de Grip, W.J., Daemen, F.J.M., Bonting, S.L.: Vision Res. **12**, 1697 (1972).

de Grip, W.J., Bonting, S.L., Daemen, F.J.M.: Biochim. biophys. Acta (Amst.) **303**, 189 (1973a).

de Grip, W.J., Daemen, F.J.M., Bonting, S.L.: Biochim. biophys. Acta (Amst.) **323**, 125 (1973b).

de Grip, W.J., van de Laar, G.L.M., Daemen, F.J.M., Bonting, S.L.: Biochim. biophys. Acta (Amst.) **325**, 315 (1973c).

Hagins, W.A.: Ann. Rev. Biophys. Bioeng. **1**, 131 (1972).

Hagins, W.A., Jennings, W.H.: Trans. Faraday Soc. **27**, 180 (1959).

Hall, M.O., Bok, D., Bacharach, A.D.E.: J. molec. Biol. **45**, 397 (1969).

Heller, J.: Biochemistry I, 2914 (1968).

Hendriks, T., Daemen, F.J.M., Bonting, S.L.: Biochim. biophys. Acta (Amst.) **345**, 468 (1974).

Hubbard, R.: J. gen. Physiol. **42**, 259 (1958).

Hubbard, R., Wald, G.: J. gen. Physiol. **36**, 269 (1952).

Korenbrot, J.I.: Exp. Eye Res. **16**, 343 (1973).

Korenbrot, J.I., Cone, R.A.: J. gen. Physiol. **60**, 20 (1972).

Liebman, P.A.: Biophys. J. **2**, 161 (1962).

Liebman, P.A., Entine, G.: Science **185**, 457 (1974).

Morton, R.A., Pitt, G.A.J.: Fortschr. Chem. Org. Naturstoffe **14**, 244 (1957).

Olive, J., Benedetti, E.L.: Molec. Biol. Repts. **1**, 245 (1974).

Ostroy, E.O., Rudney, H., Abrahamson, E.W.: Biochim. biophys. Acta (Amst.) **126**, 409 (1966).

de Pont, J., Daemen, F.J.M., Bonting, S.L.: Arch. Biochem. Biophys. **140**, 267, 275 (1970).

Rimai, L., Kilponen, R.G., Gill, D.: Biochem. Biophys. Res. Commun. **41**, 492 (1970).

de Robertis, E.: J. gen. Physiol. **43**, 1 (1960).

Rotmans, J.P., Bonting, S.L., Daemen, F.J.M.: Vision Res. **12**, 337 (1972).

Rotmans, J.P., van de Laar, G.L.M., Daemen, F.J.M., Bonting, S.L.: Vision Res. **12**, 1297 (1972).

Rotmans,J.P., Daemen,F.J.M., Bonting,S.L.: Biochim. biophys. Acta (Amst.) **357**, 151 (1974).
Schmidt,W.J.: Kolloid-Z. **85**, 137 (1938).
Tomita,T.: Quart. Rev. Biophys. **3**, 179 (1970).
Wald,G.: J. gen. Physiol. **21**, 795 (1938).
Wald,G., Brown,P.K.: J. gen. Physiol. **35**, 797 (1951).
Wald,G., Brown,P.K.: Nature (Lond.) **177**, 174 (1956).
Wald,G., Brown,P.K.: Science **127**, 222 (1958).
Yoshikami,S., Hagins,W.A.: In: Langer,H. (Ed.): Biochemistry and physiology of visual pigments, p. 245. Berlin: Springer 1973.
Young,R.W.: J. Cell Biol. **33**, 61 (1967).
Young,R.W.: J. ultrastruct. Res. **34**, 190 (1971).
Zorn,M., Futterman,S.: J. biol. Chem. **246**, 881 (1971).

Discussion

D.Brdiczka (Konstanz): I should like to ask two questions about the Ca^{2+} mechanism in retinal physiology. First: what is the mechanism of Ca^{2+} action in the cones, which have no compartments to take up, store and release Ca^{2+} ions. Second: Has anyone already studied Ca^{2+} transport and storage in the sacs from the rods? This, I think, would be fundamental for proving the Ca^{2+} hypothesis.

G.Wald (Cambridge, Mass.): If I may try to answer your first question: Yoshikami and Hagins very carefully put into their hypothesis that not only is the Ca^+ concentration high inside the disk but also in the extracellular fluid. You see the whole hypothesis comes out of experiments in which they showed that if one raises the Ca^+ concentration in the extracellular fluid outside the rods and cones that that duplicates the effects of light on the sodium current. And so is a big part of their hypothesis that the Ca^+ concentration is also high in the extracellular fluid and works equally on cones as on rods by working on the plasma membrane itself by closing off Na^+ channels through the plasma membrane. The second question you asked was, I think, how does the disk get back its Ca^+ ions — and I would say that that is an interesting question, not yet approached because you must realize — and hence Prof. Bonting's report in the finding of release of Ca^+ ions on bleaching in the membrane is very exciting — because up to that point we have a hypothesis without very much information to back it.

S.L.Bonting: In reply to Dr.Brdiczka's questions I should like to add the following remarks: Yoshikami and Hagins have observed that raising the external calcium concentration mimics the effect of light on the dark current, i.e. the presence of a high calcium concentration near the outer membrane appears to have the same effect on the sodium permeability of this membrane as the bleaching of rhodopsin. Hence they postulate that in the physiological situation the bleaching of rhodopsin would have to bring calcium ions into contact with the sodium channels in the outer membrane.

Since in cones all visual pigment molecules are located in the invaginated outer membrane, and assuming that the cytoplasmic calcium concentration is as low as in nerve and muscle ($10^{-7}-10^{-6}$ M), it is reasonable to assume that bleaching of rhodopsin would lead to a calcium influx. The calcium ions, having crossed the outer membrane, would then block sodium channels in this membrane from the inside. In rods this cannot be the major pathway, since all or virtually all rhodopsin is located in the rod sac membranes. Hence, it was proposed by YOSHIKAMI and HAGINS that the rod sacs are a calcium store, from which calcium ions are released upon bleaching of rhodopsin. Our experiments indicate that isolated outer segments have a very high calcium content (30 mmol per 1 outer segment volume), which in the lysis experiments appears to be present to a considerable extent in a rhodopsin-containing, sedimentable fraction, and that upon illumination there is a significant release of calcium from this fraction. This sedimentable fraction must represent the rod sacs, since there are not other intracellular compartments in the outer segments. While these findings seem to confirm the calcium transmitter hypothesis for the rod, no such experiments have been done with cones at this time. The problem is that animals with all-cone retinas are rare and hence bulk isolation of cone outer segments is not possible.

Dr. BRDICZKA is quite right in saying that it is essential to know how the rod sacs accumulate and store calcium. Unfortunately, here also technical problems slow down progress. There is at present no reliable and reproducible method to isolate intact rod sacs in bulk, such as has been worked out for the isolation of sarcoplasmic reticulum vesicles. Hence, we do not even know at this moment whether the stored calcium ions are present inside the rod sac or are bound to the membrane. Our finding that omitting ATP from the medium in which the outer segments are isolated reduces the calcium content by about 30% suggests, but does not prove, that the energy of ATP is needed for the accumulation process. The ATP could be utilized by a Ca^{2+}-Mg^{2+}-activated ATPase pump as occurs in the sarcoplasmic reticulum, which would imply accumulation inside the rod sacs. We have tried to establish the presence of Ca^{2+}-Mg^{2+}-activated ATPase activity in rod outer segments, but the evidence is inconclusive at this moment. Another possibility would be a Ca^{2+}-Na^+ exchange transport mediated by the Na^+-K^+-activated ATPase system present in rod sac membranes. Finally, there is the possibility of binding of calcium ions to the rod sac membrane through the phosphorylation of rhodopsin after illumination. [BOWNDS et al.: Nature (Lond.) New Biol. **237**, 125 (1972); KÜHN and DREYER: FEBS Letters **20**, 1 (1972); KÜHN et al: Biochemistry **12**, 2495 (1973)].

This possibility is, I feel, unlikely, since as many as 12 calcium ions are accumulated per rhodopsin molecules, while it appears that only one phosphate group is introduced per rhodopsin molecule. This is the present, unsatisfactory, state of our knowledge.

The Role of Protons in the Metarhodopsin I-II Transition

H. M. EMRICH[1] and R. REICH

*Max-Volmer-Inst. Phys. Chem. und Mol. Biol., Technische Universität
Berlin-West*

With 5 Figures

In isolated bovine rod outer segments metarhodopsin I—II absorption-changes are measured using rapid flash-photometry. The
formation of meta II is inhibited by increasing pH from pH 6 to
pH 8 at $2°$ C (Fig. 1a) [1]. At $23°$ C an appreciable amount of
meta II is formed also at pH 8 (Fig. 1b). This can be explained by
the following model (Fig. 2) [3].

During the meta I—II transition a conformation-change takes
place in which a base is exposed ($M_{II}*$). This "unfolded" conformation is stabilized by protonation, since the proton is too polar
to be re-enfolded into the hydrophobic core of metarhodopsin. $M_{II}*$
and $M_{II}H^+$ are assumed to have similar spectra. The pH-independent first equilibrium-constant $K* \equiv [M_{II}*]/[M_I]$ is very low at
$2°$ C (~ 0.005). The pH-dependence results from the second equilibrium, characterized by the association-constant of the exposed
base $K_B \equiv [M_{II}H^+]/[H^+][M_{II}*] \approx 10^{8.5}$.

At low temperature only increasing proton-concentrations shift
the equilibrium to meta II by stabilizing $M_{II}H^+$ (down to pH 6;
higher proton-concentrations appear to induce partial denaturation;
on the other hand in the alkaline a M_{II}-similar substance is stabilized). At $23°$ C, however, $K*$ has increased to ~ 0.4. This explains
the observation that at $23°$ C also an appreciable amount of meta II
is formed, even at pH 8. Since two equilibria are involved, $-\log K_B$
differs from the apparent pK determined directly from titrations

---

[1] Present address: Physiol. Inst. Univ. München, 8000 München 2, Pettenkoferstr. 12, Federal Republic of Germany. This work was supported by the
Deutsche Forschungsgemeinschaft.

[1, 2]. The fact that the protonation does not lead to a bathochromic shift, expected from a protonation of a Schiff-base of retinal, but to an hypsochromic shift of the absorption-band, is explained in

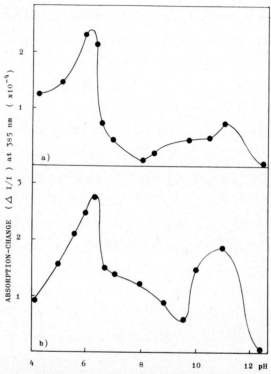

Fig. 1. Absorption-increase of meta II (385 nm) after flash photolysis of rhodopsin as a function of pH in rod outer segments, a: 2° C, b: 23° C; for details see [2, 3]

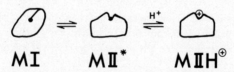

Fig. 2. Scheme of the meta I—II conformation-change with formation of an unfolded meta II structure. The dot represents the exposable base. Protonation of the base stabilizes the unfolded structure

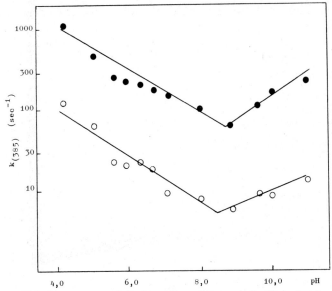

Fig. 3. Velocity constant of the formation of the meta I—II equilibrium as a function of pH (rapid and slow phase)

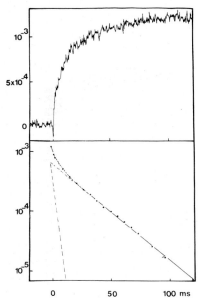

Fig. 4. Upper part: Time course of the absorption increase of meta II (385 nm) following a 10^{-5} sec flash at $t = 0$. Lower part: Half-logarithmic plot of the deviation of extinction from its equilibrium value ($t \to \infty$) as a function of time. Scheme of separation of a slow and a rapid phase

our model by the assumption that the protonated conformation-regulating base is not in the chromophoric region of rhodopsin.

Protons (and OH⁻) also have a *catalytic* effect on the meta I—II transition (Fig. 3). The characteristic deviation of the kinetics from a first-order process (Fig. 4) which often is observed can be explain-

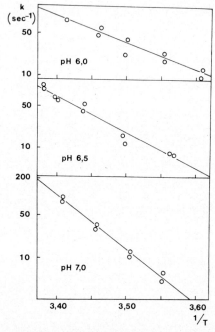

Fig. 5. Velocity constant for the adjustment of the meta I—II equilibrium (slow phase) as a function of 1/T at pH 6.0, 6.5 and 7.0

ed by an inhomogeneity of the shieldings to H^+ (and OH^-) of the catalytic centers of different rhodopsin-molecules. The catalytic and thermodynamic action of protons seems to act on different sites of metarhodopsin, since the catalytic protons should decrease the free energy of an M_IH^+-intermediate whereas the protonated base should have a high free energy in the M_I-conformation (thus stabilizing the M_{II}-conformation). Arrhenius-plots of the meta I—II kinetics (Fig. 5) show decreasing slopes with increasing proton-concentration. This finding can be explained by a decrease of activation-energy by proton-catalysis. The data cannot easily be interpreted quantitatively, since the real unidirectional $\vec{E}_A$ can only be obtained from $\vec{k}_{(T)}$ data.

References

1. MATTHEWS, R. G., HUBBARD, R., BROWN, P. K., WALD, G.: J. gen. Pysiol. **47**, 215 (1963).
2. EMRICH, H. M.: Z. Naturforsch. **26 b**, 352 (1971).
3. EMRICH, H. M., REICH, R.: Z. Naturforsch. **29 c**, 577—591 (1974).

Aktivitäten von ATPasen im Fliegen-Auge

H. LANGER

Institut für Tierphysiologie, Ruhr-Universität, 463 Bochum-Querenburg
Federal Republic of Germany

With 1 Figure

Für das Facettenauge der Insekten hatten wir — am Beispiel der Schmeißfliege *Calliphora erythrocephala* — früher zeigen können [2], daß der ATP-Spiegel durch Lichteinwirkung, also in Verbindung mit dem Sehvorgang, absinkt. Im Anschluß an diesen Befund haben wir uns in letzter Zeit den ATPasen zugewandt; die Magnesium- und die zusätzlich Natrium-Kalium-abhängige ATPase wurden von MARIA E. RIVERA [3] biochemisch charakterisiert. Eine jetzt laufende Untersuchung — gemeinsam mit Frau RIVERA — beschäftigt sich mit der Größe der Aktivität dieser ATPasen in den Augen und im Zentralnervensystem von *Calliphora* im Zusammenhang mit der Abwesenheit oder der Einwirkung von Licht. Hierfür stehen uns, neben der Wildform der Fliege mit dunkelroten Augen (*n*), gelb-(*"lemon"*) und weißäugige (*"chalky"*) Mutanten zur Verfügung, deren Augen aufgrund der Verarmung an Abschirmpigmenten eine größere Reizantwort auf einen gegebenen Lichtreiz zeigen. Die Aktivitäten wurden nach der Methode von BONTING et al. [1] bestimmt, in μmol freigesetztem P_i/Std berechnet und auf den Proteingehalt des Gewebeextraktes bezogen.

In allen Teilen des Nervensystems im Kopf der Fliege ist die Aktivität der Natrium-Kalium-ATPase höchstens gleich, meist aber deutlich niedriger als die der Magnesium-ATPase. Im Vergleich der Wildform mit den Mutanten zeigt sich, daß die Natrium-Kalium-ATPase in allen Augenfarbtypen etwa gleiche Aktivität aufweist, während die Magnesium-ATPase-Aktivität um so größer ist, je weniger Abschirmpigment die Augen enthalten: Die Aktivitäten der Natrium-Kalium-ATPase liegen um 1,5, die der Magnesium-ATPase bei *n* unter 2, bei *chalky* aber oberhalb 4 μmol

P_i/mg Protein × Std. Dadurch liegt das Verhältnis der beiden ATPase-Aktivitäten zueinander bei etwa 1 : 1 in der Wildform und bei etwa 3 : 1 in der weißäugigen Mutante. Im Zentralnervensystem derselben Tiere liegen die Aktivitäten etwas höher als in den Augen, sind aber bei den Farbtypen nicht signifikant verschieden; das Verhältnis von Magnesium-ATPase- zu Natrium-Kalium-ATPase-Aktivität beträgt ungefähr 2 : 1 (Abb. 1a).

Da die verschiedenen Stämme von Fliegen unter den gleichen Belichtungsbedingungen gehalten wurden, interpretieren wir die unterschiedlichen Aktivitäten der Magnesium-ATPase in den Augen als eine Folge der verschieden hohen effektiven Reizlichtintensität am Ort der Photoreceptorzellen in Abhängigkeit von dem Gehalt an Abschirmpigmenten.

Um die Wirkung von Licht direkt zu prüfen, wurden zwei Gruppen von Fliegen aus gleicher Zucht parallel für etwa 30 Std dunkel gehalten bzw. nach Dunkelhaltung über Nacht für 6 Std mit hellem ,,Weiß''licht (einer Hochleistungsglühlampe) bestrahlt. In diesen Versuchen wurden die optischen Ganglien und das Gehirn im engeren Sinne getrennt analysiert, weil sich gezeigt hatte, daß die Aktivitäten der beiden ATPasen in diesen Teilen des Zentralnervensystems unterschiedlich hoch sind. In den 24 Versuchen der Serie an Tieren der Mutante *chalky* (Abb. 1b) zeigte sich in den bestrahlten Augen eine signifikante Vermehrung beider ATPase-Aktivitäten. Im Zentralnervensystem war nur die Magnesium-ATPase-Aktivität der belichteten Tiere vergrößert, und zwar signifikant nur in den optischen Ganglien; dagegen blieb die Natrium-Kalium-ATPase unverändert. Ähnliche Ergebnisse wie für die Mutante *chalky* (Abb. 1b) wurden auch für die Wildform erhalten; jedoch sind die Veränderungen unter denselben Bestrahlungsbedingungen erwartungsgemäß kleiner.

Bei der Beurteilung dieser Befunde muß berücksichtigt werden, daß — wegen der Aktivitätsbestimmungen unter optimalen Bedingungen — der gefundene Anstieg eine Vermehrung des aktiven Enzyms nachweist, die während der Belichtung der Augen erfolgt sein muß. Es ist überraschend, daß von der Lichtwirkung im Auge auch die Magnesium-ATPase betroffen ist, während im Zentralnervensystem die als Transportenzym angesehene Natrium-Kalium-ATPase unbeeinflußt bleibt. Wir vermuten eine enge Beziehung der Magnesium-ATPase zum Sehprozeß; diese Erwartung

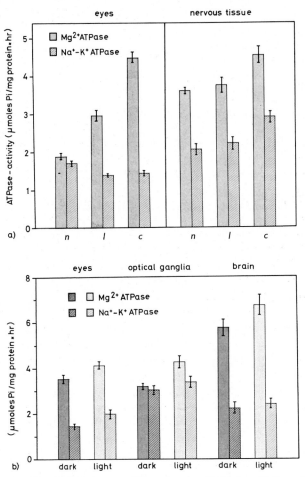

Abb. 1a und b. Aktivitäten von Magnesium- und Natrium-Kalium-ATPase in Augen und Nervengeweben des Kopfes der Schmeißfliege *Calliphora erythrocephala*. a) Vergleich von Augenfarbtypen: *n* Wildform, *l* Mutante *lemon*, *c* Mutante *chalky*. b) Vergleich von Tieren der Mutante *chalky* nach Dunkelhaltung bzw. nach 6stündiger Bestrahlung mit hellem Weißlicht. Mittelwerte aus 24 Versuchspaaren. Die senkrechten Striche am oberen Ende der Säulen stellen den zweifachen mittleren Fehler des Mittelwertes dar. Signifikanzen im *t*-Test Hell- gegen Dunkel-Tiere: Für beide Aktivitäten in Augen, für Magnesium-ATPase in optischen Ganglien $P \gtrless 0.01$; für beide Aktivitäten in Gehirn, für Natrium-Kalium-ATPase in optischen Ganglien $P \geqq 0.05$

wird durch die neuesten Befunde von K. M. WEBER [4, 5] bestärkt: Er konnte sowohl histochemisch als auch durch Zellfraktionierung nachweisen, daß diese ATPase hauptsächlich in den Rhabdomen lokalisiert ist, also den Teilen der Ommatidien, in denen der Primärprozeß des Sehens abläuft.

Literatur

1. BONTING, S. L., SIMON, K. A., HAWKINS, N. H.: Studies on sodium-potassium-activated adenosinetriphosphatase. I. Quantitative distribution in several tissues of the cat. Arch. Biochem. Biophys. **95**, 416—423 (1961).
2. LANGER, H.: Der Phosphatstoffwechsel des Facettenauges im Dunkeln und im Licht. Helgoländer Wiss. Meeresunters. **9**, 251—260 (1964).
3. RIVERA, M. E.: The ATPase system in the compound eye of the blowfly, *Calliphora erythrocephala* Meig. Comp. Biochem. Physiol. im Druck (1974).
4. WEBER, K. M.: Funktionelle Morphologie am Auge von *Calliphora erythrocephala* Meig. Habilitationsschrift, Ruhr-Universität Bochum 1974.
5. WEBER, K. M., SCHORRATH, G.: Histochemische Untersuchungen am Auge der Schmeißfliege *Calliphora erythrocephala* Meig. 2. Mitteilung: Nukleosidphosphatasen, Thiaminpyrophosphatase, unspezifische Esterase und Cholinesterase. Histochem. **30**, 131—149 (1972).

Thermal and Photic Regeneration of Rhodopsin in Perfused Frog Retina

W. SICKEL

*Institut f. normale u. pathologische Physiologie, Universität Köln, 5000 Köln
Federal Republic of Germany*

With 1 Figure

Rhodopsin, when hit by light quanta undergoes changes, one of which triggers visual excitation, but *in situ* is restored subsequently for renewed quantum catch. The "visual cycle" of the photopigment requires an energy source. This driving source has been looked for under conditions which would seem to preserve the required chemical reactions intact.

Frog retinas were isolated and, in a suitable chamber, perfused with a nutrient medium such as to maximize their electrical responses to light stimulation rather than their metabolic rates [1]. Three effects of light on retinal energy metabolism have thus been observed: i) a spurt of increased oxygen uptake in proportion to the electrical responses of the neural network of the retina, switching the light on and off; ii) a stationary decrease of metabolic rates *during* light exposure which parallels the reduction of the dark current of retinal receptor cells; and iii) an O_2-debt accruing from, and payed off only *after*, prolonged exposure to light. From circumstantial evidence this third effect has been attributed to the powering of visual pigment regeneration [2].

To this end i) it remained to be shown that regeneration of rhodopsin does occur in a perfused retina devoid of the pigment epithelium, and ii) a mechanism other than thermal regeneration, *e.g.* photoreversal, should be demonstrated as significantly contributing to the maintenance of the equilibrium state of light sensitive pigments under illumination.

Experiments [3] employing Triton X-100 extraction are presented (Fig. 1) which corroborate the above contention: In frog retinae at 20° C it took 25 min to half-restore rhodopsin thermally after a 20% bleach, but complete recovery after such bleaching was obtained immediately following irradiation with blue (Schott filter BG 12) light, well beyond the lifetimes of early photolytic intermediates. The photo-regenerated product did not differ spectrally from the parent rhodopsin.

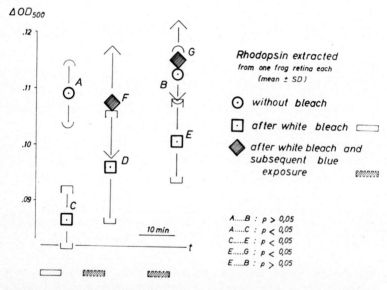

Fig. 1. *Circles A and B:* Retinae were perfused for 30 and 60 min, resp., in a recirculating flow system [2] with a nutrient medium, which was replaced at the resp. times by 4% alum for 20 min. After a brief water wash the system was filled up with 2% Triton (total volume 1 ml) which during 15 min circulation extracted approx. 70% of the rhodopsin present. Hydroxylamin was added to the extract, which was then centrifuged and scanned in a Beckman DK-2 spectrophotometer before and after total bleach. From the difference spectra the density loss at 500 nm is plotted as ordinate, referred to mg dry weight. *Square symbols:* Rhodopsin recovered immediately after exposure to white light of 10 lx for 6 min (*C*), and after another 12 (*D*) or 30 (*E*) min perfusion of the retina in the dark. *Hatched symbols:* Same exposure to white light and subsequent recovery in the dark as in *D* and *E*, resp. but with additional blue light exposure just prior to the alum treatment

References

1. SICKEL, W.: Retinal metabolism in dark and light. In: FUORTES, M. G. F. (Ed.): Handbook of sensory physiology. Vol. VII/2, pp. 667—727. Berlin-Heidelberg-New York: Springer 1972.
2. SICKEL, W.: Energy in vertebrate photoreceptor function. In: LANGER, H. (Ed.): Biochemistry and physiology of visual pigments, pp. 195—203. Berlin-Heidelberg-New York: Springer 1973.
3. In collaboration with C. CRAMER: Unpublished.

Experiments on the Isomerization of 11-*cis*-Retinal

W. Sperling, G. Nöll, and R. Meissen

Institute of Neurobiology Jülich GmbH., 5170 Jülich, Federal Republic of Germany

With 3 Figures

Two pathways for the isomerization of 11-*cis*- to all-*trans*-retinal are discussed in the literature[1]: the direct isomerization from the excited singlet state of 11-*cis* to the ground state of all-*trans* (Fig. 1, Path 7), and the isomerization *via* the triplet state (Paths 1 + 9). Figure 1 also shows other possible pathways for isomerization. For the purpose of simplification, Fig. 1 does not depict the formation

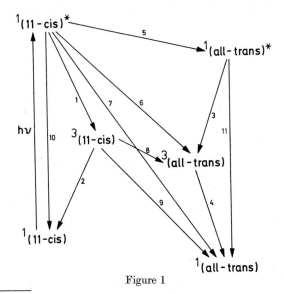

Figure 1

[1] Abrahamson, E. W. and Japar, S. M.: Principles of the interaction of light and matter. Handbook of sensory physiology, Vol. VII/1, pp. 1—32. Berlin-Heidelberg-New York: Springer 1972.

of *di-cis* compounds, and omits $^1(n, \pi^*)$ and vibrational energy states. We report experiments which help to identify the correct isomerization pathway.

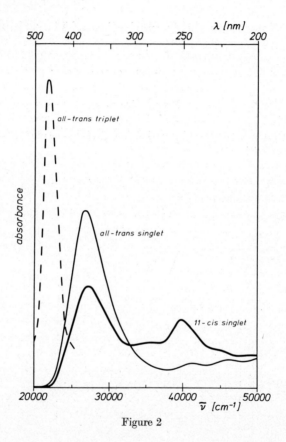

Figure 2

The singlet absorption spectra of 11-*cis*-and all-*trans*-retinal as well as the triplet spectrum of all-*trans*-retinal are given in Fig. 2. The spectra were measured in methylcyclohexane at room temperature.

A frequency-doubled ruby laser (347 nm) was used to excite retinal in methylcyclohexane solution. The time resolution of our flash light apparatus was 50 ns. Of the excited species shown in Fig. 1 only the decay times of triplet states could be resolved.

Assuming that isomerization from 11-*cis* to all-*trans* occurs only by way of Path 7, and that all the competitively formed 11-*cis* triplets (Path 1) return to the 11-*cis* ground state (Path 2), then the following absorption changes would be expected in the region of the isosbestic point (λ_i) formed by the intersection of the 11-*cis* singlet spectrum with the 11-*cis* triplet spectrum (Fig. 2 does not show the triplet spectrum of 11-*cis*, but only that of all-*trans*). At the isosbestic point only the absorbance increase reflecting the formation of all-*trans* should be seen. The transition from the 11-*cis* triplet to the 11-*cis* ground state should occur without absorbance change. However, the decay of the triplet should result in absorbance changes at wavelengths longer and shorter than the wavelength corresponding to the isosbestic point:

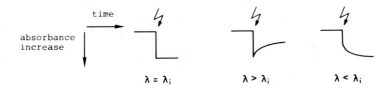

Figure 3 shows the absorption changes actually measured after a laser flash on 11-*cis*-retinal solutions in the region of the isosbestic point (*a* is a measure for the laser flash intensity; *b* depicts a 5% change in absorbance). Methylcyclohexane was used as the solvent; the temperature was maintained at 157 K. Under these conditions an isosbestic point was found at 409.5 nm (Fig. 3, $\lambda_i = 409.5$ nm). The bandwidth of the measuring beam was 1 nm.

Similar experiments with all-*trans* also revealed an isosbestic point at 409.5 nm. Other measurements on both 11-*cis*-and all-*trans*-retinal solutions demonstrated the existence of two more isosbestic points at about 275 nm and 250 nm. The wavelength positions of each of these two isosbestic points were the same for both all-*trans* and 11-*cis* solutions.

Considering that the singlet absorption spectra of 11-*cis*-and all-*trans*-retinal are quite different, one would not expect that the isosbestic points formed by the singlet and triplet all-*trans* spectra are identical within experimental error to the isosbestic points formed by the singlet and triplet 11-*cis* spectra. The coincidence of

the isobestic points suggests that the triplets originating from
11-*cis* and all-*trans* are identical. If the triplet observed after
illumination of 11-*cis* solutions is the all-*trans* triplet, then at least
some, possibly all, 11-*cis* molecules are isomerized to all-*trans* *via*
the all-*trans* triplet state. Three pathways leading to the population

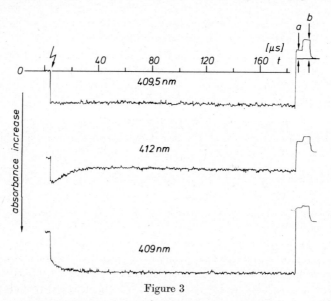

Figure 3

of the all-*trans* triplet state are conceivable (Paths 3, 6, and 8).
Path 8 implies that the 11-*cis* triplet decays to the all-*trans* triplet
more rapidly than we would measure. Additional formation of all-
trans by means of Path 7 cannot be excluded at this time.

   If the triplet observed after illumination of 11-*cis* solutions is
the 11-*cis* triplet, then isomerization of 11-*cis* molecules does not
occur by means of triplet states, but must occur directly (Path 7).
This conclusion follows from the fact that the absorption change
at the isobestic point is essentially instantaneous. The observed
slower absorption changes at longer and shorter wavelengths than
the isobestic wavelength represent the decay of the 11-*cis* triplet
to the 11-*cis* ground state (Path 2).

   Experiments are in progress to unambiguously identify the
measured triplet.

Cephalopod Retinochrome

Ruth Hubbard and Linda Sperling[1]

*Biological Laboratories of Harvard University, Cambridge, MA. 02138, USA.,
and the Marine Biological Laboratory, Woods Hole, MA. 02543, USA.*

With 6 Figures

The visual cells of vertebrates and invertebrates, though anatomically quite different from each other, contain the same kinds of visual pigment composed of a protein, opsin, to which the 11-*cis* isomer of retinal (retinaldehyde, vitamin A aldehyde) is attached as chromophore. In cattle and squid rhodopsin, the two visual pigments whose chemical composition has been examined most thoroughly, retinaldehyde forms a Schiff base (an aldimine) with the ε-amino group of an internal lysine residue in opsin (Bownds, 1967; Hagins, 1973). As might be expected from their chemical similarities, all visual pigments have similar absorption spectra with a main α-band and a much smaller β-band, both owing to absorption by the chromophore, and a narrow γ-band near 280 nm owing to absorption by the aromatic amino acid residues in opsin. The precise wavelength position of the main band is different in the different visual pigments, but in general λ_{max} lies at longer wavelengths than 440 nm. Rhodopsin, the visual pigment in vertebrate rods and in the rhabdoms of invertebrates, usually has λ_{max} near 500 nm.

There is reason to assume that in all visual pigments the chromophore is a protonated Schiff base, though this has not been proved in every instance. The reaction at the chromophoric site can be summarized:

[1] Requests for reprints should be addressed to Dr. Ruth Hubbard, Biological Laboratories, Harvard University, Cambridge, Massachusetts 02138. Linda Sperling's present address is M. R. C. Laboratory of Molecular Biology, Hills Road, Cambridge, England.

$$C_{19}H_{27} \cdot C(H) = O + H_2N \cdot R \leftrightarrows C_{19}H_{27} \cdot C(H) = N \cdot R + H_2O \qquad (1)$$

11-*cis*-retinal   opsin   Schiff base
λ_{max} 380 λ_{max} 360

$$C_{19}H_{27} \cdot C(H) = N \cdot R + H^+ \leftrightarrows C_{19}H_{27} \cdot C(H) = \overset{+}{N}(H) \cdot R \qquad (2)$$

visual pigment chromophores
$\lambda_{max} \geqq 440$

We have recently discussed the ways in which interactions between the chromophore and different opsins may affect the colors of the visual pigments (Hubbard and Sperling, 1973).

All the visual pigments contain the sterically hindered 11-*cis* isomer of retinal. Light isomerizes the 11-*cis* chromophore to all-*trans* and thereby initiates the series of events that leads to the discharge of neural transmitter at the visual cell synapse. The photoisomerization triggers intramolecular rearrangements of the visual pigment which are accompanied by measurable changes in its absorption spectrum (*cf.* Hubbard et al., 1965):

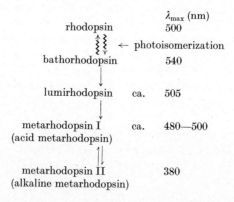

The chromophores of the intermediates are protonated until metarhodopsin I, which is homologous with acid metarhodopsin in cephalopods. Loss of the proton from the chromophoric site results in the formation of metarhodopsin II (cephalopod alkaline metarhodopsin) with λ_{max} 380 nm.

Vertebrate metarhodopsin is hydrolyzed to opsin and all-*trans*-retinal, which is subsequently reduced and stored in the eye as esters of vitamin A. The invertebrate metarhodopsins are stable and retinal remains attached to opsin (*cf.* HUBBARD and ST. GEORGE 1957—58).

Vertebrate visual pigments can be regenerated *in vitro* by mixing opsin with 11-*cis*-retinal. It is generally assumed that *in vivo* 11-*cis*-retinal is drawn from the ocular stores of all-*trans*-vitamin A esters. The sequence and precise mechanisms of the reactions by which the esters are hydrolyzed, oxidized and isomerized to 11-*cis*-retinal are not yet clear.

The only way in which invertebrate rhodopsin has been regenerated *in vitro* is by photoisomerization of the chromophores of batho-, lumi- or metarhodopsin (*cf.* YOSHIZAWA and WALD, 1964). But we do not know how invertebrates form rhodopsin in the dark.

In 1965, HARA and HARA identified retinochrome, a second photosensitive pigment in the visual cells of the Japanese squid, *Ommastrephes*, and suggested that it functions in the regeneration of rhodopsin. Retinochrome has since been found in the retinas of many other cephalopods (*cf.* HARA and HARA, 1972; SPERLING and HUBBARD, 1971). It is located between the basement membrane and the nuclei of the inner segments (HARA and HARA, 1972) in a region that contains numerous bundles of membranes that stain like rhabdomal membranes. These cytoplasmic membranes have been named myeloid or somal bodies (ZONANA, 1961; YAMAMOTO et al., 1965; COHEN, 1973) and probably contain the retinochrome. The reasons for supposing this are: (1) the cellular elements from which retinochrome is extracted float on 40% sucrose and (2) retinochrome, like rhodopsin, cannot be brought into aqueous solution without detergents such as digitonin (HARA and HARA, 1956; SPERLING and HUBBARD, 1971; SPERLING and HUBBARD, in press).

Membranous filaments occur also within the cytoplasmic core of the rhabdomal outer segments (ZONANA, 1961; SPERLING et al., unpublished experiments). HARA and HARA (personal communication) have extracted small amounts of retinochrome from outer segments and suggest that it is probably contained in these cytoplasmic membranes.

The absorption spectrum of retinochrome (Fig. 1) is similar to that of rhodopsin, with a main (α-) band with λ_{max} near 500 nm, a subsidiary β-band at about 350 nm and a narrow γ-band with λ_{max}

near 280 nm. In all species of cephalopods that have been examined, λ_{max} of the main band of retinochrome lies at somewhat longer wavelengths than that of rhodopsin (*cf.* Hara and Hara, 1972). In *Loligo pealei*, the species we have worked with, freshly prepared solutions of retinochrome have λ_{max} 500 nm and rhodopsin has λ_{max}

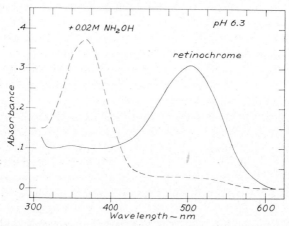

Fig. 1. Absorption spectrum of *Loligo pealei* retinochrome and of its product of bleaching by NH_2OH in the dark. To 0.5 ml of a fresh solution of retinochrome in 2% digitonin in M/15 phosphate buffer, pH 6.3, (λ_{max} 500 nm) 0.01 ml 1 M NH_2OH was added in dim red light and the spectrum was measured after 5 min at 25° C. The α- and β-bands of retinochrome are replaced by the absorption band of all-*trans* retinaldehyde oxime with
$$\lambda_{max}\ 367\ nm$$

492 nm. The most important difference between retinochrome and rhodopsin lies in the geometrical configuration of their chromophores: the chromophore of retinochrome is all-*trans* and is isomerized by light to 11-*cis* (Hara and Hara, 1967, 1973a), the opposite of the situation in rhodopsin.

Hara and Hara (1968) have suggested that retinochrome functions in the resynthesis of cephalopod rhodopsin by exchanging the 11-*cis* chromophore of its photoproduct for the all-*trans* chromophore of metarhodopsin. In this way, rhodopsin and retinochrome would be regenerated simultaneously from their respective photoproducts. There are several problems with this hypothesis. In the first place, very little retinochrome occurs in the rhabdoms, which contain a lot of rhodopsin (*cf.* HUBBARD and ST. GEORGE, 1957— 58). Photons are therefore much more likely to be absorbed by rhodopsin than by the retinochrome in the outer segments and considerably more rhodopsin will be isomerized to all-*trans* than retinochrome to 11-*cis*. Retinochrome could be isomerized in the inner segments and the photoproduct migrates into the outer segment. However, preliminary experiments suggest that little, if any, of the retinochrome in the inner segments is photoisomerized *in vivo*, probably because it is shielded from incoming light by dense layers of black screening pigment as well as by rhodopsin in the rhabdomes (SPERLING and HUBBARD, 1971; HARA and HARA, personal communication).

It is possible that the all-*trans* chromophore of retinochrome is isomerized to 11-*cis* by an unknown thermal reaction. However, cephalopod metarhodopsins in solution are stable in the presence of photoisomerized retinochrome (HARA and HARA, 1968) or even of excess 11-*cis*-retinal (HUBBARD, unpublished experiments). It is therefore difficult to see how the retinochrome chromophore could be the source of 11-*cis*-retinal for regenerating rhodopsin.

Another possibility needs to be explored. In bright light the pupil of cephalopod eyes becomes very small and a dense layer of black screening pigment moves to the tips of the outer segments. Very little light therefore reaches rhodopsin, and even in bright daylight only about 5% of it is isomerized to metarhodopsin *in vivo* (SPERLING, unpublished experiments[2]; HARA and HARA, personal communication). Perhaps the small bits of rhabdomal membrane that contain photoisomerized rhodopsin are removed from the rhabdom and replaced by pieces of somal membrane and during this exchange the entire retinochrome molecule is converted into rhodopsin.

Chemical Behavior of Retinochrome. The chemical behavior of retinochrome offers interesting parallels and differences to the chemistry of the visual pigments. We have mentioned the similarity of their absorption spectra. The retinochrome chromophore is analogous to the protonated chromophores of the visual pigments and participates in an acid-base equilibrium like that of the cephalo-

---

[2] Cited in DAW and PEARLMAN (1973—74).

pod metarhodopsins (HUBBARD and ST. GEORGE, 1957—58; HARA and HARA, 1972). This is shown in Fig. 2b. In addition, λ_{max} of the main absorption band of retinochrome varies with pH as shown in Fig. 2a and c. As the pH is raised from 6.3 to 7.8, λ_{max} shifts to

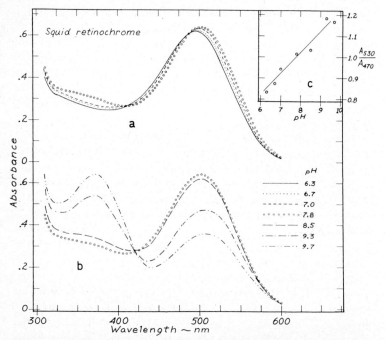

Fig. 2a—c. Changes in the absorption spectrum of *Loligo* retinochrome with pH. The pH of a solution of retinochrome in 2% digitonin in M/15 phosphate buffer was raised in steps by addition of small amounts of solid Na_2CO_3. (a) Between pH 6.3 and 7.8, λ_{max} of the α-band shifted from 495 to 503 nm and the absorption at λ_{max} increased slightly. The curves cross at 412 and 487 nm. (b) Above pH 7.8, λ_{max} of this band continued to move to longer wavelengths but its absorbance decreased as a second band appeared at shorter wavelengths, with λ_{max} 375 nm. The curves cross at 421 nm. (c) The ratio of absorbances at 530 and 470 nm (A_{530}/A_{470}) is plotted as a function of pH to show that the shift in the wavelength position of the long wavelength band is continuous. All the changes are reversed if one lowers the pH by adding small amounts of solid KH_2PO_4. Throughout this experiment, λ_{max} lies at about 5 nm shorter wavelengths than in fresh solutions, because this preparation had been stored 3 weeks at —15° C, but the same phenomena are observed with fresh retinochrome solutions

longer wavelengths and the absorbance at λ_{max} increases slightly (Fig. 2a). Above pH 7.8, λ_{max} of the main band continues to move toward the red, but its absorbance decreases and a new band appears at shorter wavelengths with λ_{max} 375 nm (Fig. 2b). These

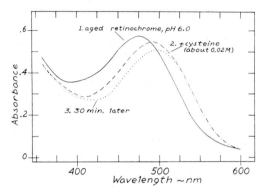

Fig. 3. Effects of ageing and of cysteine. A solution of *Loligo* retinochrome in 2% digitonin in M/15 phosphate buffer, pH 6, was stored 7 months at —15° C, at which time λ_{max} had shifted from its initial position at 500 nm to 475 nm (Curve 1). Within 2 min after addition of cysteine to a final concentration of 0.02 M, λ_{max} had shifted to 491 nm (Curve 2) and after 30 min to 496 nm (Curve 3)

changes are reversed by lowering the pH. The types of chemical interactions that may be responsible for the shift in λ_{max} of the long wavelength band have recently been discussed (HUBBARD and SPERLING, 1973).

Another change in the color of *Loligo pealei* retinochrome is shown in Fig. 3. When eyes or retinochrome solutions are stored at —15° C, λ_{max} of retinochrome shifts to shorter wavelengths. The largest displacement that we have observed is shown in Fig. 3. Curve 1 is the absorption spectrum of a solution that had been stored seven months at —15° C, during which time λ_{max} moved from 500 to 475 nm. Within 2 min of the addition of cysteine, λ_{max} shifted to 491 nm (Curve 2) and after half an hour to 496 nm (Curve 3), nearly all the way to its position in fresh solutions. Similar effects are observed when cysteine is added to less old preparations in which λ_{max} has shifted less. We have not been able to reproduce the effect of ageing by means of oxidizing agents, such as oxygen, copper sulfate or ferricyanide. However, in view of the reversibility by cysteine, it seems likely that the shift in λ_{max} is due to the oxidation of sulfhydryl groups to disulfide bridges. These groups themselves could interact with the chromophore or they could influence the conformation of opsin and so change its relationship to the chromophore (see HUBBARD and SPERLING, 1973). *Todarodes* retinochrome does not appear to change its color as it ages (HARA and HARA, personal communication).

The fact that the Schiff base linkage in retinochrome loses and adds protons depending upon the pH of the solution demonstrates its accessibility to the solvent. It suggests that in the pH invariant visual pigments and batho- and lumi-pigments, the Schiff base linkage is shielded from the solvent because it is buried in the hydrophobic portions of opsin or perhaps because it is surrounded by the phospholipid molecules that are associated with the visual pigments in the photoreceptor membranes (*cf*. CHEN and HUBBELL, 1973).

The retinochrome chromophore is accessible also to other hydrophilic molecules such as hydroxylamine (NH_2OH) and sodium borohydride ($NaBH_4$). When retinochrome is mixed in the dark with low concentrations of NH_2OH, its spectrum is replaced by that of all-*trans*-retinaldehyde oxime as shown in Fig. 1. $NaBH_4$ in the dark reduces retinochrome to N-retinyl opsin with λ_{max} near 330 nm (*cf*. HARA and HARA, 1973 b). These reactions are summarized in Eqs. (3) and (4):

$$C_{19}H_{27} \cdot C(H){=}\overset{+}{N}(H) \cdot R + NH_2OH \leftrightharpoons C_{19}H_{27} \cdot C(H){=}NOH + R \cdot \overset{+}{N}H_3 \quad (3)$$

retinochrome   retinal oxime   opsin

$$C_{19}H_{27} \cdot C(H){=}\overset{+}{N}(H) \cdot R \xrightarrow{\text{NaBH}_4} C_{19}H_{27} \cdot C(H)_2{-}\overset{+}{N}(H)_2 \cdot R \quad (4)[3]$$

retinochrome N-retinyl opsin

Another indication that the chromophoric site of retinochrome is accessible to the surrounding solvent is the fact that all-*trans*-

---

[3] Though Eqs. (3) and (4) are written with the imino nitrogens in their protonated (quaternary) form, we do not know that NH_2OH and $NaBH_4$ react with the protonated chromophores. We are merely showing that at the pH at which the reactions have been carried out, the bulk of the starting material and of the product is protonated.

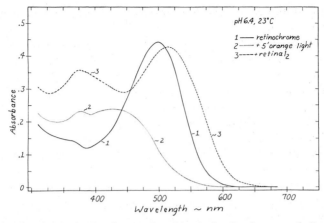

Fig. 4. Synthesis of retinochrome$_2$ from bleached retinochrome and all-*trans*-retinal$_2$. A fresh solution of *Loligo* retinochrome in 2% digitonin in M/15 phosphate buffer, pH 6.4 (Curve 1, λ_{max} 500 nm) was irradiated 5 min with orange light. The photoproduct shown in Curve 2 was incubated in the dark with the approximate molar equivalent of all-*trans* retinal$_2$. Spectrum 3 was recorded after 5 min at 23° C. It has a long wavelength band with λ_{max} 515 nm owing to absorption by retinochrome$_2$ and a short wavelength band maximal near 380 nm owing to absorption by 11-*cis*-retinal that has been displaced from the photoproduct

retinal and all-*trans*-3-dehydroretinal (retinal$_2$) can replace each other in the dark as chromophores. This type of reaction has not been observed with a visual pigment[4]. It is usual for a more firmly bound chromophore to replace the more loosely bound product of its photoisomerization. For example, after the 11-*cis* chromophore of rhodopsin has been isomerized to *trans*, it is released from opsin more rapidly if 11-*cis*-retinal is added (HUBBARD, unpublished experiments). Similarly, the 11-*cis* photoproduct of retinochrome is attacked by all-*trans*-retinal and converted to retinochrome with the release of 11-*cis*-retinal (HARA and HARA, 1968; *cf.* Fig. 4). What is unusual in the exchange reaction we are about to describe is that two molecules which are bound equally well—all-*trans*-retinal and 3-dehydroretinal—replace each other.

[4] *Note added in proof:* MATSUMOTO, TOKUNAGA and YOSHIZAWA (in press) have recently shown that the chromophore of chicken iodopsin can also be replaced in the dark.

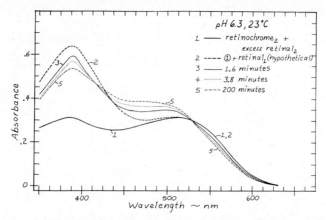

Fig. 5. Conversion of retinochrome$_2$ to retinochrome by addition of all-*trans* retinal in the dark. Retinochrome opsin, prepared as described by SPERLING and HUBBARD (in press), was incubated with an excess of all-*trans*-retinal$_2$ in the dark at room temperature. The mixture was left 1 hr to be sure that all the chromophoric sites on opsin had combined with retinal$_2$. Its spectrum was measured and the absorption spectrum of the opsin preparation sub-tracted from this and all subsequent spectra. Curve 1 is the corrected spec-trum of the synthesized retinochrome$_2$. It represents absorption by the chromophore of retinochrome$_2$ and by excess retinal$_2$ that was left over after all the opsin had been converted to retinochrome$_2$. An approximate molar equivalent of all-*trans*-retinal was added to this sample in dim red light and the calculated spectrum at the instant of mixing plotted in Curve 2. It represents the absorption spectrum of the experimental mixture at 0 time. The sample was incubated in the dark at 23° C and spectra were recorded after 1.6 min (3), 3.8 min (4) and 200 min (5). The long wavelength limb of the absorption band moves to shorter wavelengths; there is an isosbestic point at 520 nm

HARA and HARA (1968, 1973b) have shown that incubation of retinochrome opsin[5] or of the 11-*cis* photoproduct of retinochrome in the dark with an approximate molar equivalent of all-*trans*-retinal yields retinochrome with half-times of respectively about 5 sec and 30 sec at room temperature. The same is true for retinal$_2$. The synthesis of the 3-dehydro analog of retinochrome from all-

---

[5] HARA and HARA (personal communication) prefer to call the protein portion of retinochrome *"apo-retinochrome"*, in order to make it clear that we do not yet know whether the protein portions of retinochrome and rhodopsin resemble each other in their composition or tertiary structure.

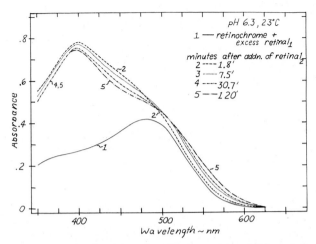

Fig. 6. Conversion of retinochrome to retinochrome$_2$ by addition of all-*trans*-retinal$_2$ in the dark. An aliquot of the opsin sample used in Fig. 5 was incubated 2 hr with a small excess of all-*trans*-retinal at pH 6.3 and room temperature to convert all the opsin to retinochrome. It was then stored 2 days at —15° C, thawed and its absorption spectrum measured. The absorption spectrum of the opsin used to synthesize the retinochrome was subtracted from this and all subsequent spectra. Curve 1 represents absorption by the retinochrome chromophore and by the excess retinal left after all the opsin had been converted to retinochrome$_2$. A 1.6 fold excess of all-*trans*-retinal$_2$ was added in dim red light and spectra were recorded after 1.8 min (2), 7.5 min (3), 30.7 min (4) and 2 hr (5) in the dark at 23° C. The long wavelength limb of the absorption band moves to longer wavelengths; there is an isosbestic point at about 505 nm

trans-retinal$_2$ and irradiated *Loligo* retinochrome is shown in Fig. 4. HARA and HARA (personal communication) have prepared such a pigment with λ_{max} 516 nm from *Todarodes* retinochrome opsin and have called it retinochrome$_2$ or 3-dehydroretinochrome.

The chromophore exchange experiments are shown in Figs. 5 and 6. When retinochrome$_2$, formed by mixing retinochrome opsin with excess all-*trans*-retinal$_2$, is mixed in the dark with approximately 1 equivalent of all-*trans*-retinal (Fig. 5) the long wavelength limb of the α-band moves to shorter wavelengths as some retinochrome$_2$ is converted to retinochrome. The changes are complete after 200 min (Curve 5). If all-*trans*-retinal$_2$ is now added in the dark, the absorption spectrum shifts back to longer wavelengths.

The reverse experiment is shown in Fig. 6. A sample of retino-chrome, synthesized by mixing retinochrome opsin with excess all-*trans*-retinal, is incubated with a small excess of all-*trans*-3-dehydro-retinal in the dark. This results in the shift of the long wavelength limb of the main absorption band to longer wavelengths. If all-*trans*-retinal is added to the mixture whose spectrum is shown in Curve 5, the long wavelength band shifts back towards shorter wavelengths.

The reactions are summarized in Eq. (5):

$$C_{19}H_{27} \cdot C(H){=}\overset{+}{N}(H) \cdot R + C_{19}H_{25} \cdot C(H){=}O \leftrightharpoons$$
retinochrome (λ_{max} 500)   retinal$_2$

$$C_{19}H_{25} \cdot C(H){=}\overset{+}{N}(H) \cdot R + C_{19}H_{27} \cdot C(H){=}O \qquad (5)$$
retinochrome$_2$ (λ_{max} 515)   retinal

They show that all-*trans*-retinal and 3-dehydroretinal, like NH_2OH, attack the chromophoric site in the dark. The reaction with NH_2OH involves the replacement of the anchoring amino group on opsin by the amino group of NH_2OH [see Eq. (3)]; the chromophore exchange, the replacement of one type of retinyl radical by the other.

Acknowledgments

This work was supported in part by grants from the National Eye Institute of the National Institutes of Health to Ruth Hubbard and to George Wald and by a grant to G. W. from the National Science Foundation.

We should like to thank Drs. Reiko and Tomiyuki Hara for many helpful discussions.

References

Bownds, D.: Site of attachment of retinal in rhodopsin. Nature (Lond.) **216**, 1178—1181 (1967).

Chen, Y. S., Hubbell, W. L.: Temperature- and light-dependent structural changes in rhodopsin-lipid membranes. Exp. Eye Res. **17**, 517—532 (1973).

Cohen, A. I.: An ultrastructural analysis of the photoreceptors of the squid and their synaptic connections. I. Photoreceptive and non-synaptic regions of the retina. J. comp. Neurol. **147**, 351—378 (1973).

Daw, N. W., Pearlman, A. L.: Pigment migration and adaptation in the eye of the squid, *Loligo pealei*. J. gen. Physiol. **63**, 22—36 (1973—74).

Hagins, F.: Purification and partial characterization of the protein component of squid rhodopsin. J. biol. Chem. **248**, 3298—3304 (1973).

HARA,T., HARA,R.: New photosensitive pigment found in the retina of the squid *Ommastrephes*. Nature (Lond.) **206**, 1331—1334 (1965).

HARA,T., HARA,R.: Rhodopsin and retinochrome in the squid retina. Nature (Lond.) **214**, 573—575 (1967).

HARA,T., HARA,R.: Regeneration of squid retinochrome. Nature (Lond.) **219**, 450—454 (1968).

HARA,T., HARA,R.: Cephalopod retinochrome. In: AUTRUM,H., JUNG,R., LOEWENSTEIN,W.R., MACKAY,D.M., TEUBER,H.L. (Eds.): Handbook of sensory physiology, Vol. VII/1. — DARTNALL,H.J.A. (Ed.): Photochemistry of vision, pp. 720—746. Berlin-Heidelberg-New York: Springer 1972.

HARA,T., HARA,R.: Isomerization of retinal catalyzed by retinochrome in the light. Nature (Lond.) **242**, 39—43 (1973a).

HARA,T., HARA,R.: Biochemical properties of retinochrome. In: LANGER,H. (Ed.): Biochemistry and physiology of visual pigments, pp. 181—191. Berlin-Heidelberg-New York: Springer 1973b.

HUBBARD,R., BOWNDS,D., YOSHIZAWA,T.: The chemistry of visual photoreception. Cold Spr. Harb. Symp. quant. Biol. **30**, 301—315 (1965).

HUBBARD,R., SPERLING,L.: The colors of the visual pigment chromophores. Exp. Eye Res. **17**, 581—589 (1973).

HUBBARD,R., ST. GEORGE,R.C.C.: The rhodopsin system of the squid. J. gen. Physiol. **41**, 501—528 (1957—58).

MATSUMOTO,H., TOKUNAGA,F., YOSHIZAWA,T.: Accesibility of the iodopsin chromophore. Nature (Lond.) in press.

SPERLING,L., HUBBARD,R.: The identification of retinochrome in *Loligo pealei*. Biol. Bull. **141**, 402 (1971).

SPERLING,L., HUBBARD,R.: Squid retinochrome. J. gen. Physiol. (in press).

YAMAMOTO,T., TASAKI,K., SUGAWARA,Y., TONOSAKI,A.: Fine structure of the octopus retina. J. Cell Biol. **25**, 345—359 (1965).

ZONANA,H.V.: Fine structure of the squid retina. Bull. Johns Hopk. Hosp. **109**, 185—205 (1961).

Discussion

E.GROSS (Bethesda, Md.): The aldehyde group of retinal terminates a conjugated system, thus activating the C=C double bond nearest it. I should like to ask Dr. HUBBARD whether this fact has been considered and — or to what extent — it is of significance for the binding of the chromophore to opsin? — In other words, does the conjugated system open the door for participation in the binding of retinal to other functional groups of the protein, *i.e.* to other groups than the ε-amino group of a lysine residue?

R.HUBBARD: I think the first thing to say is that the chromophore is a Schiff base; therefore the second double bond is much more like a carbon-carbon double bond than like a carbon-oxygen double bond. Therefore I don't think that looking at retinal itself is as useful as it might be when one is thinking about the chromophore. The other point is that we don't know what we are looking for — I mean, what type of "participation" from the protein is needed.

E. GROSS: Are the sulfhydryl groups of no further consequence than what you have indicated so far?

G. WALD: We don't really know! The point is that one could very readily add a sulfhydryl on the double bond, but that would break the conjugated system and would loose color; so we don't expect any addition reactions at that point. I think the sulfhydryl groups are playing an important role in some ways that we don't really understand as yet. I think that in part because it was so surprising when years ago PAUL BROWN and I were working on this to find those two sulfhydryl groups liberated in digitonin solutions of the rhodopsin not only in frog and cattle but also in the squid — and I hope all of you know that squids are *Tintenfische*!

Vergleichende Aspekte der Photorezeption von Retinal-Proteinkomplexen

D. Oesterhelt

Friedrich-Miescher-Laboratorium der Max-Planck-Gesellschaft, 74 Tübingen, Spemannstraße 37—39, Bundesrepublik Deutschland

Mit 19 Abbildungen

Sehpigmente waren die ersten Retinal-Proteinkomplexe, die in der Natur gefunden wurden und blieben für lange Zeit auch die einzig bekannten. Ihr gemeinsames chemisches Bauprinzip ist die Assoziation von Retinal bzw. Dehydroretinal mit einer Reihe von Proteinen, Opsine genannt, die zur Bildung tief gefärbter Chromoproteine führt[1]. Vor einigen Jahren gesellten sich zu den Sehpigmenten zwei weitere Typen von Retinal-Proteinkomplexen, die trotz ähnlicher Zusammensetzung völlig andere Funktionen besitzen: die Retinochrome und das Bacteriorhodopsin. Im folgenden sollen Unterschiede und Gemeinsamkeiten dieser drei Typen von Retinal-Proteinkomplexen diskutiert werden, wobei das Hauptgewicht auf dem Bacteriorhodopsin liegen wird, da in den vorangegangenen Vorträgen die Sehpigmente und Retinochrome bereits ausführlich zur Sprache kamen [1, 2].

Abbildung 1 zeigt schematisch den Aufbau der stäbchenförmigen Sinneszelle in der Retina des Auges. Rhodopsin, das hier als Beispiel für ein Sehpigment gewählt sei, ist zur Hauptsache in Diskmembranen enthalten, die als plattgedrückte Säckchen stapelförmig in den Außensegmenten angeordnet sind. Das Außensegment kann vom Rest der Zelle relativ leicht entfernt und Rhodopsin daraus isoliert werden. Es ist als typisches Membranprotein extrem wasserunlöslich und wird, wie auch Retinochrom, meist in wäßrigen Digitoninlösungen untersucht, in denen die Diskmem-

---

[1] Einen Überblick zum derzeitigen Stand der Kenntnis von den Sehpigmenten gibt das Buch: Biochemistry and physiology of visual pigments, Langer, H. (Ed.). Springer 1973.

branstruktur zerstört ist. Retinochrom wurde bisher nur in Invertebraten gefunden und insbesondere von Hara u. Hara an Tintenfischen untersucht [3]. Die Konstruktion der Augen dieser Tiere ist von dem höherer Tiere unterschieden [4], die Außensegmente der Sehzellen sind durch die rhodopsinhaltigen Rhabdomere ersetzt, und Retinochrom ist im inneren Teil — also dem rhodopsinfreien Teil — der Zelle lokalisiert [2, 3].

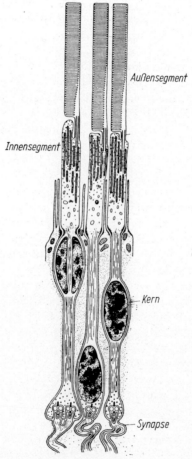

Abb. 1. Schema eines Stäbchens. (Nach Sjöstrand aus Bargmann [24])

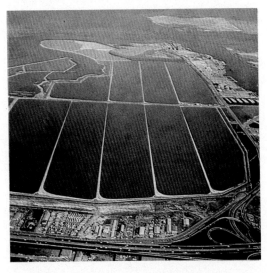

Abb. 2. Luftaufnahme einer Anlage zur Salzproduktion aus Meerwasser. Die Rotfärbung des Wassers ist hauptsächlich durch die Carotinoide von halophilen Bakterien bedingt. Aufnahme der NASA

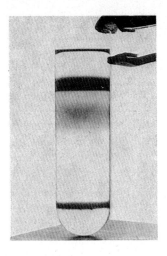

Abb. 3. Auftrennung der Zellmembranfragmente von *H. halobium* NRL $R_1 M_1$ in einem Rohrzuckergradienten (25—40%) nach 17 Std bei 100000 g. Die Farbe der drei Hauptbanden (von oben nach unten)wird durch Lycopin, β-Carotin und Bacteriorhodopsin (Retinal) verursacht

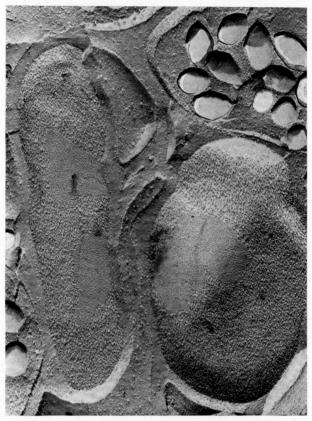

Abb. 4. Elektronenmikroskopische Aufnahme von gefriergebrochenen Zellen
von *Halobacterium halobium*. Vergrößerung ca. 50000fach (Aus [6])

Bacteriorhodopsin wurde bisher in extrem halophilen, d. h.
salzliebenden Bakterien nachgewiesen [5]. Eine Luftaufnahme
zeigt das massive Auftreten dieser Bakterien in Salinen, erkennbar
an der rötlichen Farbe ihrer Carotenoide (Abb. 2). Die Zellen
besitzen keine intracytoplasmatischen Membranen; Bacteriorhodopsin ist in der Zellmembran lokalisiert. Blickt man mit
Hilfe der Gefrierbrechtechnik durch die Zellwand auf die Zellmembran, so erkennt man Flecken dichterer Granulierung, die in
die Ebene der Zellmembran eingelagert sind (Abb. 4). In ihnen ist

Bacteriorhodopsin als das einzige Protein dieses Teiles der Zell-
membran in einer hexagonalen Gitterstruktur angeordnet [5, 6].
Die Flecken können, dank einer besonderen Eigenschaft der
Halobakterien, isoliert werden. Aus ihrem physiologischen Medium,

Name	Vorkommen	Pigment	Absorptions= maximum des Chromophors	Funktion
Sehpigmente (z.B. Rhodopsin)	Sehzellen (Vertebraten, Invertebraten)	11-cis-Retinal	500 nm	Auslösung des Sehvorganges
Retinochrom (Todarodes, pacificus)	Sehzellen (Invertebraten)	all-trans-Retinal	490 nm	Isomerisierung von Retinalen
Bacterio= rhodopsin	Purpurmembran (Halobakterien)	13-cis-Retinal all-trans-Retinal	560 nm (Purpurkomplex)	Lichtenergie- wandlung

Abb. 5. Bekannte Typen von Retinal-Proteinkomplexen

gesättigter Kochsalzlösung, in reines Wasser gebracht, lysieren
die Zellen und die Zellmembran desintegriert in Fragmente verschiedener Größe und Dichte [7], die durch Zentrifugationsver-
fahren voneinander getrennt werden können. Die Bande größter
Dichte im unteren Teil des Rohrzuckergradienten in Abb. 3 enthält
die in der elektronenmikroskopischen Aufnahme in Abb. 4 ge-
zeigten Flecken, die aus 75% Bacteriorhodopsin und 25% Lipid
bestehen. Diese Zellmembranfraktion wird aufgrund ihrer charakteristischen Farbe Purpurmembran genannt [8].

Abbildung 5 faßt in einer Übersicht das Vorkommen der drei
Retinal-Proteinkomplextypen und einige ihrer Eigenschaften
sowie ihre Funktion zusammen. Im nativen Zustand, und das
bedeutet für alle drei Photoreceptoren den Ausschluß von Licht,
enthalten Sehpigmente immer das 11-cis-Isomere, das Retinochrom all-trans-Retinal und das Bacteriorhodopsin eine Mischung
aus 13-cis- und all-trans-Retinal. Gemeinsam allen drei Typen ist
die äquimolare Stöchiometrie von Pigment und Protein sowie die
Bindung des Retinals an die Aminogruppe eines Lysinrestes im

Proteinanteil unter Bildung einer Schiffschen Base, die vermutlich protoniert ist. Das Absorptionsmaximum der Chromophore ist jedoch gegenüber protonierten Retinylidenverbindungen mit maximaler Absorption um 440 nm fast immer stark ins rotwellige Gebiet verschoben; bei den Rhodopsinen liegen die Maxima je nach Protein zwischen 500 und 560 nm, beim Retinochrom aus *Todarodes pacificus* bei 490 nm und beim Bacteriorhodopsin bei 560 nm. Die Funktion der drei Photorezeptoren ist erstaunlich verschieden. Sehpigmente sind bekanntlich verantwortlich für die Auslösung des Sehvorganges; für die Retinochrome wurde vor kurzem die lichtabhängige Katalyse der Umwandlung von Retinalen in das 11-*cis*-Retinal als Funktion vorgeschlagen [3], und Bacteriorhodopsin wandelt Lichtenergie in chemische Energie um [9—11]. Kurz ausgedrückt besitzen Sehpigmente in Gegenwart von Licht *Signalfunktion*, Retinochrome *katalytische Funktion* und Bacteriorhodopsin *energiewandelnde Funktion*.

Bei allen Retinal-Proteinkomplexen besitzt der Chromophor eine breite Absorptionsbande mit hohem molaren Extinktionskoeffizienten zwischen 40000 und 60000. Abbildung 6 zeigt stellvertretend das Absorptionsspektrum der Purpurmembran, d. h. des Bacteriorhodopsins als der einzig chromophoren Substanz der Membran mit der typischen Tryptophanabsorption bei 280 nm und der Absorptionsbande des Chromophores im Sichtbaren. Eine dritte, sehr schwache Absorptionsbande, von den Rhodopsinen her als β-Gipfel bekannt, die um 400 nm liegt, ist ebenfalls zu erkennen. Der Chromophor des Bacteriorhodopsins wird Purpurkomplex genannt und kommt in einer 13-*cis* und einer all-*trans*-Form vor, die im Dunkeln als Gleichgewichtsgemisch nebeneinander bestehen. Licht verschiebt dieses Gleichgewicht vollständig zugunsten der all-*trans*-Form, was sich in einer geringfügigen Veränderung des Absorptionsmaximums des Chromophors um 12 nm zu längeren Wellenlängen ausdrückt [12]. Es sei hier schon betont, daß diese Lichtreaktion, im Gegensatz zu Verhältnissen bei den anderen Retinal-Proteinkomplexen, für das Bacteriorhodopsin keine funktionstragende Bedeutung zu haben scheint.

Die chemische Natur der Chromophore in den Retinalproteinkomplexen ist bis heute in keinem Fall bekannt. Die kovalente

Grundstruktur einer protonierten Schiffschen Base des Retinals ist durch die Wechselwirkung mit Aminosäureseitenketten des Proteins komplexiert (Abb. 7). Der so entstehende Chromophor trägt drei charakteristische Züge: 1. Die elektronische Anregungs-

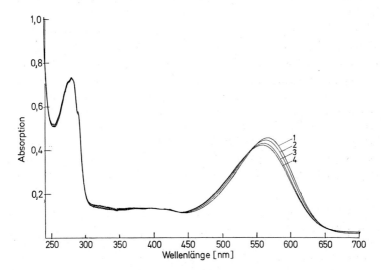

Abb. 6. Absorptionsspektrum der Purpurmembran. Die Suspension wurde belichtet und das Spektrum 1 unmittelbar darauf registriert. Spektren 2—4 wurden nach 15, 45 und 105 min aufgenommen. Die Blauverschiebung des Absorptionsmaximums im Sichtbaren und die Abnahme der Extinktion werden durch die Gleichgewichtseinstellung vom 13-*cis*- und all-*trans*-Purpurkomplex im Dunkeln verursacht (siehe auch [12])

energie ist verändert. 2. Bei gegebenem Protein passen nur bestimmte *cis/trans*-Isomere des Retinals in das Bindungszentrum des Proteins. 3. Die chemische Reaktivität der C=N-Doppelbindung ist meist verändert, was sterische Gründe haben kann, aber nicht muß.

Zur Erklärung der Rotverschiebung der Absorptionsbande, also der Erniedrigung der elektronischen Anregungsenergie, die die meisten Retinalproteinkomplexe zu Photorezeptoren sichtbaren Lichts macht, lassen sich zwei Erklärungen heranziehen; keine der beiden hat jedoch bisher eine eindeutige experimentelle Bestäti-

gung erfahren. Die erste Deutung nimmt an, daß zur Neutrali-
sierung der positiven Ladung am Stickstoff eine negativ geladene
Gruppe des Proteins dient, die in einer durch die Konformation
des jeweiligen Opsins bedingten Entfernung von der positiven

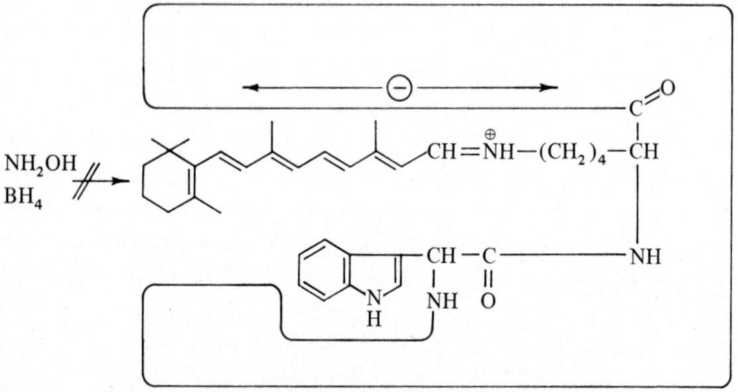

Abb. 7. Schematische Darstellung des Bindungszentrums von Retinal-
Proteinkomplexen. Die fehlende Reaktivität des Chromophors mit NH_2OH
und $NaBH_4$ gilt nicht für Retinochrom

Ladung starr fixiert ist. Molekularorbital-Berechnungen haben
gezeigt, daß mit zunehmender Entfernung der beiden Ladungen
das Absorptionsmaximum des Chromophors zu immer längeren
Wellenlängen verschoben wird und damit eine Erklärung für die
Absorption der Retinalproteinkomplexe im Sichtbaren geben
würde [13, 14]. Die zweite Deutung nimmt an, daß die protonierte
Schiffsche Base des Retinals als Elektronenakzeptor in Wechselwirkung mit Tryptophanresten als Elektronendonatoren tritt
und die Absorptionsbande der Chromophore eine charge-transfer-
Bande ist [12, 15, 16]. Chemische Untersuchungen am Bacteriorhodopsin, auf die hier nicht näher eingegangen werden soll, lassen
uns der zweiten Deutung den Vorzug geben [17].

Das Einpassen der verschiedenen Retinalisomere in die Bin-
dungszentren der verschiedenen Opsine bzw. des Retinochrom-
proteins ist eindrucksvoll spezifisch und erinnert an das Schlüssel-

Schloß-Bild von EMIL FISCHER für die sterische Beziehung von
Enzymen und ihren Substraten. Da sich aus den verschiedenen
Retinalproteinkomplexen die prothetische Gruppe durch Licht,
oder durch Licht in Verbindung mit Hydroxylamin abspalten

Retinalisomer Protein	9 - cis	11 - cis	13 - cis	all - trans
Opsin	+	+	—	—
Retinochromprotein	—	—	+	+
Bacterio-opsin	—	—	+	+

Abb. 8. Rekonstitution von Retinal-Proteinkomplexen mit verschiedenen
cis/trans-Isomeren des Retinals

läßt, kann man diese Spezifität der Proteine für bestimmte Retinalisomere direkt durch Rekonstitution der Chromoproteine be-
stimmen. Abbildung 8 zeigt den Unterschied der Rhodopsine zum
Retinochrom und dem Bacteriorhodopsin. Während nur 11-*cis*-
und 9-*cis*-Retinal mit Opsin zu Rhodopsin bzw. Isorhodopsin
reagieren, werden Retinochrom und Bacteriorhodopsin nur mit
13-*cis* und all-*trans*-Retinal zurückgebildet [3, 18]. Eine Zeitserie
von Spektren zeigt diese Rückbildung für den Fall des Bacterio-
rhodopsin-Chromophors Purpurkomplex (Abb. 9). Innerhalb weniger Minuten wird die Absorptionsbande des Chromophors prak-
tisch vollständig regeneriert, wenn man von 13-*cis*-Retinal aus-
geht, etwas länger dauert die Rekonstitution mit all-*trans*-Retinal.
In diesem Fall wird ein Zwischenprodukt mit einem Absorptionsmaximum von 460—490 nm gebildet, das auch aus Untersuchungen
der reversiblen Dissoziation des Purpurkomplexes in organischen
Lösungsmitteln bekannt ist [12]. Während sich die Absorptionsbande des Chromophors nach Zugabe von 13-*cis*-Retinal ausbildet,
ist deutlich erkennbar, daß sich das Maximum nach etwas längeren
Wellenlängen verschiebt. Dies beruht auf der bereits erwähnten

Einstellung eines Gleichgewichtsgemisches von 13-*cis*-Purpur-
komplex und all-*trans*-Purpurkomplex. Gleichzeitig muß aber die
Frage gestellt werden, wie zwei geometrisch sehr verschiedene
Retinalisomere, nämlich das gestreckte all-*trans*-Retinal- und das

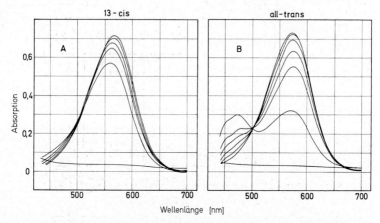

Abb. 9A u. B. Rückbildung der Absorptionsbande des Purpurkomplexes
nach Vermischen von 13-*cis*-Retinal (A) und all-*trans*- (B) mit Bacterio-
opsin im Verhältnis 1:1. Die Spektren wurden zu den Zeiten 0, 0,5, 4, 10, 25
und 25 min (A) und 0,3, 2, 4, 8, 15 und 30 min (B) nach Beginn der Reaktion
aufgezeichnet

abgewinkelte 13-*cis*-Retinalmolekül in das gleiche Bindungszentrum passen können. Die in Abb. 10 abgebildeten Kalottenmodelle zeigen, daß durch Drehen von Einfachbindungen in dem
das Retinal tragenden Lysinrest, aber unter Beibehaltung der
Atomlagen innerhalb des Polypeptidgerüstes, der 13-*cis*-Retinal-
rest in eine dem all-*trans*-Retinal sehr ähnlich räumliche Lage
geraten kann. Dies mag das gleichzeitige Auftreten beider Isomere
im Chromophor von Bacteriorhodopsin (bzw. Retinochrom)
erklären. Zu erwähnen ist, daß das Proton am Stickstoff im
untersten Kalottenmodell in Abb. 10 eine um 180° veränderte
Position gegenüber dem obersten Modell zeigt.

Weder 11-*cis*- noch 9-*cis*-Retinal rekonstituieren Bacteriorhodopsin oder Retinochrom zu nennenswertem Umfang im
Dunkeln, und es bleibt somit festzuhalten, daß diese beiden Pro-

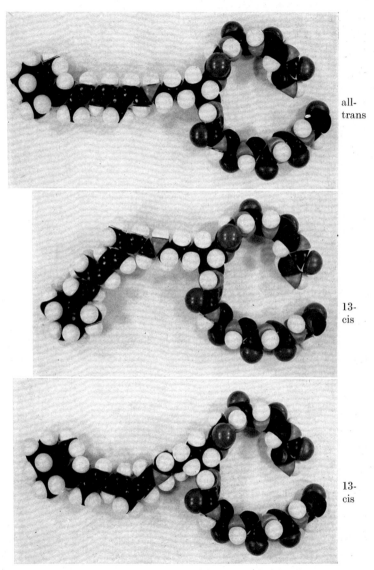

all-
trans

13-
cis

13-
cis

Abb. 10. Kalottenmodelle von protonierten Retinylidenverbindungen. In
allen drei Modellen ist Retinal über einen Lysinrest an das gleiche Poly-
peptidgerüst gebunden (ohne Aminosäureseitenketten gezeigt)

teintypen ganz offensichtlich eine ähnliche, von den Opsinen höherer Tiere aber verschiedene Geometrie ihres Bindungszentrums besitzen.

Die Wirkung von Licht auf die drei Typen von Retinal-Proteinkomplexen kann zusammengefaßt folgendermaßen beschrieben werden:

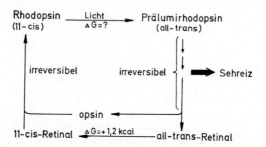

Abb. 11. Der Sehzyklus nach WALD [25]

1. Der Chromophor von Rhodopsinen wird aus der 11-*cis*-Form in die all-*trans*-Form umgewandelt und all-*trans*-Retinal spontan vom Protein abgespalten oder im Zustand des Metarhodopsins, das bei kürzeren Wellenlängen absorbiert als Rhodopsin, am Protein gebunden erhalten.

2. Der Chromophor von Retinochrom wird von der all-*trans*-Form in die 11-*cis*-Form überführt, das Absorptionsmaximum ins Blaue verschoben, und die entstandene 11-*cis*-Form kann mit frei in der Lösung befindlichen 13-*cis*-, all-*trans*- und, in geringem Umfang, 9-*cis*-Retinal durch Transiminierung austauschen.

3. Der Chromophor von Bacteriorhodopsin wird einerseits durch Licht vollständig in die all-*trans*-Form überführt und andererseits in eine kurzwellige Form umgewandelt, die spontan, also ohne weitere Lichtabsorption, sich in die langwellige Form zurückverwandelt.

Die Beschreibung der Lichtwirkung auf Rhodopsine soll kurzgefaßt werden, da sie ja bereits eingehend geschildert wurde [1]. Abbildung 11 zeigt den Sehzyklus, wie er von WALD [25] formuliert wurde. Die einzige Wirkung des Lichtes in diesem Zyklus ist die Isomerisierung des 11-*cis*-Chromophors in den all-*trans*-Chromophor. In der all-*trans*-Form, Prälumirhodopsin, zerfällt die Retinal-Proteinverbindung über eine Serie von Zwischenverbindungen in Retinal und Opsin. Während der Bildung einer der Zwischenstufen wird der Nervenreiz ausgelöst. Da im Minimum 1 Photon hierzu genügt, muß zwischen dem photochemischen Ereignis und der Bildung des Aktionspotentials eine enorme Verstärkung stattfinden, die Gegenstand verschiedener Hypothesen ist (s. diese in Fußnote S. 55). Um den Zyklus zu vollenden, wird all-*trans*-Retinal in 11-*cis*-Retinal isomerisiert und mit Opsin zu Rhodopsin zurückverwandelt. Betrachtet man die Energiebilanz des Zyklus, so stellt sich heraus, daß zwei irreversible Reaktionen, bei denen Energie frei wird, der Isomerisierung des Retinals mit einem Aufwand von 1,2 kcal gegenüberstehen [22], d. h. um die thermodynamische Bilanz des Zyklus zu erfüllen, muß in der Reaktion von Rhodopsin nach Präluminrhodopsin weit mehr Energie aufgewendet, also der absorbierten Lichtenergie von etwa 50 kcal entnommen werden, als die Umwandlung von 11-*cis*- nach all-*trans*-Retinal freisetzt, oder anders ausgedrückt: der Energieunterschied von Rhodopsin und Präluminrhodopsin muß größer sein als 1,2 kcal. Damit kann nicht der dem 11-*cis*-Retinal auferlegte sterische Zwang bei seiner Umwandlung in die all-*trans*-Form die anschließende Kaskade von Reaktionen auslösen, sondern die photochemische Primärreaktion muß, zumindest bei Raumtemperatur, auch Veränderungen im Proteinteil selbst bewirken. Ich möchte hierbei an die erwähnte Möglichkeit einer Elektronendonor-Elektronenakzeptor-Wechselwirkung erinnern, bei der im angeregten Zustand des Chromophors eine drastisch veränderte Elektronenverteilung vorläge und entsprechende Konfigurationsänderungen des Retinals (zum all-*trans*) wie auch Konformationsänderungen des Proteins erzwingen könnte. Auch spricht die Tatsache, daß Isorhodopsin mit dem sterisch ungehinderten 9-*cis*-Retinal im Chromophor ein photosensitives Pigment ist, gegen die Hypothese von sterischem Zwang im 11-*cis*-Retinal als der treibenden Kraft bei der photochemischen Primärreaktion.

Der Sehzyklus in Abb. 11 gilt für Vertebraten. Bei Invertebraten werden nach Lichtabsorption nur die ersten Reaktionsschritte durchlaufen, Retinal aber nicht vom Protein abgespalten, sondern in Form des Metarhodopsins kovalent am Protein gebunden erhalten. Erneute Absorption eines Photons regeneriert Rhodopsin.

Durch die unterschiedlichen Absorptionsmaxima von Rhodopsin
und Metarhodopsin wird, je nach der Wellenlänge des verwendeten
Lichtes, ein bestimmtes Photogleichgewicht der beiden Formen
eingestellt. Das Retinochrom verhält sich nach den Untersuchungen von
HARA u. HARA bezüglich der Retinal-*cis*/*trans*-Isomerie spiegel-

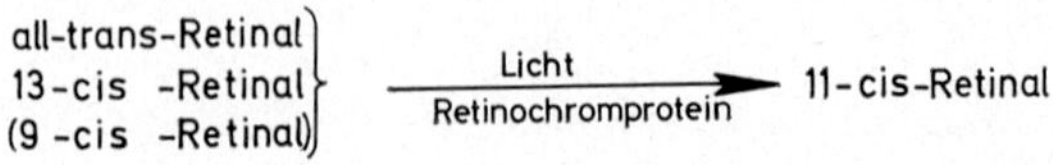

$$
\left.\begin{array}{l}
\text{all-trans-Retinal} \\
\text{13-cis -Retinal} \\
\text{(9 -cis -Retinal)}
\end{array}\right\}
\xrightarrow[\text{Retinochromprotein}]{\text{Licht}}
\text{11-cis-Retinal}
$$

Abb. 12. Mögliche Funktion des Retinochroms nach HARA u. HARA [3].
9-*cis*-Retinal kann die Reaktion nur sehr langsam ausführen

bildlich zum Invertebratenrhodopsin [3]. Wird das native Chromoprotein mit Licht der Wellenlänge seines Absorptionsmaximums
bestrahlt, so verschiebt sich dieses nach kürzeren Wellenlängen,
und die chemische Analyse zeigt, daß nunmehr der Chromophor
11-*cis*-Retinal enthält. Im Gegensatz zum Invertebraten-Meta-
rhodopsin wird jedoch durch Licht nicht mehr der ursprüngliche
Chromophor regeneriert. 11-*cis*-Retinal kann jedoch gegen all-
trans-Retinal oder 13-*cis*-Retinal durch Transiminierung ausge-
tauscht werden, mit dem Resultat, daß Retinochrom oder Iso-
retinochrom regeneriert werden. Dies ist die Basis für die von HARA
u. HARA postulierte Funktion des Retinochroms als lichtgetriebene
Retinalisomerase (Abb. 12). In Gegenwart eines Überschusses
all-*trans* - Retinal und orange Licht, das Retinochrom absorbiert,
wird all-*trans*-Retinal am Protein in 11-*cis* umgewandelt, tauscht
dann gegen ein all-*trans*-Retinalmolekül aus, das den Chromophor
regeneriert, um bei erneuter Lichtabsorption wieder ein 11-*cis*-
Retinal zu bilden. Auf diese Weise wird mit stöchiometrischen
Mengen Licht und katalytischen Mengen Retinochrom all-*trans*-
oder 13-*cis*-Retinal in 11-*cis*-Retinal umgewandelt.

Damit wäre Retinochrom die für den Sehzyklus der Vertebraten
postulierte und gesuchte Isomerase, würde sie in Vertebraten
gefunden. Invertebraten, in denen Retinochrom vorkommt,
benötigen es jedoch nicht unbedingt zur Regeneration von 11-*cis*-
Retinal, da, wie eben erwähnt, hier Rhodopsin durch Lichtabsorp-

tion regeneriert werden kann. Damit muß die Frage der biologischen Funktion der Retinochrome noch einer endgültigen Klärung überlassen werden.

Bacteriorhodopsin ist der „jüngste" Retinal-Proteinkomplex und wurde vor einigen Jahren in *Halobacterium halobium* entdeckt [5]. Zunächst sollen Untersuchungen an der isolierten

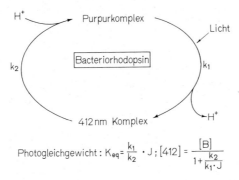

Abb. 13. Der photochemische Zyklus des Bacteriorhodopsins

Purpurmembran beschrieben werden, die vereinfacht als Bacteriorhodopsin-suspension betrachtet werden kann. In Licht gebracht und dort gehalten, wandelt sich zunächst der 13-*cis*-Anteil des Chromophors in den all-*trans*-Zustand um und wird aus ihm im Dunkel mit einer Halbwertszeit von etwa 20 min bei 35° wieder gebildet [12], so daß er als Zwischenprodukt für den photochemischen Zyklus, der im Millisekundenbereich abläuft [10, 19], kaum in Frage kommen dürfte (Abb. 13).

Funktionsvermittelnd ist eine andere Lichtreaktion, die zu einer drastischen Verschiebung des Absorptionsmaximums des Chromophors zu kürzeren Wellenlängen führt. Dieser Zustand des Chromophors wird 412-nm-Komplex genannt [20]. Er kehrt spontan ohne Lichteinwirkung in den Zustand des Purpurkomplexes zurück (Abb. 13). Wie kann dieses Zwischenprodukt, der 412-nm-Komplex, der Beobachtung zugänglich gemacht werden? Das bei konstanter Belichtung sich einstellende Photogleichgewicht hängt vom Verhältnis der beiden Geschwindigkeitskonstanten k_1 und k_2

Wellenlänge (nm)

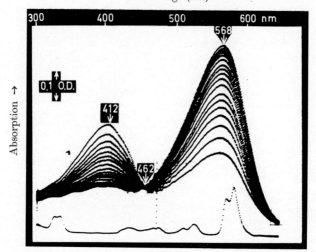

Abb. 14. Spektren des Photogleichgewichtsgemisches von 412 nm- und Purpurkomplex in einer Salz/Äthermischung und die Rückbildung des Purpurkomplexes nach Abschalten des Lichts. (Aus [20])

ab, sowie von der Lichtintensität (J), die 412-nm-Komplex-Konzentration im Photogleichgewicht außerdem noch von der Gesamtkonzentration des Bacteriorhodopsins (B). Auch bei starker Belichtung, etwa Sonnenlicht, liegen kaum meßbare Mengen des 412-nm-Komplexes vor. Durch Manipulation des Verhältnisses k_1/k_2 kann jedoch das Photogleichgewicht verschoben werden, experimentell z. B. durch die Zugabe von Kochsalz und Äther zur Reaktionsmischung. Hier macht bereits bei geringen Lichtintensitäten der 412-nm-Komplex einen erheblichen Teil des Gemisches aus (Abb. 14). Das Spektrum mit maximaler Absorption bei 412 nm und minimaler Absorption bei 568 nm ist unmittelbar nach Abschalten des Lichtes aufgenommen worden und wird gefolgt von einer Serie von Spektren, in denen sich infolge der Lichtintensität Null das Gleichgewicht vollständig zugunsten des Purpurkomplexes zurückverschiebt. Mit dieser Versuchsanordnung, in der Licht zur drastischen Verschiebung des Photogleichgewichtes benutzt werden kann, läßt sich auch die Beteiligung von Protonen

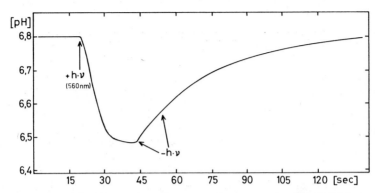

Abb. 15. pH-Änderung einer Purpurmembransuspension bei Belichtung. Suspendierendes Medium: 4.3 M Kochsalz gesättigt mit Diäthyläther; Bacteriorhodopsinkonzentration 0.1 mM. + hv und —hv bedeuten Licht an und aus

am Zyklus nachweisen (Abb. 15). Der pH-Wert des Mediums sinkt, wenn durch Belichtung der Chromophor in den 412-nm-Komplex-Zustand versetzt wird, und das pH erreicht wieder seinen Ursprungswert, wenn sich nach Abschalten des Lichtes der Purpurkomplex zurückgebildet hat. Folgende Charakteristika des photochemischen Zyklus im Bacteriorhodopsin wurden gefunden [20].

1. Die Lichtreaktion, also die Bildung des 412-nm-Komplexes, ist temperaturunabhängig; ihr Aktionsspektrum deckt sich mit der der Purpurkomplex-Absorptionsbande.

2. Die Quantenausbeute der Reaktion ist 0,79, also vergleichbar derjenigen bei anderen Retinal-Proteinkomplexen.

3. Die beiden Formen des Chromophors unterscheiden sich in ihrer Tryptophanfluorescenz, was als Zeichen für Konformationsunterschiede des Proteins gewertet werden kann.

4. Die Dunkelreaktion, also die Rückbildung des Purpurkomplexes, ist temperaturabhängig und zeigt eine Aktivierungsenergie von 11,4 kcal pro Mol.

Dieser letzte Punkt führt zu einem eleganteren Weg als dem der Verwendung von Diäthyläther, um das Photogleichgewicht zu beeinflussen. Da die Rückreaktion mit sinkender Temperatur verlangsamt wird, muß die Gleichgewichtskonzentration des 412-nm-Komplexes entsprechend steigen. Ein solches Experiment

bei Temperaturen unter 0°C, unter Verwendung von Äthylenglykol, ist in Abb. 16 für die isolierte Purpurmembran und für
intakte Zellen gezeigt. Bei Anschalten des Lichtes erreicht der
412-nm-Komplex seine temperaturabhängige Gleichgewichtskonzentration, und wird nach Abschalten des Lichtes wieder durch
den Purpurkomplex ersetzt. Experimente dieser Art bei verschiedenen Temperaturen und ihre quantitative Auswertung
bezüglich Kinetik und Gleichgewichtskonzentration erlauben die
Aussage, daß der Zyklus in Abb. 13 die Photochemie des Bacteriorhodopsins korrekt beschreibt [21]. Weitere Zwischenprodukte
konnten innerhalb des msec-Bereiches spektroskopisch nicht
nachgewiesen werden, sind aber unterhalb dieser Zeitgrenze nicht
auszuschließen. Die Abspaltung von Protonen bei der Bildung des
412-nm-Komplexes ist stöchiometrisch: Etwa 1 Proton wird für
jedes Durchlaufen des Zyklus abgegeben und wieder aufgenommen
[23].

Die entscheidende Frage ist nun, wie die Bakterienzelle sich
diesen photochemischen Zyklus nutzbar macht. Elektronenmikroskopische Untersuchungen haben gezeigt, daß die Purpurmembran
und mithin Bacteriorhodopsin asymmetrisch in die Zellmembran
eingelagert ist [6]. Dies veranschaulicht, daß der photochemische
Zyklus orientiert, d. h. vektoriell ablaufen kann. Die Protonen
werden nach einer Seite, nämlich dem Medium, abgegeben und
von der anderen Seite, dem Cytoplasma, aufgenommen. Derartige
vektorielle Prozesse sind in allen aktiven Transportvorgängen ein
wohlbekanntes Phänomen; das Besondere am Bacteriorhodopsin
ist, daß Lichtenergie diesen Transport treibt. Als experimentelle
Beobachtung findet man Ansäuerung des Mediums, wenn anaerobe
Zellsuspensionen in *H. halobium* belichtet werden (Abb. 17).
Zunächst findet eine leichte Alkalinisierung des Mediums statt,
bevor das pH sich auf ein Niveau unterhalb des Ausgangswertes
einstellt. Die vorübergehende Alkalinisierung wird bei Ausgangs-
pH-Werten unterhalb 5,2 nicht mehr gefunden; dagegen steigt
die Gesamtmenge der an das Medium abgegebenen Protonen bis
hinab zu pH-Werten um 3 noch an und erreicht das 1000fache des
zelleigenen Bacteriorhodopsins; d. h. Bacteriorhodopsin ist als
lichtgetriebene Protonenpumpe anzusprechen. Wie erwartet, wird
der von der Pumpe aufgebaute elektrochemische Gradient durch
Entkoppler, also Substanzen, die die Zellmembranen für Protonen

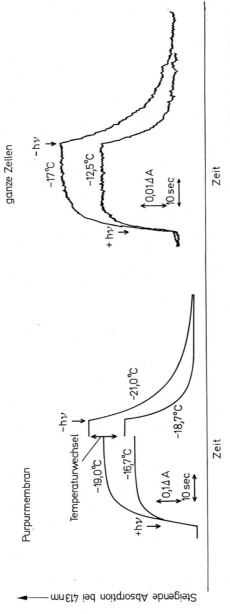

Abb. 16. Photogleichgewichtskonzentration des 412 nm-Komplexes bei Temperaturen unter 0° C. Bacteriorhodopsin-Konzentration der Purpurmembransuspension 30 μM, Titer der Zellsuspension 4×10^{10}/ml. Alle Proben enthielten 50% Äthylenglykol und wurden in der in [20] beschriebenen Versuchsanordnung belichtet

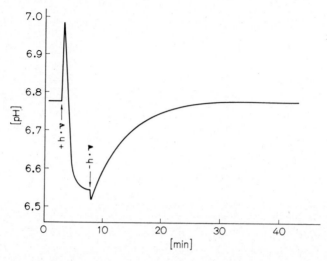

Abb. 17. pH-Änderung in einer anaeroben Zellsuspension von *H. halobium* bei Belichtung. Zellen der späten logarithmischen Phase wurden in ihrer physiologischen Salzmischung zum 5fachen der Originalkonzentration resuspendiert

durchlässig machen, zerstört, und dementsprechend kann die im Gradienten enthaltene chemische freie Energie zur Adenosintriphosphatbildung benutzt werden [10]. Im Experiment von Abb. 18 wird der relative ATP-Spiegel und das pH des Außenmediums gleichzeitig gemessen. Nach Abschalten der Sauerstoffzufuhr zur Zellsuspension sinkt der ATP-Spiegel auf 30—50% seines ursprünglichen Wertes und erreicht bei Belichtung sehr rasch wieder den unter Sauerstoffsättigung gefundenen Wert. Diese anaerobe Photophosphorylierung, die sonst in der Natur nur bei photosynthetisierenden Organismen beobachtet wird, wird, wie der elektrochemische Gradient, von entkoppelnden Agentien vollständig inhibiert, ebenso durch die Zugabe von Dicyclohexylcarbodiimid, das nach allgemeiner Anschauung das ATP-synthetisierende System in Zellen blockiert. Das Schema in Abb. 19 faßt zusammen wie die Lichtenergiewandlung in *H. halobium* stattfinden kann. Bacteriorhodopsin als lichtgetriebene Protonen-

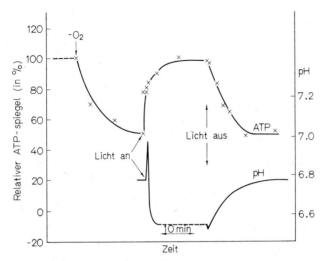

Abb. 18. Photophosphorylierung und pH-Änderung anaerober Zellsuspensionen von *H. halobium*. ATP wurde mit der Luciferin/Luciferase Methode gemessen

pumpe baut einen elektrochemischen Gradienten auf, der, wie von der chemiosmotischen Hypothese von MITCHELL beschrieben, in der Lage ist, ATP zu synthetisieren. Die passive Rückdiffusion von Protonen vermindert hierbei die Effizienz des Vorganges bzw. bringt ihn auf Null, wenn entkoppelnde Substanzen diesen Weg zum Hauptrückstrom werden lassen.

Für den Fall, daß den Zellen genügend Sauerstoff zur Verfügung steht, konkurrieren Bacteriorhodopsin und Atmung, die ja beide elektrochemische Gradienten aufbauen, um das ATP-synthetisierende System. Quantitative Messungen dieser Lichthemmung der Atmung führten zu der Aussage, daß im Minimum 24 absorbierte Quanten ausreichen, um der Zelle den Verbrauch von 1 Molekül Sauerstoff zu ersparen [11]. Dies ist von wesentlicher Bedeutung für die Halobakterienzelle, die in meist unbewegten, durch den hohen Salzgehalt sauerstoffarmen, Salinen lebt. Die Regulation der Biosynthese des Bacteriorhodopsins bestätigt die Annahme, daß das lichtenergiewandelnde System des Bacterio-

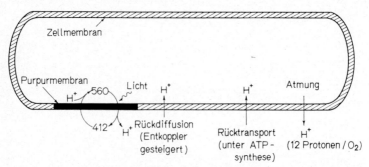

Abb. 19. Schematische Darstellung der Protonen-Translokation in *H. halobium*. Über die Beteiligung anderer Ionenarten an den dargestellten Transportprozessen ist bislang noch nichts bekannt

rhodopsins sozusagen als Sauerstoffersatz bei der Energiegewinnung dient. Nur bei Anoxie, also ungenügender Sauerstoffzufuhr und gleichzeitiger Belichtung, bilden die Zellen diesen Retinal-Proteinkomplex.

Zusammenfassend läßt sich folgendes feststellen: Sehpigmente besitzen in ihrem Proteinanteil ein Bindungszentrum, das nur 11-*cis*- und 9-*cis*-Retinal unter Bildung des charakteristischen Chromophors zu binden vermag, während Retinochrom und Bacteriorhodopsin ein solches Bindungszentrum für 13-*cis*- und all-*trans*-Retinal besitzen. Wenn ihr Chromophor Licht absorbiert, erleiden alle Retinal-Protein-Komplexe *cis/trans*-Isomerisierungen ihres Retinalteiles und Konformationsänderungen ihres Proteinteiles.

Sehpigmente und Retinochrome kehren nach den lichtbedingten Veränderungen nicht spontan in den Ausgangszustand zurück, sondern bedürfen hierzu erneuter Lichtabsorption oder chemischer Reaktion mit einem geeigneten Retinal-Isomeren. Bacteriorhodopsin dagegen stellt seinen Ausgangszustand in einer spontanen, temperaturabhängigen Dunkelreaktion wieder her.

In Gegenwart von Licht besitzen Sehpigmente signalgebende Funktion, Retinochrom wahrscheinlich katalytische Funktion und Bacteriorhodopsin energiewandelnde Funktion.

Literatur

1. Bonting, S. L., Daemen, F. J. M.: Dieses Kolloquium S. 1.
2. Hubbard, R., Sperling, L.: Dieses Kolloquium S. 41.

3. HARA,T., HARA,R.: Nature (Lond.) New Biol. **242**, 39 (1973).
4. WOLKEN,J.J.: Invertebrate photoreceptors. New York-London: Academic Press (1971).
5. OESTERHELT,D., STOECKENIUS,W.: Nature (Lond.) New Biol. **233**, 149 (1971).
6. BLAUROCK,A.E., STOECKENIUS,W.: Nature (Lond.) New Biol. **233**, 152 (1971).
7. STOECKENIUS,W., ROWEN,R.: J. Cell Biol. **34**, 365 (1967).
8. OESTERHELT,D., STOECKENIUS,W.: Methods in enzymology, Vol. 31 Biomembranes 1974 (im Druck).
9. OESTERHELT,D.: Hoppe-Seyler's Z. physiol. Chem. **353**, 1554 (1972).
10. OESTERHELT,D., STOECKENIUS,W.: Proc. nat. Acad. Sci. (Wash.) **70**, 2853 (1973).
11. OESTERHELT,D., KRIPPAHL,G.: FEBS Letters **36**, 72 (1973).
12. OESTERHELT,D., MEENTZEN,M., SCHUHMANN,L.: Europ. J. Biochem. **40**, 453 (1973).
13. BLATZ,P.E., MOHLER,J.H., NAVANGUL,H.V.: Biochemistry **11**, 848 (1972).
14. WALEH,A., INGRAHAM,L.L.: Arch. Biochem. Biophys. **156**, 261 (1973).
15. OESTERHELT,D.: Fed. Proc. **30**, 1188 (1971).
16. MENDELSOHN,R.: Nature (Lond.) **243**, 22 (1973).
17. OESTERHELT,D., SCHUHMANN,L.: Unveröffentlicht.
18. OESTERHELT,D., SCHUHMANN,L.: FEBS Letters **44**, 262 (1974).
19. OESTERHELT,D.: Int: Membrane Proteins in Transport and Phosphorylation, AZZONE,G.S.,KLINGENBERG,E.M., QUAGLIARELLO,F., SILIPRANDI, N. (Eds.), p. 79, Elsevier 1974.
20. OESTERHELT,D., HESS,B.: Europ. J. Biochem. **37**, 316 (1973).
21. HESS,B., OESTERHELT,D.: In Vorbereitung.
22. HUBBARD,R., BOWNDS,D., YOSHIZAWA,T.: Cold Spr. Harb. Symp. Quant. Biol. **30**, 301 (1965).
23. FISCHER,U.: Unveröffentlicht.
24. SJÖSTRAND,F.S.: In: BARGMANN,W. (Ed.): Histologie und mikroskopische Anatomie des Menschen. Stuttgart: Thieme 1962.
25. WALD,G.: Science (Wash.) **162**, 230 (1968).

On the Ionic Mechanisms Responsible for the Generation of the Electrical Response of Light Sensitive Cells

H. Stieve

Institute of Neurobiology, Kernforschungsanlage Jülich, 5170 Jülich, Federal Republic of Germany

With 17 Figures

The membrane potential of visual cells is determined by the concentration gradients of the ions across the cell membrane and the specific permeabilities of the cell membrane to the different ions. The membrane potentials are diffusion potentials. The light stimulus induces a transient change in permeability (conductivity)

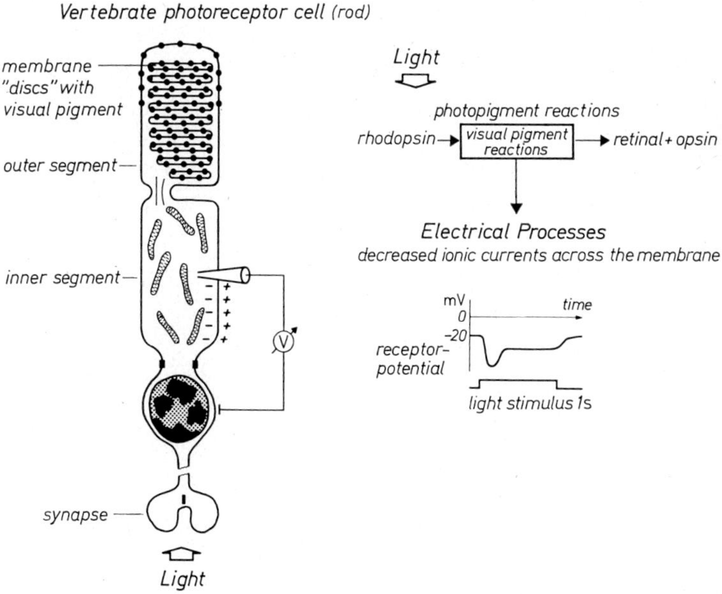

Fig. 1. Scheme of the mechanism of a vertebrate photoreceptor

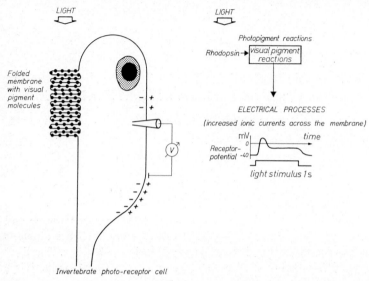

Fig. 2. Scheme of the mechanism of an invertebrate photoreceptor cell

of the cell membrane which causes a voltage signal — the receptor potential. The ions are believed to pass the cell membrane *via* pores. Up to now there exists no decisive proof of the existence of pores in excitable membranes, but a great amount of circumstantial evidence makes their existence extremely plausible.

There exist certain important differences between the photoreceptor cells of vertebrates and invertebrates (Figs. 1 and 2) [1, 58]. Therefore we have to deal with the two cases separately.

It is an important fact that the properties of the cell plasma membrane do differ in different regions of the photoreceptor cells. For instance, the ionic permeabilities in the rod outer segment membrane are quite different from those in the membrane of the rod inner segment.

As far as the ionic gradients are concerned, the same statement cannot be made with the same certainty. It does not seem unlikely, however, that the ionic gradients differ in different regions of visual cells (for instance of crustacea), especially since in several regions the extracellular spaces are extremely small [34].

Ionic Gradients

It is reasonable to assume that the cation-gradients (most important for inducing of the membrane potential) across the cell membrane of the photoreceptor cells are more or less the same in most cell types: a sodium gradient of maximally 1:10 intracellular *versus* extracellular, a potassium gradient of maximally 40:1, and a concentration gradient for free calcium ions which is considerably higher (1:10⁴). The values of these concentration gradients are uncertain, especially because some of the extracellular spaces are extremely small and might have ionic concentrations different from the usual big extracellular spaces of other tissues. Another open question is the ionic constitution of the small lumina of the discs inside the rod outer segments (see [17]).

Properties of the Cell Membrane

a) Vertebrates. According to KORENBROT and CONE [31—33], the cell membrane of the rod outer segments is selectively permeable to sodium ions in the dark but this sodium permeability seems to be vectorial. Sodium ions can enter the rod outer segment at least 100 times easier than they can leave it, possibly due to the membrane potential. The membrane of the rod outer segment seems to be almost impermeable to potassium ions in the dark. CAVAGGIONI et al. [11, 12] also described slight potassium permeability of the rod outer segment membrane in the dark. In this state, the rod inner segment is probably quite permeable to potassium ions and less permeable to sodium ions.

These different properties of the two regions of the cell membrane are the cause for a dark current between the different parts of the cell (Fig. 3).

Light causes a selective permeability decrease of the cell membrane of the rod outer segment for sodium ions [31, 32]. This is the cause of a transient decrease of the dark current [25, 49] and a hyperpolarization of the cell membrane, which is measurable intracellularly both in rod outer segments and in rod inner segments [4, 69].

The visual pigment rhodopsin seems to be situated in the outer cell membrane of the rod outer segment and also of the rod inner segment [30].

Whether or not illumination causes conductivity changes in the rod inner segment membrane is not known.

The light induced decrease in the receptor current has been experimentally demonstrated by the decreased outflow of ^{42}K caused by light [11, 12].

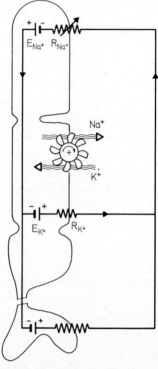

Fig. 3. Scheme of the ionic currents in a vertebrate rod according to Hagins [22]. E_{Na^+}, sodium battery, caused by the concentration gradient of sodium ions, R_{Na^+}-resistance of the cell membrane for the current carried by sodium ions. E_{K^+} and R_{K^+} resp. values for potassium

b) Invertebrates. In the invertebrate photoreceptor the existence of regions with different cell membrane properties has not as yet been conclusively demonstrated. Probably the dark potential is determined in common action by all the regions of the cell membrane, whereas the light induced permeability changes are restricted to certain areas most probably close or identical to the rhabdomeric membrane. Invertebrate photoreceptors which have been studied include those of cephalopods (squid) and of arthropods (insects, crustacea and especially the arachnid, *Limulus*). There are certain differences among the photoreceptors of these three groups of arthropods [26].

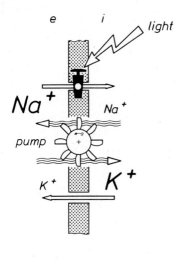

active transport

passive flow

Fig. 4. Scheme of the ionic mechanism of membrane potential in the dark and receptor potential of a photoreceptor cell of an invertebrate

In the dark the invertebrate photoreceptor cell membrane as a whole is primarily permeable for potassium ions. Light causes a permeability increase mainly for sodium ions. Therefore the receptor potential of the invertebrate photoreceptor cell has a polarity opposite to that of the vertebrates (Figs. 2 and 4).

Active Ion Transport (Ionic Pumps)

The ionic gradients are sustained by the action of active transport mechanisms (ionic pumps), which again are probably not evenly distributed over the whole cell membrane. The active transport of sodium and potassium is due to a membrane bound ATPase which is activated by sodium, potassium and magnesium ions, but inhibited by calcium ions [5, 7, 14, 54].

In the vertebrate photoreceptor the pump is probably located primarily in the membrane of the rod inner segment. The activity of the active transport is high in the dark: when the pump is blocked by ouabain, the dark current disappears within one minute. Whether the pump is electrogenic, that is, whether it exerts a transport potential by pumping an unequal number of sodium and potassium ions in opposite directions, is still open to question. The louder arguments do not favor a considerable electrogenicity [74—76]. When the pump is blocked by ouabain, then inexcitability of the photoreceptor cell by depletion of the ionic gradients is reached faster in the dark than in the light [74].

There are indications that the rod outer segment also contains an ionic pump which transports calcium ions actively across the cell membrane [44].

Invertebrate Photoreceptors: The Na^+ and K^+ transporting ionic pump is highly active, even in the dark. Under certain conditions at least, there is a partial electrogenicity causing an increase in the dark potential of 5—10 mV. If the ion pump is blocked by metabolic inhibitors or ouabain, the excitability of the visual cell is lost the faster the more the visual cell is stimulated by light [59]. In the compound eye the pump is probably concentrated close to the regions of the rhabdoms or in the rhabdomeric membranes and the pigment cells [52, 71].

The Membrane Potential of Invertebrate Photoreceptors

Dark Potential. The dark potential of the photoreceptors of invertebrates is mainly a potassium potential, as demonstrated in several experiments:

a) Those in which the ionic composition of the extracellular saline was changed by substitution [20, 55—57, 67, 72].

b) Voltage clamp experiments in which the reversal potential was measured [10, 43, 47].

Under certain conditions there is also an electrogenic component of the dark potential up to 10 mV (see above).

Response to Light: The Receptor Potential. The receptor potential is brought about by a light induced change in conductivity which primarily causes the influx of sodium ions into the visual cell. In crustacea the transient of the receptor potential is due mainly to the influx of sodium, but calcium and magnesium ions also contribute [57]. The steady state value of the receptor poten-

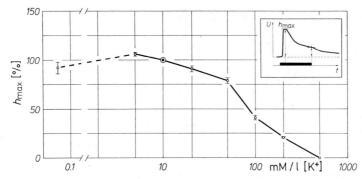

Fig. 5. The amplitude of the receptor potential of an invertebrate (hermit crab, *Eupagurus*) photoreceptor in relation to the extracellular potassium [55] (extracellular recording)

tial is increased by the action of active transport [61]. The receptor potential is gradually reduced by increasing extracellular K^+-concentration. Even at almost isotonic extracellular K^+-concentration, a small receptor potential can be elicited (Fig. 5). This behavior is typical of electrically non-excitable membranes [21].

Receptor potentials, though reduced in magnitude, still persist in sodium-free solution in crustacean and *Limulus* photoreceptors [46, 55]. No light response can be measured in sodium-free solution in squid photoreceptor cell [24]. BROWN and BLINKS [9] could demonstrate (by means of aequorin) a calcium-influx into the photoreceptor cell of the barnacle (a crustacean), but not of *Limulus*.

Perhaps the somewhat intermediate (between squid and crustacea) behavior of *Limulus* is due to the fact that all the visual cells of this species are surrounded by at least one layer of glial cells which leave only a very small extracellular space close to the visual cell membrane. Choline ions can probably partially substitute for sodium [67] and carry a light induced ion current [10].

The influence of essentially all extracellular cation substitutes on the transient of the receptor potential is different from that on the steady state value. This is mainly for two reasons:

a) Active transport is more important for the steady state value than for the height of the transient, because the small extracellular volumes probably change their ionic constitution due to the photocurrent.

b) According to a hypothesis of LISMAN and BROWN [41], the Ca^{++} influx caused by light would decrease the permeability of the cell membrane by raising the intracellular concentration of free calcium ions. The intracellular concentration of free Ca^{++} would then regulate the steady state value of the receptor potential.

The neurotoxin tetrodotoxin (TTX) has almost no influence on the receptor potential [63]. Two explanations for this may be given:

a) The pores which are activated by the light stimulus differ in nature from the pores in the nerve cell membrane.

b) The pores are topographically in a region which the TTX molecule does not reach (for instance the rhabdomeric region ?).

The receptor potential depends on the pH of the extracellular solution. In the region between neutral and acidic pH-values, the pH-dependence curve resembles somewhat that of the sodium pores of the squid axon [28, 64] (Fig. 6).

Tetraethylammonium (TEA) reduces the height of the receptor potential without influencing the decline, both as expected when the potassium permeability is decreased [63]. This could be due to the fact that the potassium pores are in different regions of the cell and not in the rhabdomeric region, where the conductivity changes caused by light probably occur.

This leads to the assumption of at least two (partially overlapping) regions of different properties of the invertebrate (crustacean) visual cell:

a) The dark potential is determined by the entire surface of the photoreceptor cell. Considerable regions of this surface, at least, are easily reached by potassium ions and probably by TEA.

b) The conductivity change caused by light is probably restricted to certain areas of the cell membrane, probably the rhabdomeric region. Sodium ions or its substitutes cannot easily reach this region.

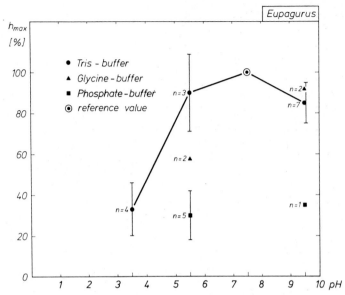

Fig. 6. The amplitude of the receptor potential of an invertebrate (hermit crab, *Eupagurus*) photoreceptor in relation to the extracellular pH [64] (extracellular recording)

c) Probably overlapping with those two regions is the area of the cell membrane in which the main activity of the Na^+-K^+ ionic pump is located. According to WEBER and ZINKLER [71], this region seems to be the rhabdomeric membrane, and it is easily reached by ouabain [59].

Ionic Fluxes across the Cell Membrane

The potassium outflow of the photoreceptor cells of crayfish can be measured using $^{86}Rb^+$ as an indicator for potassium movements, since Rb^+ behaves quite similarly to K^+. Immediately following the onset of illumination, the outflow of rubidium is at first considerably increased (Fig. 7). This increase is, however, of a transient nature, falling to a lower steady state value. In the case of *Limulus*, HOLT and BROWN [29] found that in the transient phase the potassium outflow is 10-times greater than in the steady state of the light response. The increased outflow of potassium is at least

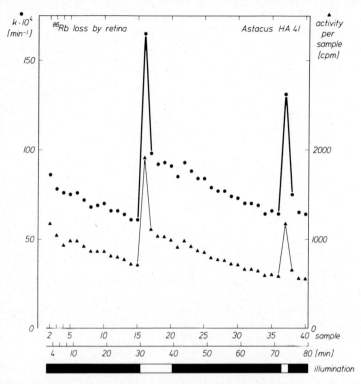

Fig. 7. The release of $^{86}Rb^+$ from preloaded crayfish (*Astacus*) retina in the dark and upon illumination. Activity of the extracellular fluid and rate constant are plotted as a function of time after loading [62]

partially due to the light induced decrease in membrane potential. Brown and Mote presented data which also indicate a light induced increase of potassium permeability in the ventral eye of *Limulus* [10]. Hagins and Adams [23] and De Pont et al. [15] also show increased potassium outflow caused by light in the squid retina.

Blocking of the Na^+-K^+ pump by ouabain application in the dark increases the K^+-outflow of the crayfish photoreceptor cell [62].

The sodium uptake of crayfish photoreceptor cells is more difficult to measure. Perhaps one of the reasons is that the sodium influx occurs in a region where ionic exchange with the perfusate can only be obtained with difficulty, as the rhabdomeric region. Table 1 shows the results of the measurements [65]. They show a significant light induced increase of sodium uptake during longer illuminations. During shorter illuminations it is smaller, and during 2

Table 1

Treatment	cpm/mg albumin eq.		ligth in % of dark	n	p
	dark	light			
20 min light	731 ± 43	869 ± 65	123 ± 6	12	0.005
2 min light	803 ± 66	856 ± 55	109 ± 9	7	0.35
20 min light OU added 40 min before light	1385 ± 103	1453 ± 99	107 ± 7	8	0.35
20 min light OU added at light begin	957 ± 82	1124 ± 99	120 ± 7	12	0.015

Uptake of $^{22}Na^+$ into *Astacus* retina during 20 min incubation in radioactive van Harreveld solution expressed in cpm pro mg albumine equivalent (mean $\pm$ S. E. of mean). Conditions of illumination:
   20 min light period:
   20 min flashing period,   0.5 sec flash duration,
   2 min light period: frequency $1 \cdot sec^{-1}$
   2 min flashing period
Applied ouabain concentration 1 mM OU.

min illuminations is no longer significant. Poisoning by ouabain shows that the Na^+-pump must already be very active in the dark; the sodium uptake in the dark is higher after the pump has been poisoned. The increase caused by light seems to be almost the same after the poisoning period. Only when ouabain is added immediately before the light period is the Na^+-uptake in the light increased significantly over the dark uptake.

The Nature of the Permeability Change

As stated above, crustacean photoreceptor cells still respond to light by producing a receptor potential when the cell is depolarized by very high external potassium concentrations (Fig. 5).

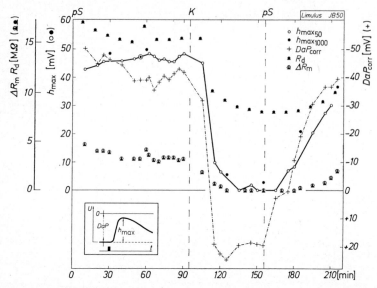

Fig. 8. A graph of electrical parameters of the photoreceptor cell membrane of an invertebrate (*Limulus*) in response to increasing the extracellular potassium concentration: dark potential (DaP); the amplitude, h_{max}, of the receptor potential; the resistance of measuring circuit (cell membrane, cell and electrode in series) in the dark R_d; the change of the membrane resistance at the maximum of the receptor potential ΔR_m; pS physiological saline (artificial sea water). At K^+ the extracellular solution was changed to a solution containing 498 mM K^+ [60]

However, when the membrane potential is decreased to zero or reversed by increasing the extracellular potassium concentration after some minutes, the light induced permeability changes and the receptor potential reversibly disappeared. As can be seen in Fig. 8, the light induced permeability changes and therefore the receptor potential disappear with some time delay following membrane depolarization. There is less time delay for the recoveries of light-induced changes of conductivity and receptor potential following the restitution of the membrane potential. The same behavior is observed when depolarization is caused by raising the extracellular potassium concentration in the presence of 10% of the normal extracellular sodium concentration.

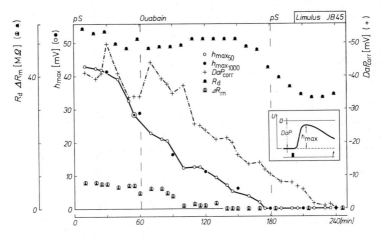

Fig. 9. A graph of electrical behavior of the photoreceptor cell membrane of an invertebrate (*Limulus*) under the influence of ouabain: at OU the extracellular solution was changed to a solution containing 1×10^{-3} M ouabain [60]. For additional explanations, see Fig. 8

When the retina is poisoned by ouabain, the receptor potential and the dark potential gradually disappear. The light-induced permeability changes, and the receptor potential disappear before the membrane potential goes to zero (Fig. 9). Those experiments are in good agreement with the experiments of BAUMANN et al. [2, 3], who blocked the visual cells of the drone by O_2 deficiency (N_2 atmosphere).

Repolarization by electrical current for a short period (several seconds) did not reestablish excitability

These results can be interpreted to mean that the dark membrane potential is necessary to induce and sustain a certain ordered structure in the membrane, which is in turn necessary for the light-induced conductance change. When the membrane potential is very low, the structure of the membrane slowly relaxes. When the membrane potential is restored, it takes some time for the membrane structure necessary for conductivity change to be reestablished.

Metabolism restores the membrane potential (and something else) which is necessary for the structure of the membrane and the condition to exert conductivity changes. In the ouabain experiments, smaller depolarizations are needed to block the light-induced changes of conductivity and the receptor potential, as compared to potassium depolarization. This could suggest, as assumed by BAUMANN and MAURO [3], that metabolic energy sustains not only the membrane potential, but another factor which is also necessary for excitation.

Calcium and the Control of Conductivity

Besides carrying a fraction of the light-induced membrane current in several photoreceptor cells (see above), calcium also plays an important role in the control of the light-induced membrane conductivity [55, 56], as it does in the nerve membrane [19].

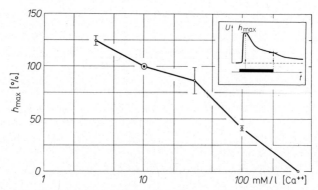

Fig. 10. The amplitude of the receptor potential of an invertebrate (hermit crab, *Eupagurus*) photoreceptor in relation to the extracellular calcium concentration [55]

The following facts support this argument for photoreceptors of invertebrates:

1. The height of the electrical response to light depends strongly on the extracellular calcium concentration (Fig. 10). The higher the calcium concentration, the smaller the response height will be. Very high extracellular calcium concentration makes the photoreceptor cells inexcitable. The rising phase of the receptor potential is not strongly influenced by the calcium concentration.

2. In calcium (and magnesium) "free" solutions the rise of the receptor potential is almost unchanged whereas the rate of decline is sharply decreased (Fig. 11).

3. When the calcium (and magnesium) concentration of the extracellular solution is further decreased by the chelating agent

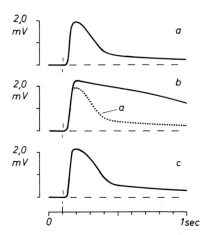

Fig. 11a—c. Receptor potential of an invertebrate (crayfish, *Astacus*) as a function of the extracellular Ca++-concentration. (a) Retina in physiological saline; (b) 70 min later than (a), after 70 min in a calcium and magnesium "free" saline; (c) 70 min later than (b), after 70 min in physiological saline [55]

EDTA (ethylene diamine tetra-acetic acid) (Fig. 12), the excitability of the visual cell is lost together with the ability of the cell membrane to exhibit light-induced conductivity changes, and the dark resistance of the cell membrane is decreased. The dark potential of the visual cell approaches about +5 mV, which is close to the sodium equilibrium potential (Fig. 12).

Those results can be explained [56] by the hypothesis that the channels in the cell membrane which are responsible for the light-induced increase in conductivity (which causes the receptor potential) are blocked in the dark by calcium. Light causes the release of calcium from those channels; the release of calcium results in the opening of the channels. Closing is induced by rebinding of calcium. When calcium is removed by binding to EDTA even without light,

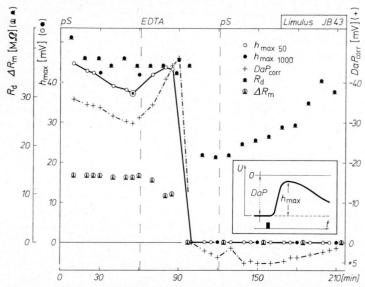

Fig. 12. A graph of electrical behavior of the photoreceptor cell membrane
of an invertebrate (*Limulus*) in response to removal of calcium ions: At EDTA
the preparation was superfused with calcium and magnesium free solution
containing 1×10^{-3} M EDTA; from 90 min on the calcium concentration
close to the cell membrane was, presumably, extremely low [60]. For additional explanation see Fig. 8

the pores are opened and the equilibrium potential for the light
response is approached.

When EGTA (ethylene glycol bis(β-amino ethyl-ether)-N,N'-
tetra-acetic acid) was used and extracellular magnesium was still
present (Table 2) the photoreceptor again became inexcitable but
the dark potential only reached about zero, which could be explained by the assumption that magnesium acts like a "weak calcium" (meaning that a much higher magnesium concentration is
needed to replace calcium in its conductivity controlling action).

To test this assumption we made experiments in which we
changed the sodium equilibrium potential by variation of the
extracellular sodium concentration [60]. In a calcium and magnesium free solution EDTA was added as before, but only 1/10 of the
extracellular sodium concentration was present, the rest was substituted by Tris or choline ions (Table 2).

Table 2. Dependence of potential and resistance of *Limulus* retinular cell membrane on extracellular Ca^{++} concentration [60]

| | Extracellular saline | | | | | | | |
	Na^+	Ca^{++}	Mg^{++}	n	DaP	ReP	ΔR_m	R_d
A^a —	500 mM	10 mM	55 mM	5	-41 ± 6 mV	43 ± 3 mV	$-\ 9 \pm 2$ MΩ	39 ± 8 MΩ
B EGTA	norm.	—	norm.	5	$+\ 3 \pm 7$ mV	0 mV	$-\ 8 \pm 8\%$	$82 \pm 7\%$
C EDTA	norm.	—	—	1	$+\ 5$ mV	0 mV	$0\ \%$	$48\ \%$
D EDTA	$10\%^b$	—	—	3	-20 ± 5 mV	23 ± 2 mV	$-20 \pm 9\%$	$73 \pm 20\%$

DaP: dark potential (membrane potential of the visual cell in the dark); ReP: receptor potential (measured as maximal amplitude of the transient); R_d: resistance of measuring circuit in the dark (sum of membrane, electrode and cell resistance); ΔR_m: change of this resistance during excitation (interpreted as change of membrane resistance); EGTA: ethylene glycol *bis* (β-amino ethyl-ether)-N,N'-tetra-acetic acid; EDTA: ethylene diamine tetra-acetic acid.

^{a} Artificial sea water.
^{b} Na-substitute: TRIS.
EGTA and EDTA 1 mM/l.

As expected, the dark potential did not decrease as much as in former experiments. It reached about -20 mV, a level in the region of the expected value of the new Na^+-equilibrium potential. But the excitability was not lost; a receptor potential and a light-induced conductivity change could still be recorded.

This unexpected sustained excitability in extremely low calcium concentration ($< 10^{-9}$ M) can be explained: Lüttgau and Niedergerke [42] found that in heart muscle the depolarization necessary to produce a given muscle concentration depends upon the relation of the concentrations between sodium and calcium. Increasing of the concentration ratio $[Ca^{++}]_e : [Na^+]_e^2$ reduces the amount of depolarization necessary to obtain a given muscle tension.

An assumption analogous to that of Lüttgau and Niedergerke [42] could explain our experimental findings, which are summarized in the following hypothesis (Fig. 13):

Under resting conditions in the dark a substance P, for instance a gating substance (rhodopsin or another protein?), exists in the state P′ with a high preference affinity to Ca^{++}. When calcium is bound to P′, the channel controlling the influx of sodium (and Ca^{++} and Mg^{++}) is closed (Fig. 13, [1]). The light stimulus turns P′ transiently into a state P″ whose affinity to sodium is increased above a lower but not negligible affinity to calcium. Calcium and sodium compete for the binding sites of P″ (Fig. 13, [2]). Under normal conditions, the sodium concentration is so much higher than that of calcium that sodium is bound. This in turn causes a conformational change of P″ resulting in the opening of the pore (Fig. 13, [3]). After some time P″ converts spontaneously to P′, which has again a much higher affinity to calcium besides a small but not negligible affinity to Na^+. Again Ca^{++} and Na^+ compete, but Ca^{++} is preferred (Fig. 13, [4]). This causes, under normal conditions, the rebinding of calcium and in turn closing of the pores (Fig. 13, [1]). In either state of P the pore is open when P has bound Na^+, and closed when Ca^{++} is bound.

To check this hypothesis we [27] started a series of experiments with the crayfish retina, in which the extracellular calcium concentration was lowered. In one set of experiments the sodium concentration was normal, and in a corresponding set the sodium concentration was lowered to such an extent that the ratio of the

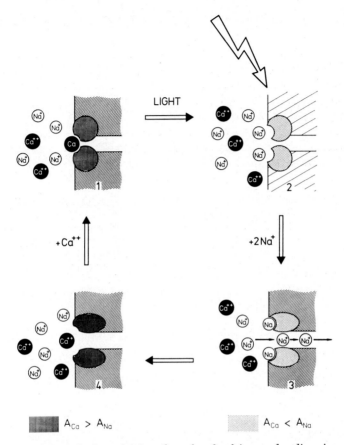

Fig. 13. A hypothesis explaining the role of calcium and sodium ions in controlling the conductivity changes of the membrane of the photoreceptor cell of an invertebrate (crayfish). 1. Initial dark conditions. The "light" channels are closed. A gating protein P has a high affinity for calcium ions and a low Na^+-affinity; the light pore is closed, since P has bound calcium. 2. Light causes P to change its affinity, which is now higher for sodium than for calcium. Sodium and calcium compete for the binding sites. Under normal conditions with high extracellular sodium, sodium is bound. 3. The binding of sodium to P causes a conformational change of P which opens the "light" channel. Now sodium (and calcium and magnesium) ions can penetrate the channel. After some time P changes its affinity spontaneously to a high preference for calcium and a low Na^+-affinity. 4. Ca^{++} and Na^+ compete for the binding site of P. Binding of calcium again causes closing of the pores [1]. $A_{Ca^{++}}$: Affinity of P for calcium; A_{Na^+}, that for sodium

concentration of calcium to the square of that of sodium was held constant.

In the first series of experiments an extracellular calcium concentration of 0.14 mM (1% of the physiological concentration) was used. So far this series is in agreement with our prediction: Changes of amplitude, latency and peak amplitude time of the receptor potential caused by solely lowering the extracellular Ca^{++}-concentration can be counteracted by additionally lowering the external sodium concentration. The decline of the receptor potential, however, seems to be controlled under the experimental conditions applied mainly by the Ca^{++}-concentration alone.

LISMAN and BROWN [41] described another possibly related sodium-calcium interaction: Their experiments suggest that the intracellular concentration of free calcium ions controls the sensitivity of the *Limulus* visual cell membrane in such a manner that the sensitivity is decreased by the calcium influx caused by light. Also, an increase of the intracellular sodium concentration (*e.g.* by the light-induced sodium influx) is assumed to lead to an increase of the intracellular concentration of free calcium ions.

The Coupling between Rhodopsin Reactions and Membrane Conductivity Changes

Still not well understood is the coupling mechanism between the rhodopsin reactions following light absorption and the permeability changes of the cell membrane of the photoreceptor. I will make only a few remarks contributing to the discussion of the processes involved. The transition from Metarhodopsin I to Metarhodopsin II in vertebrates, during which the main conformational changes of the visual pigment take place, is the reaction which is most likely responsible for the triggering of the membrane permeability changes (Fig. 14).

YOSHIKAMI and HAGINS [73] introduced a hypothesis to explain the mechanism of permeability control of the cell membrane of the vertebrate rod outer segment. Following light absorption by a rhodopsin molecule in the disc membrane, calcium ions act as transmitter for the visual excitation. The hypothesis is summarized in a simplified form in Fig. 15. For this theory it is not essential that the calcium released should come from a lumen of the disc. Calcium could also be released after being bound to the disc mem-

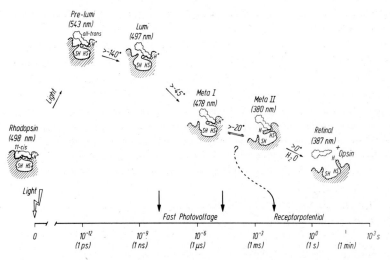

Fig. 14. Scheme of the reactions of the visual pigment (cattle rhodopsin) which follow light absorption. According to WALD [70], KROPF [36], HAGINS [22] and others

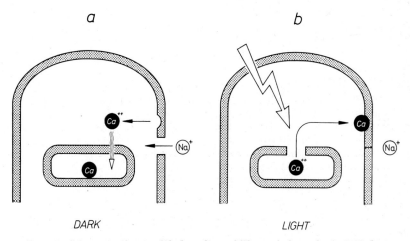

Fig. 15. Schematically simplified outline of HAGINS's hypothesis [73] describing the role of calcium ions as transmitter during the excitation of vertebrate photoreceptors (rods)

brane. Several authors have described a calcium release caused by light from discs or outer segments [6, 40, 44, 48, 50].

Using the metallochrome calcium indicator phtalein-purple NÖLL [48] found in kinetic measurements using a flash photometer that the calcium release was practically synchronous with the transition of Metarhodopsin I to Metarhodopsin II.

The kinetics of the transition from Metarhodopsin I to Metarhodopsin II does not depend on the external calcium concentration [53], even when this is decreased by chelating agents such as EDTA and EGTA [48]. Also, the regeneration of rhodopsin from opsin and 11-cis-retinal does not seem to be strongly dependent on the calcium concentration. These data make a release of calcium which was formerly stoichiometrically bound to rhodopsin improbable.

During the transition from Metarhodopsin I to Metarhodopsin II, a proton is absorbed by the rhodopsin molecule [45, 51]. KREUTZ [35] assumes that this alkalinization of the intracellular medium cooperates with the action of calcium in causing a conductivity decrease of the cell membrane.

Figure 16 shows the pH-dependence for the kinetics of the transition from Metarhodopsin I to Metarhodopsin II. The transition is slowest at physiological pH values. This result could be interpreted by the assumption that the coupling between the transition from Metarhodopsin I to Metarhodopsin II and the processes triggering the receptor potential are best at these physiological pH values.

The pH dependence of this transition does not depend on different preparations used in our experiments [66]. Only whole retinae showed a different behavior, which may suggest that our isolation technique (centrifugation in a sucrose gradient) injures the condition of the rod outer segments to a functionally important degree.

EMRICH [16] described a 30-fold time lag between the pH-change in the extracellular solution and the transition from Metarhodopsin I to Metarhodopsin II. In our preparation — isolated rod outer segments in suspension — we found only small time lags, but greater differences may exist in uninjured whole retinas [48].

Besides many results favoring the calcium hypothesis, decisive experimental proof of calcium being the transmitter between the photopigment reactions in the disc membrane and the conductivity decrease in the outer cell membrane of the rod outer segment is

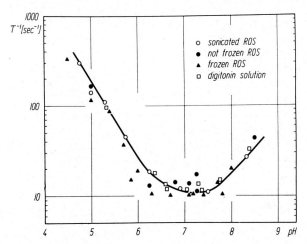

Fig. 16. The pH dependence of the reciprocal relaxation-time (τ^{-1}) of the transition from Metarhodopsin I → Metarhodopsin II at 283° K of cattle rhodopsin [66]

still lacking. However, the hypothesis leads to a number of predictions which can be tested experimentally.

In the photoreceptor cell of invertebrates, the coupling mechanism is even less known. Surely, calcium cannot here be the transmitter mediating between rhodopsin reactions and membrane conductivity changes. CONE [13] assumes that a transmitter is necessary to explain the great conductivity increase of the invertebrate photoreceptor cell membrane resulting from the bleaching of a single rhodopsin molecule.

I would like to end my talk by turning to a type of reaction which is of interest to a number of biochemists.

Phosphorylation

Following the absorption of light, the illuminated rhodopsin molecule is phosphorylated by an enzyme using ATP (Fig. 17). This reaction is relatively slow (half time about 3 min) compared to other rhodopsin reactions in the visual process (Fig. 14) [8, 18, 38, 39]. Until recently it was not clear whether the reaction is reversible or not, which made it difficult to interpret its physiological significance.

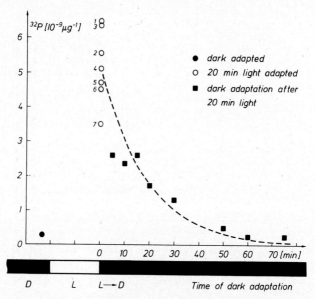

Fig. 17. Phosphorylation and dephosphorylation of rhodopsin depending on light and dark adaptation [37]

KÜHN [37] has shown recently, that in living frogs injected with ^{32}P-phosphate, rhodopsin is phosphorylated upon exposure to light 20 times faster than in the dark. During subsequent dark adaptation, the phosphorylation level decreases slowly to its original value with a time-course comparable to that of dark adaptation.

Biochemists like to think of phosphorylations as sometimes being essential in control mechanisms. Perhaps phosphorylation and dephosphorylation of rhodopsin have something to do with a control of the change in sensitivity of photoreceptor membrane in the course of light and dark adaptation.

References

1. ABRAHAMSON, E. W., FAGER, R. S., MASON, W. T.: Exp. Eye Res. 18, 51—67 (1974).
2. BAUMANN, F., BERTRAND, D., EPERON, G.: Experientia (Basel) 28, 727 (1972).
3. BAUMANN, F., MAURO, A.: Nature (Lond.) New Biol. 244, 146—148 (1973).

4. BAYLOR, D.A., FUORTES, M.G.F., O'BRYAN, P.M.: J. Physiol. (Lond.) **214**, 265—294 (1971).
5. BONTING, S.L.: In: BITTAR, E.E. (Ed.): Membranes and ion transport, Vol. I, pp. 257—363. London-New York: Wiley-Interscience 1970.
6. BONTING, S.L.: 25. Colloquium der Ges. f. Biol. Chemie in Mosbach/ Baden 1974 (these proceedings, p. 1—21).
7. BONTING, S.L., CARAVAGGIO. L.L., CANADY, M.R.: Exp. Eye Res. **3**, 47—56 (1964).
8. BOWNDS, D., DAWES, J., MILLER, J., STAHLMAN, M.: Nature (Lond.) New Biol. **237**, 125—127 (1972).
9. BROWN, J.E., BLINKS, J.R.: Spring Meeting of "The association for Research in Vision and Ophthalmology", Sarasota, Florida, p. 74 (1973).
10. BROWN, J.E., MOTE, M.I.: J. gen. Physiol. **63**, 337—350 (1974).
11. CAVAGGIONI, A., SORBI, R.T., TURINI, S.: J. Physiol. (Lond.) **222**, 427—445 (1972).
12. CAVAGGIONI, A., SORBI, R.T., TURINI, S.: J. Physiol. (Lond.) **232**, 609—620 (1973).
13. CONE, R.A.: In: LANGER, H. (Ed.): Biochemistry and physiology of visual pigments, pp. 275—282. Berlin-Heidelberg-New York: Springer 1973.
14. DE PONT, J.J.H.H.M., BONTING, S.L.: Comp. Biochem. Physiol. **39 B**, 1005—1015 (1971).
15. DE PONT, J.J.H.H.M., DUNCAN, G., BONTING, S.L.: Pflügers Arch. — Europ. J. Physiol. **322**, 278—286 (1971).
16. EMRICH, H.M.: Z. Naturforsch. **26** b, 352—356 (1971).
17. ETINGOF, R.N.: Vision Res. **12**, 929—941 (1972).
18. FRANK, R.N., CAVANAGH, H.D., KENYON, K.R.: J. biol. Chem. **248**, 596—609 (1973).
19. FRANKENHAUSER, B., HODGKIN, A.L.: J. Physiol. (Lond.) **137**, 218—244 (1957).
20. FULPIUS, B., BAUMANN, F.: J. gen. Physiol. **53**, 541—561 (1969).
21. GRUNDFEST, H.: Cold Spr. Harb. Symp. quant. Biol. **30**, 1—14 (1965).
22. HAGINS, W.A.: Ann. Rev. Biophys. Bioeng. **1**, 131—158 (1972).
23. HAGINS, W.A., ADAMS, R.G.: Biol. Bull. **119**, 316—317 (1960).
24. HAGINS, W.A., ADAMS, R.G.: Abstr. 22nd Int. Congr. Physiol. Sci. Leiden, Abstr. 970. Excerpta Medica (1962).
25. HAGINS, W.A., PENN, R.D., YOSHIKAMI, S.: Biophys. J. **10**, 380—412 (1970).
26. FUORTES, M.G.F. (Ed.): In: Handbook of sensory physiology, Vol. VII/2. Berlin-Heidelberg-New York: Springer 1972.
27. HILDEBRAND, E., STIEVE, H.: In preparation.
28. HILLE, B.: J. gen. Physiol. **51**, 221—235 (1968).
29. HOLT, C.E., BROWN, J.E.: Biochim. biophys. Acta (Amst.) **274**, 140—157 (1972).
30. JAN, L.Y., REVEL, J.-P.: J. Cell Biol. **62**, 257—273 (1974).
31. KORENBROT, J.I., CONE, R.A.: J. gen. Physiol. **60**, 20—45 (1972).
32. KORENBROT, J.I.: Exp. Eye Res. **16**, 343—355 (1973).

33. Korenbrot, J. I., Brown, D. T., Cone, R. A.: J. Cell Biol. **56**, 389—298 (1973).
34. Krebs, W.: Vision Res. **14**, 441—442 (1974).
35. Kreutz, W.: Symp. British Photobiol. Soc., London (1972).
36. Kropf, A.: VI. Int. Photobiologie-Kongreß, Bochum, p. 22 (1972).
37. Kühn, H.: Nature (Lond.) New Biol. **250** (5467), 588—590 (1974).
38. Kühn, H., Cook, J. H., Dreyer, W. J.: Biochemistry **12**, 2495—2502 (1973).
39. Kühn, H., Dreyer, W. J.: Febs Letters **20**, 1 (1971).
40. Liebman, P. A.: Spring Meeting of "The Association for Research in Vision and Ophthalmology", Sarasota, Florida, p. 21 (1973).
41. Lisman, J. E., Brown, J. E.: J. gen. Physiol. **59**, 701—719 (1972).
42. Lüttgau, H. C., Niedergerke, R.: J. Physiol. (Lond.) **143**, 486—505 (1958).
43. Mack Brown, H., Hagiwara, S., Koike, H., Meech, R. W.: J. Physiol. (Lond.) **208**, 385—413 (1970).
44. Mason, W. T., Fager, R. S., Abrahamson, E. W.: Nature (Lond.) New Biol. **247**, 562—563 (1974).
45. Matthews, R. G., Hubbard, R., Brown, P. K., Wald, G.: J. gen. Physiol. **47**, 215—239 (1963).
46. Millecchia, R., Mauro, A.: J gen. Physiol. **54**, 310—330 (1969).
47. Millecchia, R., Mauro, A.: J. gen. Physiol. **54**, 331—351 (1969).
48. Nöll, G.: Doctor thesis, Aachen (1974).
49. Penn, R. D., Hagins, W. A.: Biophys. J. **12**, 1073—1094 (1972).
50. Poo, M. M., Cone, R. A.: Exp. Eye Res. **17**, 503—510 (1973).
51. Radding, C. M., Wald, G.: J. gen. Physiol. **39**, 909—922 (1956).
52. Rivera, M. E., Langer, H.: Abstr. DFG-Rundgespräch, SPP-Rezeptorphysiologie, Bochum, p. 35a (1973).
53. Sengbusch, G. v.: Doctor thesis, Aachen (1970).
54. Skou, J. C.: In: Progress in biophysics and molecular biology, Vol. 14, pp. 133—166. Oxford: Pergamon Press 1964.
55. Stieve, H.: Z. vergl. Physiol. **47**, 457—492 (1964).
56. Stieve, H.: Cold Spr. Harb. Symp. quant. Biol. **30**, 451—456 (1965).
57. Stieve, H.: In: Langer, H. (Ed.): Biochemistry and physiology of visual pigments, pp. 237—244. Berlin-Heidelberg-New York: Springer 1973.
58. Stieve, H.: Naturwiss. Rundsch. **27**, 45—56 (1974).
59. Stieve, H., Bollmann-Fischer, H., Braun, B.: Z. Naturforsch. **27b**, 1311—1321 (1971).
60. Stieve, H., Breuer, H.: In preparation.
61. Stieve, H., Gaube, H., Malinowska, T.: Z. Naturforsch. **27b**, 1535—1546 (1972).
62. Stieve, H., Hartung, K.: In preparation.
63. Stieve, H., Malinowska, T.: Z. Naturforsch. **28c**, 149—156 (1973).
64. Stieve, H., Malinowska, T.: Z. Naturforsch. **29c**, 147—156 (1974).
65. Stieve, H., Malinowska, T., Sonnemann, D.: Z. Naturforsch., in press.
66. Stieve, H., Wilms, M., Nöll, G.: Z. Naturforsch. **28c**, 600—602 (1973).
67. Stieve, H., Wirth, Chr.: Z. Naturforsch. **26b**, 457—470 (1971).

68. TOMITA, T., MILLER, W. H., HASHIMOTO, Y., SAITO, T.: Exp. Eye Res. 16, 327—341 (1973).
69. TOYODA, J., NASAKI, H., TOMITA, T.: Vision Res. 9, 453—463 (1969).
70. WALD, G.: Nature (Lond.) 219, 800—807 (1968).
71. WEBER, K. M., ZINKLER, D.: In: LANGER, H. (Ed.): Biochemistry and physiology of visual pigments, pp. 327—334. Berlin-Heidelberg-New York: Springer 1973.
72. WULFF, V. J.: Vision Res. 13, 2309—2326 (1973).
73. YOSHIKAMI, S., HAGINS, W. A.: Biophys. Soc. Abstr. 11, 47a (1971).
74. YOSHIKAMI, S., HAGINS, W. A.: In: LANGER, H.(Ed.): Biochemistry and physiology of visual pigments, pp. 245—255 Berlin-Heidelberg-New York: Springer 1973.
75. ZUCKERMAN, R.: Nature (Lond.) New Biol. 234, 29—31 (1971).
76. ZUCKERMAN, R.: J. Physiol. (Lond.) 235, 333—354 (1973).

Chemoreception

Chemotaxis in Bacteria

JULIUS ADLER

Departments of Biochemistry and Genetics, University of Wisconsin, Madison WI 53706, USA

With 19 Figures

1. Introduction

Motile bacteria are attracted and repelled by a variety of chemicals—a phenomenon called chemotaxis (for a review, see WEIBULL, 1960). Although chemotaxis by bacteria has been recognized since the end of the 19th century, thanks to the pioneering work of ENGELMANN, PFEFFER, and other biologists, the mechanisms involved are still almost entirely unknown. How do bacteria detect the attractants? How is this sensed information translated into action; that is, how are the flagella directed?

To learn about the mechanism that bacteria use to detect attractants, it is important first to know *what* is being detected. One possibility is that the attractants themselves are detected. In that case, extensive metabolism of the attractants would not be necessary for chemotaxis. There is another possibility: the attractants themselves are not detected but, instead, some metabolite of the attractants is detected (for example, the pyruvate inside the cell); or the energy produced from the attractants, perhaps in the form of adenosine triphosphate, is detected. In these cases, metabolism of the attractants would be necessary for chemotaxis. The idea that bacteria sense the energy produced from the attractants has, in fact, gained wide acceptance for explaining chemotaxis (and also phototaxis) (CLAYTON, 1964; LINKS, 1955).

To try to determine which of these possibilities is correct, experiments were carried out with *Escherichia coli* bacteria which, we had previously shown (ADLER, 1966), exhibit chemotaxis towards various organic nutrients. The results show that extensive metabolism of the attractants is not required, or sufficient, for chemotaxis. Instead, the attractants themselves are detected.

The systems that bacteria use to detect chemicals without metabolizing them are here called "chemoreceptors". Efforts to identify the chemoreceptors are described.

2. A Quantitative Method for Studying Chemotaxis

In the 1880's, PFEFFER (1884, 1888) demonstrated chemotaxis by pushing a capillary tube containing a solution of attractant into a suspension of motile bacteria on a slide and then observing microscopically that the bacteria accumulated first near the mouth of the capillary and later inside (Fig. 1). A modification (ADLER, 1969, 1973) of this method, which permits quantitative study of chemotaxis, follows.

After incubation at 30° C for 60 min, the capillary is taken out of the bacterial suspension and the number of bacteria inside the capillary is measured by plating the contents of the capillary and counting colonies the next day (Fig. 2). Reproducibility of the

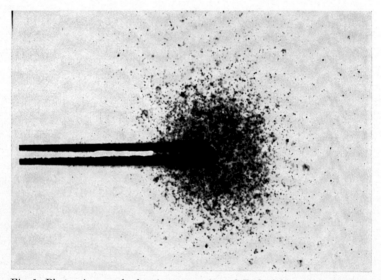

Fig. 1. Photomicrograph showing attraction of *Escherichia coli* bacteria to aspartate. The capillary tube (diameter $\sim 25\,\mu$) contained aspartate at a concentration of 2×10^{-3} M. (Photomicrograph by S. W. RAMSEY; darkfield photography) (ADLER, 1969)

CONCENCENTRATION-RESPONSE CURVE

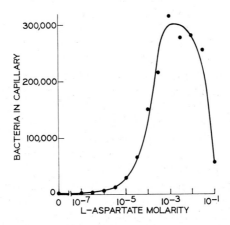

Fig. 2. The number of *E. coli* entering in 1 hr a capillary tube containing the attractant L-aspartate as a function of attractant concentration

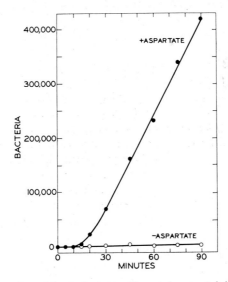

Fig. 3. The number of bacteria in capillary tubes containing L-aspartate (10^{-3} M) as a function of time. The usual assay time is 1 hr

method is $\pm 15\%$. An attractant is tested over a range of concentrations usually between 10^{-8} M and 10^{-1} M in ten-fold intervals. From such an experiment one can construct a concentration-response curve and estimate a threshold concentration for accumulation inside the capillary. Some examples of attractants are galactose, glucose, ribose, aspartate and serine. (All sugars mentioned in this paper have the D-configuration, and all amino acids the L-configuration.) For a time course, see Fig. 3.

3. Evidence that the Attractants Themselves Are Detected

The following five approaches lead to the conclusion that chemotaxis is not a consequence of the metabolism of the attractants but, rather, that the attractants themselves are detected. A more complete documentation of the data can be found elsewhere (ADLER, 1969).

a) *Some chemicals that are extensively metabolized fail to attract bacteria.* This includes galactonate, gluconate, glucuronate, glycerol (Fig. 4), α-ketoglutarate, succinate, fumarate, malate and pyruvate. This result makes it clear that metabolism of a chemical and energy production from it are not sufficient to make a chemical an attractant.

b) *Some chemicals that are essentially non-metabolizable attract bacteria.*

i) *Mutant bacteria that have lost the ability to metabolize a chemical are attracted to it.* Mutants which lack three enzymatic activities essential for the metabolism of galactose are attracted to galactose as well as wild-type bacteria (Fig. 5). Evidence has been presented (ADLER, 1969) that these mutants are 99.5% or more blocked in their metabolism of galactose, relative to a wild-type strain. A similar result for glucose taxis was obtained with a mutant defective in its ability to metabolize glucose.

ii) *Some essentially non-metabolizable analogs of metabolizable chemicals attract bacteria.* D-Fucose (6-deoxy-D-galactose) is a galactose analog that is not metabolized by *E. coli* (ADLER, 1969; BUTTIN, 1963). Nevertheless, the bacteria are attracted to it very well, although its threshold concentration for chemotaxis is higher than that of D-galactose, as might be expected for an analog (Fig. 6). The D-fucose had been purified to remove metabolizable impurities such as galactose or glucose.

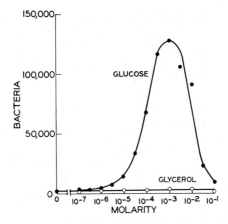

Fig. 4. Both glucose and glycerol are capable of being completely metabolized by *E. coli*, yet glucose is an attractant and glycerol is not (ADLER, 1969)

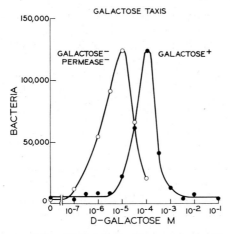

Fig. 5. Galactose taxis in wild-type bacteria (●——●) and in a mutant lacking galactose metabolism and galactose permease (○——○)

Three glucose analogs which were known to be non-metabolizable are also attractants: 2-deoxyglucose, α-methyl glucoside, and L-sorbose. The three analogs were purified before use in order to remove glucose or other contaminants.

c) *Chemicals attract bacteria even in the presence of a metabolizable chemical.* If bacteria detect metabolites of an attractant, or energy produced from it, then the addition of a metabolizable chemical should stop chemotaxis by flooding the cells with metabolites and

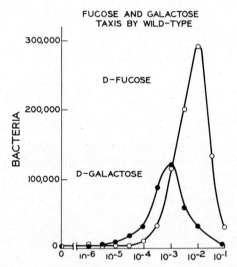

Fig. 6. D-Fucose is not metabolised, yet it is an attractant (ADLER, 1969)

energy. This was not found to be the case for either metabolizable or non-metabolizable attractants (ADLER, 1969).

d) *Attractants that are closely related in structure compete with each other, but not with structurally unrelated compounds.* This finding supports the conclusion that it is the attractants themselves that are detected, and that there exists a variety of specific receptors.

In these "competition" experiments (Fig. 7) one attractant, usually at 0.01 M, is put into the capillary tube, and another attractant at a concentration of 0.01 M is put into both the capillary and the bacterial suspension. If the two attractants use the same chemoreceptor, the response should be inhibited; if they do not, the response should not be affected. Only two examples will be presented here (see ADLER, 1969; ADLER et al. 1973; MESIBOV and ADLER, 1972 for more results).

Chemotaxis towards fucose was completely inhibited by the presence of galactose, and in the reciprocal experiment there was nearly complete inhibition. This suggests that fucose and galactose use the same chemoreceptor (the "galactose receptor").

Competition

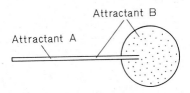

Fig. 7. The design of a competition experiment to determine if two attractants are detected by the same or different receptors

Glucose completely eliminated taxis towards galactose, but in the reciprocal experiment the inhibition was only about 60—70%, no matter how high the concentration of galactose was. This suggests that the receptor which detects galactose also detects glucose but that, in addition, there is another receptor that detects glucose but not galactose (the "glucose receptor").

e) *There are mutants which fail to carry out chemotaxis to certain attractants but are still able to metabolize them.* If there are chemoreceptors in bacteria and if they are specific, there should be mutants that are defective in their response to some attractants but not to others, because of a defect in a single receptor. Such mutants of *E. coli* have now been found (ADLER et al., 1973; MESIBOV and ADLER, 1972; HAZELBAUER et al., 1969) by use of the method shown in Fig. 8.

One mutant, defective in "serine receptor" activity, fails to be attracted to serine and shows much-reduced taxis towards glycine, alanine, and cysteine. (These residual responses result from the "aspartate receptor".) The mutant is attracted normally to aspartate and glutamate, and to galactose, glucose and ribose. It oxidizes and takes up L-serine at the same rate that its parent does.

Another mutant lacking "aspartate receptor" activity shows no chemotaxis towards aspartate and glutamate, nearly normal taxis towards serine, alanine, glycine and cysteine, and normal taxis towards galactose, glucose and ribose. The rate of oxidation and uptake of aspartate is the same for the mutant and its parent.

A third type of mutant, missing the "galactose receptor", is not attracted to galactose and fucose, and is attracted to glucose at a

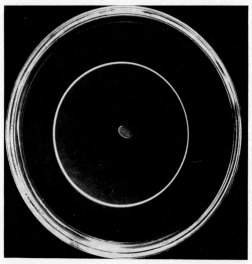

Fig. 8. The isolation of mutants lacking a specific type of chemoreceptor. A ring of wild-type bacteria form as the supply of attractant is depleted from the center, leaving at the origin those mutants lacking positive chemotaxis for the attractant (ADLER, 1966)

higher-than-normal threshold. (This residual response to glucose results from the "glucose receptor".) These mutants are normally attracted to fructose, ribose, serine and aspartate. Metabolism of galactose is normal in these mutants. In some of the mutants there is a defect in the uptake of galactose, which will be discussed below.

The existence of these three non-chemotactic mutants argues for specific receptors and provides additional support for the idea that detection of the attractants is independent of their metabolism.

4. How Many Chemoreceptors?

To determine how many kinds of chemoreceptors there are, three approaches are being used. The first is to ask whether a given

Table 1. Partial list of chemoreceptors for positive chemotaxis in
Escherichia coli

Attractant	Chemoreceptor	Threshold[a] molarity
	N-Acetyl-glucosamine receptor	
N-Acetyl-D-glucosamine		1×10^{-5}
	Fructose receptor	
D-Fructose		1×10^{-5}
	Galactose receptor	
D-Galactose		4×10^{-7}
D-Glucose		4×10^{-7}
D-Fucose		3×10^{-5}
	Glucose receptor	
D-Glucose		1×10^{-5}
D-Mannose		1×10^{-5}
	Maltose receptor	
Maltose		2×10^{-6}
	Mannitol receptor	
D-Mannitol		7×10^{-6}
	Ribose receptor	
D-Ribose		3×10^{-7}
	Sorbitol receptor	
D-Sorbitol		1×10^{-5}
	Trehalose receptor	
Trehalose		6×10^{-6}
	Aspartate receptor	
L-Aspartate		6×10^{-8}
L-Glutamate		2×10^{-5}
	Serine receptor	
L-Serine		4×10^{-7}
L-Cysteine		6×10^{-6}
L-Alanine		7×10^{-5}
Glycine		2×10^{-5}

[a] The threshold values are lower in mutants unable to take up or metabolize a chemical.

Also attractive: O_2, various inorganic ions.

Data from MESIBOV and ADLER, 1972; ADLER et al., 1973.

attractant is still effective when another attractant is present (see "competition experiments" above, p. 112, Section 3d). The second is to try to isolate mutants defective in individual receptor activities. A third approach is to study the inducibility of specific taxes (presumably the inducibility of specific receptors). For example, taxis towards galactose and fucose is inducible by galactose.

The conclusion from results obtained so far (ADLER, 1969; HAZELBAUER et al., 1969; ADLER et al., 1973; MESIBOV and ADLER, 1972) is that for positive chemotaxis there are at least the eleven chemoreceptors shown in Table 1. Oxygen is known to be an attractant for *E. coli* (ADLER, 1969), so there could be a receptor for it, but this question has not been investigated so far. A survey of other possible attractants has not been completed.

It is conceivable that, besides chemoreceptors, at least some bacteria might have receptors specialized to detect light, gravity or temperature, since all these stimuli are known to elicit tactic responses in some bacteria (WEIBULL, 1960).

5. Negative Chemotaxis

Negative chemotaxis (TSO and ADLER, 1974a) can be studied with similar techniques. Repellent is put into the bacterial suspension but not into the capillary; then bacteria "escape" into the capillary for "refuge" and they are counted (Fig. 9). Or soft agar plates containing plugs of repellent can be used (Fig. 10). Many repellent substances have been found (Table 2 contains a partial list). Competition experiments have been done, and mutants have been isolated that specifically lack the ability to be repelled by acid, indole, a group of five hydrophobic amino acids, and salicylate. On this basis and on the basis of chemical structure, the repellents can be divided into chemoreceptor classes (Table 2). Very likely there is a chemoreceptor for each class.

Most substances that act as repellents are harmful to the organism. One exception is that of leucine, probably a repellent as a result of its similarity to the toxic amino acid valine. However, the ability of a substance to harm the organism is unrelated to the mechanism of chemotaxis. Phenol is just as toxic to *E. coli* as to *Salmonella*, and mutants that do not run away from a toxic substance such as indole are equally susceptible to its toxic effects as the wild type. Chemoreceptors permit the detection of a repellent at a sufficiently low concentration to prevent its harmful effects.

Negative chemotaxis

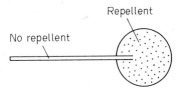

Fig. 9. Assay method for negative chemotaxis. Repellent is added to the medium containing the bacteria, and bacteria are forced to migrate into the capillary tube which lacks repellent. The concentration of bacteria within the tube is then determined

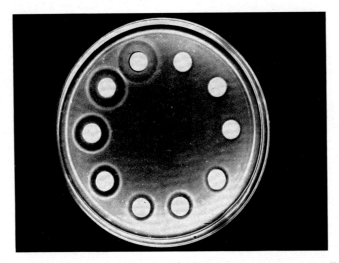

Fig. 10. Plugs of hard agar containing material to be tested as a repellent (each containing a different concentration of the repellent acetate starting with none at 1 o'clock and increasing from 3×10^{-4} to 3 M clockwise) are placed into soft agar containing the bacteria. Within one hour, the area around the plug containing a repellent will be vacated. This method can also be used for the isolation of mutants which would not flee the area (Tso and Adler, 1974a)

Table 2. Partial list of chemoreceptors for negative chemotaxis
in *Escherichia coli*

Repellent	Chemoreceptor	Threshold molarity
	Fatty acid receptor	
Acetate (C2)		3×10^{-4}
Propionate (C3)		2×10^{-4}
Butyrate, *iso*-butyrate (C4)		10^{-4}
Valerate, *iso*-valerate (C5)		10^{-4}
Caproate (C6)		10^{-4}
Heptanoate (C7)		6×10^{-3}
	Alcohol receptor	
Methanol		10^{-1}
Ethanol		10^{-3}
n-Propanol		4×10^{-3}
iso-Propanol		6×10^{-4}
iso-Butanol		10^{-3}
	Hydrophobic amino acid receptor	
Leucine		10^{-4}
Isoleucine		1.5×10^{-4}
Valine		2.5×10^{-4}
Tryptophan		10^{-3}
Phenylalanine		3×10^{-3}
Glutamine		3×10^{-3}
Histidine		5×10^{-3}
	Indole receptor	
Indole		10^{-6}
Skatole		10^{-6}
	Aromatic receptor	
Benzoate		10^{-4}
Salicylate		10^{-4}
	H^+ receptor	
Low pH		pH 6.5
	OH^- receptor	
High pH		pH 7.5
	Others	

Data from Tso and ADLER, 1974a.

6. What Is the Nature of the Chemoreceptors?

Each chemoreceptor is presumed to utilize a protein—the "recognition component"—to bind specifically the chemicals it can detect. This protein is believed to be in or associated with the cytoplasmic membrane, and to be part of a transport system. It thus serves a dual function, to sense the attractant and to bring about its transport.

A large number of mutants which lack galactose taxis have been isolated (HAZELBAUER and ADLER, 1971; ORDAL and ADLER, 1974). These are of three basic types (Fig. 11). Some either lack the galac-

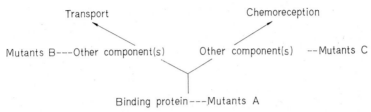

Fig. 11. Role of binding protein in chemoreception, and the relationship between chemoreception and transport (HAZELBAUER and ADLER, 1971)

tose binding protein completely, or have point mutations which result in a defective conformation incapable of binding the sugar. As a result, galactose taxis is missing, and galactose transport is also defective (Type A mutants). Type B mutants show normal galactose taxis, but are deficient in or lack the ability to transport galactose. Still a third type of mutant (Type C) specifically lacks galactose taxis, but has a normal transport mechanism for galactose and apparently contains a normal galactose binding protein. The gene involved in this Type C mutation is presumed to affect a process, or to produce a substance which is responsible for sensing the occupancy of the binding protein by galactose and then signalling this information to the chemotactic mechanism, which ultimately affects the flagella.

Mutants lacking the binding protein are not attracted by galactose (HAZELBAUER and ADLER, 1971), and both the chemotactic response and the ability to bind galactose are recovered (GOY, unpublished) following reversion of a point mutation in the structural gene for the galactose binding protein (BOOS, 1972). Other evidence for a link between chemotaxis and binding protein is the observation that, for a series of galactose analogs, the extent to which the analog acts as an attractant is directly correlated to its binding (HAZELBAUER and ADLER, 1971). A third line of evidence is that osmotically shocked bacteria lacking the binding protein are not attracted to galactose. Preliminary evidence suggests that galactose taxis can be restored by the addition of the binding protein to shocked bacteria (HAZELBAUER and ADLER, 1971); see also KALCKAR, 1971).

The galactose binding protein has been purified by ANRAKU, who discovered it, and it has a molecular weight of 35 000 (ANRAKU, 1968). Each bacterium contains 6—10 000 molecules (Boos, unpublished). The protein has no known enzymatic activity (ANRAKU, 1968). Its dissociation constant for galactose was originally reported as 10^{-6} M (ANRAKU, 1968), but later work showed that the protein actually has two dissociation constants for galactose, 10^{-7} M and 10^{-5} M (Boos et al., 1972), indicative of two binding sites per molecule. The protein had been shown to be involved in galactose transport (ANRAKU, 1968; Boos, 1972; Boos et al., 1972; Boos and GORDON, 1971).

The degree of association of chemoreceptor binding proteins to the cytoplasmic membrane varies; some are tightly associated while others are only loosely bound, if at all. This was demonstrated using an osmotic shock technique for removing the *E. coli* periplasmic proteins, *i.e.*, proteins located in the region between the cytoplasmic membrane and cell wall (HEPPEL, 1967). Binding proteins for galactose, maltose and ribose were found in the osmotic shock fluid (HAZELBAUER and ADLER, 1971), while others were not.

The binding protein for maltose has been purified from *E. coli* by SCHWARTZ et al. (unpublished thesis of KELLERMAN), and that for ribose has been purified from *Salmonella typhimurium*, and characterized and shown to serve as ribose chemoreceptor by AKSAMIT and KOSHLAND (1973, 1974).

The tightly bound (not osmotically shockable) receptors involved in sugar chemotaxis utilize a component of the phosphotransferase system that is also involved in transport processes (KUNDIG et al., 1966; SIMONI et al., 1967). The reaction sequence catalyzed by this system is:

$$\text{phosphoenolpyruvate} + \text{HPr protein} \xrightarrow{\text{Enzyme I}} \tag{1}$$
$$\text{P-HPr protein} + \text{pyruvate}$$

$$\text{P-HPr protein} + \text{sugar} \xrightarrow[\text{additional protein}]{\text{Enzyme II}} \tag{2}$$
$$\text{sugar-P} + \text{HPr protein}$$

The Enzymes II for this reaction are tightly bound to the cytoplasmic membrane and are sugar-specific, with different enzymes for fructose, mannitol and sorbitol, and two having different specificities for glucose. Mutants missing a particular Enzyme II show no taxis towards chemicals handled by that Enzyme II. Glucose taxis is absent only in mutants lacking both Enzymes II for glucose as well as the galactose receptor, which also binds glucose. The Enzymes II are thus the binding proteins for certain chemoreceptors (ADLER and EPSTEIN, 1974).

Enzyme I and the HPr protein are also required for the chemotactic response; this may be explained by (1) a requirement for transport in this case, or (2) the Enzymes II may not bind substrates well when Enzyme I and HPr are missing (ADLER and EPSTEIN, 1974). The Enzymes II are not required because the chemotactic response is dependent on metabolism of the sugar molecules: sugar phosphates do not serve as attractants even when they can be transported into the cell, and a mutant unable to metabolize glucose-6-phosphate further is still attracted to it (ADLER, 1969).

Although some of the properties of chemoreceptors have been elucidated, we do not yet understand how the chemoreceptor molecule is linked to subsequent processes. A conformational change is known to occur when galactose binds to its receptor protein (Boos et al., 1971, 1972; ROTMAN and ELLIS, 1972), and presumably such changes are sensed by the next component in the system, but little is known about this linkage. The available evidence suggests that the parameter of importance for a chemotactic response is the fraction of the binding protein that changes occupancy with time (MESIBOV et al., 1973; ORDAL and ADLER, 1974; BROWN and BERG, 1974).

7. How Do Chemoreceptors Affect Flagella?

A crucial point for determining the nature of the linkage between chemoreceptor and flagella is the location of the chemoreceptors. Although the osmotically shockable binding proteins and Enzymes II are probably distributed randomly over the cell membrane, it is theoretically possible that only those located at the base of the flagellum are involved in chemotaxis. Such a system would involve a simpler linkage than one in which all binding proteins and

Enzymes II are chemotactically active. Assuming the latter to be correct, there are several possible ways in which the receptor could be linked to the flagella: (1) release of a diffusible substance following chemoreceptor binding (see also Macnab and Koshland, 1972); (2) induction of a change in membrane potential which would propagate from the chemoreceptors to the flagella; or (3) alteration of the membrane configuration which would propagate to the flagella.

This problem is being examined using generally non-chemotactic mutants whose mutations are believed to affect the final common pathway for the transfer of information to the flagella (Fig. 12) (Armstrong et al., 1967; Adler, 1969). Such mutants either never tumble or almost always tumble (see below); they are unable to alter the basic swimming pattern sufficiently to respond to either attractants or repellents very well. Mutations which produce general non-chemotaxis have been localized to a group of four genes, suggesting that there are four components in this final common pathway (Armstrong and Adler, 1969; Parkinson and Reader, unpublished).

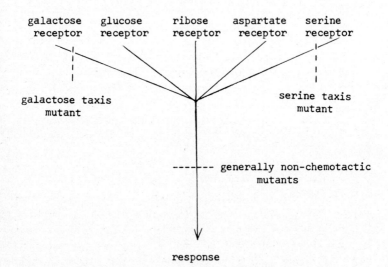

Fig. 12. Information from each of the many chemoreceptors is believed to be funnelled through a final common pathway (Adler, 1969)

One observation that may yield information about the mechanism of information transduction to the flagella is its requirement for methionine (ADLER, 1966, 1973) (Fig. 13). Bacterial swimming is quite normal in mutants that cannot synthesize methionine, except that they do not tumble in the absence of methionine. Hence

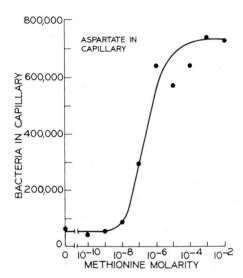

Fig. 13. Requirement for methionine to carry out chemotaxis towards 10^{-3} M aspartate in a methionine auxotroph (ADLER, 1973)

they are incapable of responding to either attractants or repellents unless methionine is added to the medium. Although the precise role of methionine in this system is not known, it is presumed to be involved in transduction through the final common pathway.

Tumbling mutants will swim smoothly when attractant is added (ASWAD and KOSHLAND, 1974). This is true even for methionine auxotrophs of tumbling mutants. However, these mutants will not return to tumbling in the absence of methionine (Fig. 14) (ORDAL et al., 1974; ASWAD and KOSHLAND, 1974). Therefore

methionine is not required for tumbling, or for the transition from
tumbling to smooth swimming, but rather for the transition from
smooth swimming to tumbling.

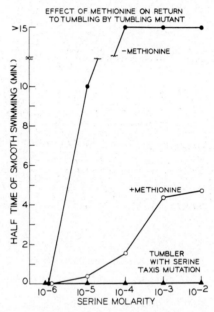

Fig. 14. Methionine auxotrophs of tumbling mutants require methionine to
return from smooth swimming to tumbling (Ordal et al., 1974)

An *E. coli* bacterium usually has about 6 flagella which may
originate anywhere on the cell surface, and they can function together as a bundle (Fig. 15). The long filament region of the flagellum had been well characterized, but little was known about the
basal portion of the *E. coli* flagellum until we isolated "intact"
flagella (Figs. 16 and 17) (DePamphilis and Adler, 1971). The
filament is attached to a hooked region, which in turn attaches to a
rod portion on which are mounted four rings; these are imbedded in
specific layers of the cell envelope (Fig. 17).

The energy for motility comes from the intermediate of oxidative
phosphorylation, not from ATP directly (Fig. 18) (Larsen et al.,
1974a). For chemotaxis, however, ATP is required in addition

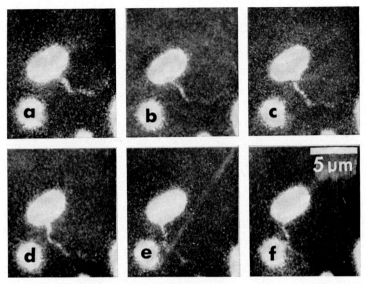

Fig. 15a—f. Flagellar bundle in *Escherichia coli* as observed by dark-field microscopy. Single frames from a 16 mm movie. The cell had become stuck and was moving its flagellar bundle about. (RAMSEY and ADLER, unpublished)

(Fig. 18) (LARSEN et al., 1974b). Work of MACNAB and KOSHLAND (1974) has led them to suggest that light-induced tumbling of *Salmonella* involves excitation of a flavin.

Without any gradient, individual bacteria swim smoothly in a straight line for about a second (a "run"), then they tumble for less than a second (a "twiddle" or series of "twiddles"), and then they go off in another run in a random direction (BERG, 1972). The movement of individuals in a gradient of attractant (BERG, 1972; MACNAB and KOSHLAND, 1972; BROWN and BERG, 1974) or a gradient of repellent (TSANG et al., 1973) has been studied. Increasing attractant concentrations cause cells to tumble less frequently, while increasing repellent concentrations cause more tumbling; on the other hand, decreasing concentrations cause the opposite effect (more tumbling for attractants and less tumbling for repellents).

Flagella are now known to rotate (BERG and ANDERSON, 1973; BERG, 1974; SILVERMAN and SIMON, 1974), and they can rotate both clockwise and counterclockwise (SILVERMAN and SIMON, 1974).

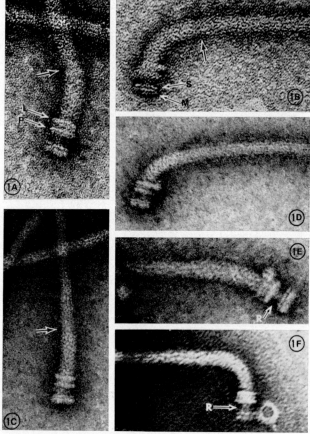

Fig. 16. Flagella isolated with both filaments and bases intact. R = rod,
L = top ring, P = next to top ring, M = bottom ring, S = next to bottom
ring. Unlabelled arrows indicate junction between hook and filament
(DePamphilis and Adler, 1971)

We have recently shown that attractants make them rotate counterclockwise, while repellents make them rotate clockwise (Larsen et al., 1974b) (Table 3). Mutants that swim but never tumble
always rotate their flagella counter-clockwise, while mutants that
almost always tumble almost always rotate their flagella clockwise
(Larsen et al., 1974b) (Table 3). Thus "runs" or smooth straight

Table 3. Effect of attractants and repellents on rotation

Strain	Addition		% Counterclockwise
Wild-type	none		73
	aspartate	2 μM	100
	serine	20 μM	100
	leucine	30 mM	9
Aspartate mutant	none		88
	aspartate	2 μM	85
Leucine mutant	none		95
	leucine	30 mM	93
Smooth mutant	none		100
	leucine	30 mM	100
Tumbling mutant	none		2
	serine	20 μM	100

Data from LARSEN et al., 1974b.

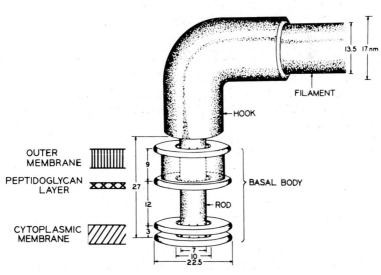

Fig. 17. A model of the flagellar base (DePAMPHILIS and ADLER, 1971)

swimming results from counterclockwise rotation of flagella, which allows an effective bundle, and "twiddling" or tumbling from clockwise rotation, which results in the bundle coming apart (LARSEN et al., 1974b). This all fits in with changes in tumbling frequency produced by changes in concentration of attractant (BERG and

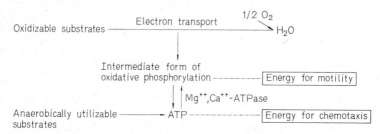

Fig. 18. The energy supply for motility and chemotaxis in *E. coli*

BROWN, 1972; MACNAB and KOSHLAND, 1972; BROWN and BERG, 1974) or repellent (TSANG et al., 1973). TAYLOR and KOSHLAND (1974) have reported on rotation of flagella in monotrichous bacteria undergoing reversal of swimming direction as a result of changes in attractant or repellent concentrations.

8. Conclusions

Extensive metabolism of chemicals is neither required, nor sufficient, for attraction of bacteria to the chemicals. Instead, the bacteria detect the attractants themselves. The systems that carry out this detection are called "chemoreceptors". There are mutants that fail to be attracted to one particular chemical or to a group of closely related chemicals but still metabolize these chemicals normally. These mutants are regarded as being defective in the activity of specific chemoreceptors. Data obtained so far indicate that there are at least eleven different chemoreceptors for positive chemotaxis in *Escherichia coli*. Negative chemotaxis has also been studied. A large number of repellents have been identified and classified into chemoreceptor groups.

The chemoreceptors are not the enzymes that catalyze the metabolism of the attractants; nor are they certain parts of the permeases and related transport systems, and uptake itself is not required or sufficient for chemotaxis towards at least certain attractants (galactose, maltose). In the case of certain chemoreceptors (galactose, ribose, maltose) an osmotically shockable binding protein is the component that recognizes the attractants; in the case of others, it is the Enzyme II of the phosphotransferase system.

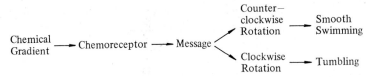

Fig. 19. Summary scheme

In summary, bacteria have receptors (chemoreceptor proteins) and effectors (rotating flagella) connected by a yet unknown transmission system (see Fig. 19), which might be considered as the "brain" of *E. coli*; this system decides whether to act on an input message, how to act on it, and what to do if there are competing messages such as the simultaneous presence of attractants and repellents (TSANG et al., 1973; Tso and ADLER, 1974b). The nature of the message sent by the chemoreceptors to the flagella is still unknown.

Acknowledgments

The research discussed was supported by a grant from the U.S. National Institutes of Health. I thank M. DAHL for having carried out many of the experiments mentioned here, and my various students and postdoctoral fellows for major contributions.

References

ADLER, J.: Science **153**, 708—716 (1966).
ADLER, J.: Science **166**, 1588—1597 (1969).
ADLER, J.: J. gen. Microbiol. **74**, 77—91 (1973).
ADLER, J., EPSTEIN, W.: Proc. nat. Acad. Sci. (Wash.) **71**, 2895—2899 (1974).
ADLER, J., HAZELBAUER, G. L., DAHL, M. M.: J. Bacteriol. **115**, 824—847 (1973).

AKSAMIT, R. R., KOSHLAND, D. E., JR.: Biochem. Biophys. Res. Commun. **48**, 1348—1353 (1972).

AKSAMIT, R. R., KOSHLAND, D. E., JR.: Biochemistry **13** (in press) (1974).

ANRAKU, Y.: J. biol. Chem. **243**, 3116—3122 (1968).

ARMSTRONG, J. B., ADLER, J.: Genetics **61**, 61—66 (1969).

ARMSTRONG, J. B., ADLER, J.: J. Bacteriol. **97**, 156—161 (1969).

ARMSTRONG, J. B., ADLER, J., DAHL, M. M.: J. Bacteriol. **93**, 390—398 (1967).

ASWAD, D., KOSHLAND, D. E., JR.: J. Bacteriol. **118**, 640—645 (1974).

BERG, H. C.: Nature (Lond.) **249**, 77—79 (1974).

BERG, H. C., ANDERSON, R. A.: Nature (Lond.) **245**, 380—382 (1973).

BERG, H. C., BROWN, D. A.: Nature (Lond.) **239**, 500—504 (1972).

BOOS, W.: Europ. J. Biochem. **10**, 66—73 (1969).

BOOS, W.: J. biol. Chem. **247**, 5414—5424 (1972).

BOOS, W., GORDON, A. S.: J. biol. Chem. **246**, 621—628 (1971).

BOOS, W., GORDON, A. S., HALL, R. E., PRICE, H. D.: J. biol. Chem. **247**, 917—924 (1972).

BROWN, D. A., BERG, H. C.: Proc. nat. Acad. Sci. (Wash.) **71**, 1388—1392 (1974).

BUTTIN, G.: J. molec. Biol. **7**, 164—182 (1963).

CLAYTON, R. K.: In: GIESE, A. C. (Ed.): Photophysiology, Vol. 2, p. 51. New York: Academic Press 1964.

DEPAMPHILIS, M. L., ADLER, J.: J. Bacteriol. **105**, 396—407 (1971).

HAZELBAUER, G. L., ADLER, J.: Nature (Lond.) New Biol. **30** (12), 101—104 (1971).

HAZELBAUER, G. L., MESIBOV, R. E., ADLER, J.: Proc. nat. Acad. Sci. (Wash.) **64**, 1300—1307 (1969).

HEPPEL, L. A.: Science **156**, 1451—1455 (1967).

KALCKAR, H. M.: Science **174**, 557—565 (1971).

KUNDIG, W., KUNDIG, F. D., ANDERSON, B., ROSEMAN, S.: J. biol. Chem. **241**, 3243—3246 (1966).

LARSEN, S. H., ADLER, J., GARGUS, JAY J., HOGG, R. W.: Proc. nat. Acad. Sci. (Wash.) **71**, 1239—1243 (1974a).

LARSEN, S. H., READER, R. W., KORT, E. N., TSO, W.-W., ADLER, J.: Nature (Lond.) **249**, 74—77 (1974b).

LINKS, J.: Thesis, University of Leiden (in Dutch, summary in English) (1955).

MACNAB, R. M., KOSHLAND, D. E., JR.: Proc. nat. Acad. Sci. (Wash.) **69**, 2509—2512 (1972).

MACNAB, R. M., KOSHLAND, D. E., JR.: J. molec. Biol. **84**, 399—406 (1974).

MESIBOV, R., ADLER, J.: J. Bacteriol. **112**, 315—326 (1972).

MESIBOV, R., ORDAL, G. W., ADLER, J.: J. gen. Physiol. **62**, 202—223 (1973).

ORDAL, G. W., ADLER, J.: J. Bacteriol. **117**, 517—526 (1974).

ORDAL, G. W., READER, R. W., KORT, E. N., TSO, W.-W., LARSEN, S. H., ADLER, J.: In press (1974).

PFEFFER, W.: Untersuch. Botan. Inst. Tübingen **1**, 363—482 (1884).

PFEFFER, W.: Untersuch. Botan. Inst. Tübingen **2**, 582—661 (1888).

ROTMAN, B., ELLIS, J. H.: J. Bacteriol. **111**, 791—796 (1972).

ROTMAN, B., GANESAN, A. K., GUZMAN, R.: J. molec. Biol. **36**, 247—260 (1968).

SILVERMAN, M. R., SIMON, M. I.: Nature (Lond.) **249**, 73—74 (1974).

SIMONI, R. D., LEVINTHAL, M., KUNDIG, F. D., KUNDIG, W., ANDERSON, B., HARTMAN, P. E., ROSEMAN, S.: Proc. nat. Acad. Sci. (Wash.) **58**, 1963—1970 (1967).

TSANG, N., MACNAB, R., KOSHLAND, D. E., JR.: Science **181**, 60—63 (1973).

TSO, W.-W., ADLER, J.: J. Bacteriol. **118**, 560—576 (1974a).

TSO, W.-W., ADLER, J.: Science **184**, 1292—1294 (1974b).

WEIBULL, C.: In: GUNSALUS, I. C., STANIER, R. Y. (Eds.): The bacteria, Vol. 1, pp. 153—205. New York: Academic Press 1960.

The Chemotactic Response in Bacteria

Daniel E. Koshland Jr.

Biochemistry Department, University of California Berkeley, CA 94720, USA

With 9 Figures

Es ist eine große Freude für mich, vor einem Auditorium der Gesellschaft für Biologische Chemie zu sprechen. Jeder Biochemiker der Welt wird geehrt sein, das Land zu besuchen, in dem Fischer, Warburg, Buchner, Meyerhof und viele andere legendäre Persönlichkeiten der Biochemie ihre Laboratorien hatten. Und es ist insbesondere stimulierend, da die gegenwärtigen Beiträge Deutschlands zur Biochemie diese gute, feine Tradition fortsetzen.

Ich möchte heute die Verhaltensweise von Bakterien diskutieren, die einen kurzen Weg zurücklegen, ins Taumeln geraten, hilflos mit den Flagellen wedeln und sich dann, hoffentlich, in einer neuen Richtung weiterbewegen.

Unglücklicherweise beschreibt das auch etwa meinen Umgang mit der deutschen Sprache. Vor vielen Jahren habe ich als Student Deutsch noch mäßig gut gesprochen, aber durch Mangel an Praxis ist meine Erinnerung verblaßt. Wie Sie heute hören werden, ist auch das Gedächtnis von Bakterien kurz. Aber ich hoffe, Sie werden erkennen, daß sie nicht vergeßlicher sind als ihre Erforscher selbst.

Um Ihnen zu helfen und um die deutsche Sprache zu schützen, möchte ich in Englisch fortfahren . . .

Introduction

The sensing of chemical gradients by bacteria has been known since the 1880s following the classical work of Engelmann [1] and Pfeffer [2]. Such a simple system may at first glance seem very distant from sensory systems in higher organisms, yet the essential unity of biochemical processes suggests that they will be related. Each species modifies basic biochemical mechanisms to its own advantage, but fundamental principles are utilized again and again over the range of differing biological organisms. That primitive organisms have precisely the same neurotransmitters as man, for example, seems unlikely, since different tissues in mammalian systems use different neurotransmitters. What does seem likely is that the principle of signal processing and information transmittal may have similarities in a wide variety of systems. Therefore it is our hope that the fundamental principles of the bacterial system will have relevance to other, perhaps all, sensory systems.

In Fig. 1 the bacterial sensing system has been broken down into its components. Evidence for these components will be present-

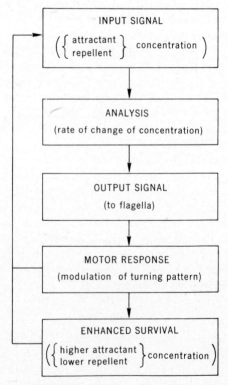

Fig. 1. A schematic outline of the components of the bacterial sensing system. The input signal is analyzed, generates an output signal causing a motor response which leads to the behavioral pattern of the organism

ed below, but a glance at the figure shows the analogy to other sensory systems. Receptors are present to detect an environmental condition, in this case an attractant or repellent. Binding of the attractant or repellent stimulates a signal which is analyzed in terms of a change in concentration over time. The sensory system, probably involving the level of a regulator molecule, transmits the signal to the flagella. The motor response of the bacteria is altered by reversal of flagellar rotation or by a suppression of this reversal. As a result the net direction of bacterial migration is controlled. The net bacterial migration is a behavioral response to allow the bacteria to move to higher concentrations of attractant (usually nutrients) and away from higher concentrations of repellents (signal of toxic or unfavorable conditions). Thus, an environmental stimulus is converted into a behavioral response.

The Biased Random Walk

The bacteria which have gathered most attention in recent time have been *E. coli* and *Salmonella*, which differ from each other in very minor ways. Both are approximately $2\mu m$ long, usually have 5 to 8 flagella located over the surface of the bacterium, and the flagella usually stream behind the bacteria in a bundle when they are swimming. If one examines the motile bacteria in a microscope, they seem to swim in a relatively straight line for moderate intervals, 0.3 to 2 sec, and then change direction abruptly, an event which is referred to as a "tumble" or a "twiddle" or a "turn". This behavior led early investigators to speculate that bacteria migrated by a biased random walk process (*cf.* [3]). A mechanism which might explain the bias is one in which the velocity was modulated by the absolute concentration of attractant. The bacteria would then migrate from low concentrations and accumulate at high concentrations. Early studies of PFEFFER suggested bacteria respond to ratios [2], and observations of DAHLQUIST and LOVELY in a migration apparatus clearly excluded a response to absolute levels of attractant [4]. These studies in well defined gradients demonstrated that bacteria sense ratios, but only to a first approximation. MESIBOV and ADLER [5] also demonstrated a limited dependence on WEBER's law.

Early suggestions were made that the chemotactic bacteria bias their random walk process by a device similar to phobotaxis, *i.e.* they tend to flee unfavorable circumstances rather than be attracted to favorable environment [3]. This was proven not to be the case by the experiments of Berg and Brown [6], who devised a bacterial tracker to record the detailed motion of bacteria. This tracking device confirmed that the bacteria did proceed by biased random walk and described their motion in mathematical detail. The lengths of runs, the frequency and direction of turns followed a Poissonian pattern. The average angle of the turn was 62° not 90°, as would be calculated for a completely random turn. Furthermore, the runs in the positive direction of the gradient, *i.e.* towards higher attractant concentrations were greater than normal, whereas runs in unfavorable directions were approximately normal. Such a biased walk would lead to a net migration up an attractant gradient by suppression of tumbling in a favorable direction rather than increased tumbling in the unfavorable direction.

Bacterial Memory

Two types of mechanisms can be envisioned for the control of tumbling. The first we might call an instantaneous spatial sensing in which an instantaneous comparison of concentration is made by sensors at the head and tails of the bacteria. When the sensors are in a gradient, they will send different signals to some central analytical device and hence can distinguish a gradient from a uniform distribution of attractant. An alternate mechanism would be a temporal sensing mechanism in which a record over time is used.

The receptors could be distributed uniformly around the membrane and would record direction because the bacteria are moving through the gradient. Since the signals received would record over an interval and since the concentration varies with time, such a system would indicate whether the bacterium was travelling up or down the gradient. Sensory stimuli based on time dependence are known for other organisms such as phototactic bacteria [7] as well as higher species, and the same is true of spatial sensing mechanisms.

To distinguish between these two for chemical sensing, R. Mac-nab devised an apparatus [8] (Fig. 2a) which was based on a sudden change in the bacterial environment in a very short interval of time. A schematic diagram of this type of change is shown in Fig. 2b. The bacteria are thrust through a rapid change in concentration

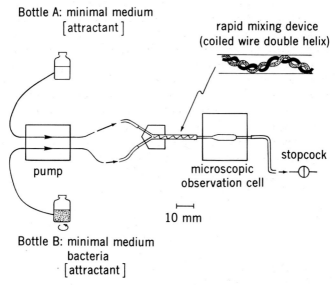

Fig. 2a. The temporal gradient apparatus. Attractant concentrations or repellent concentrations can be placed in bottles A and B to yield increased gradients, decreased gradients or zero gradients. The bacteria are suddenly mixed in the mixing chamber and projected into a microscopic observation cell. At the time of observation they are in a uniform distribution of attractant following a mixing time of approximately 200 msec

and are examined only after they have achieved a uniform environment.

Hence they should show a normal tumbling pattern if they were sensing only instantaneous differences at their head and tail. On the other hand, they will act as if they were travelling through a gradient if they use temporal sensing device, *i.e.* if they compare their past with their present environment over a time interval. It was found that indeed the latter was the correct mechanism. A control with zero gradients established that the mixing apparatus did not introduce artifacts, since the bacteria swam normally. When they were subjected to a decrease in concentration in approximately 200 msec, they tumbled almost continuously on initial examination (Fig. 3). In a few seconds tumbling started to decrease and the bacteria gradually "relaxed" back to normal tumbling patterns. On the other hand, if they were subjected to a sudden increase in concentration, their tumbling was suppressed and for an initial interval practically no bacteria tumble at all if the gradient is steep

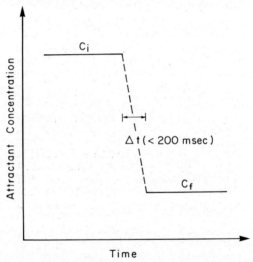

Fig. 2b. Rationale of the temporal gradient apparatus. Bacteria in a uniform concentration of attactant C_i are suddenly mixed and find themselves in a uniform concentration of attractant C_f which in this example is less the C_i. They have thus experienced a temporal decreased gradient equivalent to swimming down a spatial gradient of attractant. They are observed, however, in a uniform environment of attractant

Fig. 3a—c. Motility tracks of *S. typhimurium*, taken in the time interval 27 sec after subjecting bacteria to a sudden (200 msec) change in attractant (serine) concentration in the temporal gradient apparatus. (a) $C_i = 0$, $C_f = 7.6 \times 10^{-4}$ M. Smooth, linear trajectories. (b) $C_i = C_f = 0$ (control). Some changes in direction; bodies often show "wobble" as they travel. Bright spots indicate tumbling or non-motile bacteria. (c) $C_i = 10^{-3}$, $C_f = 2.4 \times 10^{-4}$ M. Poor coordination; frequent tumbles and erratic changes in direction. (Photomicrographs were taken in dark field with a stroboscopic lamp operating at 5 pulses sec^{-1}. Instantaneous velocity of bacteria in straight line trajectories is of the order of 30 μm/sec)

Attractants

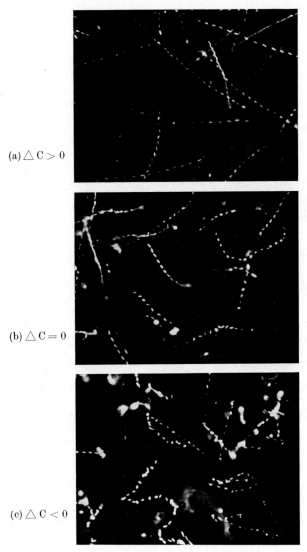

(a) $\triangle C > 0$

(b) $\triangle C = 0$

(c) $\triangle C < 0$

Fig. 3a—c. (Legend see p. 138)

enough. After several seconds or in some cases several minutes, bacteria started tumbling and gradually "relaxed" back to a normal pattern. Thus, the artificial device mimicked the changes in concentration that a bacterium would experience in travelling down or up a gradient of attractant, but the device eliminated the ambiguity of the interpretation by examining them only in a uniform concentration. The results show bacteria must posses a "memory" which allows them to compare a past with a present environment.

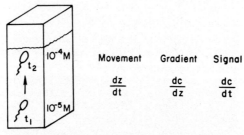

Fig. 4. Relationship of the bacterial memory to the actual observation of the spatial gradients. Bacteria travelling up or down a spatial gradient travel through a gradient over space dc/dz. They travel at a velocity dz/dt which is roughly uniform. The signal thus becomes a function of dc/dt, which is analyzed by the temporal sensing devices

The temporal memory allows the bacteria to detect a spatial gradient, as shown in Fig. 4. Its movement through space (dz/dt) causes it to see the spatial gradient (dc/dz) as a function of time (dc/dt). The precise functions are not yet known (the population studies suggest a $d \ln c/dt$ function over short intervals).

What kind of biochemical system could suppress or accelerate tumbling and provide some type of memory ? A number of mechanisms can be envisioned, the simplest of which involves a stimulus proportional to the number of receptor molecules containing bound attractant. Although the number of attractant molecules bound to receptor must enter into the mechanism, a little thought shows that this system is too simple. For example, uniform attractant concentrations of 10^{-5} M ribose, 10^{-4} M ribose and 10^{-3} M ribose all lead to normal swimming patterns, whereas changes by a factor of 2 within this concentration range causes abnormal swimming. Hence the bacteria are not responding to an absolute concentration of attractant in the medium, but to some more complicated function which compares this in past and present. One potential mechanism is outlined in Fig. 5, but it is symbolic of a type of mechanism rather than a unique answer. The amount of attractant bound to receptor controls the level of compound X. The compound X then regulates flagella function. Compound X would have some obvious similarities to neurotransmitter substances.

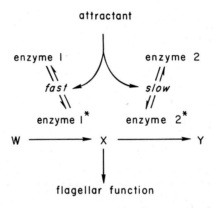

Fig. 5. Schematic illustration of one possible time dependent mechanism. Attractant alters conformation of enzymes 1 and 2 to catalytically more active forms, enzyme 1 rapidly and enzyme 2 slowly. The compound X, which controls flagellar function, therefore tends to increase in positive gradients decrease in negative gradients; remain unchanged in zero gradients

Our studies in the temporal-gradient apparatus showed that attractant could increase tumbling when the gradient was negative and decrease tumbling when the gradient was positive. The length of responses in these two cases were, however, quite different. A sharp positive gradient suppressed tumbling in some cases for as long as thirty minutes. Sharp negative gradients caused increased tumbling for as long as thirty seconds, but never as long as thirty minutes. Part of the difference in response times, of course, is caused by difficulty in producing very large negative gradients. In a positive gradient one can go from zero to a high concentration of attractant, an infinite ratio. In a negative gradient dilution by factors of 2—4 are typical, but it is difficult to dilute much more than that. In equally steep temporal gradients, however, there is a more distinct asymmetry in the response to a positive gradient than to a negative one, the negative one being for shorter duration. These results fit in very well with the findings of BERG and BROWN described above, in which the main quantitative effect is in the suppression of tumbling. In the gradient apparatus, gradients much larger than could be experienced by bacterial motion are realized. Hence one can exaggerate effects and detect properties which are difficult to detect otherwise but which are not physiological. With shallow temporal gradients response, times consistent with bacterial motion experiments are obtained.

„Useful Memory"

The existence of bacterial "memory", albeit a short one, raises the question of whether memory is real or merely a semantic relation to higher species. The memory in this case allows the bacterium to select its movement in a gradient situation in such a way as to optimize biological properties. Not only can it travel to a more efficient nutrient, but it flees a hostile environment. Hence there is little doubt the memory is real and designed for survival value to the organism.

It could next be asked why a memory mechanism is preferred to spatial sensors which provide an instantaneous analysis of differing concentrations at the head and the tail. Certainly depth perception in humans operates through the latter mechanism. For the bacterium, however, a different challenge arises. The length of the bacterium is only 2 μm, and gradients which give a ready response show a concentration difference between the head and the tail of the bacterium of 1 part in 10^4. Even a highly sophisticated analytical system will have difficulty providing such accuracy. A memory which allows the bacterium to move through space by 10 or 100 body lengths would allow the bacterium to measure the concentration difference which it must detect. Moreover, by integrating over time it could level out statistical fluctuations. Hence a more accurate assessment of the true gradient situation could be obtained with a less sensitive analytical system. This would argue for a relatively long memory.

On the other hand, there is a problem since the bacterium tumbles spontaneously in a uniform environment. If the memory is too long it will perhaps receive the information from a previous run when it is headed in a new direction. This would argue that memory time should be limited so that the signal transmitted to the flagella occurs as soon as possible after the stimulus is received.

Obviously the organism is going to have to compromise between these extremes, and some detailed analyses have been performed [9]. These lead to the conclusion that the memory time in normal processing is of the order of 1—10 sec in *Salmonella*. *E. coli* may have a shorter "memory". The precise number cannot be fixed yet and will perhaps be difficult to define in any case. Nevertheless, this allows *Salmonella* to integrate information over the equivalent of many body lengths in space. This is long enough to obtain information in a more precise way than it could by sensors at its head and tail, and yet not so long that the information is processed after it has ceased having any value. The bacteria, therefore, have a "useful memory" span, and this may, indeed, have its counterpart in higher species. We are all aware of short term and long-term memory. In higher systems also, a permanent memory which records all stimuli in detail would not have survival value.

Integration of Stimuli

It has long been known that bacteria are repelled by certain compounds [10] just as they are attracted by others. Moreover, Tso and ADLER have made an extensive study of repellents, showing that they fall into classes suggestive of receptor molecules [11]. We therefore examined whether repellents acted in the same way as attractants, and if they contributed to the same signalling system [12].

As a first step the repellents were subjected to the same temporal sensing apparatus as the attractants, and the same effects were observed except that they were opposite in sign. Thus, an increase in repellent concentration caused increased tumbling and a decrease in repellent concentration caused repression of tumbling (*cf.* Fig. 6). Hence, the bacteria will travel down gradients of repellents because their tumbling is suppressed. The quantitative relations were the same as for attractants except for an inverse sign [12].

Additivity experiments were then performed. A concentration of repellent which would tend to drive the bacteria to the bottom

Repellents

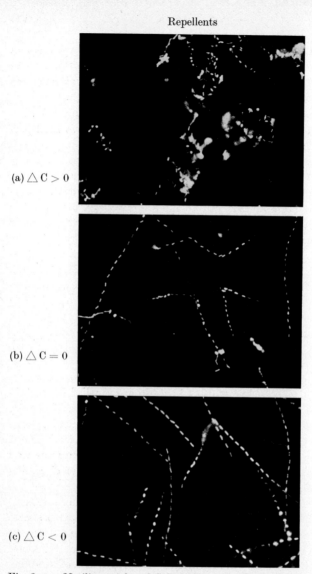

(a) $\triangle C > 0$

(b) $\triangle C = 0$

(c) $\triangle C < 0$

Fig. 6a—c. Motility tracks of *Salmonella* in the interval of 2—7 sec after subjecting bacteria to a sudden (200 msec) change in repellent (phenol) concentration in the temporal gradient apparatus. (a) Phenol increased from 0 to 7.5×10^{-4} M, (b) no concentration change (control), (c) phenol decreased from 3×10^{-4} to 7.5×10^{-5} M. Photomicrographs were taken in dark field with a stroboscopic lamp operating at 5 pulses sec^{-1}. Instantaneous velocity of bacteria in straigth trajectories is of the order of 30 μm/sec

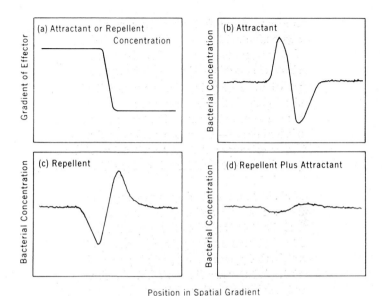

Fig. 7a—d. Demonstration of integration of stimuli. Bacteria were studied in the population migration apparatus of DAHLQUIST, LOVELY, and KOSH-LAND. When subjected to an effector gradient of the type shown in (a), the bacteria migrate towards higher concentrations of attractant (b) and towards lower concentrations of repellent (c). If the gradients of attractant and repellent are now superimposed on each other, they essentially nullify and there is little net migration of the bacteria (d)

of the cell was superimposed on a gradient of attractant which would tend to attract the bacteria to the top. Other permutations arranged repellents and attractants in opposite directions. In all of these cases the quantitative behavior was that of a system which integrated the signals from the repellent and attractant to produce a net effect. If, for example, a gradient of serine attractant in which bacteria migrated at a velocity of 2.8 μm/sec towards the top of the cell was superimposed on a phenol gradient which repelled them to the bottom of the cell at a migration velocity 3 μm/sec, the two gradients essentially cancel out and bacteria show little tendency to migrate (Fig. 7).

The simplest and most likely explanation for this phenomenon is that the receptors for repellents operate as the precise inverse as receptors for attractants. In a mechanism such as that of Fig. 5, repellents and attractants activate enzymes 1 and 2 in such a way that the level of compound X is an integrated average of all the stimuli. Then the net information is achieved by the pool level of X, and repellent and attractant gradients can be additive or subtractive depending on experimental design. Such was found to be the case. This conclusion is relevant to the understanding of the inhibitory and excitatory neurons where again the individual cells seem to integrate the signal, probably by a chemical mechanism of the type described above.

Receptor Molecules

Evidence that chemoreceptors are involved in chemotaxis has been obtained by extensive specificity, inhibition and genetic studies of ADLER and his colleagues [13]. The first receptor isolated was the galactose binding protein of *E. coli*. ANRAKU [14] obtained this protein by the shock procedure of HEPPEL [15]. A mutant was discovered by WU, BOOS, and KALCKAR [16] which lacked this protein and was deficient in transport. This mutant was tested by HAZELBAUER and ADLER [17] and found to be deficient in chemotaxis to galactose, but not other attractants.

This identification is given strong support by Dr. AKSAMIT's studies on the ribose binding protein of *Salmonella* [18]. In this case the same procedure of osmotic shock was followed until a ribose binding protein which was homogeneously pure was isolated. The isolated protein was shown to have the characteristics of the biological response, *e.g.* the specificity of a wide variety of substrates shown in Table 1 was the same for the pure protein and the chemotactic response. Only one other compound, allose, binds to pure protein and only this causes the chemotactic response. Moreover, the quantitative relationship between the binding of ribose and allose to the pure protein is maintained in the chemotactic response. Allose binds far less well to the pure protein (K_D of 10^{-4} *vs.* A ribose K_D of 10^{-7}) and requires much higher concentrations (10^3 fold) to generate the chemotactic response.

The final evidence that this ribose binding protein is the true receptor was obtained through genetic tests. To produce a mutant lacking the ribose protein, selection procedures were devised for

Table 1. The specificity of the ribose receptor

D—ribose   D—allose

Position	Ribose modification	Binding to ribose binding protein
C1	-OH replaced by	no
	-H	
	-OH	
	-OPO$_3$H^{--}	no
C2	epimer	no
	-OH replaced by	
	-H	no
C3	epimer	no
	-OH replaced by	
	-H	no
	-OCH^3	no
C4	epimer	no
C5	-H replaced by	
	-CH$_2$OH (allose)	yes

ribose transport, and these mutants were then tested for ribose
binding protein. An organism was obtained that lacked ribose
chemotaxis and also lacked ribose binding protein. However, this
type of genetic information, although strongly suggestive, is not
definitive. It can be shown statistically that the probability of
having one mutation on such a selection procedure is very remote,
and therefore the statistical possibility remains that a second gene
has been altered which may be responsible for the loss in the chemotactic response. To eliminate this possibility, revertants were isolated, and the new organisms gave a chemotactic response to ribose
and also contained a functional ribose binding protein (AKSAMIT
and KOSHLAND, Biochemistry, in press). Hence there seems no
doubt that this protein molecule is indeed the receptor for ribose

chemotaxis. It is a pure protein of 29000 Daltons, binds with one molecule of ribose at saturation and exists in the periplasmic space.

The Motor Response

How is the flagellar motion altered ? Two general mechanisms for propulsion of bacteria have gained the most support in recent years. On of these involves an induced conformational change which propagates through the length of the flagella, creating a thrust in the forward direction [3]. The second by STOCKER [19] and DOETSCH [20] postulates that the bacterial flagella are relatively rigid helical structures which rotate like a propeller. Recently, evidence has appeared which strongly favors the rotation hypothesis. SIMON and SILVERMAN have attached antibodies to flagella and to glass surfaces and have observed the rotation of the cell body [21, 22]. BERG and coworkers [23, 24] have analyzed the various lines of evidence in theoretical terms, measured velocities of rotation and rotation reversal with their tracking apparatus. ADLER and his coworker have added repellents and attractant and observed reversals of flagellar rotation [25].

In pursuing high intensity light experiments which allowed Dr. MACNAB to see individual flagella [26], we could see the flagella fly apart during the tumbling process. One could also see an apparent clockwise rotation of flagella bundle during swimming. One possible explanation for both processes is that the flagella rotate synchronously in a bundle during a run, but reverse rotation and fly apart during a tumble [26]. The degree of the reversal would therefore determine the degree of the tumble. Whether the bacteria hesitated, made a small turn or a massive tumble would depend on the duration of reversal of the flagella rotation.

To explore this possiblity further, a monoflagellated *Pseudomomas* was examined by Dr. TAYLOR. Since this organism has only a single flagellum, its movement was easier to analyze and it was found that it indeed went forward and backed up under various stimuli. In some cases the backing up involved a reversal in direction of 180 degrees without tumbling of the bacterial body (Fig. 8). This and other evidence leads us to conclude that flagella rotation reversal is the means of achieving directional changes, occurring spontaneously or under the influence of gradients. It can also be induced by light [26]. In the monoflagellated organism it can cause

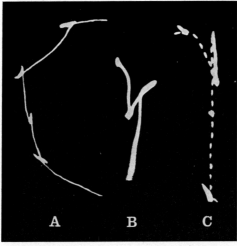

Fig. 8 A—C. The trajectories of the *Pseudomonas citronellolis* bacteria indicating reversals of flagella as a device for altering direction. A stroboscopic light was used with a 16 flash sec/interval in (A). The bacterium is seen to move in roughly straight lines and sometimes reverses at essentially 180° from the starting direction. After a short reversal it starts forward again. The forward and reverse thrusts are not always precisely 180°, and therefore a net random walk behavior occurs. A similar trajectory is shown in (B). The wider tracks being caused by the bacterium being slightly out of focus. Because the flashes are frequent, the bacterium does not cover more than one body length between flashes and the trajectory therefore appears as a continuous line. If the interval between flashes is increased (5 flashes/sec) the trajectory in (C) is observed, the dotted line indicating the forward movement of a bacteria which then reverses at an almost 180° angle. The backward velocity is lower than the forward velocity, hence leading to the appearance of a solid line. The bacterium then resumes its forward direction at much the original velocity

single "backing up"; in the peritrichously flagellated it causes tumbling. In either case the results show that the sensory signals need produce only a very simple on-off motor response in order to control migration of the bacteria.

Role of Methionine

The regulation of the level of compound X may involve many factors. One of the most interesting relationships is that of methionine. ADLER and DAHL observed [27] that a methionine auxotroph of *E. coli* was non-chemotactic towards all attractants tested when starved for methionine. The effect of methionine starvation does not result from lack of protein synthesis, since starvation for other amino acids such as threonine or leucine had no effect on chemotaxis. Moreover, methionine starvation does not lead to loss of motility. Studies on the effect of methionine starvation on normal and chemotactically defective strains of *Salmonella typhimurium* allowed Dr ASWAD to gain some insight into the nature of this phenomenon [28].

Methionine starved cultures of *Salmonella typhimurium* are motile, but there is a striking difference between their motility and that of non-starved cultures. The absence of methionine shown in Fig. 9 causes the trajectories of the bacteria to be much smoother. Although the bacteria do not swim in precisely straight lines, vigorously motile individual bacteria were not observed to display a *bona fide* tumble for up to a minute of continuous observation. The same impression is gained from looking at a field of bacteria (20—50 in view at any one time). Thus, in normally motile cells tumbling is completely suppressed by methionine starvation.

Since normal bacteria exhibit only smooth motility in the absence of methionine, it seemed of interest to see whether methionine starvation would alter the motility pattern of an uncoordinated mutant. This mutant, SL 4041, is non-chemotactic because of constant tumbling or uncoordination, with no smooth coordinated swimming. Five methionine auxotrophs were independently derived from SL 4041 and their motility examined both in the presence and absence of methionine. In all five cases the continuous tumbling was unaffected by methionine starvation.

The observation that ST4, a mutant of SL4041 which was converted to a methionine auxotroph, continues to tumble in the absence of methionine suggests one of two possibilities. The first is that SL4041 contains a mutation which allows tumbling to occur in the absence of methionine, and the second is that the abnormal motility pattern of SL4041 is not the result of continuous tumbling but rather the result of a defective flagellar apparatus. In the first alternative the mutation is assumed to affect the regulation of tumbling, *i.e.* the flagella are capable of coordinating properly, but they are constantly receiving signals which prevent smooth swimming. In the second alternative the flagella are receiving the proper

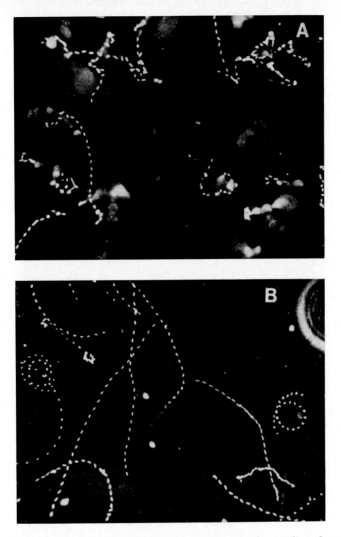

Fig. 9 A and B. The effect of methionine starvation on the motility of strain ST 41. Bacteria were washed and then diluted to a cell density of about 2×10^7 cells/ml in VBC-glycerol containing 1×10^{-5} M L-histidine, 1×10^{-5} M L-tryptophan and 1×10^{-5} M L-methionine, (A), or the same without methionine(B). In the presence of methionine (A), the motility tracks consist of relatively smooth gently curved segments in which the bacterial soma is oriented along the direction of the track interrupted by "tumbles" where the bacterial soma shows random orientation. In the absence of methionine (B), tumbling is virtually absent and the motility tracks are nearly all smooth

signals, but they are unable to coordinate their flagella properly, regardless of which signals are being received.

To choose between these alternatives, ST4 was subjected to a positive temporal gradient of serine. Normally, chemotactic bacteria subjected to such a temporal increase in attractant concentration respond by suppressing tumbling for several minutes. Inhibition of tumbling was observed in 90% of the bacteria. These bacteria swam in a coordinated manner with a linear velocity typical of normal strains. This period of smooth motility died away in a few minutes, giving rise to the tumbling pattern characteristic of this mutant strain. These observations prove that the flagella of ST4 are capable of normal coordinated motility for a prolonged period of time, and hence the defect is in the tumble regulation and not in the flagellar apparatus.

Although our results show that a supply of methionine is necessary for tumbling in normal strains, the experiments with ST4 indicate that mutants can be isolated which continue to tumble in the absence of methionine. This puts severe restrictions on the possible role of methionine in relation to tumble regulation. Any mechanism in which methionine or a methionine derived metabolite is a substrate for a tumble generating reaction seems eliminated. A hypothetical example of such a mechanism would involve S-adenosylmethionine donating a methyl group to a protein in the basal region of the flagella, which would perturb the orientation of the flagella and result in a tumble. Methionine starvation would deplete the supply of SAM and turn off the tumble generating reaction. If bacteria operated by this mechanism, a mutant which tumbled in the absence of methionine could not occur. ST4, an uncoordinated mutant, does just that, eliminating this hypothesis.

An alternative is that methionine (or its metabolite) has some less direct, perhaps regulatory role in the control of tumbling. The data of Table 2 suggest that this regulatory role is to create a biochemical environment which turns off the smooth response. In the presence of methionine, ST4 showed a smooth response in the temporal gradient apparatus of only 1.5 min, whereas in the absence of methionine, the response duration is increased six-fold to a value of roughly 10 min. Thus, the presence of methionine in the cell is necessary for rapid return to a condition which allows tumbling.

Table 2. The effect of amino acid starvation on duration of the smooth response

Strain	Starvation conditions	Response duration[a] (min)
St42 (che+, control)	—histidine	2.3 ± 0.3
	—tryptophan	2.5 ± 0.3
	—methionine	[b]
ST4 (uncoordinated)	—histidine	1.2 ± 0.3
	—tryptophan	1.5 ± 0.3
	—methionine	10 ± 2.0

[a] Stimulus is a temporal gradient of $0 \to 1$ mM L-aspartate generated in the apparatus described by MACNAB and KOSHLAND (9).

[b] No response listed because methionine-starved che+ strains always swim in a smooth, coordinated manner.

At present little is known how tumbles are regulated at the molecular level. Presumably there exists within the cell some parameter (compound X was used in the possible mechanism cited earlier), e.g. metabolite concentration, ion concentration or membrane potential, which serves to integrate information from chemoreceptors and modify motility. When a stimulus is encountered, the value of this parameter changes but must return to its steady state level soon after the stimulus has ended. Methionine may serve to correct the level of the tumble regulatory parameter to its steady state value.

The observation on the wild-type and mutant strains agree with this hypothesis. In wild-type bacteria, this regulatory parameter is apparently delicately balanced so that only sporadic tumbling occurs. A slight perturbation in its steady state level caused by methionine starvation would thus effectively eliminate tumbling. ST4, however, has a much higher frequency of spontaneous tumbling. In this case methionine starvation could decrease the probability of tumbling without eliminating it.

In recent publications, ARMSTRONG [29, 30] has presented evidence that in E. coli the methionine effect reflects a need for S-adenosylmethionine in chemotaxis. Experiments in our laboratory with Salmonella concur with this conclusion. Thus, the methionine requirement probably reflects a need for S-adenosylmethionine or one of its metabolites in turning off the smooth response.

Relation of Chemotaxis to Higher Neural Systems

The signalling process in these bacteria is certainly not as complex as in higher species with a central nervous system, but it could quite possibly use similar biochemical principles. The information is received at receptors on the surface, as in higher species. The signal is processed and transmitted to the motor organs as in higher species. The distance the signal must travel is much shorter, but the stimulus is transmitted and does elicit a behavioral response. The response to specific chemicals is analogous to the specific responses in higher organisms, e.g. odor in man and pheromones in insects. The high specificity of the response indicates a protein molecule as the receptor, and such a molecule has been isolated. The response does not require the metabolism of the attractant, as is also true in higher species. An exactly parallel and inverse relationship is seen in repellents. The bacteria obey WEBER's law roughly over short ranges of stimulus and deviate significantly from it over wide ranges, again as seen in higher species.

The bacteria utilize "memory" in the sense that it allows the bacterium to compare its past with its present. This memory is very short, but it requires a biochemical mechanism which allows an integration over time. Quite obviously, this is a long way from the memory of more complex species, but the bacteria have no need of such an intricate system.

The level of some chemical or membrane potential seems critical for the signal to the flagella. Moreover, the inputs to this level from a variety of attractant and repellents act as a summation process. Such levels could logically be related to equivalent levels in a neuron. In that case the state of polarization of the nerve depends on additive and subtractive relationship of stimuli from chemicals, dendrites and hormones.

If new interneuron connections are to be initiated or reinforced by the synthesis of new proteins or are to be deleted by hydrolysis of old proteins, some chemical levels should change. Small molecules such as cyclic AMP, inducers or repressors, initiate protein synthesis or inhibit protein breakdown. A change in the level of compound X could therefore trigger other more permanent chemical changes as well as being involved with the firing of an individual neuron. Learing and memory may well be products of a common primary biochemical event. The analogies exist. Their usefulness in evaluating sensory systems will depend on these and future studies.

References

1. ENGELMANN, T. W.: Pflügers Arch. ges. Physiol. **57**, 375—390 (1902).
2. PFEFFER, W.: Untersuch. Botan. Inst. Tübingen **2**, 582—589 (1888).
3. WEIBULL, C.: The bacteria, Vol. I, pp. 153—202. GUNSALUS, I. C., STANIER, R. Y. (Eds.) New York: Academic Press 1960.
4. DAHLQUIST, F. W., LOVELY, P., KOSHLAND, D. E., JR.: Nature (Lond.) New Biology **236**, 120—123 (1972).
5. MESIBOV, R. E., ORDAL, G. W., ADLER, J.: J. gen. Physiol. **62**, 203 (1973).
6. BERG, H. C., BROWN, D. A.: Nature (Lond.) New Biol. **239**, 500 (1972).
7. CLAYTON, R. K.: Arch. Mikrobiol. **19**, 141 (1953).
8. MACNAB, R. M., KOSHLAND, D. E., JR.: Proc. nat. Acad. Sci. (Wash.) **69**, 2509—2512 (1972).
9. MACNAB, R. M., KOSHLAND, D. E., JR.: J. Mechanochem. (in press) (1974).
10. LEDERBERG, J.: Genetics **41**, 845 (1956).
11. TSO, W. W., ADLER, J.: J. Bacteriol. **118**, 560 (1974).
12. TSANG, N. R., MACNAB, R., KOSHLAND, D. E., JR.: Science **181**, 60—63 (1973).
13. ADLER, J.: Science **166**, 1588 (1969).
14. ANRAKU, Y.: J. biol. Chem. **243**, 3116—3122 (1968).
15. HEPPEL, L. A.: Science **156**, 1451—1455 (1967).
16. WU, H. C. P., BOOS, W., KALCKAR, H. M.: J. molec. Biol. **41**, 109—120 (1969).
17. HAZELBAUER, G. L., ADLER, J.: Nature (Lond.) New Biol. **230**, 101—104 (1971).
18. AKSAMIT, R., KOSHLAND, D. E., JR.: Biochem. Biophys. Res. Commun. **48**, 1348—1353 (1972).
19. STOCKER, B. A. D.: Symp. Soc. Gen. Microbiol. **6**, 19—40 (1956).
20. DOETSCH, R. N.: J. theoret. Biol. **11**, 411—417 (1966).
21. SILVERMAN, M. R., SIMON, M. I.: J. Bacteriol. **112**, 986—993 (1972).
22. SILVERMAN, M. R., SIMON, M. I.: Nature (Lond.) New Biol. **249**, 73 (1974).
23. BERG, H. C., ANDERSON, R. A.: Nature (Lond.) New Biol. **249**, 77 (1974).
24. BERG, H. C.: Nature (Lond.) New Biol. (in press) (1974).
25. LARSEN, S. H., READER, R. W., KORT, E. N., TSO, W. W., ADLER, J.: Nature (Lond.) **249**, 74 (1974).
26. MACNAB, R., KOSHLAND, D. E., JR.: J. molec. Biol. **84**, 399 (1974).
27. ADLER, J., DAHL, M. M.: J. gen. Microbiol. **46**, 161—173 (1967).
28. ASWAD, D., KOSHLAND, D. E., JR.: J. Bacteriol. **118**, 640 (1974).
29. ARMSTRONG, J. B.: Can. J. Microbiol. **18**, 591 (1972).
30. ARMSTRONG, J. B.: Can. J. Microbiol. **18**, 1695 (1972).

Discussion

G. WALD (Cambridge, Mass.): I used to tell students that living organisms have developed every type of mechanical device but the wheel. Now it turns out that flagella of *E. coli* turn on wheels. All our mechanical technology tends to develop as projections of organs. Perhaps the lack of wheel-like organs is why the wheel was not invented in Eurasia until about 3000 B.C., and was never used in the Western Hemisphere. What a moving thought — that this profound lesson could have been learned from man's most intimate companion *E. coli.*! But what mechanism in a cell — any cell — can turn a wheel?

J. ADLER: Right. We don't know the mechanism — we'll have to find the spokes, hub, axel, moving power, etc.

G. WALD: I would like to ask Dr. ADLER a question about that beautiful ring experiment that you showed us. The thing that puzzles me is that it depends on the capacity to metabolize the thing being tried, so it is not just attractant, it is also, and it must be, coupled with metabolism — is that right?

J. ADLER: That is correct.

H. M. KALCKAR (Boston, Mass.): Metabolism is a necessary set-up for this device?

J. ADLER: Metabolism is not necessary for chemotaxis; metabolism is necessary for achieving that ring. If one uses an attractant that cannot be metabolized — then no ring is achieved.

B. HESS (Dortmund): The dynamic phenomena of chemotactic activities with its temporal sensing device of chemical gradients in space as well as the flagellar motion described by Drs. ADLER and KOSHLAND raise the question whether they all or in part result from the function of one or more biochemical oscillators. Such a kinetic mechanism is even more attractive because the general kinetic properties of allosteric enzymes that are part of Dr. KOSHLAND's hypothetical mechanism of sensing and flagellar motion are quite appropriate to generate chemical oscillations [see GOLDBETER, A.: Proc. nat. Acad. Sci. (Wash.) **70**, 3255—3259 (1973)]. Indeed, as will be shown later in this symposium, periodic activities can well be demonstrated in the more complex *Dictyostelium* cells which generate periodic chemical signals and responses to chemotaxis as part of their life-cycle [see discussion GERISCH, and GERISCH, G., and HESS, B.: Proc. nat. Acad. Sci. (Wash.) **71**, 2118—2122 (1974)]. Perhaps it is appropriate to point out in this symposium that the nonlinear chemical and biochemical oscillators which have been observed more recently are quite useful for such a function on the basis of their properties to generate temporal and spatial patterns. They might well serve as devices to measure time, or even to measure and remember chemicals or synchronize cellular activities. The greater sensitivity of oscillating receptors and enzymes relies on the fact that the number of variables needed to receive and transmit chemical concentration changes in increased because the presence of n chemicals in an oscillating system leads to additional time dependent variables,

which are given by n chemicals $+ 1$ period $+ (n-1)$ phases. Furthermore, non
linear oscillators have the properties to synchronize to external periodic action,
to generate subharmonics of the driving frequency, to react to stochastic
signal input, to amplify incoming signals and to couple non-linear oscillators
present in a given cellular system [see HESS, B., BOITEUX, A.: Ann. Rev.
Biochem. **40**, 237—258 (1971); — HEMKER, H. C., HESS, B.: Analysis and
simulation of biochemical systems. Amsterdam: North-Holland Publ. Co.
1972; — NICOLIS, G., PORTNOW, J.: Chem. Rev. **73**, 365—384 (1973); —
HESS, B., GOLDBETER, A., BOITEUX, A.: Unpublished observations]. I am
just wondering whether your system is not driven by such an internal timing
device, which would be necessary to do all this. And if you add methionine,
it very much looks to me as if you synchronize your wheel which turns the
flagella in one direction. I don't see any reason why this couldn't be coupled
to respiration, because we know that respiration is a perfect system to generate oscillatory phenomena. So I'd like to ask Dr. KOSHLAND, with respect to
the allosteric systems which certainly could amplify and give the amplification factor you were talking about, and Dr. ADLER, what he thinks about
synchronization as part of the phenomena of tumbling and non-tumbling?

J. ADLER: HOWARD BERG [Nature (Lond.) New Biol. **239**, 500—504 (1972)]
has called your oscillator the "twiddle generator" — aside from that aspect
of nomenclature, I don't know anything to say to your question.

D. E. KOSHLAND, JR.: An oscillating system has some great attractions.
BERG has studied the turning frequency of the bacterium and found it to
follow a Poissonian distribution. An oscillating system could easily cause a
Poissonian distribution of tumbling patterns. Moreover, it is quite easy, as
Dr. HESS said, to alter such an oscillating system to give the kind of suppression of tumbling that is observed. There is no doubt that it would be intriguing if the chemotactic response and the motility of bacteria could readily
be identified with an intermediate in the electron transport system. In
studies in our laboratory, Dr. MACNAB has found that tumbling can be
generated by light with an absorption spectrum of a flavin which has fasci-
nated us. — Dr. ADLER's laboratory has shown that interruptions of the
electron transport pathway can prevent motility. Finally, we have shown
that a methionine derivative, possibly S-adenosyl methionine, does have
an influence on the rate at which perturabtions are returned to the normal
value. S-adenosyl methionine is itself a high energy compound in many
reactions.

B. HESS: May I add one point to this? Maybe it is not known that Dr.
KOSHLAND's enzyme oscillates over a wide range of concentrations — and
even the frequency of a very large range of enzyme concentrations can be
varied almost linearly. This has been shown recently in numerical analysis
of your system.

T. JOVIN (Göttingen): A more prosaic mechanism than that proposed by
Dr. HESS might be responsible for the memory phase and the „clock". Is it
not possible that the "memory phenomenon" exhibited by the bacteria is

due to the binding process itself ? In the case of a good attractant like aspartate, threshold concentration of ca. 10^{-7} M was reported by Dr. ADLER. Assuming an admittedly modest recombination rate constant of 10^6 M sec^{-1}, the corresponding dissociation rate constant would be 10^{-1} sec. Thus, the life time of the complex between attractant and receptor protein would be about 10 sec, a value which is in the range of the persistence time cited by Dr. KOSHLAND. If we further assume that the response elicited by the bacteria traversing a concentration gradient reflects the binding function or, in the case of an allosteric system, a state function, then the temporal behavior will show a lag due to the convolution of the binding process with the concentration gradient; that is, the response at any moment, *i.e.* locus, would correspond partially to a concentration at a prior point in space and thus time. The lag would be accentuated if the rate limiting conformational transitions, for example, existed in the sequence of reactions between binding and final flagellar response. Such a mechanism could be regarded not so much as "memory" but rather as the "inability to forget". Experimentally, I would predict that different attractants and repellents and thus receptor systems might demonstrate different persistence times.

D. E. KOSHLAND, JR.: That is quite correct. All that we know at the moment in regard to memory is that it must be a time dependent response which compares two situations. The kinds of differential rates which you mentioned are certainly ways of building in a comparison system, if the constants are chosen correctly. A further possibility is a mechanism in which some receptors are on the outside and some are on the inside of the membrane. Then, of course, the outside receptors are in instantaneous equilibrium with the environment, whereas the inside ones lag behind the environmental concentration by the length of time it takes to diffuse across the membrane. Moreover, one can superimpose conformational changes on this geographical distribution. Thus there are a number of potential systems, but each of them must have some kind of time dependent process. An enzyme is appealing because there is a simple way to amplify this system.

V. NANJUNDIAH (Tübingen): You said the chemotactic response was proportional to the change in the fraction of bound protein whith time. What precisely does that mean ?

D. E. KOSHLAND: That is a rough statement which indicates that the chemotactic response depends upon binding of the attractant to a receptor molecule and the amount bound is typical of the kind of saturation curve we find with pure proteins. The mathematics of the behavior is certainly more complicated than that. At the moment we are studying this with various quantitative techniques. It is clear that if you go to very low concentrations of the attractant you don't get any response, and if you go to very high concentrations, you get saturation. In between the response corresponds to a typical binding curve, but only on a very rough way.

V. NANJUNDIAH: Does this depend on the precise spatial geometry of the situation in which the experiment is done ?

D. E. KOSHLAND: The answer to that, I believe, is "no" if I understand your question precisely. I mentioned that the bacterium does need to have the receptors located around its periphery in any particular geometry. Its motion through space is what gives it a sense of direction. On the other hand, geometry of the gradient has a great influence on the way the bacterium responds.

E. GROSS (Bethesda, Md.): Would you be prepared to equate the role of methionine with protein biosynthesis as an element necessary to generate the response of the microorganisms?

D. E. KOSHLAND, JR.: Methionine has a special effect on chemotaxis which is not related to protein synthesis. The time element would be against it. The methionine can be washed out in a matter of minutes, and then in a matter of seconds the behavior pattern can be observed. This is too fast for any significant depletion or synthesis of proteins. Moreover, other amino acids can be left out without getting an effect equivalent to that of methionine. Finally, the methionine can be washed out and chloramphenicol added during the addition of methionine. The methionine effect if still observed. Hence, whatever the phenomenon, it is not involved with protein synthesis.

L. JAENICKE (Köln): Hearing methionine, an old one-carbon hand thinks of folates and pteridines. Is it known what happens to chemotaxis in bacteria and particularly to tumbling mutants in the presence of antifolates? Furthermore, pteridines have a spectrum not unlike that of flavins and are also light-sensitive. Might the photo-effect you observe not be due to destruction of a pteridine cofactor?

D. E. KOSHLAND, JR.: That is an excellent question. We have not done the experiment and have not considered the ramifications, but it is an excellent thing to do because serine has a special property and is also involved with one-carbon metabolism. The role of folic acid in such a scheme has particular appeal. — There appear to be two light-sensitive pigments. One has the action spectrum of a flavin, as I mentioned in my talk [MACNAB and KOSHLAND: J. molec. Biol. **84**, 399—406 (1974)]. A second molecule absorbs in the green light region and acts as a phototactic receptor. (TAYLOR and KOSHLAND, in preparation). It tends to cause an opposite response to the flavin-like molecule. Both molecules appear to be light sensitive, and can be destroyed by excess light for prolonged periods.

R. SCHMITT (Erlangen): How is the lefthandedness of the flagellar helix of *E. coli* related to the counter-clockwise rotation with regard to forward motion? Would a right-handed helix require clockwise rotation for bundle formation and forward motion?

D. E. KOSHLAND, JR.: It seems quite clear that the flagellum is an inert protein. It has been shown that the flagellum is a single peptide chain and it looks as it the whole mechanism is what JULIUS ADLER described: The hook region right connected to the peptidoglycan layer. So it really is like a propeller. It is a stiff piece of machinery that is being cranked. I don't think it will go to the right.

R. SCHMITT: Is left-handedness a general feature of the helix of bacterial flagella or is it only confined to *E. coli*?

D. E. KOSHLAND, JR.: In a *Pseudomonas* we found it was the same as in *E. coli* and *Salmonella*. I don't known about others. Do you know that?

ADLER, J.: Yes, I have read that some are right-handed [WEIBULL, C.: In: GUNSALUS, I. C., STANIER, R. Y. (Eds).: The Bacteria, Vol. 1, pp. 153 to 205, esp. p. 167. New York: Academic Press 1960].

R. SCHMITT: We have characterized complex flagella in *Pseudomonas rhodos* [SCHMITT, R. RASKA, I., MAYER, F.: J. Bacteriol. **117**, 844—857 (1974)] and *Rhizobium lupini* [SCHMITT, R.: Intern. Congr. IAMS (Tokyo) 1974] with a right - handed superimposed triple helix. I wonder if this handedness could explain the unusual spinning and oscillating motions which we observe in these species.

G. WALD: As I remember, ENGELMANN discussed a wholly different mechanism for concentrating bacteria and motile algae: Stasis by the presence or absence of some agent in the medium. Thus if oxygen is needed for motion, a region lacking oxygen acts as a trap, since all organisms entering it stop swimming and so cannot leave such a region. The presence of any agent that slows or stops swimming would act similarly!

J. ADLER: That is correct. Any agent that will stop the motion of the bacteria will also collect the bacteria. However, in the situation that I described stasis by the presence of an agent is excluded, since for every attractant or repellent we showed that there is no response by the generally non-chemotactic (but fully motile) mutants [ADLER: Science **166**, 1588—1597 (1969); Tso and ADLER: J. Bacteriol. **118**, 560—576 (1974); remainder unpublished]. Also, stasis by the absence of an agent has been excluded by microbiological observations (unpublished).

H. M. EMRICH (München): Have you any idea how the mechanism of rotation of the flagella could be constructed? A muscle fiber normally produces only contraction, but no rotation.

J. ADLER: No idea! — In the case of muscle, there are cross-bridges. However, HOWARD BERG's article [Nature (Lond.) New Biol. **249**, 77—79 (1974)] points to the unlikelihood of cross-bridges turning the bacterial flagellum. I may add another point: In the case of muscle, the energy source is ATP directly; in the case of the swimming of the bacteria ATP directly is not the energy source; rather it is the intermediate of oxidative phosporylation. [LARSEN et. al.: Proc. nat. Acad. Sci. (Wash.) **71**, 1239—1243 (1974)]. So here is another difference compared with the mechanism of rotation of flagella.

Functions of Bacteriorhodopsin

N. Dencher

*Institut für Neurobiologie der Kernforschungsanlage Jülich GmbH
5170 Jülich, Federal Republic of Germany*

With 2 Figures

Our results indicate that the bacteriorhodopsin in *Halobacterium halobium* has not only an energy-converting function as reported by Oesterhelt (see p. 69 ff), but also a photosensory function comparable with the photoreception in animals (Hildebrand and Dencher, in preparation).

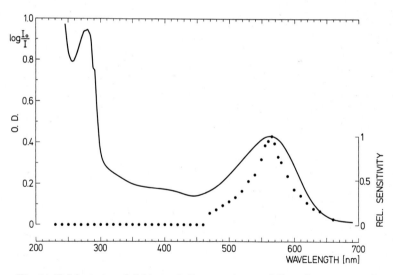

Fig. 1. *Halobacterium halobium:* Action spectrum of the *off*-response and absorption spectrum of isolated purple membrane containing bacteriorhodopsin. · · · spectral sensitivity [sec/hν], defined as reciprocal value of the number of photons per time at each wavelength triggering the reaction of the bacterium at threshold, ———— absorption spectrum

For a typical behavior reaction after a light stimulus we found two different photosystems in the bacterium:

1. Photosystem$_{565}$ which is responsible for the *off*-response, the reaction to a sudden decrease of light intensity (inverse photophobic reaction). The action spectrum of this *off*-response and the absorption spectrum of bacteriorhodopsin both have their maximum at 565 nm (Fig. 1). From this and other results we suppose bacteriorhodopsin to be the pigment of the photosystem$_{565}$. By means of this photosystem the bacterium can find optimal light conditions (intensity and wavelength) for the bacteriorhodopsin-dependent ATP synthesis and stay there. Preliminary results indicate that the quantum efficiency in this system is considerably lower than in the photoreceptor cells of animals. Approximately $2 \cdot 10^{11}$ h$\nu \cdot$ sec$^{-1} \cdot$ mm^{-2} ($= 6 \cdot 10^5$ hν/bacterium $\cdot$ sec or about 1.7 hν/pigment molecule $\cdot$ sec) at 565 nm trigger the reaction. There is no measurable light adaptation.

2. Photosystem$_{370}$ which is responsible for the *on*-response, the reaction to a sudden increase of light intensity or a short light flash

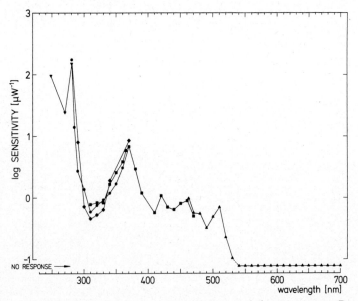

Fig. 2. *Halobacterium halobium:* Action spectrum of the *on*-response. Log sensitivity see Fig. 1, but in units of [μW^{-1}]

(direct photophobic reaction). The action spectrum of this *on*-response shows two main maxima at 280 nm and 370 nm (Fig. 2). The pigment, most probably a chromoprotein, has not yet been identified. The action spectrum resembles the absorption spectrum of a retinylidenprotein ($\lambda_{max} = 285$—290 nm and 365 nm). The sensitivity of the photosystem$_{370}$ is higher than the sensitivity of the photosystem [565]; at 370 nm about 15 times, at 280 nm about 400 times that of the photosystem [565] at 565 nm.

My question to Dr. KOSHLAND: Please can you say something about action spectrum of the light effect on the tumbling reaction you have reported.

D. E. KOSHLAND: We have indeed looked for the rhodopsin-like molecule and have found a molecule which acts opposite to that of the flavin. It could be a rhodopsin-like molecule having the same effects, and we are currently working on this very intensively.

The Role of the Escherichia Coli Galactose-Binding Protein in Galactose Transport and Chemotaxis

T. J. Silhavy, W. Boos, and H. M. Kalckar

Department of Biological Chemistry, Harvard Medical School and the Biochemical Research Laboratory, Massachusetts General Hospital, Boston, MA. 02114, USA

With 18 Figures

Introduction

The galactose-binding protein (GBP) was first isolated by Anraku, and he suggested that GBP was involved in galactose transport in *Escherichia coli* (Anraku, 1968). The study of galactose transport in this organism is complicated by the existence of at least six transport systems with specificity for galactose (Kalckar, 1971; Rotman et al., 1968). This overlap made the design of selection procedures needed to obtain well defined mutants rather complex. Since no well characterized mutants were available, and since no other galactose derivatives were checked for binding, it was not possible at this time to tell which transport system required GBP.

Early genetic studies by Ganesan and Rotman (1966) had shown that a mutation responsible for the defect in the β-methylgalactoside (MeGal) transport system in strain W4345 mapped in the *mgl* locus, which was closely linked to the *his* operon. Closer examination of this strain revealed a lack of GBP (Boos, 1969). Mating studies performed with this strain strongly suggested that the gene coding for GBP was closely linked, if not identical with the genes determining the MeGal transport system (Boos and Sarvas, 1970). In addition, Lengeler et al. (1971) were able to show that synthesis of GBP and the MeGal transport system were coregulated. Although these studies suggested a close relationship between GBP and the MeGal transport system, they also introduced another complicating factor. A survey of *E. coli* strains showed that all mgl^+ strains tested produced GBP (Boos and Sarvas, 1970). However, the reverse was found not to be the case. The mgl strains fell into two categories; those which contain no detectable GBP and those which are still able to synthesize it in normal amounts. From these results, one must conclude that the MeGal transport system is coded for by more than one gene. In this respect, the MeGal transport differs from other transport systems such as the lactose transport system, which is known to be coded for by a single gene (Kennedy, 1970). This extra complexity appears to be common to other transport systems which contain shock releasable binding proteins (Boos, 1974).

Fluorescence studies with purified GBP showed that galactose and other substrates produced a characteristic increase in the fluorescence of the protein (Boos et al., 1972). This proved to be a valuable tool. A mutant was found, EH 3039, which produced a defective but immunologically cross reactive binding protein (Boos, 1972). When GBP was purified from this strain and examined by fluorescence, it too showed a characteristic increase in the emission spectra. However, in this case, approximately 7000 times more substrate was required in order to see this fluorescence increase. This mutant strain was reverted to a transport positive phenotype. Subsequent examination of the purified GBP from this revertant showed that it had acquired the fluorescence properties of the wild-type protein. This simultaneous alteration in the structure and activity of GBP upon mutation to transport negative and reversion to transport positive phenotypes clearly demonstrates the essential role of GBP in the MeGal transport system.

It is now known that a second role for GBP exists in *E. coli*. The recent studies of Ordal and Adler using episomes carrying wild-type and a variety of mutant genes in respect to mgl have shown conclusively that GBP is also required for galactose chemotaxis (Ordal and Adler, 1974). Although the phenomenon of chemotaxis in bacteria has been known for nearly 100 years (Pfeffer, 1884), little progress has been made in this field until recently. This phenomenon has proven to be even more difficult to study than is transport. Since chemotaxis involves the actual movement of bacteria, even simply measuring this process has proven to be quite difficult. A big step forward was taken when Adler and his colleagues developed a semiquantitative assay for chemotaxis (ADLER, 1973). This technique has allowed them to distinguish between different chemoreceptors and to determine the relative specificity of each (MESIBOV and ADLER, 1972; ADLER et al., 1973). HAZELBAUER and ADLER (1971) have developed methods which enable selection and characterization of mutants defective in general chemotaxis, as well as mutants defective in taxis towards attractants which belong to a single chemoreceptor. Along other lines, the studies of DAHLQUIST et al. (1971) and BERG and BROWN (1972) suggest that bacteria are only able to recognize movement up a gradient, not down. On the other hand, MACNAB and KOSHLAND (1972) have found that bacteria react to both increased and decreased attractant concentrations.

Despite these advances, little is actually known about the molecular mechanism of chemotaxis and efforts were, therefore, concentrated on the elucidation of the first step, the recognition of the attractant by the chemoreceptor. KALCKAR (1971) pointed out possible correlations between galactose chemotaxis and the presence or absence of GBP in various strains. On this basis, he proposed that GBP may be the galactose chemoreceptor. HAZELBAUER and ADLER (1971) were able to demonstrate a striking similarity between the properties of the galactose chemoreceptor *in vivo* and the properties of purified GBP *in vitro*. As was previously mentioned, ORDAL and ADLER (1974) have now shown conclusively that GBP is required for galactose chemotaxis.

An important study by MESIBOV, ORDAL and ADLER (MESIBOV et al., 1973) compares the chemotactic responses of *E. coli* towards two types of non-metabolizable substrates, β-methylaspartate and galactose (in mglP and galK mutants). The chemotactic response to galactose (treshold, K_D, optimum responses, saturation and inhibition at excess concentrations of galactose) bear more resemblance to the kinetic parameters of the higt affinity site of GBP than to those of the low affinity site. The demand for steep gradients of galactose in order to achieve a significant chemotactic response, is presumably also rooted in the strong preferential retention of galactose by GBP (see later sections). Likewise, the marked interference of galactose chemotaxis by the presence of glucose or galactose in background concentrations as low as 10^{-8} M, matches the strong tendency to retention of glucose or galactose by GBP

(HAZELBAUER and ADLER 1971; KALCKAR 1971; MESIBOV et al.
1973; PARNES and BOOS 1973).

In this article, we would like to discuss in some detail the properties of GBP in regard to its function in both transport and chemotaxis. In addition, we would like to propose a mechanism for the interaction of GBP with its respective recognition site on the cytoplasmic membrane, the step following the recognition of substrate by GBP.

The Galactose-Binding Protein
Isolation

GBP is most commonly isolated from *E. coli* by the cold osmotic shock procedure of NEU and HEPPEL (1965). This procedure involves plasmolysis of the cell with a hypertonic sucrose-*Tris*-EDTA solution, followed by osmotic shock with an ice cold, low ionic strength $MgSO_4$ solution. This procedure liberates a number of proteins from the cell envelope including other binding proteins and enzymes such as alkaline phosphatase. Cell lysis does not occur and, in fact, essentially none of the cytoplasmic enzymes (β-galactosidase, glucose-6-P dehydrogenase) are lost (HEPPEL, 1971). The proteins released by this procedure have come to be called "periplasmic proteins", since they seem to be located in the "periplasm". The periplasm is defined as the space between the cytoplasmic membrane and the cell wall of gram-negative bacteria (MITCHELL, 1961). The periplasmic proteins are all water soluble, and for this reason it would seem as though they exist in this state in the periplasm. This, however, is difficult to show, since they could just as easily be weakly bound to the cytoplasmic membrane. In either event, a number of experiments have been done which strongly indicate that the periplasmic proteins are located outside the osmotic barrier of the cell, the cytoplasmic membrane (HEPPEL, 1971).

Properties

When purified GBP is subjected to analytical polyacrylamide gel electrophoresis in the presence of sodium docecyl sulfate, a single band corresponding to a molecular weight of 36500 is observed (BOOS and GORDON, 1971). Values obtained for the native protein by other procedures such as molecular sieve chromatography and sedimentation equilibrium give similar values (BOOS et al.,

1972). These results indicate that GBP exists in solution as a monomer. Except for a complete lack of cysteine, the amino acid composition of the protein is uninformative (ANRAKU, 1968). Little is known about the native structure of the protein; however, ORD/CD studies indicate an unusually high content of β-structure and a near absence of any α-helical regions (Boos et al., 1972). The protein is remarkably stable and is unaffected by brief exposure to temperatures as high as 80° C or pH changes from 5–9 (ANRAKU, 1968; McGowan et al., 1974).

Conformational Change

Boos and GORDON (1971) observed that purified GBP showed two bands on polyacrylamide gels at pH 8.4. When electrophoresis was run on gels that had been equilibrated with 0.1 μM ^{3}H-galactose, it was found that both components were capable of binding galactose. Furthermore, it was found that re-electrophoresis of either component resulted in the appearance of the same two bands. On the basis of these experiments, it was proposed that GBP existed in two conformational states. Further examination into this phenomenon revealed that the altered electrophoretic mobility was substrate dependent. The simultaneous appearance of two bands on these gels in the absence of substrate was due to the presence of sucrose in the incubation mixture. If, instead of 20% sucrose, 20% non-polymerized acrylamide was used to increase the density of the protein sample, only one band was observed. However, the presence of as little as 1 μM galactose in the gel and the electrode buffer did cause an increase in the electrophoretic mobility of the protein. Figure 1 gives an account of this phenomenon with a purified as well as crude preparation of GBP.

Other known substrates such as glucose or 2R-glyceryl-β-D-galactopyranoside (glycerylgalactoside) also altered the electrophoretic mobility of GBP while other compounds, not substrates of GBP, did not (Boos et al., 1972).

Techniques such as sedimentation velocity, sedimentation equilibrium, ORD, CD and infrared spectroscopy did not show any change in GBP upon the addition of substrate (Boos et al., 1972). However, indication that the two forms differed in charge was obtained by electrofocussing. This technique separated GBP into two species with a pI of 5.3 and 5.4, respectively (Boos, 1972).

A thorough examination of the binding properties of GBP by equilibrium dialysis provided further evidence for the substrate-induced conformational change. The Lineweaver-Burk plot of these data was biphasic, and extrapolation yielded dissociation constants of 0.1 and 10 µM, Fig. 2 (Boos et al., 1972). When the data were plotted according to SCATCHARD (1949), the heterogeneous behavior was even more pronounced, Fig. 3. Extrapolation of this plot to high galactose concentrations clearly indicates that two moles of galactose are bound per mole of GBP (36000 molecular weight).

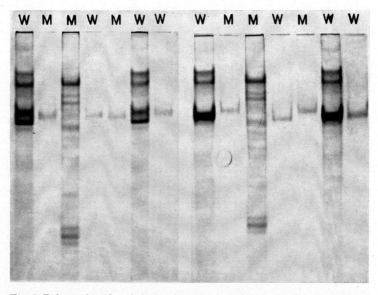

Fig. 1. Polyacrylamide gel electrophoresis of a galactose binding protein preparation of a transport-positive and a transport negative strain of *Escherichia coli* in the presence and absence of 0.1 mM galactose. The gel slabs (4 × 120 × 160 mm) contained 10% acrylamide, 0.375% bisacrylamide, 0.1 M *tris*-borate, pH 8.4 and 0.002 M EDTA. The gel shown on the right also contained 0.1 mM galactose. In this case, the electrode buffer also contained 0.1 mM galactose. The electrophoresis was run for 5 hr at 300 V with a final current of 50 ma. The gels were stained in Coomassie blue. The following preparations were applied: 1. Sephadex G-100-treated shock fluid from the transport-positive strain W3092cy⁻ (ATCC 25939). 2. Purified binding protein from strain W3092cy⁻. 3. Sephadex G-100-treated shock fluid from the transport-negative strain AW550. 4. Purified binding protein from strain AW550.
(Boos et al., 1972)

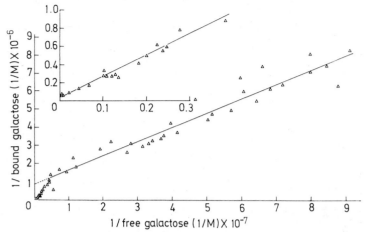

Fig. 2. Galactose-binding activity of the galactose-binding protein as a function of galactose concentration measured by equilibrium dialysis. Double chambers of 100 μl volume separated by dialysis tubing were filled with 90 μl of galactose-binding protein (0.4 mg per ml) in 0.01 M *Tris*-HCl, pH 7.3 and 90 μl of [1-^{14}C]galactose or [1-^{3}H]galactose in the same buffer. The dialysis was performed at 4° for at least 12 hrs. Fifty microliters from each chamber were counted for radioactivity. (Boos et al., 1972)

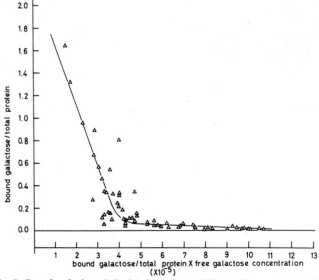

Fig. 3. Scatchard plot of the binding data of Fig. 2. (Boos et al., 1972)

Other investigators have also provided evidence consistent with the existence of more than one conformation in GBP. Kepes and Richarme (1972) have reported that GBP binds more galactose during equilibrium dialysis than when precipitated with 80%

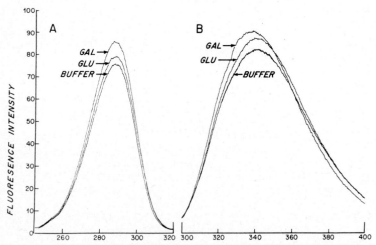

Fig. 4 A and B. Fluorescence spectra (uncorrected) of galactose-binding protein in the presence and absence of 0.1 mM galactose and glucose. Galactose-binding protein (16.7 µg per ml) in 0.01 M *Tris*-HCl, pH 7.3; excitation slit, 10 nm; emission slit, 8 nm. (A) Excitation spectra. Emission wavelength was 330 nm. (B) Emission spectra. Excitation wavelength was 290 nm. Temperature was 24°. (Boos et al., 1972)

ammonium sulfate. Rotman and Ellis (1972) have shown that the binding activity of GBP can be increased by the presence of specific antibodies. This latter result, in particular, indicates that affinity can be increased by altering the conformation *(vide infra)*.

As was previously mentioned, GBP exhibits a characteristic increase in fluorescence in the presence of substrate. Figure 4 shows the emission spectra of GBP, which is characterized by a broad maximum at 340 nm. Galactose increases the intensity by as much as 13.5% (at 330 nm), and it causes a 2 nm blue shift in the emission maximum. Glucose causes a similar increase, but no shift in the emission maximum. The increase in fluorescence intensity occurs at wavelengths which correspond to tryptophan fluorescence.

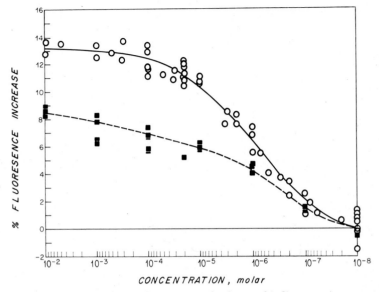

Fig. 5. Per cent increase in fluorescence of galactose-binding protein versus total sugar concentration. ○----○, galactose; ■----■, glucose. Excitation: 290; emission: 330. Excitation slit was 4 nm; emission slit was 10 nm. Protein concentration was 16.7 μg per ml. Temperature was 24°. (Boos et al., 1972)

Furthermore, the emission spectra remain unchanged in shape when the protein is excited at 280 or 295 nm. These results clearly indicate the involvement of a tryptophan residue(s) (UDENFRIEND, 1962). The differences in the fluorescence changes caused by galactose and glucose suggested that these two sugars might be bound at different sites. This was shown not to be the case, since the fluorescence increase in the presence of both sugars is not additive (Boos et al., 1972).

Figure 5 shows the dependence of the fluorescence increase of GBP on the total concentrations of glucose and galactose. The half-maximal effects are observed at total concentrations of 1 μM for both sugars. Since the protein concentration in these experiments was approximately 0.5 μM, a considerable amount of the total sugar present is bound. Thus, the actual half-maximal values are some-what less than indicated, and in good agreement with the disso-ciation constants as determined by equilibrium dialysis. The specifi-

Table 1. Effect of different sugars on entry and exit of galactose and on
          fluorescence of galactose-binding protein

Concentration of sugar 0.1 mM	Inhibition of galactose uptake at an initial concentration of 0.5 µM [1-^{14}C]-galactose (%)	Galactose exit at steady state accumulation of 1 mM internal [1-^{14}C]galactose concentration[a] (%)	Maximal fluorescence increase of the purified galactose-binding protein (%)
Glycerolgalactoside	96	93	88
L-Arabinose	54	63	59
Fucose	24	104	48
Methyl-1-β-D-galactopyranoside	22	41	29
Xylose	22		41
TMG	1	< 4	1
(2-Glyceryl)-1-β-D-galacto paranoside	< 1	< 4	< 1
β-D-Galactosyl-1-thio-β-D-galactopyranoside	< 1	< 4	< 1
Melibiose	< 1	< 4	< 1
Lactose	< 1	< 4	< 1
IPTG	< 1	< 4	< 1

[a] Exit is initiated by inhibiting recapture of galactose.

city of the response is demonstrated by Table 1, which shows the
inhibition of galactose transport produced by various sugars in
comparison to the fluorescence increase caused by that particular
sugar. As can be seen, there is a direct correlation between these
two effects (PARNES and BOOS, 1973).

Although the fluorescence increase produced by the addition of
substrate clearly involves a tryptophan residue(s), the nature of
this involvement is not clear and it could be interpreted in several
ways:

1. There is a tryptophan residue(s) present in the binding site,
and the microenvironment of this residue is altered by direct interaction with the substrate itself.

2. The tryptophan residue(s) itself is not located in the binding
site, but rather, it is located in such a way as to undergo a change

in its microenvironment as a result of a substrate-induced conformational change.

3. Both processes may be occurring.

Addition of galactose to GBP results in the production of an ultraviolet (uv) difference spectrum which closely resembles the solvent perturbation difference spectra of N-acetyltryptophan ethyl

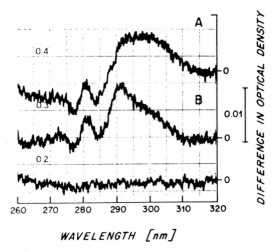

Fig. 6A and B. Ultraviolet difference spectra of galactose-binding protein caused by galactose and glucose. Protein solution (1 ml; 16 μM in 0.01 M *Tris*-HCl, pH 7.3) was placed in two matched quartz cuvets. A base line was obtained from 320—260 nm. Glucose (10 μl) (A) or galactose (10 μl) (B), final concentration 10 mM, was added to the sample cell and 10 μl of water was added to the reference cell and the resultant spectrum was recorded. (McGowan et al., 1974)

ester, Fig. 6. This figure also shows the uv difference spectra produced by the addition of glucose. Figure 7 shows that this alteration in the difference spectra is specific and saturable. At a protein concentration of 18 μM, no further increase in the 291 nm peak was observed above 100 μM galactose. Assuming that only one of the two binding sites was occupied below substrate concentration of 1 μM, one can calculate that the half-maximal response occurs at a free substrate concentration of 1 μM. Both spectra have positive absorbance above 295 nm, higher than that observed with model tryptophan compounds, but similar to that observed with lyozyme in the presence of its substrate analog glycol chitin. In this case, the difference spectra was shown to result from the interaction of the substrate analog with a specific tryptophan residue removing it

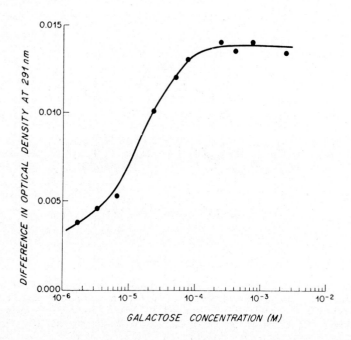

Fig. 7. Concentration dependence of the galactose-induced spectral change. The protein solution was prepared as in Fig. 1. Galactose was added in 1—5 µl aliquots of 10 mM to 1 M solutions to the sample cell and an equal volume of water was added to the reference cell. The increase in ΔA_{291nm} was determined. (McGOWAN et al., 1974)

from contact with the aqueous environment (HAYASHI et al., 1963). The similarity, but nonidentity of the uv difference spectra obtained with GBP and glucose and galactose respectively suggests that a tryptophan residue in the active site is being affected somewhat differently by the two sugars. Addition of freshly prepared α-galactose to a solution of GBP results in the production of a difference spectrum, Fig. 8, markedly different from that seen with equilibrated (70% β) galactose. The time dependent increase in the 291 nm maximum is seen by comparing the spectra obtained at 2, 15, and 25 min. Spectrum C is the same as that obtained with equilibrated

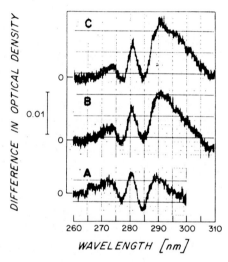

Fig. 8 A—C. Dependence of the spectral change on the anomeric state of galactose. Protein (18 µM) was prepared as in Fig. 1. Freshly prepared α-galactose was added to the sample cell at a final concentration of 80 µM. Spectra were obtained 2 min (A), 15 min (B), and 25 min (C) after dissolving the galactose. (McGowan et al., 1974)

galactose. This result indicates that both forms of galactose are bound by the protein and that the configuration of the C-1 hydroxyl group affects the absorbance of a tryptophan residue in the active site. Since it is unlikely that such small structural alterations in the substrate (compare α-galactose, equilibrated galactose and glucose) could affect the chemical environment of a tryptophan residue not present in the active site, it was concluded that at least part of the substrate induced difference spectra was due to a direct interaction between the substrate and a tryptophan residue in the active site (McGowan et al., 1974).

Solvent perturbation spectroscopy was used in order to investigate the possibility that an additional tryptophan may experience a change in its environment due to a conformational change in the protein. This technique allows the determination of the relative extent of exposure of chromophoric groups in the protein (HERSKOVITS and LASKOWSKI, 1960, 1962). If the binding of substrate causes a refolding of the peptide chain with a concomitant alteration in the exposure of one or more external tryptophan residues, then the solvent perturbation difference spectrum should be altered when obtained in the presence of substrate. CROWDER et al. (1973) have recently done such experiments with aldolase. They found that the solvent perturbation difference spectra of this enzyme were markedly different, depending on the presence or absence of the competitive inhibitor D-arabinitol-1,5-diphosphate. They concluded that a conformational change occurs upon binding of the inhibitor which results in increased exposure of tryptophan to the solvent at a point removed from the binding site.

Figure 9 shows the solvent perturbation difference spectrum of GBP (McGOWAN et al., 1974) produced by the addition of 20% dimethyl sulfoxide. By using the model compound data of HERSKOVITS and SORENSEN (1968), it was found that 2 of the 5 tryptophan and 4—5 of the 7 tyrosine residues are accessible to this solvent. Similar results were obtained with other perturbants such as methanol and ethylene glycol. The smallest perturbant available (90% deuterium oxide) perturbed 2 additional tryptophan residues. The solvent perturbation difference spectra are further enhanced by the addition of subtrate to the protein in the sample cell alone, Fig. 10. Manual substraction of the two curves shown in Fig. 10A and B indicated that the observed alteration was identical with the galactose induced difference spectrum in the absence of perturbant, Fig. 6. It should be noted that this was found to be true with all perturbants tested, even dimethyl sulfoxide and deuterium oxide which cause perturbation in the plus and minus sense, respectively. Subsequently, it was found that the substrate induced difference spectra with GBP prepared in the presence of various perturbants were identical with those obtained with GBP in buffer alone, Fig. 6. Conversely, it was found that the solvent perturbation difference spectra of the protein and the protein in the presence of substrate are identical. These experiments clearly show that the binding of substrate does not alter the exposure of any accessible chromophores, and this result further substantiates the contention that the substrate induced difference spectrum is due to a direct interaction between the sugar and a tryptophan residue in the active site. Since deuterium oxide perturbs all four remaining tryptophan residues, the possibility of a buried tryptophan undergoing a change in its environment can be excluded.

Another more subtle conclusion can be drawn from these studies which might be discussed better with the aid of a model, Fig. 11. GBP exists in solution in two different states, I and II, which are in equilibrium with each other such that $II/I \ll 1$. The addition of galactose shifts this equilibrium to the right by combining with the

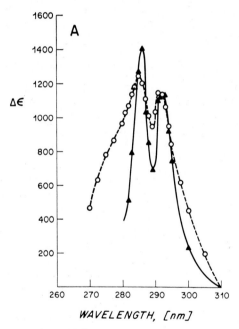

Fig. 9. Solvent perturbation different spectra of the galactose-binding protein. (A) Protein (20 μM in 0.01 M Tris-HCl, pH 7.3) was prepared in the presence and absence of 20% (v/v) dimethyl sulfoxide as described by HERSKOVITS and LASKOWSKI (1960, 1962). (▲) Best fit (5 tyrosine, 2 tryptophan residues) calculated from the model compound data of HERSKOVITS and SORENSEN (1968); (○) observed spectrum. (McGOWAN et al., 1974)

State II conformation. The active site tryptophan is here designated as T_1; the remaining tryptophan residues are designated $T_2 - T_5$. In light of the previously mentioned studies which show that substrate alters the electrophoretic mobility of the protein, the charge of the State II conformation is more negative than I. The second low-affinity binding site is known to exist when galactose occupies

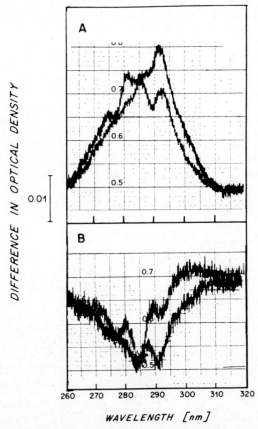

Fig. 10A and B. Solvent perturbation spectra of the galactose-binding protein in the presence and absence of galactose (A) Protein (20 µM) was perturbed by 20% (v/v) dimethyl sulfoxide (lower spectrum), then 0.1 mM galactose was added to the sample solution (upper spectrum). (B) The protein (44 µM) was perturbed by 90% (v/v) D_2O (lower spectrum), then 0.1 mM galactose was added (upper spectrum). (MCGOWAN et al., 1974)

the high affinity site A. However, our present knowledge does not allow a decision on whether or not this site exists in the State I conformation or even in State II in the absence of galactose. It is, therefore, designated by a dotted line.

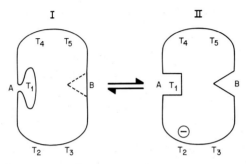

Fig. 11. Model of the conformational change occurring upon addition of galactose to the protein. (A) High-affinity binding site, active only in State II; (B) low-affinity binding site; T_1, tryptophan in the active site; T_2, T_3, external tryptophan residues accessible to all perturbants; T_2 is located close to an electrical charge, which is different in state I and II; T_4 and T_5, tryptophan residues not accessible to dimethyl sulfoxide, ethylene glycol or methanol, but accessible to D_2O. (McGowan et al., 1974)

The solvent perturbation studies showed that the substrate-induced perturbation of the active site tryptophan residue is unaffected by the presence of various solvent perturbants. Furthermore, the solvent perturbation difference spectra were found to be unaffected by the presence of substrate. Since the different refractive indices of the various solvent mixtures (particularly in the case of deuterium oxide, Fig. 10) do not give rise to different values of the substrate-induced absorbance change, it must be concluded that the active site tryptophan residue is not accessible to any of the employed perturbants either in the presence of absence of substrate. In the model (Fig. 11), this is designated a "closed" active site in the State I conformation. Once galactose is bound, it prevents the approach of perturbant in the State II conformation.

Another method that is used to detect conformational changes is the technique of fluorescence perturbation spectroscopy (LEHRER, 1967). This technique makes use of the fluorescence quenching properties of KI and as such, it is another useful method of determining the relative exposure of chromophoric groups. In some cases, the addition of substrate has resulted in decreased quenching (protection), and has been used as evidence of conformational

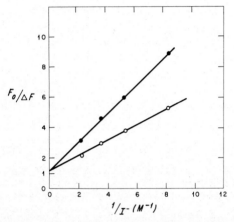

Fig. 12. Quenching of protein fluorescence emission by KI. To wild-type galactose-binding protein (0.5 μM in 0.01 M *tris*-HCl, pH 7.3) in the presence and absence of 10 μM galactose, increasing amounts of 6 M KI were added. A control cuvet obtained increasing amounts of 6 M NaCl. F_0, fluorescence in the NaCl-containing control cuvet; ΔF, difference in fluorescence of sample and control cuvet. $1/I^-$ was calculated using the proper dilution factor. The emission wavelength was monitored at 330 nm. Excitation was 290 nm. Open symbols, quenching in the absence of galactose; closed symbols, quenching in the presence of galactose. (McGOWAN et al., 1974)

change (LEHRER, 1971; LAIKEN et al., 1972). As can be seen in Fig. 12, KI quenches the fluorescence emission of GBP and the amount of quenching was proportional to the concentration KI. When galactose was present at 1 μM or above in the protein solution, the quenching by KI was decreased, as shown by the increased slope of the $F_0/\Delta F$ vs. $1/[KI]$ plot (LEHRER, 1971). (F_0, fluorescence in the absence of KI; ΔF, change in the fluorescence produced by KI.) It is obvious that if all chromophores were accessible to KI, F_0 would equal ΔF and, therefore, extrapolation to infinite [KI] should equal 1. Since this is not observed, it was concluded that not all tryptophan residues were accessible to quencher either in the presence or absence of substrate (McGowan et al., 1974). These studies clearly indicate that substrate alters GBP in some way as to protect it from the quenching effects of KI. However, as was previously discussed, the solvent perturbation studies indicated that substrate had no effect on the exposure of the chromophoric groups. This protective effect of substrate must be the result of something other than the burial of a chromophore. Lehrer (1971) has demonstrated that quenching by KI can be affected by charged residues near the tryptophan residue in the tertiary structure of the polypeptide chain. It was, therefore, concluded that the alteration in the surface charge of GBP shown to accompany the binding of substrate causes this differential quenching of an external tryptophan. Two observations support this conclusion:

1. Fluorescence perturbation studies performed on the mutant GBP isolated from strain EH3039 show only a small protective effect of galactose (see Fig. 13). This is paralleled by the observation that the mutant protein does not alter its surface charge upon the binding of substrate *(vide supra)*.

2. Both the galactose and glucose induced difference spectra of GBP show marked positive absorbance above 295 nm. Ananthan-

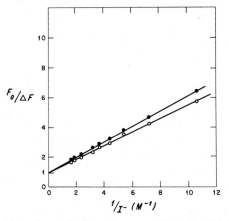

Fig. 13. Quenching of protein fluorescence emission by KI. Same experiment as Fig. 12. except mutant galactose-binding protein was useed (strain EH3039) and the galactose concentration was 10 mM. Open symbols, quenching in the absence of galactose; closed symbols, quenching in the presence of galactose Mc Gowan et al. 1974)

Arayanan and Bigelow (1969) have studied the difference spectra of tryptophan model compounds and proteins. They concluded that a more negative environment in the vicinity of a tryptophan residue results in a positive increase of the absorbance at 300 nm.

Thus, it seems most likely that the decreased quenching observed with KI in the presence of substrate is due to repulsion of the iodide ion from tryptophan T_2 by the increased negative charge characteristic of the State II conformation (see Fig. 11). T_1, which is not accessible to the perturbant deuterium oxide, is not accessible to KI, either in the presence of absence of substrate, and thus, extrapolation of Fig. 12 to infinite [KI] yields values greater than 1.

In this section, we have presented conclusive evidence that a conformational change accompanies the binding of substrate to GBP. This change does not involve a major refolding of the peptide backbone, but is rather confined to small alterations that seem to involve the active site region of the molecule. Another property of GBP which could conceivably be important is the existence of a second, low-affinity galactose-binding site. Although neither the conformational change nor the existence of a second substrate site appears to be common to all binding proteins (Boos, 1974), we feel that these properties are crucial for the normal functioning of GBP in the β-methylgalactoside transport system.

The Role of GBP in Transport and Chemotaxis

The Carrier Hypothesis

From the combination of biochemical and genetic analysis, it is clear that GBP is an essential component for galactose transport (via the MeGal transport system) as well as for galactose chemotaxis. However, these studies do not reveal the molecular mechanism by which GBP participates in these two physiological processes.

Several attempts have been made to implicate a direct membrane translocating function to GBP as well as other periplasmic substrate binding proteins.

1. It has been reported that purified binding proteins are able to restore, to varying degrees, transport in shocked cells (Anraku, 1968; Medveczky and Rosenberg, 1970; Wilson and Holden, 1969; Iwashima et al., 1971). In the case of galactose transport, a crude fraction of the shock fluid, not containing binding protein,

was shown to increase the restoration of transport. However, these reports could not be reproduced in all cases and have since been questioned (ROSEN, 1973; HEPPEL et al., 1972; PARDEE, 1970). Difficulties in the interpretation of restoration studies might arise from the incomplete removal of binding proteins by the shock procedure and restoration of energy supply after incubation of shocked cells in the transport assay system, rather than restoration of exogenous binding protein. Indeed, it has recently been demonstrated that lipids and long chain fatty acids (found in crude osmotic shock fluid) were able to stimulate active transport of lactose in an *E. coli* mutant energy-uncoupled for the lactose transport system, and to a minor degree also in the wild-type strain (WONG et al., 1973). Thus, restoration studies are only valid under strictly controlled conditions, as far as energy sources are concerned, and should only be performed in mutants defective in transport due to a mutation in the respective binding protein.

2. Over the past years, models of active transport in bacteria have invariably postulated the existence of two or more conformational states of the transport carrier protein (KENNEDY, 1970; KEPES, 1971; MITCHELL, 1970; KABACK and BARNES, 1971). The functional properties of these conformational states was either to alter the binding affinity or the rate of translocation of the carrier molecule upon input of energy. This would result in association of substrate on the outside of the membrane and dissociation on the inside, and thus generate active transport. The demonstration of reversible conformational changes would, therefore, be indicative of the translocational properties of transport associated proteins. As discussed before, substrate-dependent conformational changes have, indeed, been observed with GBP. Experiments with other periplasmic binding proteins are consistent with conformational changes as well. Studies with the leucine-binding protein of *E. coli* (PENROSE et al., 1970; BERMAN and BOYER, 1972) have shown that this protein does not exhibit substrate dependent alteration of the studied parameters, even though reversibility of denaturation was interpreted as integral property of the protein to easily undergo conformational changes. However, substrate-dependent fluorescence changes have been reported for the glutamine- (WEINER and HEPPEL, 1971), the sulfate- (LANGRIDE et al., 1970) and the arabinose-binding proteins (PARSONS and HOGG, 1973). Also, it has been

noted that the elution profile of a phenylalanine-binding protein of *Comomonas* changes in the presence of substrate (KUZUYA et al., 1971). Moreover, the cystein-binding protein *(E. coli)* can be eluted from a DEAE column at two different positions (BERGER and HEPPEL, 1972), as can the arabinose-binding protein *(E. coli)* on polyacrylamide gel electrophoresis (PARSON and HOGG, 1973). ROTMAN and ELLIS (1972) reported an increase in "binding activity" when specific antibodies were present in the binding assay. The order of additions was important for this increase. Galactose had to be added first to react with the GBP before addition of the antibodies. An explanation, other than a trivial trapping of bound galactose by formation of the antigen-antibody precipitate is again that GBP exists in two different (substrate dependent) conformations which are fixed by the interaction with the specific antibodies. Based on this observation, ROTMAN and ELLIS have postulated the existence of a membrane bound high molecular weight effector whose role *in vivo* is similar to that of specific antibodies *in vitro*. The sequence of events in transport would be as follows: GBP upon contract with the external substrate changes its conformation. This change puts GBP in contact with the high molecular weight effector in the membrane which, in turn, causes two effects: it translocates the binding site of the protein and lowers its affinity for substrate, upon which the substrate is released into the cytoplasm. The release of substrate then reverses the process and allows the binding protein to go back to its original conformation. Again, the important features of this model are the direct participation of GBP in the translocation step and accumulation of substrate based on the energy dependent alteration of binding affinity.

However, several lines of evidence indicate that GBP does not, in fact operate as a membrane penetrating carrier. Most of this evidence is derived from the unidirectional transport activity associated with GBP. From the similarity of uptake specificity *in vivo* and the binding specificity of the galactose-binding protein *in vitro*, it is clear that the binding protein must be involved in the entry process. To determine whether the exit process is also mediated by the galactose-binding protein, we attempted to measure a K_m value for exit of galactose stimulated by glucose. Figure 14 shows the dependence of the rate of exit upon the inside concentration

[¹⁴C]galactose. The rate of exit does not reach saturation even at an internal concentration of 20 mM. Therefore, no K_m of exit can be measured, and it is very unlikely that the galactose-binding protein (estimated $K_{diss's}$ 0.1 μM and 10 μM) (Boos et al., 1972)

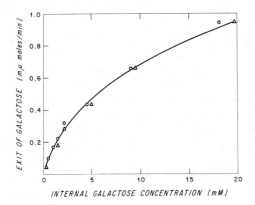

Fig. 14. The initial rate of galactose exit at different internal galactose concentrations. The cell suspension prepared for the transport assay was incubated with different [1-¹⁴C]galactose concentrations (from 10 nM to 0.1 mM) at 23°. After equilibrium state of accumulation had been reached, the cells were transferred to 15° for 2 min and unlabeled glucose, 1 mM final concentration, was added. Aliquots (0.5 ml) were filtered as fast as possible through Millipore filters (0.65 μ pore size). Each filtrate (0.2 ml) was counted in a scintillation counter. The rate of exit was calculated by interpolation of the first three time points. The results are given in nanomoles per min per 2.5 × 10⁸ cells. Δ----Δ, rate of exit with untreated cells; ○----○, rate of exit in the additional presence of 30 mM sodium azide. (PARNES and BOOS, 1973)

establishes the recognition site for exit on the inside of the cytoplasmic membrane. This conclusion is corroborated by measuring entry and exit in an *mgl* mutant, possessing a structurally defective galactose-binding protein (Boos, 1972). Under the standard transport assay conditions, this mutant exhibits only 6% of the initial rate of uptake in comparison to the wild type, while the rate of exit from preloaded cells is identical with that found in the wild type (PARNES and BOOS, 1973).

At present, it cannot be decided whether galactose exit is mediated by an entirely different transport system or by components of the MeGal transport system other than the galactose-binding protein. The former possibility has, indeed, been suggested by earlier studies on galactose transport in *E. coli* (Horecker et al., 1960), at a time when periplasmic binding proteins were not yet discovered. Also, the unilateral transmembranal stimulation of exit observed with the MeGal system (Parnes and Boos, 1973) indicates that the carrier for exit is different from that of entry: transmembranal stimulation (exchange diffusion) should be observed for both entry and exit on a carrier catalyzing both reactions (Heinz and Geck, 1972).

On the other hand, there is also evidence for the possibility that galactose exit is mediated by components of the MeGal system other than the galactose-binding protein:

1. Entry and exit are inhibited by *p*-hydroxymercuribenzoate in a time dependent reaction for which the half-time of inactivation is identical (Parnes and Boos, 1973). This would indicate that a common component exists for entry and exit, or possibly for the energy coupling of both fluxes.

2. Transmembranal stimulation of exit occurs only with substrates of the MeGal system, though not with all of them, and it is dependent on a functional galactose-binding protein.

Similar observations of unidirectional transport activity in a substrate-binding protein mediated transport system have been made by Halpern et al. (1973). From the asymmetric location of the galactose-binding protein in the periplasmic space of gram negative bacteria, one is tempted to predict an asymmetric transport activity for all substrate-binding protein mediated transport systems.

The Diffusion-Facilitator Hypothesis

Periplasmatic binding proteins are easily released from the cell surface by a mild osmotic shock. Therefore, it has been argued that these proteins could hardly be involved in a function intimately connected to the hydrophobic environment of the cytoplasmic membrane. And, indeed, thus far, attempts to demonstrate directly the interaction of radioactively labeled GBP with isolated membrane vesicles or even shocked cells have failed. Consequently, it has been proposed that periplasmic binding proteins might facilitate transport of exogenous substrate through the periplasmic space and deliver it to the "permease proper" located in the cytoplasmic membrane (OXENDER, 1972). This would be in analogy to the ability of the O_2 binding protein, hemoglobin, to drastically increase the rate of O_2 diffusion through an aqueous compartment (SCHOLANDER, 1960). In an attempt to demonstrate such a model for GBP,

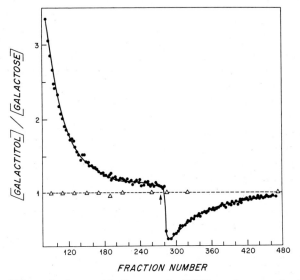

Fig. 15. Effect of galactose-binding protein (GBP) on the rate of galactose diffusion through a small aqueous compartment. GBP at a concentration of 2.6 mg/ml was placed in a $200\,\mu$l compartment between two dialysis membranes of 1.5 cm diameter. The reservoir above the upper membrane contained 5 ml of 10 mM $Tris$-HCl, pH 7.3, 0.1 mM [1-^{14}C]galactose and 0.1mM [6-^{3}H]galactitol. Buffer was pumped through the lower chamber at a flow rate of 0.144 ml/min. Five drop fractions were collected and counted. The arrow indicates the addition of 0.5 ml of 1 M glucose

we devised the following experimental setup: GBP at a concentration of 2.6 mg/ml (7.2×10^{-5} M) was placed into a small ($200\,\mu$l) compartment between two dialysis membranes of 1.5 cm diameter. Above the upper membrane, we placed 5 ml of a buffer solution containing 5×10^{-4}M galactitol and galactose labeled with different isotopes. While galactitol has the same molecular dimensions as galactose, only the latter is a substrate for GBP. We then followed the time dependent appearance of the two carbohydrates and their relative amounts. Figure 15 shows the ratio of galactitol over galactose as they passed through the compartment containing GBP. As can be seen initially, galactitol preferentially passes through until equilibrium is reached. At no time, even after equilibrium has been reached, is galactose facilitated in its diffusion through the GBP containing layer. However, when unlabeled glucose is added, which is an excellent substrate of GBP, the ratio of galactitol over galactose declines temporarily, presumably caused by an increase of free galactose in the GBP containing chamber. This demonstrates that the preferential retention of galactose at the beginning of the experiment is not an artifact and strongly indicates that GBP is not able to increase the rate of diffusion of galactose through the periplasmic space. In contrast, the concentration of free galactose in the periplasmic space is only *reduced* by the presence of GBP. This experiment thus clearly demonstrates that it is the galactose-GBP complex and not free galactose itself that must be recognized by the cytoplasmic membrane for its subsequent steps in transport or chemotaxis.

The Auxiliary or "K_m Factor" Hypothesis

Another proposal for the function of periplasmic substrate binding proteins was that of a "K_m factor". The transport system would operate continously, but addition of periplasmic binding protein would greatly increase the system's affinity for substrate (OXENDER, 1972; MINER and FRANK, 1974). This conclusion seemed to be corroborated by the finding that membrane vesicles of *E. coli* also exhibited transport activity for leucine-isoleucine-valine, histidine, glutamic acid and lysine (LOMBARDI and KABACK, 1972), amino acids for which binding proteins had been isolated (PENROSE et al., 1968; LEVER, 1972; ROSEN and VASINGTON, 1971; BARASH and HALPERN, 1971; ROSEN, 1973). Uptake of these amino acids occurs in membrane vesicles, even though the periplasmic binding proteins supposedly were removed during their preparation (KABACK, 1972). Yet for all of the above amino acids, more than one transport system has been reported in whole cells (AMES and LEVER, 1970; ROSEN, 1971; RAHMANIAN et al., 1973; HALPERN and EVEN-SHOSHEN, 1967), and one might argue that transport systems operating in membrane vesicles are unrelated to transport systems mediated by periplasmic binding proteins. Therefore, any argumentation for an auxiliary function of periplasmic binding proteins for membrane-bound systems has to be restricted to homogeneous systems. At the present time, this is true only for the uptake of glutamine (WEINER and HEPPEL, 1971), diaminopimelic acid *via* the cystine general system (BERGER and HEPPEL, 1972) and arginine *via* the arginine specific system (ROSEN, 1973). Indeed, no transport activity for these amino acids can be found in membrane vesicles (LOMBARDI and KABACK, 1972). Similar correlations can be made in regard to cells subjected to the cold osmotic shock treatment of NEU and HEPPEL (1965): amino acids whose uptake is not reduced upon the shock treatment such as proline, glycine or alanine (HEPPEL et al., 1972) are very well transported by membrane vesicles. No soluble periplasmic binding protein has been found for this class of amino acids. Other amino acids such as leucine-isoleucine-valine, glutamic acid and lysine, for which binding proteins have been isolated and which are still transported in membrane vesicles, show a partial reduction in the ability to be transported by shocked cells (HEPPEL et al., 1972). But in contrast, uptake in shocked cells is reduced more than 90% for glutamine (WEINER and HEPPEL, 1971), diaminopimelic acid (BERGER and HEPPEL, 1972) and arginine [via the arginine specific system (ROSEN, 1973),] paralleled by the finding that these amino acids are not taken up in membrane vesicles either.

These observations strongly suggest that the binding protein mediated transport of glutamine, diaminopimelic acid and arginine is entirely different and independent from the transport systems observed in membrane vesicles. It is highly likely that this is also true for other binding protein related systems, such as the MeGal system. Indeed, membrane vesicles of a *lac Y* strain which take up galactose do not transport MeGal (KERWAR et al., 1972), which in this mutant is only transported by the GBP mediated MeGal system.

From this consideration, it is clear that typical periplasmic binding proteins do not simply have the role of K_m factors for membrane bound transport systems, but are essential for translocation as well.

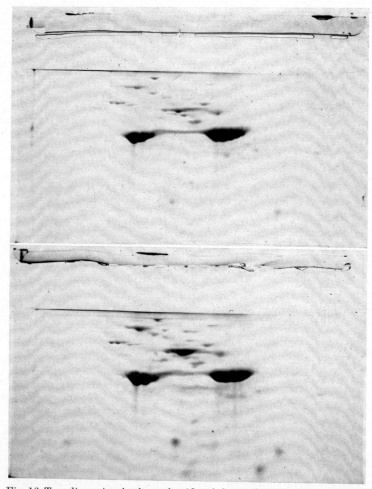

Fig. 16. Two-dimensional polyacrylamide gel electrophoresis of the membrane fraction of a D-fucose-induced (bottom) and an uninduced (top) culture of strain M188—777. 500 ml cultures were grown to stationary phase. The cells were collected by centrifugation and broken in a French pressure cell. The membrane fraction was isolated by centrifugation and was solubilized with 6 M guanidine thiocyanate. The solubilized fraction was dialyzed against 6 M urea, and then approximately 300 μg of protein was applied to the first dimension gel. The first dimension gel contained 6 M urea and was run at pH 8.5. This gel was then fused to a polyacrylamide slab gel and the second dimension was run in 0.2% sodium dodecyl sulfate. This first dimension

The Membrane-Bound Components of the MeGal Transport System

Numerous genetic studies with transport systems mediated by periplasmic substrate binding proteins have clearly established that these proteins are essential but not sufficient for a functional system, and that additional components are required. In the case of the MeGal transport system, it has recently been demonstrated by complementation studies that three adjacent genes, *mglA*, *B*, and *C* are required for an intact transport system where GBP is coded for by *mglB* (ORDAL and ADLER, 1974).

We have tried to identify the gene products of *mglA* and *C* by analyzing the membrane fraction of cells grown in the presence and absence of D-fucose as inducer with a two-dimensional polyacrylamide gel electrophoresis technique. Figure 16 shows the results of such an experiment. Induction of this strain causes a noticeable increase in two spots. These two membrane-bound proteins, which we have designated MTA α and γ (Membrane Transport Associated), have molecular weights of approximately 80 000 and 50 000 respectively under denaturing conditions. Although these results are encouraging they are only preliminary, and we are at present conducting similar experiments with isogenic transport mutants in order to provide more conclusive evidence for the relationship between MTA α and γ and the MeGal transport system.

In any event, the function of the *mglA* and *C* gene products in the MeGal transport system is not as yet clear. Besides trying to determine their possible binding activity for galactose, it may be more important in our view, to try to examine their postulated interaction with GBP or the GBP-galactose complex.

GBP-Membrane Interaction

It is clear from the results presented that GBP is a component of the MeGal transport system. Since GBP is not involved in exit through this system, it seems very likely that GBP is not the trans-

---

separates horizontally, the second separates vertically. The cathode is at the top and left, respectively. The two spots near the center of the gel above the heavy horizontal band of outer membrane proteins are clearly fucose inducible and have been designated MTA α and γ. (JOHNSEN et al., un-published)

locating protein, *i.e.*, the protein which is physically responsible for carrying the substrate through the cytoplasmic membrane. The complementation studies by ORDAL and ADLER (1974) indicate that there are two other structural genes in the presumed *mgl* operon which code for proteins of the MeGal transport systems. We have tentatively identified the respective gene products of *mglA* and *C*, MTA α and γ (see above p. 193). The genetic studies indicate that there are no other structural genes in this "operon" and therefore, MTA α and γ are likely candidates for the translocating or energy coupling proteins.

At the present time, the most interesting problem in the study of the MeGal transport system is how GBP could recognize these membrane bound components, MTA α and γ, and accomplish translocation. There are several properties of GBP which could conceivably be involved in the interaction with the membrane bound components MTA α and γ. The first of these is the alteration in surface charge of the protein which has been shown to accompany substrate binding. GBP becomes more negative when substrate is bound, and the previously mentioned fluorescence perturbation studies indicate that this alteration in charge occurs in a small defined region of the protein. Indeed, the transport negative mutant EH3039 contains a binding protein which does not show the alteration in surface charge upon substrate binding. Furthermore, GBP isolated from a transport positive revertant of this strain has regained this substrate dependent alteration in surface charge.

The second possibility is, of course, the conformational change itself. Unfortunately, this term has come to mean a wide variety of changes and it is commonly used to describe all kinds of interactions, especially those which are poorly understood. The conformational change which occurs in GBP is confined to the binding site region and does not appear to involve any major refolding of the peptide chain. So far, no indications other than the prediction by transport models give support to the idea that the observed conformational change is directly involved in recognition of GBP by the membrane or MTA α or γ.

A third possibility is based on the yet somewhat puzzling characteristic of GBP, the appearance of a second low affinity binding site (Site B in Fig. 11). This does not seem to be a feature common to other binding proteins. In fact, to the best of our knowledge, no other bacterial periplasmic binding protein has been found to exhibit more than one substrate binding site[1]. It is, therefore, difficult to imagine what essential function this second site could have. In search of an explanation for this second site, our interest in the GBP-MTA α,γ interaction lead us to suspect that this second site might not be a substrate site but rather a binding site for a membrane bound carbohydrate, possibly in the form of a glycoprotein. This might then imply that MTA α or γ, or both, are glycoproteins.

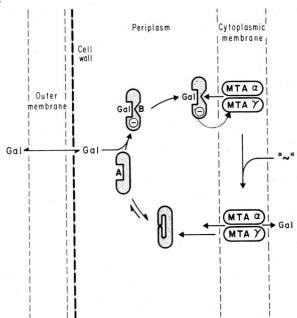

Fig. 17A and B. Model for the galactose-binding protein (GBP)-membrane interaction. The conformational states of GBP are as indicated in Fig. 11. The GBP-membrane interaction is seen to occur through binding of a carbohydrate portion of either MTA α or, γ or both (designated by a triangle) to low-affinity site of GBP (Site B). The energy input required for translocation is designated by "$\sim$". See text for details on these models

[1] Recently, a maltose binding protein from *E. coli* has been isolated and data indicate that it can exist in two states differing by their affinity to maltose [O. KELLERMANN and S. SZMELCMAN: Eur. J. Biochem. **47**, 139—149 (1974). The protein is also involved in maltose chemotaxis (HAZELBAUER, unpubl.)].

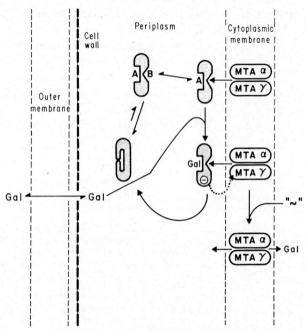

Fig. 17B. Legend see p. 195

Figure 17a indicates how one could illustrate the State I and II GBP equilibrium and the interaction with MTA α and γ might be integrated in the energy dependent uptake of substrate. Galactose diffuses through the outer membrane and the cell wall to the periplasm. Once here, it combines with the State II (see Fig. 11), removing this conformation from the pre-existing equilibrium and opening the low-affinity second site. When this site is available, binding to MTA α or γ occurs via the carbohydrate portion of these glycoproteins. Energy input then results in the reformation of State I GBP, translocation of galactose, and finally release of State I GBP into the periplasm ensues. Again, as galactose is removed from GBP by energy input (through MTA α or γ), GBP reverts to the State I conformation. As was previously mentioned, this conformation is characterized by a "closed" binding site. Since the tryptophan residue present in the binding site is not accessible to even deuterium oxide, it is very unlikely that this conformation binds galactose at all. This, then, could explain why GBP does not seem to be involved in substrate exit.

There is as yet no way to examine Site B without interference from Site A and because of this, it is not possible to tell in which GBP conformation Site B first appears. As a result, other models can be drawn; for example, Fig. 17 B. In this model, Site B is available before galactose binding. Therefore, GBP will exist loosely-bound to the cytoplasmic membrane in the absence of galactose, since binding at Site B will shift the State I − State II equilibrium. An additional change must now be proposed in order to signal galactose binding at Site A. A number of factors could serve as this signal, but we have chosen to represent this "trigger" for the trans-location event by the alteration in surface charge that accompanies galactose binding. The other events portrayed in this figure are similar to those of Fig. 17 A.

One of the predictions of this model would be that sugars which bind to Site B would inhibit transport. It has been shown that galactose binds to Site B. If Site B is not a substrate binding site but is rather the MTA α, γ site, then it follows that high galactose concentrations should inhibit the MeGal transport system. Figure 18 shows the results of a study conducted by Wu (1967). The galactose transport seen in the mgl mutant is most likely due to the galactose permease. The mgl^+ strain shows much higher transport activity than the mgl strain but only at low galactose concentrations. However, at galactose concentrations around 1 mM transport in the two strains is nearly identical, indicating that the MeGal system has become inoperative. At intermediate galactose concentrations of approximately 10 μM, transport in the mgl^+ strain is less than would normally be expected. This is especially interesting in view of the fact that the K_{diss} of galactose for Site B is about 10 μM. Similar results have also been obtained by Wilson (1974). He observed that the galactose transport in several K 12 strains did not fit a model in which galactose uptake is due to two independent trans-port systems, $i.e.$ the MeGal transport system and the galactose permease. Again, it was found that galactose uptake was less than expected at concentrations above 10 μM. These results are con-sistent with our model and are explainable by inhibition of the GBP-MTA α or γ interaction by substrate.

The phenomenon of galactose chemotaxis must also be mediated by a GBP-membrane interaction. The work of ORDAL and ADLER (1974) shows conclusively that other components besides GBP are required and, furthermore, they show that *mglA* and *C* (MTA α and γ) are not involved in this process. We would propose that the membrane-bound component of this chemotaxis system is also a glycoprotein. The GBP-glycoprotein interaction would be similar

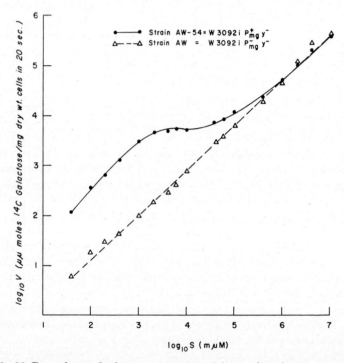

Fig. 18. Dependence of galactose transport activity on the substrate concentration in strain AW *(galK lacY mgl)* as compared with strain 54 *(galK lacY mgl+)*. Uninduced cells of strain AW and strain 54 were incubated at 20° C with differing concentration of [14C]galactose. Samples of 0.5 ml were taken at 20 sec after the addition of [14C]substrate for measurements of radioactivity. The abscissa represents the logarithm (log₁₀) of the galactose concentration in mμmoles/l (nM); the ordinate represents the logarithm of the galactose concentration in the cells in μμmoles (pmoles) [14C]galactose/mg dry wt of cells at 20 sec after the addition of [14C]galactose to cell suspensions. --●--●--, strain 54; --Δ--Δ--, strain AW. (WU, 1967)

to that shown in Fig. 17 A and B, except that here the interaction would influence flagella rotation (LARSEN et al., 1974) instead of substrate translocation. Again, our model would predict that carbohydrates which bind to Site B would inhibit chemotaxis as well as transport by preventing the GBP-membrane interaction. Indeed, the previously mentioned study by MESIBOV et al. (1973) clearly indicate that galactose chemotaxis is strongly inhibited at galactose concentrations around 1 mM. The aspartate system did not respond in the same way, the moderate inhibition seen above saturating concentrations of β-methylaspartate (10−100 mM) might well be explained by loss of polarity as well as mere physico-chemical non-biological effects. In contrast, striking inhibition of the galactose chemotaxis system is clearly expressed at 0.1−1 mM galactose concentrations. In this context it seems important to emphasize that inhibitors of the latter system need not be sub-strates of the MeGal transport system or the galactose chemo-receptor. ADLER et al. (1973) have examined the inhibitory effects of a number of sugars on galactose chemotaxis. They found tre-halose (at 10 mM) to be a powerful inhibitor, and they suggested that this inhibition was due to glucose production by the enzyme trehalase. This explanation is not entirely satisfactory because it was also found that trehalose did not inhibit glucose chemotaxis in a galactose chemoreceptor mutant.

Accordingly, we have examined the effects of trehalose on galac-tose transport via the MeGal transport system. At 10 mM, trehalose causes a 35−40% inhibition of galactose transport. However, there are complications; for example, if trehalose is incubated with cells for 5 min before the addition of (^{14}C)galactose, no inhibition can be detected. We believe that this is due to glucose production in the cytoplasm resulting in an increase in the available energy of the cells. Since this 5 min incubation does not lead to inhibition of the MeGal transport system, we feel that it is very unlikely that any glucose appears in the periplasm. Since trehalose does inhibit both transport and chemotaxis and since glucose does not appear to be involved in this effect, we believe that trehalose is causing inhibition by binding to Site B. To further support this claim, we have ex-amined the effect of trehalose on the fluorescence emission spectra of GBP. No increase is observed in the fluorescence emission upon the addition of 10 mM trehalose to GBP and, furthermore, this concentration of trehalose does not inhibit the galactose (at 0.1 mM) induced increase. These results indicate that trehalose inhibits both transport and chemotaxis without binding to Site A.

Conclusion

Both galactose chemotaxis and transport via the MeGal transport system have been shown to be mediated by GBP. In both instances, substrate recognition by GBP is the first step. Evidence that has been accumulated by several investigators makes it appear likely that the next step for both chemotaxis and transport involves a GBP-membrane interaction and, accordingly, we have examined the properties of GBP in order to obtain some clue as to how this interaction might occur.

GBP exists in solution as a monomer of 36000 molecular weight. Its amino acid composition is typical of any soluble protein except for the absence of cysteine, and it is remarkably stable to heat or to changes in pH. There are, however, three characteristic properties of the protein which occur upon substrate binding and which could conceivably be important for the GBP-membrane interaction:

1. Conformational change.

2. Alteration in surface charge.

3. Appearance of a second low-affinity galactose binding site.

The conformational change that occurs upon the binding of substrate has been studied in detail. The results of these studies show that this conformational change does not involve an extensive refolding of the polypeptide backbone and, furthermore, it does not lead to alteration in the exposure of surface chromophores. It seems rather to involve only small changes in the binding site region of the protein. The substrate dependent alteration in surface charge seems to be important for normal function, but it is probably not the major factor in the GBP-membrane interaction. This brings us to the second low-affinity binding site (Site B). Since its discovery, the second binding site has been a puzzle to us. No other bacterial binding protein is known to have more than one binding site, and so this does not seem to be a general feature of periplasmic binding proteins. Another feature of the MeGal transport system which has caused us some concern is the apparent inhibition caused by high substrate concentrations. These two observations lead us to suspect that the second site was not really a substrate binding site, but rather a recognition site for a membrane-bound glycoprotein. We have expanded this idea into a model which is shown in some detail in Fig. 17 A and B. The basic premise of this model is that the GBP-membrane interaction is mediated through Site B and that one of the other components of the MeGal transport or the galactose chemotaxis systems is a glycoprotein.

This model is consistent with the observation that high galactose concentrations inhibit the MeGal transport system (WU, 1967; WILSON, 1974). This inhibition is seen to occur by galactose binding to Site B, thus preventing the GBP-membrane interaction. In addition, the model makes several experimentally testable predictions. If Site B is really a glycoprotein-recognizing site, then one should be able to find other carbohydrates which would inhibit transport or chemotaxis without themselves being substrates of these respective systems. We have examined a variety of sugars with the hope of obtaining such an inhibitor. Unfortunately, our results are often unclear. The high-affinity site (Site A) binds galactose and glucose very tightly, and most likely Site B specific candidates contain one or the other as a possible contaminant. However, the disaccharide trehalose causes a marked inhibition of both transport and chemotaxis without any detectable binding to Site A. These results, although consistent with the model, will require further study in order to clarify the nature of trehalose inhibition.

As was previously mentioned, we have utilized a two-dimensional polyacrylamide gel electrophoresis technique in order to locate the remaining components of the MeGal transport system (Fig. 16). Our model would predict that at least one of the proteins (MTA α or γ) should be a glycoprotein. Experiments are currently in progress in which we hope to be able to label MTA α or γ, or both with [^{14}C]N-acetylglucosamine, or other radioactive carbohydrates contained in bacterial glycoproteins.

Even if this model proves to be correct, much remains to be done. The nature of the translocation event in transport and the mechanism of chemotaxis remain a virtual mystery. Efforts are currently directed towards isolating and characterizing the membrane bound components (MTA α and γ) of the MeGal transport system. We are hopeful that the study of these components will provide an answer to the third and final step in transport, the translocation step.

Acknowledgements

The research performed in this laboratory was supported by grants from the NIH (GM-18498), the USPHS (AM05507), the NSF (GB30785X), the American Cancer Society (BC-120) and the Milton Fund. T.J. SILHAVY was supported by a National Institutes of General Medical Siences Training Grant (GM-00451). W. Boos was a recipient of the Solomon A. Berson Research and Development Award of the American Diabetes Association. We would like to express our thanks to the following publishers for allowing us to reproduce many of the figures used in this text: The American Society of Biological Chemists, Inc., the American Chemical Society, and Academic Press Inc. (London) Ltd.

References

ADLER,J.: J. General Microbiol. (Great Brit.) **74**, 77—91 (1973).

ADLER,J., HAZELBAUER,G.L., DAHL,M.M.: J. Bacteriol. **115**, 824—847 (1973).

AMES,G.F., LEVER,J.E.: Proc. nat. Acad. Sci. (Wash.) **66**, 1096—1103 (1970).

ANANTHANARAYANAN,V.S., BIGELOW,C.C.: Biochemistry **8**, 3717—3728 (1969).

ANRAKU,Y.: J. biol. Chem. **243**, 3116—3135 (1968).

BARASH,H., HALPERN,Y.S.: Biochem. Biophys. Res. Commun. **45**, 681—688 (1971).

BERG,H.C., BROWN,D.A.: Nature (Lond.) New Biol. **239**, 500—504 (1972).

BERGER,E.A., HEPPEL,L.A.: J. biol. Chem. **247**, 7684—7694 (1972).

BERMAN,K., BOYER,P.D.: Biochemistry **11**, 4650—4657 (1972).

Boos,W.: Eur. J. Biochem. **10**, 66—73 (1969).

Boos,W.: J. biol. Chem. **247**, 5414—4324 (1972).

Boos,W.: Ann. Rev. Biochem. **43**, 123—146 (1974).

Boos,W., GORDON,A.S.: J. biol. Chem. **246**, 621—628 (1971).

Boos,W., GORDON,A.S., HALL,R.E., PRICE,H.D.: J. biol. Chem. **247**, 917—924 (1972).

Boos,W., SARVAS,M.O.: Europ. Biochem. **13**, 526—533 (1970).

CROWDER,III,A.L., BARKER,R., SWENSON,C.A.: Biochemistry **12**, 2078—2082 (1973).

DAHLQUIST,F.W., LOVELY,P., KOSHLAND,D.E.,JR.: Nature (Lond.) New Biol. **236**, 120—123 (1972).

GANESAN,A.K., ROTMAN,B.: J. Mol. Biol. **16**, 42—50 (1966).

HALPERN,Y.S., EVEN-SHOSHAN,A.: J. Bacteriol. **93**, 1009—1016 (1967).

HALPERN,Y.S., BARASH,H., DRUCK,K.: J. Bacteriol. **113**, 51—57 (1973).

HAYASHI,K., IMOTO,T., FUNATSU,M.: J. Biochem. (Tokyo) **54**, 381 (1963).

HAZELBAUER,G.L., ADLER,J.: Nature (Lond.) New Biol. **230**, 101—104 (1971).

HEINZ,E., GECK,P.: Biochim. biophys. Acta (Amst.) **255**, 442—461 (1972).

HEPPEL, L. A.: In: ROTHFIELD, L. I. (Ed.): Structure and function of biological membranes, pp. 224—247. New York: Academic Press 1971.
HEPPEL, L. A., ROSEN, B. P., FRIEDBERG, I., BERGER, E. A., WEINER, J. H.: In: WOESSNER, J. F., HUIJING, F. (Eds.): The molecular basis of biological transport, pp. 133—149. New York: Academic Press 1972.
HORECKER, B. L., THOMAS, J., MONOD, J.: J. biol. Chem. 235, 1586—1590 (1960).
HERSKOVITS, T. T., LASKOWSKI, M., JR.: J. biol. Chem. 235, PC56 (1960).
HERSKOVITS, T. T., LASKOWSKI, M., JR.: J. biol. Chem. 237, 2481—2492 (1962).
HERSKOVITS, T. T., SORENSEN, M.: Biochemistry 7, 2523—2532 (1968).
IWASHIMA, A., MATSUURA, A., NOSE, Y.: J. Bacteriol. 108, 1419—1421 (1971).
KABACK, H. R., BARNES, E. M., JR.: J. biol. Chem. 246, 5523—5531 (1971).
KABACK, H. R.: Biochim. biophys. Acta (Amst.) 265, 367—416 (1972).
KALCKAR, H. M.: Science 174, 557—565 (1971).
KENNEDY, E. P.: In: BECKWITH, J. R., ZIPSER, D. (Eds.): The lactose operon, pp. 49—92. Cold Spr. Harb. Laboratory 1970.
KEPES, A.: J. Membrane Biol. 4, 87—112 (1971).
KEPES, A., RICHARME, G.: Fed. Europ. Biochem. Soc. Proc. 28, 327—339 (1972).
KERWAR, G. K., GORDON, A. S., KABACK, H. R.: J. biol. Chem. 247, 291—297 (1972).
KUZUYA, H., BROMWELL, K., GUROFF, G.: J. biol. Chem. 246, 6371—6380 (1971).
LAIKEN, S. L., GROSS, C. A., VON HIPPEL, P. H.: J. molec. Biol. 66, 143—155 (1972).
LANGRIDGE, R., SHINAGAWA, H., PARDEE, A. B.: Science 169, 59—61 (1970).
LARSEN, S. H., READER, R. W., KORT, E. N., TSO, W.-W., ADLER, J.: Nature (Lond.) 249, 74—77 (1974).
LEHRER, S. S.: Biochem. Biophys. Res. Commun. 29, 767—772 (1967).
LEHRER, S. S.: Biochemistry 10, 3254—3263 (1971).
LENGELER, J., HERMANN, K. O., UNSÖLD, H. J., BOOS, W.: Europ. J. Biochem. 19, 457—470 (1971).
LEVER, J. E.: J. biol. Chem. 247, 4317—4326 (1972).
LOMBARDI, F. J., KABACK, H. R.: J. biol. Chem. 247, 7844—7857 (1972).
MACNAB, R. M., KOSHLAND, D. E.: Proc. nat. Acad. Sci. (Wash.) 69, 2509—2512 (1972).
MCGOWAN, E., SILHAVY, T., BOOS, W.: Biochemistry 13, 993—999 (1974).
MEDVECZKY, N., ROSENBERG, H.: Biochim. biophys. Acta (Wash.) 211, 158—168 (1970).
MESIBOV, R., ADLER, J.: J. Bacteriol. 112, 315—326 (1972).
MESIBOV, R., ORDAL, G. W., ADLER, J.: J. gen. Physiol. 62, 293—215 (1973).
MINER, K. M., FRANK, L.: J. Bacteriol. 117, 1093—1098 (1974).
MITCHELL, P.: In: GOODWIN, T. W., LINDBERG, O. (Eds.): Biological structure and function, Vol. II, pp. 581—603. New York: Academic Press 1961.
MITCHELL, P.: Symp. Soc. Gen. Microbiol. 20, 121—166 (1970).
NEU, H. C., HEPPEL, L. A.: J. biol. Chem. 240, 3685—3692 (1965).
ORDAL, G. W., ADLER, J.: J. Bacteriol. 117, 509—526 (1974).

OXENDER, D. L.: Ann. Rev. Biochem. **41**, 777—814 (1972).

PARDEE, A. B.: In: Bolis, L., KATCHALSKY, A., KEYNES, R. D., LOEWENSTEIN, W. R., PETHICA, B. A. (Eds.): Permeability and function of biological membranes, pp. 86—93. Amsterdam: North-Holland Publishing Co. 1970.

PARNES, J. R., BOOS, W.: J. biol. Chem. **248**, 4436—4445 (1973).

PARSON, R. G., HOGG, R. W.: J. Biol. Chem. **249**, 3608—3614 (1974).

PENROSE, W. R., NICHOALDS, G. E., PIPERNO, J. R., OXENDER, D. L.: J. biol. Chem. **243**, 5921—5928 (1968).

PENROSE, W. R., ZAND, R., OXENDER, D. L.: J. biol. Chem. **245**, 1432—1437 (1970).

PFEFFER, W.: Untersuch. Botan. Inst. Tübingen **1**, 363 (1884).

RAHMANIAN, M., CLAUS, D. R., OXENDER, D. L.: J. Bacteriol. **116**, 1258—1266 (1973).

ROSEN, B. P.: J. biol. Chem. **246**, 3653—3662 (1971).

ROSEN, B. P.: J. biol. Chem. **248**, 1211—1218 (1973).

ROSEN, B. P., VASINGTON, F. D.: J. Biol. Chem. **246**, 5351—5360 (1971).

ROTMAN, B., ELLIS, J. H.: J. Bacteriol. **111**, 791—796 (1972), Am. Society for Microbiology.

ROTMAN, B., GANESAN, A. K., GUZMAN, R.: J. Mol. Biol. **36**, 247—260 (1968).

SCATCHARD, G.: Ann. N. Y. Acad. Sci. **51**, 660—672 (1949).

SCHOLANDER, P. F.: Science **131**, 585—590 (1960).

UDENFRIEND, S.: Fluorescence assay in biology and medicine. New York: Academic Press 1962.

WEINER, J. H., HEPPEL, L. A.: J. biol. Chem. **246**, 6933—6941 (1971).

WILSON, D. B.: J. biol. Chem. **249**, 553—558 (1974).

WILSON, O. H., HOLDEN, J. T.: J. biol. Chem. **244**, 2743—2749 (1969).

WONG, P. T. S., MACLENNAN, D. H.: Can. J. Biochem. **51**, 538—549 (1973).

WU, H. C. P.: J. molec. Biol. **24**, 213—223 (1967).

Discussion

K.-E. KAISSLING (Seewiesen): We have seen the complicated wall structure of the bacterium. Has it been investigated in which part of the wall, in which layer, these proteins are bound?

H. M. KALCKAR: Well, actually, PARDEE has already worried about the topography of the sulfate binding protein. Is it really floating around in the space or is it bound on the outside of the inner membrane? SHEN and BOOS [Proc. nat. Acad. Sci. (Wash.) **70**, 1481—1485 (1973)] did an interesting study on a mutant which has a temperature-sensitive division mechanism, so that at 41 °C it grows to very long "snakes", and studies on this mutant indicate that the galactose binding protein (GBP) may be synthesized around the septum: If there is no septum formed, no renewal of this protein is detectable. The binding protein has a rather long half-life, hence there seems to be a marked decrease in the *de novo* synthesis in the absence of cell division. Also, the concentration of GBP in this space has to be high, in the order of magnitude of 10^{-3} to 10^{-2} M to bring about this highly effective transport. I may also remind you that ORDAL and ADLER [J. Bacteriol.

117, 509—526 (1974)] find three genes involved in this high affinity galactose transport, A, B, and C; B programmes GBP, the galactose receptor protein. Genes A and C programme certain membrane proteins involved in translocation of galactose. As mentioned, the membrane proteins for translocation of galactose ("MTA α" and "MTA γ") may be spotted by techniques being tried in our laboratory (in "Abteilung Boos".)

K.-E. KAISSLING: Is it known whether the activity of this receptor protein is high near the base of the flagella, or whether it is distributed all around the bacterium?

H. M. KALCKAR: I mentioned that its biosynthesis does depend on cell division and that the GBP concentration at the end of a cell division may be higher around the septum. In the study by ORDAL and ADLER to which I referred, they invoke the existence of a specific membrane protein which they call a "signaller" which is supposed to transmit conformational changes from GBP to the flagella system. GBP is the only protein common for galactose transport as well as for galactose chemotaxis. The membrane proteins are different for the two functions.

G. HARTMANN (München): The electrophoretic mobility of galactose binding protein is changed by binding the neutral molecule of galactose Are there other examples for this phenomenon?

H. M. KALCKAR: I think DAN KOSHLAND could give us some good examples.

D. E. KOSHLAND, JR. (Berkeley): I think there are now a number of examples. Dr. HOLZER just mentioned oxygen hemoglobin; this is one, and in electrofocussing apparatus you can now find neutral substances like glucose that will change the pH of a group nearby. And, actually, you can see it easily.

H. M. KALCKAR: Oxygen hemoglobin is a good example. In regard to this parable, permit me to remind you of some striking kinetic differences. The galactose binding protein is very disinclined to catalyze any exchange unless it is fully saturated. And this may explain why the high affinity galactose transport system (unlike the lactose system) does not show any specific exit.

α-Glucosidases as Sugar Receptor Proteins in Flies

KAI HANSEN

*Fachbereich Biologie der Universität, 84 Regensburg,
Federal Republic of Germany*

With 7 Figures

Insects are capable of discriminating between water and sugar solutions. The responsible sensory organs, the taste hairs, densely populate the surface of their legs (Fig. 2) and mouthparts, and are characterized by the following properties:

1. The taste hairs always show a simple morphological construction; the whole sense organ consists of only eight cells, five primary bipolar receptor cells and three sheath cells (Section 1).

2. Each receptor cell is sensitive to one class of substances only. So one cell is specifically stimulated by carbohydrates, while others react to salts and water (Section 3).

3. The activity of the sugar receptor cell in hungry flies is strongly coupled with a feeding response (Section 2).

In contrast to taste hairs, the taste buds of the vertebrate tongue consist of 30—80 secondary receptor cells. Each cell reacts to several substances of different classes. Furthermore, a direct electrophysiological recording of the spike activity of a single receptor cell as it can be done in taste hairs (Section 3) is not possible with the cells of the taste bud.

Due to their more simple organization and properties as well as their accessibility to several technical methods, the taste hairs of insects seem to be a more favorable object for studying basic sensory processes than the corresponding vertebrate organs. A similar situation is met in the physiology of olfaction, where SCHNEIDER and coworker emphasized the advantages of the insect olfactory hairs (SCHNEIDER and HECKER, 1956; SCHNEIDER, 1971; KAISSLING, 1971 and this issue p. 243).

This paper reviews new biochemical attempts to identify and to characterize the receptor protein of the fly's sugar receptor cell. In 1969 Hansen presented the hypothesis that this receptor protein should possess enzymatic properties and might be identical with an α-glucosidase found in taste hair-rich segments. New biochemical evidence in favor of this hypothesis is discussed in relation to electrophysiological and behavioral studies on sugar reception.

The sugar receptor proteins of insects and vertebrates have no features in common. The literature concerning the latter proteins is summarized in the papers of Price (1974), Dastoli (1974), and of Hiji and Sato (1972, 1973).

1. Organization and General Physiology of Taste Hairs

The structural organization of a taste hair is shown schematically in Fig. 1 A and explained in the legend.

How does the taste hair work ? The wet hair tip continuously takes very small samples of soluble material out of the environment. These molecules diffuse through the fluid-filled pore (Fig. 3) at the hair tip to the distal ends of the dendrites (Fig. 1 B). Each dendrite contains as part of the membrane its specific receptor protein. In the case of a stimulating sugar, reversible complexes are formed between the receptor protein molecule and the sugar in a ratio of 1:1, as may be assumed for a simple case. It has yet to be shown how the complexes effect an opening of the ion channels and thus give rise to a decrease of membrane permeability. The membrane area involved in the primary process is in the range of one μm^2. Due to the resistance change a receptor current through the dendrite results that controls the firing rate of the spike generator. The spike generating membrane being localized in the proximal region of the receptor cell body is separated from the site of the primary process by a distance of about $50-450\,\mu m$. The voltage source for this current seems to be the system of folded membranes of the outer sheath cells (Thurm, 1970, and this issue p. 367). This circuit is completed by Canal II as low resistance path with the hair tip. The lymph cavity I is assumed to deliver the ionic milieu of Canal I surrounding the distal parts of the dendrites.

The different receptor cells of one hair accepting either salts or sugars operate according to the same reaction sequence (Fig. 1 C).

However, each cell has its own type of receptor protein. Furthermore the spike frequencies of the different receptor cells trigger antagonistic behavioral responses; in the case of sugar receptor

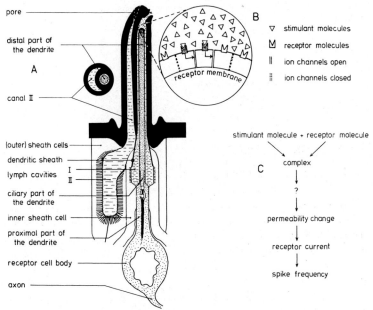

Fig. 1. (A) Schematic organization of an insect taste hair. For reasons of clarity only one receptor cell is shown instead of five; the outlines of the sheath cells are only partly shown. The receptor cell parts are: the axon connected to the central nervous system, the cell body with the nucleus and the dendrite. The latter is divided into a proximal, a ciliary and a distal part. The distal part is a modified cilium and contains microtubules as the only cytoplasmatic structure. In the largest labellar taste hairs, its real length is about 400 μm, and its diameter is about 0.3 μm. It first passes through the tubelike dendritic sheath, then through Canal I of the hair shaft and reaches the pore at the hair tip. The Canal II of the hairshaft seems to be connected to the outside of the hair by tiny pores (GAFFAL, unpublished). The receptor cells are surrounded concentrically by three sheath cells. The space between the inner sheath cell and the dendrites gives rise to lymph Cavity I, and the space between the two outer and the inner sheath cells forms lymph Cavity II. No connection exists between Cavity I and II. Cavity II is distinguished by a well developed system of folded membranes (modified from HANSEN and HEUMANN, 1971). (B) Schematic representation of the primary process at the molecular level (see text). (C) Sequence of processes in the receptor cell (see text)

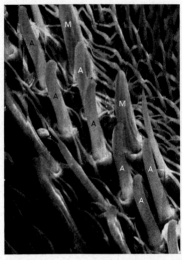

Fig. 2. Scanning electron micrograph of the lower side of the 3rd tarsomere of a fly's foreleg. A: taste hairs of the A-type; on the right side of each hair tip the wall surrounding the pore is seen as a small projection. The length of the hair shaft is about 40 μm, its diameter at the base about 3.5 μm. M: mechanoreceptive hairs

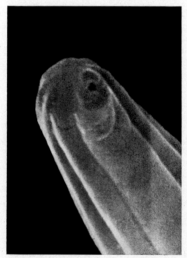

Fig. 3. The hair tip of an A-hair showing the pore of 0.1 μm in diameter

activity, a feeding response — extention of the proboscis —, in the case of salt receptor activity an avoidance response — retraction of the proboscis. Thus the feeding response of the fly supplies specific information about interferences between sugar molecules and the sugar receptor protein.

2. Behavioral Threshold Pattern as Properties of the Receptor Proteins

According to the statement in Section 1, the feeding response to a certain sugar reflects the formation of a complex between sugar and receptor protein. Thus we can test various sugars and qualitatively ensure whether or not they form complexes. Furthermore we can determine semiquantitatively the behavioral thresholds by testing which minimal concentration of a sugar is necessary for a reaction. This informs us that one sugar is bound better than another one, and indirectly that the dissociation constant of the complex is small for a low threshold value, but large for a higher one. In a similar way all investigations of the relation between molecular structure and stimulating effectiveness reflect the structural demands of the receptor protein to the sugar.

Since determinations of the behavioral thresholds are easy to undertake, much more information could be obtained, in this manner than by the electrophysiological method. The most favored objects are flies (Haslinger, 1935; Hassett, Dethier, and Gans, 1950; Dethier, 1955; Evans, 1963; Salama, 1966; Pflumm, 1971a, 1972; Jakinovich et al., 1971), but also other insects have been investigated (e.g. the honey bee, v. Frisch, 1935; ants, Schmidt, 1938; butterflies, Weiss, 1930). Altogether about 170 carbohydrates have been tested. For the concept of this paper, those sugars were selected (see Table 1, Columns 1—3) for which the threshold values are of special interest. These sugars belong to the class of the di- and trisaccharides, methyl- and nitrophenylglycosides. For comparative purposes the monosaccharides representing the glycosidic components of the others are also included (Nos. 21 to 25).

Comparing the threshold values, the following conclusions can be drawn (for details see Evans, 1963; Pflumm, 1971; Jakinovich et al., 1971; Shimada et al., 1974):

Table 1. Threshold values and electrophysiological data of dipteran sugar receptors and substrate pattern of the tarsal glucosidase activities for various sugars

| | | | Behavioral thresholds millimolar conc. | | | Electrophysiological data | | | | Hydrolysis |
| | | | Phormia | | Aedes | Sarcophaga | Boettcherisca | | | Phormia |
			1	2	3	4 f_{max}	5 K_b	6 f_{max}	7 n_H	8
1	Sucrose	Glc α1-2 β Fruf	10	10	23	1.43	60	=1.00	1	+
2	Turanose	Glc α1-3 Frup	11	10	58					+
3	Palatinose	Glc α1-6 Fru		10						+
4	Maltose	Glc α1-4 Glc	4	10	51					+
5	Cellobiose	Glc β1-4 Glc	5000[a]	100- 500						—
6	Lactose	Gal β1-4 Glc	—		1000[a]					—
7	Gentiobiose	Glc β1-6 Glc		1000-3000						—
8	Trehalose	Glc α1-1 Glc	133	100- 200						(+)
9	Melibiose	Gal α1-6 Glc		1000-3000	1100					—
10	Raffinose	Gal α1-6 Glc α1-2 β Fruf	200	100- 200	445					—
11	Melezitose	Glc α1-3 Fruf β2-1 α Glc	64	20	113					+
12	Methyl-α-glucopyranoside		69	25	213	1.1	73	0.71	1.11	—
13	Methyl-β-glucopyranoside			100- 200	771	0.5	280	0.27	2	—
14	Methyl-β-fructofuranoside				—	—				
15	Methyl-α-mannopyranoside			—						
16	Methyl-α-galactopyranoside					—				
17	Methyl-α-xylopyranoside					0.5				
18	4-Nitrophenyl-α-glucopyranoside		1				1,9	0.21	1.0	+
19	4-Nitrophenyl-β-glucopyranoside		200- 500							—
20	4-Nitrophenyl-α-mannopyranoside		1000							—

No.	Sugar	1	2	3	4	5	6	7
21	α/β-Glucose, equilibrium mixture	132	50 - 100	108	= 1.0			
	α-Glucose (Glc-)				1.11	150	0.74	
	β-Glucose				1.73	150	0.66	
22	Galactose (Gal-)	500	100 - 200	916				
23	Mannose (Man-)	7600[a]	1000	1000				
24	Xylose (Xyl-)	440	1000	294				
25	Fructose (Fru-)	6	20	20	0.77			

Behind the trivial names of the di- and trisaccharides, the monosaccharide components (for explanation see the symbols behind the monosaccharides 21—25) and the types of linkage are denoted. All sugars belong to the D-series.

Column 1: The tarsal threshold values of *Phormia regina* (HASSETT et al. 1950; DETHIER, 1955). "Threshold" represents that concentration of the test sugar, to which 50% of a population of hungry flies respond, calculated by the Probit Plot. Values marked by [a] are extrapolated from the plot.

Column 2: The tarsal threshold values of *Phormia terraenovae* (PFLUMM, 1971, 1972). In his paper, PFLUMM gives relative threshold values determined with single flies in many trials; the sucrose threshold was set to unity, the thresholds of the other sugars is expressed as a factor < 1 for the less and > 1 for the more effective sugars; for better comparison the unity value of sucrose is given a value equal to 10 mM; e.g. 100 mM in this table corresponds to a relative effectiveness of 0.1 in the original paper.

Column 3: Threshold values of the proboscidal taste receptors of the mosquito *Aedes aegypti* (SALAMA, 1966) determined by the method of HASSETT et al. (1950).

In the Columns 1—3 the Symbol (—) indicates that the sugar is not effective, even at high concentrations.

Column 4: Electrophysiologically determined maximal spike frequencies (f_{max}) of the labellar sugar receptor of the fly *Sarcophaga bullata*, relative to the f_{max} (glucose) set to unity (JAKINOVICH et al., 1971).

Columns 5—7: Parameter of the response concentration curves of the largest labellar taste hairs (terminology after WILCZEK, 1967) of the fly *Boettcherisca* (MORITA and SHIRAISHI, 1968; HANAMORI et al., 1972). K_b: The inflection point of the curve defines the sugar concentration at which the half maximal response is obtained. Additionally, AMAKAWA and MORITA (cited by AMAKAWA et al., 1972) give a K_b value of 67 mM for the labellar taste hairs of *Phormia regina* with sucrose as stimulant; SHIRAISHI (cited by MORITA, 1972) reports a K_b value of 120 mM for the marginal hairs of *Boettcherisca* stimulated with sucrose; the curve he got shows a greater steepness than usually found. f_{max}: relative maximal response to high sugar concentrations (4-nitrophenyl-α-glucoside 20 mM, all other sugars 2 M, the maximal rseponse to sucrose is set to unity. n_H: Hill coefficient.

Column 6: The Symbol (+) indicates that the sugar is split by crude extracts of tarsi, the Symbol (—) that no splitting occurs (HANSEN, 1969).

1. Influence of the Type of Linkage. Comparing maltose (4) with cellobiose (5), methyl-α-(12) with -β-glucoside (13) and nitrophenyl-α- (18) with -β-glucoside (19) it is evident that the α-glucosides are more stimulating than the corresponding β-compounds. The α-glucosides have lower thresholds than glucose (21) itself. α- and β-glucose exhibit the same threshold in behavioral tests (Evans, 1963), but differ in the concentration response curves (see Columns 6 and 7, Section 3).

2. Modification of the Glycosidic Component. Substitution at the glycosidic glucose moiety often leads to a diminuition or a complete loss of the stimulating effectiveness, e. g. the inversion of the equatorial hydroxyl group into an axial one at C-4 [melibiose (9), methyl-α-galactoside (16), see Column 4] or at C-2 [methyl-α-mannoside (20)]. On the other hand, substitution at C-6 or its elimination can be tolerated, as may be seen in the cases of raffinose (10), a sucrose substituted at C-6 by a galactoside, and the methyl-α-xyloside (17, see Column 4).

3. Classification of the Effective α-Glucosides. a) In disaccharides, the nature of the non-glycosidic sugar influences the threshold only slightly: For the fructofuranose (sucrose, 1), the fructopyranose (turanose, 2) or the glucopyranose (maltose, 4), the threshold values lie in the same order of magnitude, no matter how the sugar is structured.

b) The non-glycosidic sugars may be linked by different C-atoms to the glucose. In the case of fructose, the linkage at C-2 (sucrose), C-3 (turanose, 2) or C-6 (palatinose, 3) makes no essential difference to the threshold value. For glucose the binding at C-4 (maltose) results in a slightly more effective disaccharide than at C-6 (isomaltose). This could be shown for the sugar receptor of the cotton stainer *Dysdercus* (Bresch, 1973) and it may be valid in flies too, but is seen only in the case of β-linked sugars cellobiose (5) and gentiobiose (7). Trehalose (8) with its more stable C-1 linkage shows an elevated threshold concentration.

c) Sucrose seems to be accepted as an α-glucoside, because methyl-β-fructofuranoside is not stimulating in contrast to methyl-α-glucoside. Hassett et al. (1950) emphasized that this threshold pattern parallels the sugar specificity of α-glucosidases. These authors compared the thresholds with the nutritive value of the same sugars, and stated that all those disaccharides were perceived at low thresholds that could also be split by intestinal α-glucosidases. Further examples for this relation are known. Aside from the α- and β-anomers of methyl-glucoside, methyl-α-xyloside (17) is the only methyl glycoside accepted, whereas both glucose and xylose are competitive inhibitors of glucosidases (HANSEN, 1968). Moreover, p-nitrophenyl glycosides always show smaller dissociation constants than corresponding disaccharides [e.g. glucosidases of yeasts (HALVORSON and ELIAS, 1958), β-galactosidase of E. coli (WALLENFELS, 1972]). Trehalose is an exception in both systems; it exhibits a higher threshold than all other α-glucosides and is generally not split by α-glucosidases.

3. Electrophysiological Data of the Sugar Receptor

In 1932 MINNICH observed in behavioral tests that flies can distinguish sugar solutions from pure water or salt solutions with their tarsal taste hairs. Only since the development of electrophysiological recording techniques about 1955 it became clear that contact-chemoreceptor cells of insects specifically respond only to one class of chemically related substances, e.g. carbohydrates (HODGSON et al., 1955; HODGSON, 1965; WOLBARSHT, 1965; MORITA, 1969; SCHNEIDER, 1971).

The technical arrangement utilizes a glass microelectrode with a cut tip and filled with the test solution. This electrode is put over the hair tip and so functions simultaneously as recording electrode as well as stimulating device. The several receptor cells of a taste hair are discernable by their different spike amplitudes. In a more elaborated technique, MORITA pierced the hair wall on the side of Canal II (Fig. 3) near the tip with a needle, replaced the needle with a saline-filled recording electrode and used a second glass capillary for stimulation.

MORITA and SHIRAISHI (1968) and HANAMORI et al. (1972) recorded responses from the same hair to a sequence of stimulating solutions of different concentrations. Thus they succeeded in determining the exact concentration dependency of the response. The curves obtained (Fig. 4, characteristic data in Table 1, Columns 5 to 7) reveal several essential aspects:

1. The curves for sucrose, 4-nitrophenyl-α-glucoside, methyl-α-glucoside and α-glucose as well as for maltose and ethyl-α-glucoside, both not shown in Fig. 4, can be described by a formalism

identical with that of the Michaelis-Menten equation. The K_b and the maximal response vary independently. The curves are completely characterized by these two values.

2. The maximal responses are different, as was also shown for the sugar receptor of *Sarcophaga* (Jakinovich et al., 1971, Table 1,

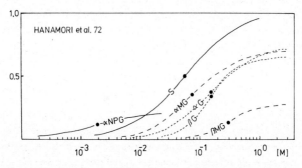

Fig. 4. Concentration dependency of the relative response of the sugar receptor for different sugars (largest labellar hairs of the fly *Boettcherisca*). The response is equal to the number of spikes during a period from 0.15 to 0.35 sec after the beginning of the stimulus. The maximal response for sucrose is set to unity. The maximal responses were determined at 2 M sugar concentrations except for 4-nitrophenyl-α-glucoside, which was tested at the concentration of 20 mM because of its low solubility. The K_b-values are marked by black points, they correspond to the sugar concentrations that give half maximal responses. Abbreviations: α-G:α-D-glucopyranose; β-G:β-D-glucopyranose, αMG:methyl-α-D-glucopyranoside, βMG:methyl-β-D-glucopyranoside, α-NPG:4-nitrophenyl-α-D-glucopyranoside, S:sucrose. (Modified after Hanamori et al., 1972)

Column 4). Therefore the maximal responses do not reflect the electrical properties of the membrane, but characteristic properties of the receptor protein.

3. As Morita (1969) and Kaissling (1971) evaluated theoretically for the special case of taste hair dendrites, the true dissociation curves of the receptor protein-sugar-complexes have the same shape as the curves shown here, but are shifted towards the higher concentrations. Consequently the constants of isolated receptor proteins must be greater or equal, but not smaller than the K_b-values.

4. Methyl-α-glucoside shows a smaller K_b than methyl-β-glucoside, generally expected for α-glucosides from the behavioral data. Additionally, methyl-β-glucoside as well as β-glucose exhibit curves with steeper slopes at the K_b. These curves do not fit the Michaelis-Menten equation. Correspondently, the Hill coefficients lying near unity for α-glucosides deviate towards higher values for β-glucosides. This fact, well known from allosteric enzymes, indicates that cooperative effects exist between at least two sites. Similar curves with Hill coefficients >1 are for 1-naphthyl-β-glucoside at the glycoside receptor of a caterpillar (WIECZOREK, 1974), for turanose and sorbose at the sugar receptor of the cotton stainer *Dysdercus* (Hemiptera) (BRESCH, 1973) and at the electroplax membrane for carbamylcholine and its antagonists (CHANGEUX and PODLESKI, 1968).

5. The sucrose curve of Fig. 4 is idealized according to the Michaelis-Menten equation. In reality, MORITA and SHIRAISHI (1968) observed a slight deviation towards higher response in the range between 3 and 30 mM. This deviation is not obtained with maltose. MORITA (1971) suggests that two receptor proteins may exist having two K_b values, one smaller and the other greater than 60 mM. The latter would coincide with the K_b value of the receptors of the marginal hairs. Similar effects are known when sinigrine is used to stimulate the above mentioned glycoside receptor (WIECZOREK, 1974), and from the binding curves of the isolated acetylcholine receptor (RAFTERY, this issue p. 541) and from curves of the galactose binding protein of *E. coli* (BOOS, 1972; SILHAVY, BOOS, and KALCKAR, this issue p. 165).

6. By comparing the behavioral thresholds of Table 1 with the receptor response obtained at the same concentration, it becomes clear that the behavioral thresholds are nearly identical with those of the receptors in hungry flies (thereby it is presumed that the labellar sugar receptors of *Phormia* are consistent with those of *Boettcherisca*). Due to the different maximal responses and to the different shapes of curves, the proportions of behavioral thresholds give only rough information as to the proportion of the K_b and K_{diss} values, resp. Furthermore, the behavioral thresholds usually obtained from many hairs of different types reflect only the receptor with the smallest K_b value.

4. The Glucosidase Activities in Crude Extracts of Taste Hair-Bearing Leg Segments: Their Distribution and Properties

All investigations on the relation between taste hairs and glucosidase were initiated by Dethier's (1955a) observation that the legs of the blowfly *Phormia* contain an enzymatic activity capable of hydrolyzing disaccharides. It was surprising that Dethier did not discuss the functional meaning of this activity, although in the same year, reviewing the physiology of contact chemoreceptors, he indicated the significance of the α-glucosidic linkage of disaccarides in stimulating the tarsal taste hairs. Wiesmann (1960), studying the house fly *Musca*, confirmed the existence of those enzyme activities in homogenates of tarsi and wrote; "it could not be excluded that these enzymes might be involved in the sensing of sugars by the tarsal sense organs".

Investigations by Hansen (1963, 1967—1969) on the legs and proboscis of *Phormia* revealed the following correlations between (1) the distribution of the glucosidase activity and the taste hairs and (2) between the properties of the enzyme(s) and the sugar receptor(s).

1a) The tarsi of the first leg contain three times more activity (mU/mg protein, sucrose as substrate) than the tibia and eight times more than the femora. The tarsi have 25 times more taste hairs [per mg protein] than the tibiae, whilst the femora are without any taste hairs [the taste hairs were counted by Grabowski and Dethier (1954)]. Thus high activities are always correlated to high densities of taste hairs, even though constant quotients of activity to the number of taste hairs were not obtained. The activity of the femur was thought to be of muscular origin, as has been described by Sacktor (1955) and van Handel (1968).

(1b) The taste hairs of the tarsomeres 2—5 are numerically divided between the lower and upper halves 85 and 15% respectively; similarly, 75—85% of the absolute glucosidase activity is found in the upper halves, but only 15—25% in the lower halves.

(1c) The distal parts of the fly's proboscis, the labella, show four times higher activities (mU/mg dry weight) than more proximally lying parts.

Further investigations revealed the existence of analogous activity gradients in various insects and in one spider (Hansen, 1968). In the bugs

Picromerus and *Rhaphigaster* [Hemiptera], the tarsi have 7—10 times higher activities than tibia. The presence of taste hairs in these bugs has been described, but the distribution and number of the hairs are not known.

In the spider *Araneus sclopetarius*, the tarsi of the 1st and 2nd leg contain 10 times higher activities than metatarsi, whilst tibiae, patellae and femora show no or only a slight activity. If the situation of *Aranea diadematus* is considered for comparison, rather good correspondence exists between the activity pattern and the distribution of the chemosensitive hairs (FOELIX, 1970). High numbers of hairs are found in the distal and low ones in the proximal segments of the leg. Activity gradients analogous to that of *Phormia* are further found in *Eristalis* (Dipt.), *Vanessa jo* (2nd and 3rd leg, Lepidopt.) and *Stenobothrys bicolor* (Orthopt.).

The legs of cockroaches possess no tarsal taste hairs; the glucosidase activity they contain is accordingly not distributed in a gradient pattern.

(2a) As shown in Column 8 of Table 1, the tarsal extracts of *Phormia* only split di- and trisaccharides or glucosides, that contain D-glucose as glycosidic component in an α-glycosidic linkage. This is a typical feature of all α-glucosidases (E.C. 3.2.1.20), *e.g.* those of the vertebrate intestine (SEMENZA, 1968) or those of microbiological origin (HALVORSON and ELLIAS, 1958). Methyl-α-glucoside is not split by the tarsal glucosidase activity. Trehalose, easily hydrolysed by tarsal extracts, is not hydrolysed by the α-glucosidase, but by a specific trehalase (E.C.3.2.1.28). Other glycosidase activities are lacking (β-glucosidase, α-mannosidase, α-, and β-galactosidase). Comparing the substrate specificity of the glucosidase with the threshold values (Columns 1 and 2), the following correlation results: the substrates of the glucosidase have low threshold values (1—4, 11, 18), sugars not acting as substrates (5—10, 12, 13, 19, 20) have high values.

(2b) The apparent K_m-values of the glucosidase in the crude extracts show a rough parallel to the behavioral thresholds for five substrates.

(2c) The rejection thresholds of the sugar receptor and the apparent inhibition constants of the glucosidase for aliphatic alcohols (methanol to *n*-octanol) decrease logarithmically with increasing chain length (inhibition of the sugar receptor: DETHIER and CHADWICK, 1948; STEINHARDT et al., 1966; inhibition of the glucosidase: HANSEN, 1968).

Based on these parallels, HANSEN (1969) proposed the following hypothesis: The glucosidase could act as the receptor protein of the sugar receptor cells in flies. Therefore the initial process of reception might be identical with the formation of a sugar glucosidase complex which controls the membrane permeability.

5. Chromatographic Separation of the Glucosidases

The linearity of the Lineweawer-Burk-plots for several substrates seemed to be an indication that the crude tarsal extracts contained only one glucosidase. But gel-chromatographic controls to prove the suggested homogeneity led to the detection of at least three different peaks (Hansen and Kühner, 1972). Two of the peaks were only partially separated, but could be clearly distinguished due to their different substrate patterns. Simultaneously, Morita (1972; Amakawa et al., 1972) separated the labellar glucosidases of *Phormia* by chromatography on DEAE-Sephadex. They too obtained three peaks which differed in their K_m-values for sucrose, 4-nitrophenyl-α-glucoside and turanose. Kühner and Hansen (1975) then used DEAE-cellulose to further separate the tarsal glucosidases. In addition, they characterized the five peaks obtained by using the substrates maltose, melezitose and palatinose. These sugars were split at a different, rate, typical for each peak. Thereby it was shown that each peak corresponded to an individual enzyme. The peak pattern obtained with 4-nitrophenyl-α-glucoside as substrate and the K_m-values conformed with those described by Morita and coworkers for the labellar extracts. Figures 5–7 illustrate separations of the glucosidases of the labella, the tarsomeres 2–5 of the first leg and the tibiae of the third leg. The technique is a slight modification of that of Kühner and Hansen and gives rise to about nine peaks. (Bührer and Hansen, unpublished.)

Table 2 shows the substrate specificity and the K_m-values of the different peaks. Furthermore, it can be seen which of the peaks — although differently numbered by the investigators — are identical. The peaks were numbered according to their elution sequence from the DEAE-cellulose column and exhibit the following properties:

Peak I is not adsorbed by DEAE-cellulose; it always hydrolyses sucrose three to four times faster than 4-nitrophenyl-α-glucoside. Its specificity is relatively, broad.

Peak II splits sucrose only and with a high K_m-value. It's activity in the labella is smaller than in the tarsomers.

Within the same fractions another activity is eluted that splits 4-nitrophenyl-α-glucoside and maltose. Because of its very low activity it is only seen in the tibial profile, but is also present in the tarsomeres as well as in the labella.

The Peak-III-group contains three components. Peak III_1 is clearly visible in the tarsomeres, it exists as a shoulder of Peak III_2

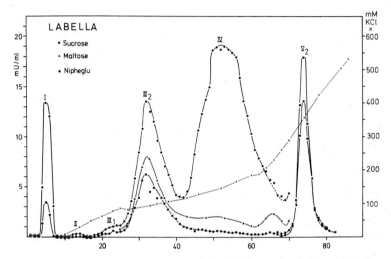

Fig. 5. Chromatographic separation of the labellar α-glucosidases. 650 labella were homogenized in 1 ml barbital-Na-HCl-buffer (25 mM), pH 6.9 containing 2 mM EDTA and 0.2 M mannitol. After an extraction period of 5 hr at 5° C the homogenate was centrifuged (1 hr, 50000 g). The supernatant, containing 60% of the total activity, was applied on a column (0.6 × 6 cm) of DEAE-cellulose ion exchanger (Whatman DE-52). The starting buffer was the same as above, but without mannitol. The KCl-gradient begins at Fraction 8, its profile is marked by (×), see right ordinate (volume of the gradient: 53 ml, divided into fractions of 0.65 ml). Peak I leaves the column unadsorbed. The sucrose profile corresponds to maximal velocities (except the labellar Peak IV): pH 5.5: Peak I 100 mM, Peak II to Fraction 70 400 mM sucrose; pH 5.9: Peak V_2 40 mM sucrose. With sucrose and maltose as substrates, the liberated glucose was determined enzymatically by the glucose oxidase method; using 4-nitrophenyl-α-glucoside (Peak I-Fraction 70: 14 mM, Peak V_2: 3.5 mM) the liberated 4-nitrophenol was measured at 410nm in alkaline solution. The activities (ordinates) of the Figs. 5—7 were calculated for 10 mg tissue including chitin (dry weight). The total activity of each peak was calculated by summing the activities of all fractions belonging to it (BÜHRER and HANSEN, unpublished)

Table 2. Glucosidases of taste hair-bearing segments

| Peak numbers | | | | Substrate specificity + well split — not or poorly split | | | | | | Michaelis constants[a] (mM) | | Ratio of activities tarsomeres/tibiae | Visible in Fig. |
this paper	Amakawa et al.	Kühner and Hansen	Hansen and Kühner	Sucrose	Turanose	Palatinose	Maltose	Melezitose	4-nitrophenyl-α-glucoside	Sucrose	4-Nitrophenyl-α-glucoside		
I	I	I		+	+	+	+		+	~ 30	0.3	3.3	5—7
II		II		+	−	−	−	−	−	~ 120	—	~ 100	6
III$_1$				+		+	+		+				6
III$_2$	II	III	III	+	+	−	+	+	+	~ 60	10	40	5—7
III$_3$				+									7
IV		IV	I?	+	−	−	+		−	~ 120	—	25	5—7
(×)							+		+				5
V$_1$				+					−				6
V$_2$	III	V	II	+	+	−	+	+	+	~ 12	0.3	4.8	5—7
tip enzyme				+	+		+		+	~ 50			

[a] Kühner and Hansen

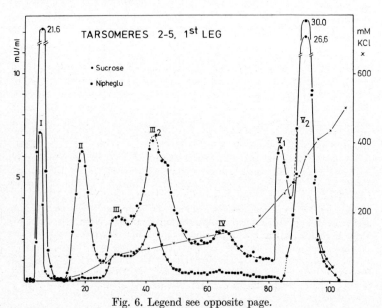

Fig. 6. Legend see opposite page.

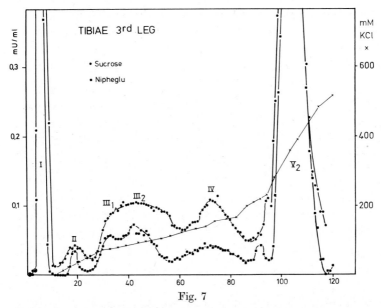

Fig. 7

Figs. 6 and 7. Chromatographic separation of the glucosidases of tarsomeres 2—5 of the first leg and of tibiae of the third leg. 600 tarsomeres 2—5 (70% of the activity in the supernatant) and 980 tibiae (50% of the activity in the supernatant) were used; the gradients begin at the Fractions 12 and 11 respectively. The maxima of the Peaks I and V_2 (tibiae) lie at 4.7 and 5.8 mU/ml respectively. All other experimental data are the same as in Fig. 5. Note that the ordinate scales of activity differ by the factor 33! (BÜHRER and HANSEN, unpublished)

in the labellar profile, but is not separated from Peak III_2 in the tibia. The Peaks III_1 and III_2 differ in the ability to split palatinose: at 30 mM the activity of Peak III_1 is several times higher than that of III_2, and it was thus possible to identify Peak III_1 in the tibial profile. In the tarsomeres and labella, III_2 has the highest activity of the Peak-III-group, whilst in the tibia all three exhibit nearly the same small activity. Peak III_3 is seen only as shoulder of Peak III_2 in the sucrose profile of tibia and tarsomeres, but, has not yet been further characterized.

Peak IV favors sucrose as substrate and resembles Peak II, but splits maltose and, very slowly, 4-nitrophenyl-α-glucoside. Its homogeneity is questionable for several reasons (broad elution profile of irregular shape, broad pH-optimum), especially in the labella, where it contains a component of unusually high K_m-value (0.5 M).

For the separation of Peaks III and IV we used an elution buffer of pH 6.90. At slightly higher pH-values (7.2), as used by AMAKAWA et al., we observed an overlap of the peaks that might be an explanation for the finding of these authors that 4-nitrophenyl-α-glucoside is split only with 21% of the maximal velocity of sucrose.

A small unnumbered peak (x) is found in the maltose profile between Peaks IV and V_1. The activity of this peak is specific for maltose and 4-nitrophenyl-α-glucoside, whereas sucrose is hydrolysed slowly or not at all.

The tarsomeres and tibiae contain the peak V_1 that splits sucrose but not 4-nitrophenyl-α-glucoside, but it is absent or very weak in the labella. Peak V_2 splits 4-nitrophenyl-α-glucoside slightly faster than sucrose. Low K_m-values and a pronounced substrate inhibition are typical for it.

6. Which of the Separated Glucosidases Can Be Denoted as the Receptor Protein?

This question may be answered by the two following different kinds of experiments:

1. One can compare the properties of the glucosidase peaks with those of the sugar receptor. Properties in common indicate that the peak in question may function as receptor protein. MORITA (1972) and AMAKAWA et al. (1972) found that the K_m-values for sucrose (50—100 mM) and 4-nitrophenyl-α-glucoside (10—25 mM) of Peak II (equal to III_2 + IV in our separations) coincide with the K_b-values (67 mM and 3 mM) of the sugar receptor of the largest labellar taste hairs. Therefore, this peak "could be a candidate for the sugar receptor protein of the blowfly". This is further established by the findings of KIJIMA et al. (1973), who report that the tip enzyme (see Section 7) has a K_m of about 55 mM for sucrose.

Concerning the Peaks I and V_2, the authors made the following statement: "Provided that only one receptor protein exists and that the K_m values *in vitro* correspond to those *in vivo*, the Peaks I and V_2 having low K_m values should be excluded as receptor proteins because the relation $K_b < K_m$ must be kept."

The marginal hairs of the labella show a K_b-value of 120 mM (SHIRAISHI, cited by MORITA, 1972). At present it is not clear whether the labellar Peak IV contains, in addition to a component with a high K_m-value, a component corresponding to Peak IV of the tarsi and tibiae with a K_m of about 120 mM.

2. Because of the great technical difficulties encountered in measuring concentration response curves for the small tarsal taste hairs of the A- and B-type, we are restricted here to the following experiments. We started to compare the activity of the different peaks in tarsomeres rich in taste hairs with that of tibiae poor in taste hairs, as demonstrated in the Figs. 6 and 7.

Considering the number of taste hairs counted by GRABOWSKI and DETHIER (1954), we can calculate that an extract of 10 mg tarsomeres 2−5 contains 130000 A-hairs, 80000 B-hairs and 18000 C- and D-hairs. An extract of 10 mg tibiae of the third leg contains 1600 B-hairs only. Thus the extract of tarsomeres contains 50 times more B-hairs than that of the tibiae.

The activities of the five main peaks of the tibiae are smaller by different factors than those of the tarsomeres. Two groups can be distinguished. One group – the Peaks I and V_2 – exhibits the factors 3 and 5 (see Table 2); the other group – the Peaks I, III_{1-3}, and IV – shows much greater factors: 100, 50, and 25 respectively.

We can now conclude:

a) Because the factors of Peaks I and V_2 are very small compared with the proportions of taste hairs in tarsomeres and tibiae, these peaks are not specifically localized within the taste hairs.

b) Peaks corresponding to the A-, C-, and D-hairs of the tarsomeres should be completely absent in the tibia. In fact, Peak II is reduced by more than the factor 100 because the activity found in the same fractions belongs mainly to another peak which also splits 4-nitrophenyl-α-glucoside. Thus Peak II may not represent the receptor protein of the B-hair sugar receptor.

c) The reduction factors of the Peaks III and IV correspond roughly to the factor 50 of the B-hairs; in this respect both peaks therefore may be the appropriate receptor proteins of the B-hair sugar receptors.

7. *In vivo* Determination of Glucosidase Activity at the Hair Tip

Investigations by Koizumi et al. (1973) revealed that whole, living labella and legs of *Phormia* and *Boettcherica*, dipped after washing into a buffered 4-nitrophenyl-α-glucoside solution, have a glucosidase activity on the outside surface which is not solubilized into the medium during incubation. Since the legs seem to have no other pores except those at the tip of the taste hairs, the authors assume the glucosidase to be bound to the dendritic membrane and to take part in some way in sugar reception.

Kijima et al. (1972) performed very sophisticated experiments demonstrating a glucosidase activity at the tip of taste hairs. They put a glass capillary containing the buffered substrate solution over a pair of the largest labellar taste hairs. After an incubation time of one hour, the glucose formed was measured with a radio-active ultra-micromethod (glucose was converted to its 6-phosphate with ^{32}P-ATP and hexokinase, the 6-phosphate was then separated and counted, Chick and Like, 1969). The activity of a single hair was found to be 10^{-8} units, and the K_m about 50 mM for sucrose as substrate. 4-Nitrophenyl-α-glucoside, maltose, turanose and trehalose were split, too, but not raffinose and lactose. The activity was bound strictly to the taste hair tip. Other spines and tactile hairs showed no activity. If, however, the hair tip was cut, a very active and soluble glucosidase appeared. This glucosidase has a low K_m-value of 2.2 mM and is not yet known in the chromatographic pattern. According to these results the authors assume that this membrane bound tip enzyme — corresponding to their Peak II with respect to the K_m — should be the receptor protein. In addition to this enzyme, another one not involved in reception exists in the taste hairs.

Very recently the same authors (Koizumi et al., 1974) report the following similarities between the further evaluated properties of the tip enzyme and electrophysiological data of the sugar receptor which are, however, partially inconsistent with the properties of their Peak II enzyme (Peak III$_2$ of our terminology):

1. The activity of the tip enzyme is not dependent on pH in the range from pH 3 to 8. In an earlier paper Shiraishi and Morita (1969b) found the spike frequency also to be independent of pH (4–10). In contrast to this feature of tip enzyme and receptor

cell, the activity of Peak II enzyme follows a very steep pH curve with an optimum about pH 6.0.

2. Tris inhibits the tip enzyme and the sugar receptor with a similar inhibition constant K_i, which is (with sucrose as substrate) about two orders of magnitude greater than the K_i of the Peak II enzyme (with 4-nitrophenyl-α-glucoside as substrate, KAWABATA et al., 1973).

3. Ca^{++} ions (5 mM) inhibit the tip glucosidase and the sugar receptor, but activate the Peak II enzyme (KAWABATA et al., 1973).

KOIZUMI et al. (1974) discuss three possible explanations for these differences. The membrane bound tip enzyme may have other properties than in the solubilized state; the "homeostatic micro-environment" of the enzyme in the dendritic membrane may have an influence on its properties, or finally the hair tip enzyme may be a new glucosidase not yet found in the chromatographic pattern.

In my opinion the arguments of KOIZUMI et al. against the identity of the Peak II enzyme with the sugar receptor protein should not be over-emphasized. Determining pH profiles under these conditions, it should be kept in mind that the buffer solution is mixed with the perhaps not unbuffered medium surrounding the dendrites; thus, the pH at the membrane may be shifted considerably. Furthermore, it has not been checked whether *Tris* exhibits the same inhibition constant for different substrates.

8. Are the Glucosidases *in vivo* Bound to Membranes or Not?

For the chromatographic separation the glucosidases must be solubilized during the extraction procedure. Therefore it should be insured, that the peaks identical with the receptor proteins are not located in the cytoplasma, *in vivo* for this would be in contrast to their function controlling the membrane permeability.

Before tissue can be extracted, the chitinous cuticle of the tarsi, tibiae and labella must be crushed by vigorous grinding in a mortar either with quartz sand or in the presence of liquid nitrogen. This handling makes it impossible to extract the soluble proteins from the intact tarsi or labella by previous mild mechanical and chemical treatment. After grinding and short extraction with buffer at low pH (5.5) and low ionic strenght, only 20−30% of the total activity was solubilized and obtained in the Supernatant I after centrifugation. In an early separation experiment of Super-natant I the Peaks I, and III + IV (not separated), but not V_2

were visible. If thereafter the pellet is extracted for several hours with buffer at pH 7.0, further 40–60% of the activity is solubilized in Supernatant II, and 20–40% remains in the pellet. As a preliminary result it can be concluded that *in vivo*, at least, the greater part of the Peaks I and III + IV and all of V_2 is structurally bound, as they appear predominantly after the second extraction step in the Supernatant II.

Concluding Remarks

This paper outlines the present state of investigations. There is no doubt that an α-glucosidase is involved in the reception process of the sugar receptor. The K_m values of the Peak III_2 enzyme for two sugars resemble on the one hand those of the tip enzyme, and on the other hand the K_b-values of the receptor cell. These corresponding properties indicate that the glucosidase acts as the receptor protein.

Several pieces of evidence suggest that more than one sugar receptor protein exists. Different hair types seem to contain different receptor proteins. Furthermore, even one receptor cell may have several receptor proteins, or at least several sites working independently or cooperatively.

At present three important questions remain unresolved:

1. Does the glucosidase act as receptor protein for monosaccharides, too? The first positive indication was obtained by SHIMADA et al., 1974. They found that sucrose and maltose combine with the PCMB-sensitive hexopyranose site.

2. Is the catalytic step of the glucosidase reaction involved in the primary process? The formation of a protein-sugar-complex is a condition for the control of the membrane permeability as well as for the splitting of the glycosidic linkage. As yet nothing is known about the connection between the catalytic process and the permeability control.

3. By which mechanism does the protein-sugar-complex control the opening of the ion channels?

Acknowledgement

These investigations have been generously supported by the Deutsche Forschungsgemeinschaft (Schwerpunktprogramm Rezeptorphysiologie).

References

AMAKAWA, T., KAWABATA, K., KIJIMA, H., MORITA, H.: Isozymes of α-glucosidase in the proboscis and legs of flies. J. Insect Physiol. **18**, 541—553 (1972).

BOOS, W.: Structurally defective galactose-binding protein isolated from a mutant negative in the α-methylgalactoside transport system of *Escherichia coli*. J. biol. Chem. **247**, 5414—5425 (1972).

BRESCH, W.-E.: Der Zuckerrezeptor eines Rüsselhaares der Baumwollwanze *Dysdercus intermedius*, eine elektrophysiologische Untersuchung. Diss. Univ. Heidelberg 1973.

CHANGEUX, J.-P., PODLESKI, TH. R.: On the excitability and cooperativity of the electroplax membrane. Proc. nat. Acad. Sci. (Wash.) **59**, 944 (1968).

CHICK, W., LIKE, A.: Ultramicro method for determination of glycogen and glucose by enzymic labeling with adenosine triphosphate-γ-^{32}P. Anal. Biochem. **32**, 340—347 (1969).

DASTOLI, F. R.: Taste receptor proteins. Life Sciences **14**, 1417—1426 (1974).

DETHIER, V. G.: The physiology and histology of the contact chemoreceptors of the blowfly. Quart. Rev. Biol. **30**, 348—371 (1955a).

DETHIER, V. G.: Mode of action of sugar-baited fly-traps. J. econ. Entomol. **48**, 235—239 (1955b).

DETHIER, V. G., CHADWICK, L. E.: An analysis of the relationship between solubility and stimulating effect in tarsal chemoreception. J. gen. Physiol. **33**, 589—599 (1950).

EVANS, D. R.: Chemical structure and stimulation by carbohydrates. In: ZOTTERMANN (Ed.): I. Intern. Symp. Olfaction and Taste, pp. 165—176. New York: Pergamon Press 1973.

FOELIX, R. F.: Chemosensitive hairs in spiders. J. Morph. **132**, 313—334 (1970).

v. FRISCH, K.: Über den Geschmackssinn der Biene. Ein Beitrag zur vergleichenden Physiologie des Geschmacks. Z. vergl. Physiol. **21**, 1—155 (1935).

GRABOWSKI, C. T., DETHIER, V. G.: The structure of the tarsal chemoreceptors of the blowfly, *Phormia regina* MEIG. J. Morph. **94**, 1—20 (1954).

HALVORSON, H., ELLIAS, L.: The purification and properties of an α-glucosidase of *Saccharomyces italicus*. Biochim. biophys. Acta (Amst.) **30**, 28—40 (1958).

HANAMORI, T., SHIRAISHI, A., KIJIMA, H., MORITA, H.: Stimulation of labellar sugar receptors of the fleshfly by glycosides. Z. vergl. Physiol. **76**, 115—129 (1972).

VAN HANDEL, E.: Utilization of injected maltose and sucrose by insects, evidence for non-intestinal oligosaccharidases. Comp. Biochem. Physiol. **24**, 537—541 (1968).

HANSEN, K.: Über Carbohydrasen in den Tarsen von *Calliphora* und *Phormia*. Verh. Deutsch. Zool. Ges. München 1963, Zool. Anz. Suppl. **27**, 628—634 (1964).

HANSEN, K.: Zur kompetitiven Hemmung der tarsalen Glucosidase und der Zuckerrezeptoren bei *Phormia regina* Meig. durch Amine. Verh. Deutsch. Zool. Ges. Heidelberg 1967, Zool. Anz. Suppl. **31**, 558—564 (1968).

HANSEN, K.: Untersuchungen über den Mechanismus der Zucker-Perzeption bei Fliegen. Habilitationsschrift der Universität Heidelberg (1968).

HANSEN, K.: The mechanism of insect sugar reception, a biochemical investigation. In: PFAFFMANN, C. (Ed.): III. Intern. Symp. Olfaction and Taste, pp. 382—391 (1968). New York: Rockefeller Univ. Press 1969.

HANSEN, K., HEUMANN, H.-G.: Die Feinstruktur der tarsalen Schmeckhaare der Fliege *Phormia terraenovae* Rob.-Desv. Z. Zellforsch. **117**, 419—442 (1971).

HANSEN, K., KÜHNER, J.: Properties of a possible acceptor protein of the fly's sugar receptor. In: SCHNEIDER, D. (Ed.): IV. Intern. Symp. Olfaction and Taste, Starnberg 1971, pp. 350—356. Stuttgart: Wiss. Verlagsges. 1972.

HASLINGER, F.: Über den Geschmackssinn von *Calliphora erythrocephala* Meig. und über die Verwertung von Zuckern und Zuckeralkoholen durch diese Fliege. Z. vergl. Physiol. **22**, 614—640 (1935).

HASSETT, C. C., DETHIER, V. G., GANS, J.: A comparison of nutritive values and taste thresholds of carbohydrates for the blowfly. Biol. Bull. **99**, 446—453 (1950).

HIJI, Y., SATO, M.: Properties of sweet-sensitive protein extracted from the rat tongue. In: SCHNEIDER, D. (Ed.): IV. Intern. Symp. Olfaction and Taste, Starnberg 1971, pp. 221—225. Stuttgart: Wiss. Verlagsges. 1972.

HIJI, Y., SATO, M.: Isolation of the sugar-binding protein from rat taste buds. Nature (Lond.) New Biol. **244**, 91—93 (1973).

HODGSON, E. S., LETTVIN, J. Y., ROEDER, K. D.: Physiology of a primary chemoreceptor unit. Science **122**, 417—418 (1955).

HODGSON, E. S.: The chemical senses and changing viewpoints in sensory physiology. Viewpoints in Biol. **4**, 83—1124 (1965).

JAKINOVICH, W., GOLDSTEIN, I. J., VON BAUMGARTEN, R. J., AGRANOFF, B. W.: Sugar receptor specificity in the fleshfly, *Sarcophaga bullata*. Brain Res. **35** 369—378 (1971).

KAISSLING, K.-E.: Insect olfaction. In: BEIDLER (Ed.): Handbook of sensory physiology, IV/1, pp. 351—431. Berlin-Heidelberg-New York: Springer 1971.

KAWABATA, K., KIJIMA, H., SHIRAISHI, A., MORITA, H.: α-Glucosidase isozymes and the labellar sugar receptor of the blowfly. J. Insect Physiol. **19**, 337—348 (1973).

KIJIMA, H., KOIZUMI, O., MORITA, H.: α-Glucosidase at the tip of the contact chemosensory seta of the blowfly, *Phormia regina*. J. Insect Physiol. **19**, 1351—1362.

KOIZUMI, O., KIJIMA, H., KAWABATA, K., MORITA, H.: α-Glucosidase activity on the outside of the labella and legs of the fly. Comp. Biochem. Physiol. **44** B, 347—356 (1973).

KOIZUMI,O., KIJIMA,H., MORITA,H.: Characterization of α-glucosidase at the tips of the chemosensory setae of the fly, *Phormia regina*. J. Insect Physiol. **20**, 925—934 (1974).

KÜHNER,J., HANSEN,K.: Die Isolierung von α-Glucosidasen aus den schmeckhaarreichen Tarsen der Fliege *Phormia terraenovae* Meigen (submitted for publication in J. comp. Physiol.).

MINNICH,D.E.: The chemical senses of insects. Quart. Rev. Biol. **4**, 100—112 (1929).

MORITA,H.: Electrical signs of taste receptor activity. In: PFAFFMANN,C. (Ed.): III. Intern. Symp. Olfaction and Taste, New York 1968, pp. 370 to 381. Rockefeller Univ. Press 1969.

MORITA,H.: Properties of the sugar receptor site of the blowfly. In: SCHNEIDER,D. (Ed.): IV. Intern. Symp. Olfaction and Taste, Starnberg 1971, pp. 357—363. Stuttgart: Wiss. Verlagsges. 1972.

MORITA,H., SHIRAISHI,A.: Stimulation of the labellar sugar receptor of the fleshfly by mono- and disaccharides. J. gen. Physiol. **52**, 559—583 (1968).

PFLUMM,W.: Zur Reizwirksamkeit von Monosacchariden bei der Fliege *Phormia terraenovae*. Z. vergl. Physiol. **74**, 411—426 (1971).

PFLUMM,W.: Molecular structure and stimulating effectiveness of oligosaccharides and glycosides. In: SCHNEIDER,D. (Ed.): IV. Intern. Symp. Olfaction and Taste, Starnberg 1971, pp. 364—370. Stuttgart: Wiss. Verlagsges. 1972.

PRICE,S.: Chemoreceptor proteins in taste cell stimulation. In: POYNDER,T. M. (Ed.): Transduction Mechanisms in Chemoreception, pp. 177—184. London: Information Retrieval Ltd. 1974.

SACKTOR,B.: Cell structure and the metabolism of insect flight muscle. J. Biophys. Biochem. Cytol. **1**, 29—46 (1955).

SALAMA,H.S.: The function of mosquito taste receptors. J. Insect Physiol. **12**, 1051—1060 (1966).

SCHMIDT,A.: Geschmacksphysiologische Untersuchungen an Ameisen. Z. vergl. Physiol. **25**, 351—378 (1938).

SCHNEIDER,D.: Molekulare Grundlagen der chemischen Sinne bei Insekten. Naturwissenschaften **58**, 194—200 (1971).

SCHNEIDER,D., HECKER,E.: Zur Elektrophysiologie der Antenne des Seidenspinners *Bombyx mori* bei Reizung mit angereicherten Extrakten des Sexuallockstoffes. Z. Naturforsch. **11**b, 121—124 (1956).

SEMENZA,G.: Intestinal oligosaccharidases and disaccharidases. In: CODE, C.F. (Ed.): Handbook of physiology, Section 6.3, pp. 2543—2566. Washington: American Physiological Soc. 1968.

SHIMADA,I., SHIRAISHI,A., KIJIMA,H., MORITA,H.: Separation of two receptor sites in a single labellar sugar receptor of the fleshfly by treatment with p-chloromercuribenzoate. J. Insect Physiol. **20**, 605—621 (1974).

SHIRAISHI,A., MORITA,H.: The effects of pH on the labellar sugar receptor of the fleshfly. J. gen. Physiol. **53**, 450—470 (1969).

STEINHARDT,R.A., MORITA,H., HODGSON,E.S.: Mode of action of straight chain hydrocarbons on primary chemoreceptors of the blowfly *Phormia regina*. J. Cell Comp. Physiol. **67**, 53—62 (1966).

Thurm, U.: Untersuchungen zur funktionellen Organisation sensorischer Zellverbände. In: Rathmayer (Ed.): Verh. Deutsch. Zool. Ges., Köln 1970, pp. 79—88. Stuttgart: Fischer 1970.

Wallenfels, K., Weil, R.: β-Galactosidase. In: Boyer (Ed.): The enzymes VII, 3rd. ed., pp. 618—663. New York: Academic Press 1972.

Weis, I.: Versuche über die Geschmacksrezeption durch die Tarsen des Admirals, *Pyrameis atalanta* L. Z. vergl. Physiol. **12**, 206—248 (1930).

Wieczorek, H.: Eigenschaften des Glykosidrezeptors der Kohleulenraupe. In: Rathmayer (Ed.): Verh. Dtsch. Zool. Ges. Bochum 1974. Stuttgart: Fischer (in press).

Wiesmann, R.: Zum Nahrungsproblem der freilebenden Stubenfliegen, *Musca domestica* L. Z. angew. Zool. **47**, 159—182 (1960).

Wilczek, M.: The distribution and neuroanatomy of the labellar sense organs of the blowfly *Phormia regina* Meigen. J. Morph. **122**, 175—202 (1967).

Wolbarsht, M. L.: Receptor sites in insect chemoreceptors. Cold Spr. Harb. Symp. quant. Biol. **30**, 281—288 (1965).

Discussion

E. Gross (Bethesda, Md.): Could the p-nitrophenol liberated possibly inhibit your glucosidase?

K. Hansen: Nitrophenol is indeed a competitive inhibitor of glucosidases. However, since in control experiments with yeast glucosidase the inhibition constant of nitrophenol had the value 3.5 mM (Bührer, unpublished), its inhibitory effect should be negligible in our assay for activity determination. The maximal concentration of nitrophenol reaches only about 0.1 mM.

P. Karlson (Marburg): Is it possible to detect binding proteins in the chemosensory hairs, e. g. by radioautographic methods?

K. Hansen: At the time being this possibility is limited. Affinity labeling agents are lacking and the autoradiographic resolution lies in the same order of magnitude as the structures in the hair tip.

B. Hamprecht (München): Couldn't it be possible that the sugar receptor and the glucosidase are two different proteins, in analogy to the acetylcholine system?

K. Hansen: Nothing is known of the mechanism freeing the receptor of the stimulant molecules after stimulation. So the possibility cannot be fully excluded that the glucosidase functions in analogy to acetylcholine esterase; but it does not seem very probable for the following reasons:

(i) if the high specific activity (12000 U/mg) and the small K_m (0.1 mM) of acetylcholine esterase are necessary for its synaptic function, the glucosidases do not seem to be very well suited for this purpose, because their activities are smaller and the K_m-values higher;

(ii) the hydrolysis of disaccharides would be less effective than the splitting of acetylcholine since one product, viz. glucose, retains an affinity towards the receptor;

(iii) since the dissociation constants of a certain glucosidase and the sugar receptor are the same, the simplest conclusion is to assume identity of the glucosidase with the sugar receptor.

Thaumatin and Monellin, the Intensely Sweet-Tasting Proteins from Tropical African Fruits

H. van der Wel

Unilever Research, Vlaardingen, The Netherlands

With 1 Figure

Introduction

The discovery of the sweet-tasting proteins thaumatin I, thaumatin II (Van der Wel and Loeve, 1972) and monellin (Morris and Cagan, 1972; Van der Wel, 1972; Morris et al., 1973; Van der Wel and Loeve, 1973) of plant origin shows us the first macromolecules evoking a specific taste sensation. These proteins are isolated in an electrophoretically pure form by means of water extraction, ultrafiltration, gel filtration and ion-exchange chromatography from the fruits of *Thaumatococcus daniellii* Benth and *Dioscoreophyllum cumminsii* Diels respectively, two fruits from tropical Africa.

Thaumatin I and II and monellin are basic proteins with isoelectric points of 12.12 and 9.03 and molecular weights if 21000, 20400, and 11500 (Van der Wel and Loeve, 1972; Van der Wel and Loeve, 1973). The sweetness intensity of these proteins on a molar basis are 1×10^5, 1×10^5, and 8.4×10^4 times that of sucrose. So far, these proteins are the sweetest compounds known, although very recently Fujino et al. (1973) published the synthesis of L-aspartyl-aminomalonic-O_1-methyl, O_2-fenchyl diester, which compound has a sweetness intensity of 2.2×10^4 times that of sucrose on a molar basis.

Structural investigations show that the proteins in question are single polypeptide chains with very little, if any, α-helix configuration in the molecules, as indicated by circular dichroism measurements and supported by nuclear magnetic resonance studies (Korver et al., 1973). The detailed structure of the NMR spectrum shows characteristics of amino acid residues in a non-rigid protein structure. The high field methyl signals, however, indicate that at least part of the molecules possess a well defined tertiary structure.

Psychophysical experiments (VAN DER WEL and LOEVE, 1973) reveal that the sweetness of the proteins is temperature- and pH-dependent. Above a certain temperature, the sweetness disappears completely (see Table 1). It also disappears after cleavage of the

Table 1. pH-dependent temperatures (°C) at which a heat-induced conformational irreversible transition occurs in correlation with the loss of sweetness

pH	Temperatures (°C)		
	Thaumatin I	Thaumatin II	Monellin
3.0	55	55	50
5.0	75	75	65
7.2	65	65	55

disulphide bonds in the proteins. All these facts point to the importance of the role of the tertiary structure in the taste activity. We are, therefore, paying special attention to thet hree-dimensional conformation of these proteins and the possible conformational alterations which accompany their biological activity. Circular dichroism measurements already showed (KORVER et al., 1973) that there is a correlation between the sweetness dependence of the proteins on the temperature and pH, and the conformational changes in the protein structures.

The sweetness intensity of both proteins on a molar basis is nearly the same. This is a reason to suppose that the proteins contain similar sites responsible for the sweetness and the similarities in their CD spectra in correlation with their sweetness, indicating that the groups underlying the conformational change are also operative in generating the sweet taste.

Circular Dichroism

Circular dichroism spectra of the thaumatins and of monellin were recorded at varying temperatures and pH's (KORVER et al., 1973). The spectra measured at pH 7.2, 5.0, and 3.0 at 25° C show negative peaks at 295, 287, 280, and 206 nm for the proteins.

Moreover, the thaumatins show positive bands at 228 and 245 nm and monellin a negative shoulder at 228 nm, a positive band at 234 nm and a negative peak at 268 nm. Figure 1 shows the CD spectra at pH 7.2 and 25° C. The negative peaks exhibited by the thaumatins and monellin at 295 and 287 nm are due to electronic transitions of the amino acid residues of tryptophan and tyrosine, at 280 nm to a tyrosine residue and at 206 nm to the peptide bonds of the backbone conformation of the proteins. The conclusion that the 280 nm peak is due to a tyrosine residue is based on a study of

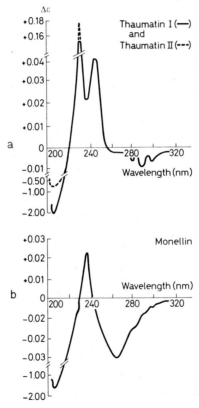

Fig. 1a and b. CD-spectrum of the sweet-tasting proteins between 200 and 300 nm at pH 7.2 and 25° C. (a) Thaumatin I (————) and Thaumatin II (- - - -), (b) Monellin

Beychok and Breslow (1968) on oxytocin and several oxytocin analogues.

For the assignment of the positive bands of the thaumatins at 245 and 228 nm it is worthwhile looking at the similarity between the thaumatin spectra and the spectrum of oxytocin. Urrey et al. (1968) and Beychok and Breslow (1968) assigned the positive long-wavelength band at 250 nm in oxytocin to the electronic transition of the disulfide group corresponding to a disulfide dihedral angle close to 90°. They arrived at this assignment on the basis of the fact that the disulfide chromophore has a long-wavelength absorption band depending on the dihedral angle φ, exhibiting either one band at roughly 245—250 nm for $\varphi = \pm 90°$ or two bands of opposite sign that are positionally symmetrical on each side of this value for $\varphi \neq 90°$ as confirmed later on by Donzel et al., 1972. The positive short-wavelength band at 225 nm is assigned, by the same investigators, to a tyrosine chromophore. On the basis of these studies, it is plausible to assign the positive peaks of the thaumatins at 245 and 228 nm to a disulfide chromophore and a tyrosine residue.

The same authors indicated that a negative band at 228 nm is due to a disulfide moiety; thus the shoulder at 228 nm in monellin is likely to be due to a disulfide bond. The other peaks in monellin, the positive 234 nm band and the negative 268 nm band, are due to the disulfide chromophore with a dihedral angle $\varphi \neq \pm 90°$, as is supported by model experiments of Ludescher and Schwyzer (1971) and Donzel et al. (1972). For instance, [2,7-cystine]-gramicidin S, a cyclic decapeptide fixed in the P-helical configuration with $\varphi \cong + 120°$, exhibits essentially bands arising from disulfide-inherent optical activity, negative at 271 nm and positive at 230 nm. Another support for these assumptions is the striking resemblance between the shifts in the CD-spectra on heating the proteins. Similar effects are observed when the medium is changed from water to the less polar solvent water/dioxan. Both in oxytocin and in the thaumatins the intensity of the positive band at 228 nm decreases and a negative peak appears at 235 nm. Similarly, in monellin the 268 nm peak decreases.

This temperature effect is pH-dependent for thaumatin and monellin and is largely reversible. For instance, the heat-induced conformational changes for Thaumatin I and II are reversible up to 75° C at pH 5.0, even when this temperature is maintained for two hours. On cooling to 25° C, the negative peak disappears and the positive band increases to the original level. Above 75° and pH 5.0 the thaumatins denature irreversibly with a complete loss of sweetness (see Table 1). Chemical modification of the proteins as succinylation of the amino groups or esterification of the carboxylic groups destroy the sweet taste, which is in agreement with the disappearance of the characteristic CD-spectrum.

Support for a transition in the disulfide bridges is provided by proton magnetic resonance measurements on the thaumatins in that the intensity of the signal from methylene groups adjacent to hetero-atoms at $\delta = 2.95$ in a 30% acetonitrile/^{2}H$_2$O mixture increases compared with that in water. This is an indication that the methylene groups adjacent to sulfur become more mobile. Another support is given by an ultraviolet difference spectroscopic measurement using the thermal perturbation technique, where a positive band at 260 nm arises from a change in the environment of the disulfide group.

Discussion

It is not clear from the CD results whether the tyrosine chromophore is actually involved in the conformational transition or whether only a compensation effect occurs in the form of enhancement of the negative disulfide signal. Model experiments with oxytocin and related compounds made URREY et al. (1968) assign the negative 235 nm band to the disulfide chromophore; they explain it in terms of valence bond description, viz. that the 90° dihedral angle results from a repulsion between unshared electron pairs on each sulfur atom, the repulsion constituting a rotational barrier. This barrier can be overcome by heating the solvent medium or by making it less polar. The resulting distortion of the skewed asymmetric spatial arrangement of S-S linkage gives then rise to the negative CD band at about 235 nm.

Experiments by CARMACK and NEUBERT (1967) and LUDESCHER and SCHWYZER (1971) provide correlations between the chirality of cystine disulfide groups and the sign of the two Cotton effects observed in the regions 250—300 nm and 230—250 nm using model compounds of known asymmetry and with dihedral angles φ of $[0°] < [\varphi] < [90°]$. In this angle range (*cis*), the positive helical sense (P) is related to a positive Cotton effect at $\lambda > 250$ nm and a negative Cotton effect at λ between 230 and 250 nm (*vice versa* for a left-handed helical (M) arrangement). The signs of the bands in chiral disulfides with dihedral angles φ of $|90°| < |\varphi| < 180°|$ (*trans*) will be opposite of those from the *cisoid* system. These and other experiments show, as demonstrated by Donzel et al. (1972), that knowledge of the dihedral angle (*cisoid* or *transoid*) is necessary for an unequivocal assignment of helicity.

In spite of the remarkable similarities between the CD-spectra of oxytocin and the sweet tasting proteins, a different spatial arrangement exists because the long-wavelength band in oxytocin is > 250 nm in the thaumatins < 250 nm, both with a positive sign; and in monellin > 250 nm, with a negative sign. So, if we assume a *cisoid* system in oxytocin, the proteins must have a *transoid* system or vice versa.

The conclusion from the spectroscopic study of the sweet-tasting proteins thaumatin I, thaumatin II, and monellin is that they are flexible molecules and that a temperature dependent, reversible conformational change occurs involving a disulfide chromophore and probably a tyrosine residue and that the irreversible heat-induced conformational transition is responsible for the loss of sweetness.

The disulfide bond present in the molecule is probably necessary to stabilize the high degree of order in the protein, since this results from a very large number of weak interactions involving secondary valence forces and entropy effects due to the surrounding water. This high degree of order can be necessary for the protein to form a stable complex with the receptor, since the persistence of the effects of thaumatin and monellin raises the possibility that these proteins are firmly bound to taste receptor cells. As shown in Table 1, monellin is less stable to heating then the thaumatins. An explanation for this phenomenon can be the difference in the dihedral angle φ. The assumption, based on model experiments of Lude-scher and Schwyzer (1971), Donzel et al. (1972), and Urrey et al. (1968), is that in thaumatin the dihedral angle is close to $90°$ and in monellin $\neq 90°$, so the barrier to rotation about the S-S bond is higher for the thaumatins than for monellin. Only X-ray analysis can give us more detailed information on the dihedral angle φ. One of the possibilities for the binding strength is a number of hydrogen bonds, if SHALLENBERGER'S (1969) proposal that the sweet-tasting substances form complexes with the receptor by means of AH, B systems (proton donator and proton acceptor), is valid. From a number of independent studies, KIER (1973) concluded that, beside the AH, B system, a third binding site in a molecule is necessary for evoking a sweet taste sensation. In the proteins, the aromatic side chains of the amino acids tryptophan, tyrosine and phenylalanine are electron-rich. For instance, the 2-position in the indole is a π-π charge transfer donor, as is supported by molecular orbital calculations, and the phenyl ring in phenylalanine and tyrosine are susceptible to electrophilic attack. So these moieties of the molecule would probably play an important role as a third binding site, involving an electron-rich position capable of undergoing electrophilic attack, engaging in localized charge transfer. Finally, it may be expected that elucidation of the tertiary structures of these proteins will give more information to explain the mechanism of sweet-taste perception.

References

BEYCHOK, S., BRESLOW, E.: Circular dichroism of oxytocin and several oxytocin analogues. J. biol. Chem. **243**, 151—154 (1968).

CARMACK, M., NEUBERT, L. A.: Circular dichroism and the absolute configuration of the chiral disulfide group. J. Amer. chem. Soc. **89**, 7134—7136 (1967).

DONZEL, B., KAMBER, B., WÜTHRICH, K., SCHWYZER, R.: A chiral cystine disulfide group without inherent-optical activity in the long-wavelength region. Helv. chim. Acta. **55**, 947—961 (1972).

FUJINO, M., WAKIMASU, M., TANAKA, K., AOKI, H., NAKAJIMA, N.: L-aspartylamino malonic acid diesters. Naturwissenschaften **60**, 351 (1973).

KIER, L. B.: A molecular theory of sweet-taste. J. Pharm. Sci. **61**, 1394—1397 (1972).

KORVER, O., VAN GORKOM, M., VAN DER WEL, H.: Spectrometric investigation of Thaumatin I and II, two sweet-tasting proteins from *Thaumatococcus daniellii* Benth. Europ. J. Biochem. **35**, 554—558 (1973).

LUDESCHER, U., SCHWYZER, R.: On the chirality of the cystine disulfide group. Helv. chim. Acta. **54**, 1637—1644 (1971).

MORRIS, J. A., CAGAN, R. H.: Purification of monellin, the sweet principle of *Dioscoreophyllum cumminsii*. Biochem. biophys. Acta **261**, 114—122 (1972).

MORRIS, J. A., MARTENSON, R., DEIBLER, G., CAGAN, R. H.: Characterization of monellin, a protein that tastes sweet. J. biol. Chem. **248**, 534—539 (1973).

SHALLENBERGER, R. S., ACREE, T. E., LEE, C. Y.: Sweet taste of D- and L-sugars and amino acids and the steric nature of their chemo-receptor site. Nature (Lond.) **221**, 555—556 (1969).

URREY, D. W., QUADRIFOGLIO, F., WALTER, R., SCHWARTZ, I. L.: Conformational studies on neurohypophyseal hormones: the disulfide bridge of oxytocin. Proc. nat. Acad. Sci. (Wash.) **60**, 967—974 (1968).

VAN DER WEL, H.: Isolation and characterization of the sweet principle from *Dioscoreophyllum cumminsii* (Stapf) Diels. FEBS Letters **21**, 88—90 (1972).

VAN DER WEL, H., LOEVE, K.: Isolation and characterization of Thaumatin I and II, the sweet-tasting proteins from *Thaumatococcus daniellii* Benth. Europ. J. Biochem. **31**, 221—225 (1972).

VAN DER WEL, H., LOEVE, K.: Characterization of the sweet-tasting protein from *Dioscoreophyllum cumminsii* (Staph) Diels. FEBS Letters **29**, 181—184 (1973).

Discussion

E. GROSS (Bethesda, Md.): Dr. VAN DER WEL, would you please give the structure of the sweetest of sweet peptides which you mentioned in your presentation?

H. VAN DER WEL: The structure of this peptide is:

There are many other sweet-tasting dipeptide-O-esters like L-aspartyl-L-phenylalanine methylester with a sweetness intensity 100—200 times that of sucrose on a weight basis published by MAZUR et al. [MAZUR, R. H., SCHLATTER, J. M., GOLDKAMP, H. A.: J. Amer. chem. Soc. **91**, 2684 (1969). MAZUR, R. H., GOLDKAMP, H. A., JAMES, P. A., SCHLATTER, J. M.: J. med. Chem. **13**, 1217 (1970)].

L. JAENICKE (Köln): Do bacteria or insects taste the sweet protein?

H. VAN DER WEL: Until now, chemotaxis in bacteria has not been studied with respect to the sweet-tasting proteins. Neither have taste experiments been done with insects. Electrophysiological studies reveal that thaumatin and monellin elicit a significant response in the monkey, showing several characteristics that can be related to psychophysical observations in man. In the guinea pig and the rat little or no response was recorded in the *chorda tympani* and glossopharyngeal nerves [BROUWER, J. N., HELLEKANT, H., KASAHARA, Y., VAN DER WEL, H., ZOTTERMANN, Y.: Acta physiol. scand. **89**, 550 (1973)].

Sensory Transduction in Insect Olfactory Receptors*

KARL-ERNST KAISSLING

*Max-Planck-Institut für Verhaltensphysiologie, Seewiesen und Erling-Andechs,
8131 Seewiesen, Federal Republic of Germany*

With 16 Figures

Sensory transduction means the conversion of a physical or chemical stimulus into the excitation of a sensory (or receptor) cell. This process involves a number of steps which can be fully understood only by a combined effort of biophysicists, biochemists, morphologists and physiologists. To study sensory transduction it is also worthwhile to compare sensory systems adapted to different stimulus modalities, since the receptor organs differ considerably depending on their adequate form of stimulus energy.

Insects provide two main advantages for studying the transduction of olfactory stimuli: First, certain species of insects have many tens of thousands of receptor cells of one or a few types, each with a relatively uniform chemical specificity. This means that although each cell type usually responds to a number of chemical compounds, it responds maximally to a biologically important compound, *e.g.* a sexual pheromone. Secondly, the response of single insect olfactory receptor cells can be relatively easily recorded by electrophysiological methods.

The chemical analysis of bombykol, the sexual pheromone produced by the female of the silkmoth *Bombyx mori* (BUTENANDT et al., 1959, 1962; TRUSCHEIT and EITER, 1962), was followed by the identification of a large number of insect pheromones (for references see JACOBSON, 1972; PRIESNER, 1973). It also stimulated sensory physiologists to work on the mechanism of odor perception and

---

* Dedicated to PETER KARLSON, who chaired this lecture. Almost 20 years ago in Tübingen on the Neckar, he introduced his neighbour DIETRICH SCHNEIDER to ADOLF BUTENANDT and his group, thereby igniting the cooperation between a sensory physiologist and biochemists.

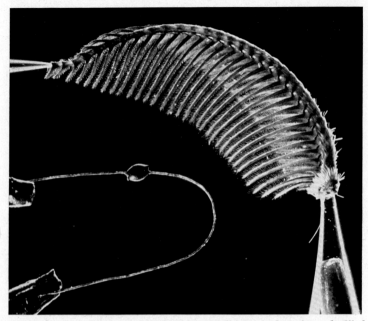

Fig. 1. Recording of the electroantennogram (EAG). A glass electrode filled with Ringer solution is inserted into each end of the antenna of *Bombyx mori*. The long olfactory hairs (sensilla trichodea, 17000 per antenna) are seen on the antennal branches. Only those on the antennal stem contribute to the EAG. The thermistor is used to measure the air stream velocity. Length of the antenna: 6 mm (original photograph)

discrimination in insects (SCHNEIDER, 1957; for references see KAISSLING, 1971). Here we will try to summarize the present state of knowledge and the hypotheses about the olfactory transducer process, illustrated mainly by studies of the male silkmoth *Bombyx mori* (see also KAISSLING, in press).

The olfactory receptor cells of insects are located on their antennae (Fig. 1) which are covered by olfactory hairs, each having an external wall surrounding the receptor lymph space and the dendritic processes of the receptor cells. The cuticular hair wall protects the dendrites from mechanical distortion, prevents water loss of the hair and allows the passage of odor molecules, probably via the numerous pores and extracellular channels connecting the outer hair surface with the receptor cell membrane (Fig. 2). Often

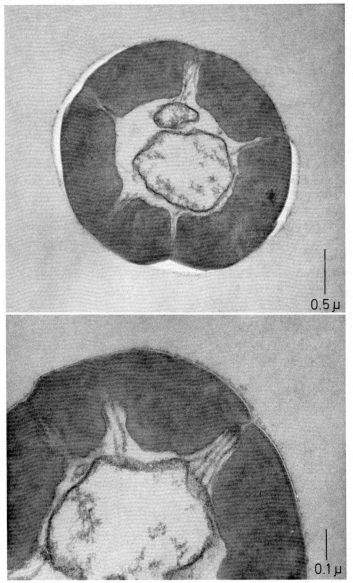

Fig. 2. Cross section of olfactory hairs of male *Bombyx mori*. The hair wall has several outer layers and contains pores and tubules (12 000 per hair) connecting with the dendrites of two receptor cells. The receptor cells are surrounded by the receptor lymph. Both cells respond to bombykol with different sensitivity. [Electron micrographs from STEINBRECHT and MÜLLER (1971)]

several receptor cells with different chemical specificities send their
dendrites into the same hair, suggesting that the hypothetical
receptor molecules (or acceptors) originate from each cell and are
probably located at the cell membrane (Schneider et al., 1964;
Kaissling, 1969; Kafka, 1970; Vareschi, 1971). In *Bombyx mori*
males, both receptor cells of the long hairs respond to bombykol.
There is no reason to assume other types of receptor molecules than
those for bombykol in these highly specialized hairs.

The interaction of the stimulus molecules with the receptor
molecules is supposed to control (probably increase) the ion conductance of the cell membrane, thereby producing a receptor
potential. The initial depolarization of a dendritic region by the
stimulus is usually thought to spread electrotonically (= passively) towards the impulse generating zone near the cell soma, where it
triggers impulse firing (Kaissling, 1971).

The transduction of the odor stimulus to the receptor potential
must involve *at least* six steps:

(1)   Adsorption. S_{gas} $\rightarrow S_{surface}$

(2)   Diffusion. $S_{surface}$ $\rightleftharpoons S_{at\ receptor\ molecules}$

(3)   Binding. $A + S_{at\ receptor\ molecules}$ $\rightleftharpoons AS$

(4)   Activation. $AS \rightleftharpoons A'S$

(5)   Increase of $A'S$ induces $\Delta G_{membrane}$
      conductance.

(6)   Early
      inactivation. $\left.\begin{array}{l} S_{surface} \\ S_{at\ receptor\ molecules} \end{array}\right\} \rightleftharpoons S_{inactive}$

In (1), the stimulus molecule is adsorbed from the air onto the
outer surface of the hair wall. The molecule then diffuses through
the channels of the hair wall (2) and binds to a receptor molecule
(A) on the cell membrane (3). It is assumed that this binding can
lead to an activation of the receptor (A'), *e.g.* a change in the state
of its conformation (4), and that this altered state induces further
changes leading to an increase in membrane conductance (5) and,
in turn, to local depolarization of the membrane. We will explain

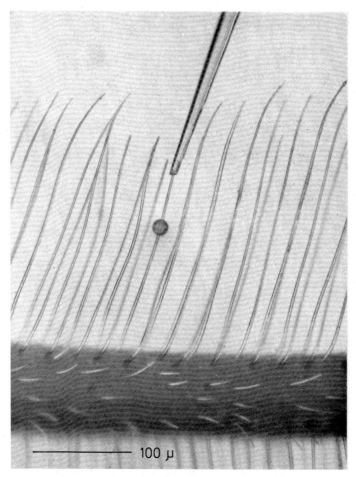

Fig. 3. Long olfactory hairs on an antennal branch of *Telea polyphemus* (Saturniidae). The tips of 5 hairs are cut off in order to get electrical contact with the Ringer solution in the capillary electrode which is slipped over one of the hairs. The odor can be locally applied through another capillary. Its mouth can be seen near the middle of the one hair. (Original photograph). This arrangement enables one to record from the two or three cells within the hair. Each of the three cells responds with maximum sensitivity to a different key compound. Correspondingly, the female seems to have at least two pheromone compounds (KAISSLING, unpublished)

below that, in addition, we must assume a fairly rapid ("early") inactivation of the odor molecule (6).

The essential metabolic destruction of the odor molecule, found by KASANG (1971), is a comparatively slow process ("late" inactivation), and is not considered as a step in the transduction. Bombykol is changed into probably two acid and at least six ester fractions (KASANG and WEISS, 1974). This process is very likely catalyzed by enzymes, and also converts 10-*trans*-hexadecenol and hexadecanol at a similar rate (50% in about 3—4 min, KASANG and KAISSLING, 1972). The breakdown of all of these compounds also occurs on female antennae which are insensitive to bombykol. A chemical conversion of odorants has been reported for other species as well (FERKO-VICH, et al., 1972, 1973; KASANG et al., 1974).

In the following part we shall discuss the experimental evidence for some of the six steps, and ask how the characteristic properties

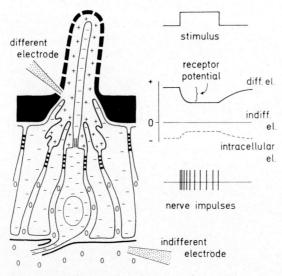

Fig. 4. Schematic diagram of an olfactory sensillum. The receptor cell is a modified epithelial cell. Its odor-sensitive outer segment is separated from the inner one by a ciliary structure. The cell (with the nucleus) sends its axon directly into the brain. The receptor cell is surrounded by auxiliary cells which generate a positive potential of the receptor lymph versus the haemolymph (THURM, 1970, 1972, 1973). Septate junctions between all the cells of the epithelium provide a high electrical resistance across the epithelium. The different electrode must have contact with the receptor lymph and records a negative receptor potential. The nerve impulses are generated near the cell soma

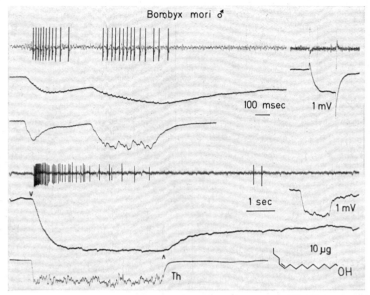

Fig. 5. Nerve impulses (Lines 1 and 4) and receptor potentials (Lines 2 and 5) of bombykol receptor cells. Airstream velocity recorded by a thermistor (Lines 3 and 6). Upper and lower experiments with two cells of the same type. Stimulus: 10 μg of 10-*cis*-tetradecen-1-ol on the odor source

of the receptor potential could be interpreted in terms of the various processes. It seems particularly interesting to discuss which of the processes could account for the compound-specific effects observed on a given type of receptor cell. The chemical specificity of a receptor cell is reflected in the stimulus-response curves which show the steady amplitude of the receptor potential *versus* the stimulus intensity for the effective compounds. Additional information on the specificity can be obtained from the time course of the receptor potential after application of stimuli with standard time course.

The stimulus, given in an air current, requires about 50 to 100 msec to reach a constant odor concentration and a somewhat shorter time to go to zero (= fresh air current) at the end of stimulation. The receptor potential starts with a minimum reaction time of about 10 msec, reaches a steady state after 50—1000 msec (depending on the stimulus intensity), and declines with a half-time of about 1 sec after the end of stimulation (Figs. 3—5). The half-time of the decline is relatively independent of the stimulus intensity but increases drastically at very high stimulus concentrations (see p. 253 and Fig. 7).

Adsorption

Tritium-labelled bombykol (10-*trans*, 12-*cis*-hexadecadien-1-ol) and 10-*trans*-hexadecen-1-ol (KASANG, 1968) as well as ^{14}C-labelled hexadecan-1-ol (Amersham) adsorb at similar rates on the antennae, whereas their effectiveness in terms of cell response differ by many $\log_{10}$ units (KASANG and KAISSLING, 1972). Therefore, adsorption is a relatively unspecific process. The number of adsorbed molecules increases in proportion to duration and concentration of the stimulus. No detectable desorption takes place within 30 min after exposure. The lack of desorption was confirmed up to the greatest stimulus concentrations used, which are more than 10^3-fold below the concentration of saturated vapor of hexadecanol (≈ 0.015 Torr at $20°$ C). At least 80% of the adsorbed molecules are caught by the antennal hairs (STEINBRECHT and KASANG, 1972), which was predicted on the basis of diffusion laws and the geometry of the hairs (ADAM and DELBRÜCK, 1968). This system is capable of concentrating the odorant by a factor of about $1.5 \cdot 10^5$ times over the concentration in the surrounding air during 1 sec of stimulation in an air current of 60 cm/sec. For this calculation we assumed homogeneous distribution of the adsorbed molecules over the total hair volume of $5 \cdot 10^{-3}$ mm^3 per antenna. Probably, the concentration is $10-100$ times higher in the outer layers of the hair wall. Capillary condensation might further increase the expected concentration in the pore tubules.

Diffusion

Molecules adsorbed on the hair wall could reach the pores by 2-dimensional surface diffusion and the cell membrane by 1-dimensional diffusion through the pore tubules. There are, so far, two ways of estimating a diffusion coefficient of bombykol on the hairs. STEINBRECHT and KASANG (1972) cut off the hairs after exposure to labelled bombykol and found a shift of the radioactivity from the hairs towards the antennal branches along the concentration gradient. This gradient is about $240 : 1$, as calculated from the initial ratio of adsorbed molecules (about $80:20$) on hairs and branches and their volume ratio (1:60). Half of the molecules left the hairs after 40 sec. This result would imply a diffusion coefficient of $5 \cdot 10^{-7} \, cm^2 \cdot sec^{-1}$. Accordingly, a molecule adsorbed at the outer hair surface should reach the dendritic membrane in an average time of about 5 msec (STEINBRECHT, 1973). It remains, however, an open question whether this value, determined at very high stimulus concentrations ($5 \cdot 10^6$ to $5 \cdot 10^7$ molecules per hair; KASANG, 1973), is valid for the thermal motion of single molecules on the hair surface. It is also not certain whether the measured shift of radioactivity occurred on the surface or within the hairs.

Another possible method of estimating diffusion time is to measure the reaction time of nerve impulses at very low stimulus concentrations; the estimate depends on the report that a single molecule should be capable of eliciting a nerve impulse (KAISSLING and PRIESNER, 1970). The average reaction time of the impulses was about 500 msec with stimuli of 1 sec duration. New experiments with brief stimuli of 100 msec revealed an average reaction time of about 200 msec. The elementary receptor potential triggering one impulse seems to start not earlier than 50 msec before the impulse (see p. 262 and Fig. 14). These results suggest $10-100$ times smaller diffusion coefficients for single molecules. The long reaction time might, however, include a considerable portion of time needed for the processes occurring between the arrival of the molecule at the end of the tubule and the opening of ion gates, *i.e.* the time necessary for finding the receptor molecule and for the intermediate steps of interaction. Even visual cells of insects can have reaction times as large as 100 msec (see p. 262).

The minimum delay of 10 msec between the onset of a strong stimulus and that of the receptor potential mentioned earlier (and found in many other sensory receptor cells) can be neglected in this context but indicates, again, unknown steps of sensory transduction.

It remains to be noted that differences in the diffusion coefficients probably do not contribute to a large extent to the specificity of the cell response, since the stimulus compounds have similar molecular weight.

Binding, Activation and Early Inactivation

These processes are still of hypothetical nature, but it is interesting to ask whether they could underly the kinetics of the receptor potential. *Binding* of stimulus molecules to receptor sites according to the mass action law was considered by BEIDLER (1954) as a basic process in chemoreception. A change of dissociation constant $[A \cdot S/(AS + A'S)]$ would shift the semilogarithmic stimulus-response curve of the receptor potential parallel to the abscissa. The ratio of inactive and *activated* receptor molecules $[AS/A'S]$ could account for differences of the saturation amplitude of the stimulus-response curve, found in olfactory organs (Fig. 8) as well as in insect taste receptors (MORITA, 1969, 1972). The early *inactivation* (Step 6) was proposed in order to explain the steady amplitude of the receptor potential during constant stimulation while the amount of adsorbed odor increases on the antenna (Fig. 6). Correspondingly, this process could explain the decay of the receptor potential after the end of the stimulus during the few seconds while the odor molecules remain on the antenna and even on the hairs (KAISSLING, 1969, 1972; KAFKA, 1970).

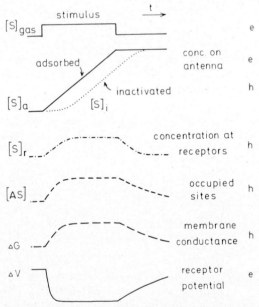

Fig. 6. Schematic time course of different parameters of some of the hypothesized (*h*) and eyperimentally verified (*e*) transducer processes in insect olfaction. For further explanation see text

This early inactivation might be a physical process, for example a translocation of the odor molecules into the receptor lymph or into the inside of
the dendrites. The odor molecules could also become bound to a carrier and
still be able to diffuse from the hairs. No chemical conversion of bombykol
could be found on isolated hairs (KASANG, 1973). An isomerization of bombykol into the less active stereo-isomers seems improbable since the isomers
themselves have to undergo inactivation,—i.e., they produce receptor
potentials similar to those of bombykol.

The mechanism of early inactivation seems to fail or become "overloaded"
if the number of molecules adsorbed on the antenna reaches a critical range
for a given stimulus compound. The half-time of the decline of the receptor
potential increases strongly for bombykol and many other compounds at
similar stimulus intensities (source of $1000\,\mu g$) if one extends the time of
stimulation to 1 sec or more (KAISSLING, 1971, 1972 and Fig. 7). This corresponds to about 10^3 or more molecules adsorbed per tubule. The prolonged

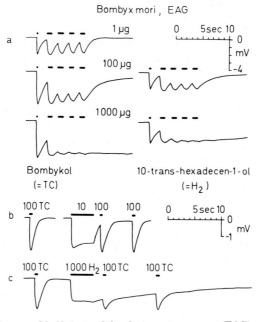

Fig. 7. (a) Increased half-times of the electroantennogram (EAG) after strong
stimulation (black bars = sequence of 5 stimuli). (b) Stimuli with 10 and
$100\,\mu g$ of bombykol (TC). (c) Stimuli with $100\,\mu g$ of bombykol on top of a
slow decline after a strong stimulus with a less effective compound ("H_2")
(a)—(c) from three antennae. The lower two traces have different mV scales.
(c) Indicates that different compounds are inactivated independently

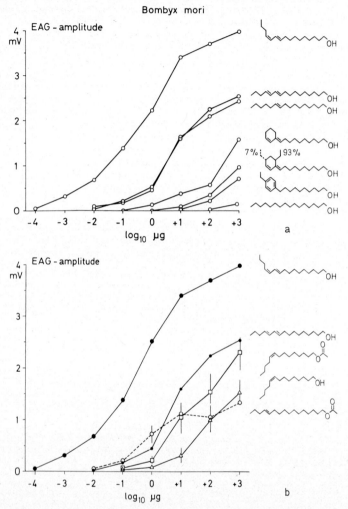

Fig. 8a and b. Stimulus-response curves of bombyx pheromone receptors to bombykol and some analogues. Ordinate: Steady amplitude of summated receptor potentials (EAG = electroantennogram). Abscissa: Stimulus intensity as load of the odor source. The release of molecules was found by means of tritium-labeled bombykol to be proportional to the load between —2 and +3. The vertical lines in (b) indicate the range of 2—10 measurements. In (a) and (b) the top curve is the response to bombykol. This curve was measured first (in mV) and was taken as a standard. The responses to the other

decline could be interpreted by way of a reversible early inactivation which gives a significant backward reaction only with strong stimuli.

Figure 7 c shows that a bombykol stimulus produces about the same total depolarization and half-time of decline, whether it is given alone or on top of

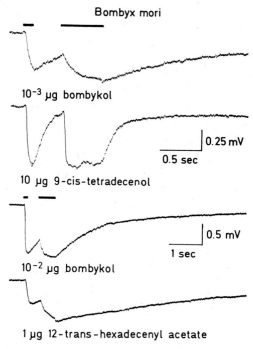

Bombyx mori

10^{-3} µg bombykol

0.25 mV
0.5 sec

10 µg 9-cis-tetradecenol

0.5 mV
1 sec

10^{-2} µg bombykol

1 µg 12-trans-hexadecenyl acetate

Fig. 9. EAG's of one antenna showing different half-times of the decline after the end of stimulus (black bar = stimulus). This may suggest compound-specific velocities of the early inactivation. Upper and lower two traces with different scales. The reaction times and time courses of the EAG's are qualitatively similar to those of the receptor potentials in single cell recordings, but show significant differences especially for weak stimuli with bombykol (compare Fig. 12)

---

compounds were always compared with alternated bombykol responses and normalized to the standard curve. The cyclic compounds (called cyclo-bombykols) were prepared by Dr. SCHUDEL et al. from Givaudan-Esrolko in Zürich, Switzerland. Dr. E. PRIESNER kindly provided me with the 3 additional compounds in (b). The structural formulae are given in the same order as the maximum responses, respectively

the slow decline after a very strong stimulus of 10-*trans*-hexadecenol. Consequently, the two compounds seem to act competitively at the receptors and to be inactivated independently. Many analogs of bombykol behave similarly. Other compounds stimulate the cell and inhibit responses to bombykol stimuli (*e.g.* some amines, see KAISSLING, 1972). Such compounds also produce "normal" receptor potentials (and nerve impulses, unpublished) and, therefore, would undergo early inactivation. This fact and the above-mentioned independence of different compounds with respect to their inactivation could be explained if the early inactivation is a translocation of the odorant away from the receptors by diffusion.

All three processes discussed above (binding, activation, inactivation) seem to have their own specificity to the stimulus compounds. We see considerable shifts of the stimulus response curves parallel to the abscissa and curves with smaller saturation maxima (Fig. 8). There are compounds giving shorter or longer lifetimes of the receptor potential in the electroantennogram (EAG) (ROELOFS and COMEAU, 1972 b), as well as in single-cell recordings possibly indicating different velocities of the inactivation process (Figs. 9 and 12).

Quantitative Interpretation of the Receptor Potential

In interpreting receptor potentials as controlled by molecular processes, one has to keep in mind the nonlinear relationship between conductance and voltage to be expected in chemoreceptors as in other sense or nerve cells (MORITA, 1969). Theoretically, a stimulus response curve can be hyperbolic, having thus the same shape as the underlying binding curve in the semilogarithmic plot, but must have its half-saturation at stimulus concentrations lower than necessary for half-maximal binding. The stimulus-response curve can have, in addition, a flatter shape due to intensity-dependent changes of the cable properties of the long olfactory dendrite (KAISSLING, 1971) and due to spatial nonuniformities (THORSON and BIEDERMANN-THORSON, 1974). Indeed, most of the olfactory stimulus response curves show a flatter shape than the hyperbolic function (or adsorption isotherm, Fig. 10). In this context one might recall that, similarly, half bleaching of rhodopsin occurs at much higher light intensities than the half-maximum amplitude of the receptor potential in visual receptor cells (CONE, 1965; DÖRR-SCHEIDT-KÄFER, 1972). Considering the unknown electrical parameters of the olfactory cells, it seems impossible at present to determine quantitatively how binding, activation and early in-activation processes would each contribute to the response charac-teristics of olfactory cells for a given stimulus compound.

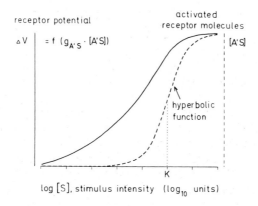

Fig. 10. Shows that the receptor potential of chemoreceptors reaches half-saturation at stimulus concentrations lower than those needed for half-saturation of receptor molecules. The stimulus-response of olfactory receptors is often found to be flatter than the hyperbolic binding curve. This could partially be explained by a change of cable properties during stimulation (see KAISSLING, 1971)

Because of these complications we can give only a rough estimate of the odor concentration at the receptors necessary for half-maximum saturation $(A = AS + A'S = A_{\text{tot}}/2)$. We assume that the rate of early inactivation $(k_i \cdot S_R)$ equals the adsorption rate per volume $(N_{\text{eff}a} \cdot f \cdot v_h^{-1} \cdot \sec^{-1})$ under steady state conditions *i.e.* with constant stimulus concentration and constant receptor potential amplitude. The following equation allows to calculate the odor concentration S_R at the receptor molecules:

$$S_R = \frac{N_{\text{eff}a} \cdot f}{\sec \cdot v_h \cdot k_i}$$

k_i is the velocity of the early inactivation $(S_R \xrightarrow{k_i} S_{\text{inactive}})$ which can be estimated from the decay of the receptor potential as to be $2.3 \cdot \sec^{-1}$ (KAISSLING, in press)

$N_{\text{eff}a} \cdot \sec^{-1}$ is the number of molecules absorbed by the 17 000 hairs per antenna and per sec

v_h is the total volume of the hairs of $5 \cdot 10^{-3}$ mm^3

f is the factor by which S_R is higher than with homogeneous distribution of the adsorbed molecules over the hair. We set $f = 100$ (compare p . . .).

Half maximum receptor potential (EAG) is reached with about $5 \cdot 10^{-1}$ µg of bombykol (Fig. 8). This corresponds to $N_{eff_a} = 1.1 \cdot 10^8$ for one sec according to measurements with radioactively labeled bombykol (KAISSLING and PRIESNER, 1970; KAISSLING, 1971). We arrive at $S_R = 1.6 \cdot 10^{-6}$ Mol $\cdot$ l^{-1} for half maximum response. The odor concentration necessary for half-maximal saturation of the receptors might even be higher than this value (KAISSLING, in press). This rough estimation shows that the extraordinary sensitivity of olfactory cells could be reached with dissociation constants similar to those found in other systems, e.g. the enzyme-substrate reaction.

Very briefly we want to mention that various attempts have been made to correlate molecular parameters of the stimulus molecules with their effectiveness. Figures 8 a and b show that alterations with respect to the double bonds, to the functional group and to the non-polar portion of the molecule change the stimulus response curve in various ways.

In noctuid moths, systematic alterations in chain length and double bond position of mono-unsaturated acetates produce relatively small changes in effectiveness (Fig. 11) and indicate, for example, that the distance from the double bond to the nonpolar end of the molecule is more critical for the EAG-response than the distance to the polar portion (PRIESNER, 1973). Similar data from another noctuid species have been used to generate a model for the binding of the odorant to the receptor molecule, assuming a three-point attachment by weak, non-covalent interactions (NEUWIRTH, 1973; KAFKA, in press). The purpose of this model was to explain quantitatively the specificity of the molecular binding, assuming that the relative stimulus concentrations needed for a standard EAG-response correspond to the relative dissociation constants of the odorant-receptor complexes.

Other investigators have proposed a four-point attachment for the red-banded leaf roller pheromone (cis-11-tetradecenyl acetate), based on behavioral and EAG data (ROELOFS and COMEAU, 1971 a and b). A striking example that suggests binding mainly at certain regions (e.g. the two ends) of the odor molecule is the alarm-pheromone undecane, which is about 10^3 times as effective as decane or dodecane for olfactory cells of the ant Lasius fuliginosus (DUM-PERT, 1972; KAFKA, in press).

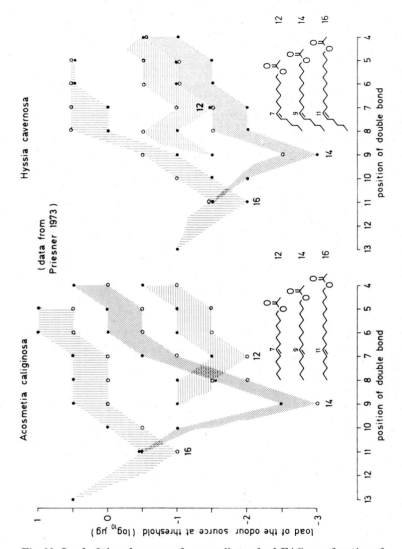

Fig. 11. Load of the odor source for a small standard EAG as a function of double bond position in a 12, 14, and 16 carbon chain. The compounds are *cis*-(●) and *trans*-(o) isomers of mono-unsaturated acetates. The structural formula of the most effective compound is given for each chain length. From EAG measurements in two species of moths. (Data from PRIESNER, JACOBSON and BESTMANN, cited in PRIESNER, 1973)

Membrane Conductance

It was suggested earlier that a change in the amount of membrane conductance per activated receptor molecule ($g_{A'S}$) would also change the stimulus-response curve and could, therefore, contribute to the specificity of the cell response (KAISSLING, 1972).

This effect is obvious for the simplest model of conductance increase ($\Delta G_{\text{membrane}}$), which could be described for the steady response amplitude by

$$\Delta G_{\text{membrane}} = g_{A'S} \cdot A'S .$$

Recent experiments suggest that, indeed, $g_{A'S}$ can be compound-specific. With weak stimuli ($10^{-2}\,\mu g$ on the odor source) of bombykol, there results a very irregular time course of the receptor potential and, correspondingly, irregular impulse firing. These fluctu-

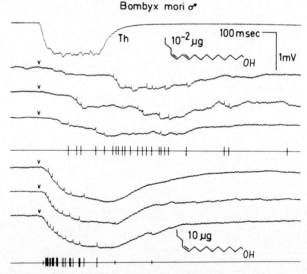

Bombyx mori ♂

Fig. 12. Single cell recording of receptor potentials and nerve impulses. Upper line (Th): Airstream velocity recorded by a thermistor. The upper three traces show three fluctuating responses and irregular impulse firing to bombykol. The lower three traces show smooth receptor potentials and more regular impulse firing with a 1000 times stronger stimulus of 10-*cis*-tetradecen-1-ol. The impulses of each group of three traces are added on a separate line, respectively

ations may be produced by elementary receptor potentials induced by single molecules. The same cell shows a similarly fluctuating response pattern with a 10^4 times stronger stimulus of cyclo-bombykol, but a very smooth receptor potential and regular spike firing with a 10^3-fold concentrated stimulus of cis-10-tetradecen-1-ol (Fig. 12). The small effectiveness of cyclobombykol could, for example, be due to a small affinity for the receptor molecule or a smaller fraction of occupied receptors switching into the activated state $A'S$ while the $g_{A'S}$ remains "normal". The smooth time course of the (small) cis-10-tetradecenol response, however, could be explained by a high affinity and numerous activated receptor molecules but a small conductance change per activated receptor $g_{A'S}$. The large number of small superimposed elementary receptor potentials would, of course, smooth out the receptor potential.

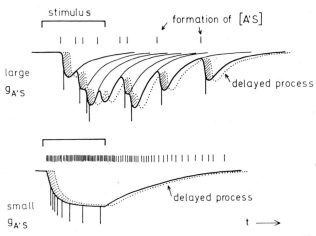

Fig. 13. Schematic diagram of the two response types shown in Fig. 12. Above: a few $A'S$-complexes are formed, and each produces a large elementary receptor potential capable of eliciting a nerve impulse. Below: Many $A'S$-complexes are formed due to higher stimulus concentration, higher binding affinity or more activation. Each $A'S$-complex elicits only a small elementary receptor potential (not shown in the diagram). Many superimposed potentials produce a smooth time course. A delayed process could explain the differentiation between receptor potential and impulse frequency often found in sensory receptors

More regular responses can also be obtained with bombykol at high stimulus concentrations. The intervals between nerve impulses vary less where the smooth type of receptor potential is observed (Figs. 12 and 13).

The elementary receptor potential could theoretically be briefer or smaller, or both, depending on the life-time or the extent of opening of ion gates. KATZ and MILEDI (1972, 1973) showed that the life-times of single ion channels in motor endplates differ for various transmitter analogues.

Small transient potential changes as recorded in *Bombyx mori* and saturniid moths often occur along with a single nerve impulse and can be considered as elementary receptor potentials (Fig. 14). The amplitude reaches $200-300\mu$V, and the duration is about 100 msec or more. Elementary potentials of $0.5-2.5$ mV and about $30-40$ msec half-width have been found in retinula cells of locusts and flies (SCHOLES, 1965; KIRSCHFELD, 1966). These "bumps" occurred with a considerable latency of $20-150$ msec in the locust and about 20 msec in the fly, after a brief light flash containing single or a few quanta per visual cell. These sensory potentials differ markedly from the minute depolarizations of muscle end-plates, the latter being about $0.3\,\mu$V in amplitude and 1 msec in duration (KATZ and MILEDI, 1972). In spite of these differences, the conductance increase per ion channel seems to be of the same order — about $10^{-10}\,\Omega^{-1}$ in sensory as well as in end-plate potentials. We recalculated this value using a cable equation for the olfactory cell (derived by J. THORSON, see KAISSLING, 1971 and Appendix).

Values of the order of $10^{-10}\,\Omega^{-1}$ have also been given for sodium gates in lobster axons (HILLE, 1970) and for lipid bilayers modified by the bacterial protein EIM (BEAN et al., 1969). One may conclude from all of these estimates that the conductance is much more constant than the life-time in such systems. This "elementary" conductance change could suggest similar dimensions of molecular ion gates. Some pores have variable conductances (BOHEIM, 1974).

It seems worth mentioning that the reaction times of the various elementary responses vary in correspondence with the durations of the respective potentials—that is, from 1 msec in synapses to the order of 10 msec or even a hundred msec in sensory cells.

Fluctuating and smooth olfactory receptor potentials have also been found in saturniid moths by using only slightly altered molecules (KAISSLING, unpublished). By assaying over many stimulus compounds, one should be able to distinguish between those molecular properties of the ligand more important for the binding to the receptor molecule and those controlling its activation and, consequently, the conductance mechanism. For instance, different intramolecular distances of the stimulus compound could

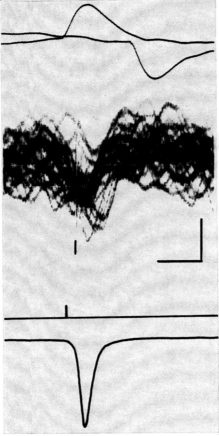

Fig. 14. Middle: 30 photographically superimposed elementary olfactory receptor potentials, triggered by means of the elicited nerve impulse (at the small vertical bar). Scale 100 msec, 100 μV. AC-recording from *Telea poly-phemus* (cf. Fig. 3). Above: Two traces produced each by a rectangular voltage step for showing the distortion of the signal by the AC-amplification. Below: Averaged elementary receptor potentials of a retinula cell of the fly *Musca* (0.5—2.5 mV amplitude and same time scale as middle and above). The stimulus was a light flash of 6—8 μsec (vertical bar on the horizontal line). (After KIRSCHFELD, 1966)

be differently involved in binding and activation. The molecule
could, for example, first be attached by two particular points to the
appropriate sites of the receptor and then induce activation by
attracting a third site. Such speculations are invited by the idea
of a few-point attachment between ligand and receptor, and might
justify further experiments in this direction.

This few-point idea was established for the enzyme-substrate interaction
(OGSTON, 1948). The above-mentioned suggestion that binding and increase
of conductance could depend on different parts of the ligand molecule recalls
the findings on the specificity of purified horse-liver carboxylesterase (WEBB,
1966). The substrates were saturated straight-chain esters with systematically
altered chain length of the alkyl and acyl groups. An optimum of reactivity
(measured as maximum velocity of the enzyme reaction) was obtained with
4 carbons in the acyl group for esters with a total number of 7, 8, 9, and
10 carbon atoms. The affinity, however, was largely independent of the
reactivity. This example shows clearly that different molecular properties of
the ligand can control different steps of the interaction with a macromolecule.

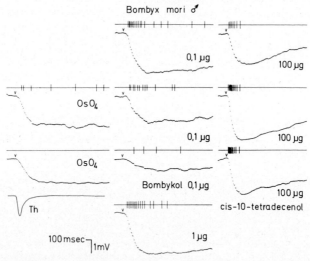

Fig. 15. 9 responses of a single bombykol receptor, nerve impulses and receptor potentials. Above: Two control stimuli of bombykol and *cis*-10 tetradecen-
1-ol. Second row: 0.1 sec vapor of OsO_4 and the two compounds. Third
row the same sequence repeated. The OsO_4 blocks preferentially the response
to bombykol. After OsO_4, 1 µg of bombykol elicits a response similar to that
of 0.1 µg in the beginning. Stimulus duration 0.1 sec. Air stream velocity was
registered by a thermistor (Th)

In addition to varying the structure of the stimulus compounds, one could try to find appropriate inhibitors for the olfactory response. A very brief exposure of the antenna to the vapor of OsO_4 reduces preferentially the response to bombykol but leaves unchanged the response to 10-*cis*-tetradecenol (Fig. 15). Likewise, the response of female olfactory cells in *Bombyx* to linalool found by Priesner (cited in Boeckh et al., 1965) belongs to the smooth type and is relatively insensitive to OsO_4. Therefore, the working hypothesis is proposed that there are inhibitors which act specifically on the conductance changing mechanism.

The transduction of olfactory stimuli into physiological excitation appears as a cascade of molecular events each having different specificity. This system seems to be appropriate to improve the degree of chemical specificity of the cell response.

Summary

A minimum of six steps must be considered within the transduction of the olfactory stimulus to the receptor potential: 1) adsorption on the antennal surface, 2) diffusion to receptor molecules, 3) binding, and 4) activation (*e.g.* a conformational change) of the receptor molecule, 5) change of membrane conductance and 6) early inactivation of the odor molecule (Fig. 16). Adsorption and diffusion seem to be rather unspecific with respect to the stimulus compound. All other steps may be compound-specific and contribute in various proportions to the chemical specificity of the cell response. This is suggested by differences of the stimulus-response curves as well as of the time course of the receptor potential. Elementary receptor potentials occurring along with single nerve impulses can be observed during weak stimulation with some compounds (amplitude $200-300\,\mu V$, duration about 100 msec). These depolarizations correspond to a change of membrane conductance of the order of $10^{-10}\,\Omega^{-1}$ as found in various ion gating systems, including end-plates. The time course of the receptor potential can fluctuate or appear relatively smooth. Such differences probably depend on larger or smaller sizes and numbers of elementary responses specific to the stimulus compound.

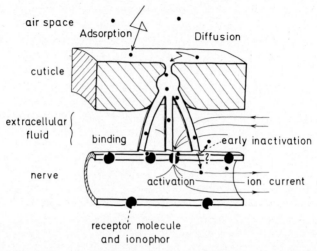

Fig. 16. Schematic view of the structures involved in sensory transduction in an olfactory hair. It may be possible for the molecules to reach the nerve membrane without leaving the lipophilic phase, which could be continued from the outer surface *via* the pore tubules. The early inactivation might be a diffusion into the extracellular receptor lymph. The picture shows 11 molecules adsorbed per three pore tubules. This would correspond to a stimulus of 1 sec using about 3 μg bombykol on the odor source (compare Fig. 8). Nothing is known so far about the nature, number and distribution of receptor molecules and about the ion gating mechanism and its connection with the receptor molecules

Acknowledgements

I would like to thank Miss TRAUDL RIMBECK and URSULA RAGER for technical help, Mrs. CAMILLA ZACK, Dr. GÜNTER GROSS, Dr. ERNST KRAMER, Dr. HERMANN, Z. LEVINSON, Dr. D. SCHNEIDER and, especially, Dr. JOHN THORSON for their critical comments on the manuscript.

References

ADAM, G., DELBRÜCK, M.: Reduction of dimensionality in biological diffusion processes. In: RICH, A., DAVIDSON, N. (Eds.): Struct. chem. and molec. biology, pp. 198—215. San Francisco-London: Freeman Co. 1968.

BEAN, R. C., SHEPHARD, W. C., CLAN, H., EICHNER, J.: Discrete conductance fluctuations in lipid bilayer protein membranes. J. gen. Physiol. **53**, 741—757 (1969).

BEIDLER, L. M.: A theory of taste stimulation. J. gen. Physiol. **38**, 133—139 (1954).

BOECKH, J., KAISSLING, K.-E., SCHNEIDER, D.: Insect olfactory receptors. Cold Spr. Harb. Symp. quant. Biol. **30**, 263—280 (1965).

BOHEIM, G.: Statistical analysis of alamethicin channels in black lipid membranes. J. Membrane Biol. (1974, in press).

BUTENANDT, A., BECKMANN, R., STAMM, D., HECKER, E.: Über den Sexuallockstoff des Seidenspinners *Bombyx mori*. Reindarstellung und Konstitution. Z. Naturforsch. **14** b, 283—284 (1959).

BUTENANDT, A., HECKER, E., KOCH, W.: Über den Sexuallockstoff des Seidenspinners. IV. Liebigs Ann. Chem. **658**, 39—64 (1962).

CONE, R. A.: The early receptor potential of the vertebrate eye. Cold Spr. Harb. Symp. quant. Biol. **30**, 483—491 (1965).

DÖRRSCHEIDT-KÄFER, M.: Die Empfindlichkeit einzelner Photoreceptoren im Komplexauge von *Calliphora erythrocephala*. J. comp. Physiol. **81**, 309—340 (1972).

DUMPERT, K.: Alarmstoffrezeptoren auf der Antenne von *Lasius fuliginosus* (Latr.) (Hymenoptera, Formicidae). Z. vergl. Physiol. **76**, 403—425 (1972).

FERKOVICH, S. M., MAYER, M. S., RUTTER, R. R.: Conversion of the sex pheromone of the cabbage looper. Nature (Lond.) New Biol. **242**, 53—55 (1972).

FERKOVICH, S. M., MAYER, M. S., RUTTER, R. R.: Sex pheromone of the cabbage looper: Reactions with antennal proteins *in vitro*. J. Insect Physiol. **19**, 2231—2243 (1973).

HILLE, B.: Ionic channels in nerve membranes. Progr. Biophys. molec. Biol. **21**, 1—32 (1970).

JACOBSON, M.: Insect sex pheromones, p. 382. New York: Academic Press 1972.

KAFKA, W. A.: Physiochemical aspects of odor recognition in insects. Ann. N. Y. Acad. Sci. (in press). See also this volume.

KAFKA, W. A.: Analyse der molekularen Wechselwirkung bei der Erregung einzelner Riechzellen. Z. vergl. Physiol. **70**, 105—143 (1970).

KAISSLING, K.-E.: Kinetics of olfactory receptor potentials. In: PFAFFMANN (Ed.): III. Int. Symp. Olfaction and Taste, pp. 52—70. New York: Rockefeller Univ. Press 1969.

KAISSLING, K.-E.: Insect olfaction. In: BEIDLER, L. M. (Ed.): Handbook of sensory physiology IV/1, pp. 351—431. Berlin-Heidelberg-New York: Springer 1971.

KAISSLING, K.-E.: Kinetic studies on olfactory receptors of *Bombyx mori*. In: SCHNEIDER, D. (Ed.): Intern. Symp. Olfaction and Taste, pp. 207—213. Stuttgart: Wiss. Verlagsges. 1972.

KAISSLING, K.-E.: Chemoreception in the olfactory system. In: SCHMITT, F. O. (Ed.): Functional linkage in biomolecular system New York: Raven Press (in press).

KAISSLING, K.-E.: Sensorische Transduktion bei Riechzellen von Insekten. 68. Verh. Deutsche Zool. Ges., RATHMEYER, W. (Ed.), (1974, in press).

KAISSLING, K.-E., PRIESNER, E.: Die Riechschwelle des Seidenspinners. Naturwissenschaften **57**, 23—28(1970).

KASANG, G.: Tritium-Markierung des Sexuallockstoffes Bombykol. Z. Naturforsch. **23** b, 1331—1335 (1968).

KASANG,G.: Bombykol reception and metabolism on the antennae of the silkmoth *Bombyx mori*. In: OHLOFF,G., THOMAS,A.F. (Eds.): Gustation and olfaction, pp. 245—250. London-New York: Academic Press 1971.

KASANG,G.: Physikochemische Vorgänge beim Riechen des Seidenspinners. Naturwissenschaften **60**, 95—101 (1973).

KASANG,G., KAISSLING,K.-E.: Specificity of primary and secondary olfactory processes in *Bombyx* antennae. In: SCHNEIDER,D. (Ed.): IV. Intern. Symp. Olfaction and Taste, pp. 200—206. Stuttgart: Wiss. Verlagsges. 1972.

KASANG,G., KNAUER,B., BEROZA,M.: Uptake of the sex attractant ^{3}H-disparlure by male gypsy moth antennae (*Lymantria dispar = Porthetria dispar*). Experientia (Basel) **30**, 147 (1974).

KASANG,G., WEISS,N.: Dünnschichtchromatographische Analyse radioaktiv markierter Insektenpheromone. Metaboliten des ^{3}H-Bombykols. J. Chromatog. **92**, 401—417 (1974).

KATZ,B., MILEDI,R.: The statistical nature of the acetylcholine potential and its molecular components. J. Physiol. (Lond.) **224**, 665—699 (1972).

KATZ,B., MILEDI,R.: The characteristics of "end-plate noise" produced by different depolarizing drugs. J. Physiol. (Lond.) **230**, 707—717 (1973).

KIRSCHFELD,K.: Discrete and graded receptor potentials in the compound eye of the fly (*Musca*). Proc. Int. Symp. The Functional Organization of the Compound Eye, pp. 291—307. Oxford: Pergamon Press 1966.

MORITA,H.: Electrical signs of taste receptor activity. In: PFAFFMANN,C. (Ed.): III. Intern. Symp. Olfaction and Taste, pp. 370—381. New York: Rockefeller Univ. Press 1969.

MORITA,H.: Properties of the sugar receptor site of the blowfly. In: SCHNEIDER,D. (Ed.): IV. Intern. Symp. Olfaction and Taste, pp. 357—363. Stuttgart: Wiss. Verlagsges. 1972.

NEUWIRTH,J.: Multiple-site Wechselwirkung zwischen Duftmolekülen und Akzeptoren. Diplomarbeit an der Technischen Univ. München, Physik-Department. E 10, 60 p. (1973).

OGSTON,A.G.: Interpretation of experiments on metabolic processes, using isotopic tracer elements. Nature (Lond.) **162**, 963 (1948).

PRIESNER,E.: Artspezifität und Funktion einiger Insektenpheromone. Fortschr. Zool. **22**, 49—135 (1973).

PRIESNER,E., JACOBSON,M., BESTMANN,H.J.: Structure and electrophysiological activity of noctuid sex pheromones and analogues—an introductory report. Z. Naturforsch., in press.

ROELOFS,W.L., COMEAU,A.: Sex pheromone perception: Synergists and inhibitors for the red-banded leaf roller attractant. J. Insect Physiol. **17**, 435—448 (1971a).

ROELOFS,W.L., COMEAU,A.: Sex pheromone perception:Electroantennogram response of the red-banded leaf roller moth. J. Insect Physiol. **17**, 1969—1982 (1971b).

SCHNEIDER,D.: Elektrophysiologische Untersuchungen von Chemo- und Mechanorezeptoren der Antenne des Seidenspinners *Bombyx mori* L. Z. vergl. Physiol. **40**, 8—41 (1957).

SCHNEIDER, D., LACHER, V., KAISSLING, K.-E.: Die Reaktionsweise und das Reaktionsspektrum von Riechzellen bei *Antheraea pernyi* (Lepidoptera, Saturniidae). Z. vergl. Physiol. **48**, 632—662 (1964).

SCHOLES, J.: Discontinuity of the excitation process in locust visual cells. Cold Spr. Harb. Symp. quant. Biol. **30**, 517—527 (1965).

STEINBRECHT, R. A.: Der Feinbau olfaktorischer Sensillen des Seidenspinners (Insecta, Lepidoptera). Z. Zellforsch. **139**, 533—565 (1973).

STEINBRECHT, R. A., MÜLLER, B.: On the stimulus conducting structures in insect olfactory receptors. Z. Zellforsch. **117**, 570—575 (1971).

STEINBRECHT, R. A., KASANG, G.: Capture and conveyance of odour molecules in an insect olfactory receptor. In: SCHNEIDER, D. (Ed.): IV. Intern. Symp. Olfaction and Taste, pp. 193—199. Stuttgart: Wiss. Verlagsges. 1972.

THORSON, J., BIEDERMAN-THORSON, M.: Distributed relaxation processes in sensory adaptation. Science **183**, 161—172 (1974).

THURM, U.: Untersuchungen zur funktionellen Organisation sensorischer Zellverbände. Verh. dtsch. Zool. Ges. Köln, 79—88 (1970).

THURM, U.: The generation of receptor potentials in epithelial receptors. In: SCHNEIDER, D. (Ed.): IV. Symp. Olfaction and taste, pp. 95—101. Stuttgart: Wiss. Verlagsges. 1972.

THURM, U.: Basics of the generation of receptor potentials in epidermal mechanoreceptors on insects. "Mechanoreception" Symposium, Bochum SCHWARTZKOPFF, J. (Ed.): Abh. d. Rhein. Westfäl. Akademie der Wiss. Opladen: Westdeutscher Verlag (1974, in press).

TRUSCHEIT, E., EITER, K.: Synthese der vier isomeren Hexadecadien-(10, 12)-ole-(1). Liebigs Ann. Chem. **658**, 65—90 (1962).

VARESCHI, E.: Duftunterscheidung bei der Honigbiene—Einzelzell-Ableitungen und Verhaltensreaktionen. Z. vergl. Physiol. **75**, 143—173 (1971).

WEBB, E. C.: Cited in DIXON, M., WEBB, E. C.: Enzymes, p. 218ff. London: Longmans, Green & Co. 1966.

Appendix

Calculation of the Increase in Membrane Conductance $g_{A's}$ Produced by a Single Bombykol Molecule

The following cable equation allowing the calculation of $g_{A's}$ was derived by THORSON on the basis of the receptor cell model of THURM (1970, 1972, 1973) (see KAISSLING, 1971). The outer and inner dendrites of the receptor cell are represented by the cylindric cables 1 and 2. ΔV and ΔV_{max} are receptor potentials at the junction of the two cables

$$\frac{\Delta V}{\Delta V_{max}} = 1 - \frac{\dfrac{1}{r_1 \cdot \lambda_{1r}} \cdot \tanh\left(\dfrac{l_1}{\lambda_{1r}}\right) + \dfrac{1}{r_2 \cdot \lambda_2 + R_a}}{\dfrac{1}{r_1 \cdot \lambda_{1e}} \cdot \tanh\left(\dfrac{l_1}{\lambda_{1e}}\right) + \dfrac{1}{r_2 \cdot \lambda_2 + R_a}}.$$

The following equations have been used:

$$r_1 = \frac{\varrho_p}{\pi\, a_1^2} \cdot \frac{a_1'^2}{(a_1'^2 - a_1^2)} \qquad r_2 = \frac{\varrho_p}{\pi\, a_2^2} \quad [\Omega \cdot \mathrm{cm}^{-1}]$$

$$\lambda_{1r} = \sqrt{\frac{a_1}{2}\left(1 - \frac{a_1^2}{a_1'^2}\right)\frac{1}{\varrho_p \cdot G_m}} \qquad \lambda_2 = \sqrt{\frac{a_2}{2 \cdot \varrho_p \cdot G_m}} \quad [\mathrm{cm}]$$

$$\lambda_{1e} = \sqrt{\frac{a_1}{2}\left(1 - \frac{a_1^2}{a_1'^2}\right)\frac{1}{\varrho_p \cdot \left(G_m + \frac{g_{A'S}}{2\,\pi\, a_1\, l_1}\right)}} \quad [\mathrm{cm}]$$

$$\varrho_p = \frac{R_h}{l_1}\,\pi\,(a_1'^2 - a_1^2) \qquad\qquad [\Omega \cdot \mathrm{cm}].$$

ϱp was calculated from R_h, l_1, a_1, and a'_1 for the receptor lymph. All other specific plasma and lymph resistances were assumed to be equal to ϱp (75 Ωcm).

The following parameters have been used for the calculation:

ΔV $= 200-300\,\mu\mathrm{V}$ amplitude of the elementary receptor potential,

$\Delta V_{\max} = 20-30\,\mathrm{mV}$ maximum amplitude of the receptor potential,

R_h $\approx 2 \cdot 10^8\,\Omega$ extracellulary resistance of the hair from tip to base,

R_a $\approx 2 \cdot 10^8\,\Omega$ resistance from the hair base across the epithelium,

G_m $= 10^{-3}\,\Omega^{-1}\,\mathrm{cm}^{-2}$ assumed specific conductance of the cell membranes,

l_1 $= 100\,\mu$ length | of the outer dendrite
$2a_1$ $= 0.4\,\mu$ diameter ∫ (Cable 1),

l_2 $= \infty$ length | approximations for the inner
$2a_2$ $= 1.1\,\mu$ diameter ∫ dendrite (Cable 2),

$2a'_1$ $= 0.8\,\mu$ inner diameter of the hair.

[l_1, a_1, a_2, a'_1 are based on measurements from STEINBRECHT (1973)].

Discussion

H. E. HUMMEL (Urbana, Ill.): Dr. KAISSLING, in the abstract of your paper [Hoppe-Sayler's Z. Physiol. Chem. **355**, 108 (1974) you mention electrophysiological observations, suggesting the two geometrical isomers of the female *Pectinophora gossypiella* sex pheromone gossyplure interact with different sensory cell types on the male antenna.

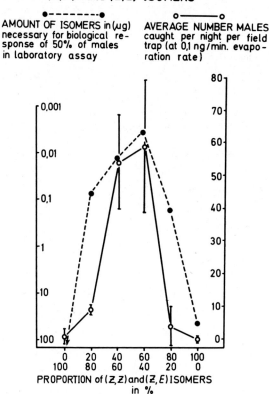

Behavioral bioassays performed in collaboration with the research groups of Dr. SHOREY and Dr. SILVERSTEIN [see HUMMEL et al.: Science **181**, 873—875 (1973); Chemical Ecology **1** (1975) (in press)] indicate relatively low behavioral activity in response to stimulation with the pure 7,11-(Z,Z)-and

7,11-(Z,E)-hexadecadienyl acetate (Isomers 1 and 2, respectively) alone (see Fig. 1). However, when Isomer 1 and 2 are combined in various proportions, significantly enhanced biological activity of 4 powers of ten and more is observed with the maximum effect in the vicinity of a 50:50 isomer ratio. Biological responses of 50% of the male moths were observed ($\bar{x} = 10$ experiments with 10 males each) with a pheromone stimulus as low as 5×10^{-3} μg. In the cotton field, in a series of 8 nights, 60 ± 20 males were caught per night per trap at 0.1 nanogram evaporation rate per min. Although the laboratory bioassay measures close-range sexual activation of caged pink bollworm males, and the field traps evaluate long-range flight attraction of males towards the sex pheromone source, both assay techniques yield curves of surprisingly similar shape.

Could you observe a similar proportion-dependent enhancement effect with the electrophysiological assay technique and, if so, at what level of pheromone concentration? Would you, in order to explain this effect mechanistically, rather favour the assumption that discrimination of Isomers 1 and 2 occurs exclusively at the antennal receptor level?

Could one, at the present time, rule out the existence of two (or more) independently firing information channels with possible integration steps build in at the CNS level? A more general view of this matter would be helpful in understanding similar phenomena most recently described for other insect species as well [see for example KLUN et al.: Sience 181, 661—663 (1973)].

K.-E. KAISSLING: Many thoroughly investigated species of insects do not produce only one pheromone compound, but rather a mixture of two or more chemically similar compounds. Only a certain ratio of the compound in the mixture fully attracts the males of a given species [see for instance TAMAKI et al.: Kontyu 39, 338—340, (1971); KLUN et al.: Ann. Entomol. Soc, Amer. 65, 11337—1340, (1972); MEIJER et al.: Science 175, 1469—1470, (1972); HUMMEL et al.: Science 181, 873—875, (1973)]. Single cell recordings in two species of Saturniid moths (*Telea plyphemus* and *Antheraea pernyi*; KAISSLING, unpublished) and in the Tortricid moth *Adoxophyes orana* (DEN OTTER, unpublished) show that the male insect has two or more types of receptor cells which respond maximally to two (or more) respective pheromone compounds. These experiments support the suggestion that the effects of several pheromone components are integrated by the CNS. An integration by the same receptor cell seems improbable if stimuli in the order of one or less moleculess adsorbed per cell are sufficient to elicit behavioral responses.

P. KARLSON (Marburg): This could also be a question of evolution. One may consider a specialized system such as the bombykol system as incapable of further evolution, because this would require simultaneous mutations of the synthetic *and* the receptor systems. It is extremely improbable that this would occur and lead to an improved pheromone.

P. SUNDER-PLASSMANN (Münster): How are the afferent olfactory fibres centrally connected? Is there a topical representation of the sense as found in the optic system?

K.-E. KAISSLING: The olfactory receptor cells of insects as in the vertebrates are primary sensory which send their axons directly into the brain. Topical representation is only reported for the gustatory system of vertebrates. On the central connections of the olfactory fibres in insects see PARETO: Z. Zellforsch. **131**, 109—140, (1972); BOECKH: J. comp. Physiol. **90**, 183—205, (1974).

P. KARLSON (Marburg): I should like to draw your attention to an analogy that might be useful, *i.e.* the so-called "symport" of organic molecules and ions (mainly Na^+). If the sex attractant is "symported" into the cell, this could account for Na^+ influx and potential changes as well as removal of bombykol from its site of action without a chemical reaction — that means in a much shorter time. — From an evolutionary point of view it could be visualized that the very specific chemoreceptor mechanisms may have evolved from the much less specific and sensitive transport mechanisms.

K.-E.KAISSLING: In this context we should also consider the enormous ion current of 10^6 charges within 100 msec, which is triggered by a single odor molecule and could be conducted through a single "ion channel".

A Formalism on Selective Molecular Interactions

Wolf A. Kafka

Max-Planck-Institut für Verhaltensphysiologie
8131 Seewiesen, Federal Republic of Germany

With 3 Figures

Structure-activity relationships between odor molecules and their hypothetical acceptors in insects may be used as a model mechanism for selective molecular interactions.

In collaboration with Neuwirth [2, 3, 8, 17], an attempt has been made to describe such mechanisms of interaction by means of a mathematical-physical formalism. Well-supported by electro-physiological data from single olfactory receptor cells in insects in response to stimulus molecules systematically altered in shape, flexibility, rotational characteristics and position and nature of single or combined functional groups, this concept is based in essence on the following assumptions:

1. The interaction between stimulus molecules and acceptors is not due to a homogeneously-distributed binding over the full length of the binding partners, but is dependent on discrete ordered binding sites on both binding partners, as shown schematically in Fig. 1.

2. These interactions are of the weak chemical type resulting from dispersion and dipole forces in these positions [4].

3. The geometrical arrangement of the binding sites in the acceptor reflects the position of functional groups of the most effective compound in its lowest-energy conformation.

4. By these interactions the acceptors become switched into distinct (presumably, but not necessarily [7], conformational) states which trigger the electrical processes of the cell responses [3, 4]. These changes appear to be brought about by a cooperative activation of the binding sites on the acceptor.

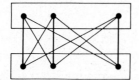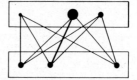

Fig. 1. Selective interaction mechanism between stimulus molecule (above) and acceptor (below) by means of a multiple (here three) point interaction. A successful attachment —here to be seen in terms of triggering the response of olfactory receptor cells — depends both on spatial distribution of the interacting sites and on appropriate magnitudes of electron polarizabilities and submolecular dipole moments as indicated by the dimensions of the full circles. (The strength of binding is reflected by the thickness of the conjugating lines.) As shown on the right, with different proportions of binding energies, the chances for triggering the responses are lowered, even if higher total binding energies would be given (Fig. 2) [2]

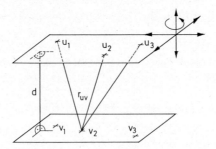

$$U_{tot} = \sum_{u,v} (U^p_{u,v} + U^a_{u,v})$$

$$U^p_{u,v} = -\frac{f_1\, p_u\, p_v}{r^3_{u,v}} - \frac{f_2\, p_u^2\, p_v^2}{4\,K\,T\,r^6_{u,v}} \qquad\qquad \frac{c_m}{c_s} = \frac{k_s}{k_m} = \exp\left(\frac{{}^sU_{tot} - {}^mU_{tot}}{K\ T}\right)$$

$$U^a_{u,v} = -\frac{3\,J\,a_u\,a_v}{4\,r^6_{u,v}}$$

Fig. 2. Multiple point interaction between u positions of the odor molecule and v positions of a hypothetical acceptor. Each position is characterized by an electron polarizability a_u, a_v, dipole moment p_u, p_v, and its relative distances $r_{u,v}$. The binding energies U_{tot} are the sum of the binding energies U^a_{uv} and U^p_{uv} between each position. The numbers of molecules c_s, c_m necessary to elicit equal cell responses are correlated with the Boltzmann-factors k_s, $k_m \cdot f_1$ and f_2 account for intramolecular rotations of dipoles. J Ionizing potential, K Boltzmann konstant, $T\,°$Kelvin [2, 3]. When tracing $U_{tot,\,max}$, the "stimulus molecule" is moved over the model acceptor as indicated by the arrow

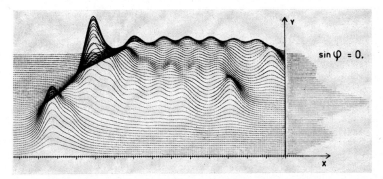

Fig. 3. Binding energy U_{tot} between odor molecule (*cis*-9-tetradecen-1-yl acetate) and its acceptor of the noctuid moth *Apamea rubrirena* as a function of (7000) different x, y positions (0.2 Å steps, at a constant angle of rotation) according to Fig. 2. U_{tot} is projected in arbitary units in direction of the y-axis. The maximum for each y-series is projected in direction of x-axis one of which is $U_{tot,\ max}$. The other peaks arise from binding energies U_{tot}, when, according to the movements in Fig. 2, only one or two of the discrete binding positions are in opposition. The small hills reveal interactions of the C—H bonds of the stimulus molecule with the three acceptor binding positions. [2, 3]

5. In view of this cooperative multiple-point interaction, selectivity of cell responses depends on whether different molecules (*e.g.* indicated by *s* or *m*) may undergo formation of such complexes (Fig. 1) [5]. These chances may be expressed in terms of the Boltzmann statistics and the inherent binding energies (Fig. 2). Thus, the magnitude of cell excitation may reflect the duration of the appropriate attachments, or in other words the number of momentarily existent odor molecule-acceptor complexes.

It should be noted that the proportions of the energies transferred at the binding sites must not necessarily be the same as those required to activate the acceptor. Similar to stereoselectivity of (*e.g.*) enzyme- [1, 9, 10] and drug-action [11, 14, 15, 16] it is reasonable to assume that among them the far-ranging and strong intermolecular forces are in part involved in keeping the odor molecule oriented in the acceptor field during a necessary minimum of time [3]. In addition, these binding forces might also be involved in arranging the acceptor binding sites before the final attachment occurs.

Electrophysiological data on specificity of pheromone receptors, kindly provided by PRIESNER ([12, 13], see also [6]) were applied to test this model, and to calculate unknown acceptor polarizabilities a_v, dipole moments p_v and distances r_{uv} by means of a mathematical fitting procedure (Figs. 2 and 3). Using these values, activity values for further pheromone analogues could be predicted [2, 3]. Despite the inevitable simplifications the predicted values are fully consistent with the experimental data.

References

1. HIRSCHMANN, H.J.: J. biol. Chem. **235**, 2762 (1960).
2. KAFKA, W.A.: Ann. N. Y. Acad. Sci. 1974.
3. KAFKA, W.A., NEUWIRTH, J.: In press.
4. KAFKA, W.A.: Z. vergl. Physiol. **70**, 105 (1970).
5. KAFKA, W.A.: Umschau **13**, 464 (1971).
6. KAISSLING, K.-E.: This issue.
7. LING, G.N.: Tex. Rep. Biol. and Med. **22**, 244 (1964).
8. NEUWIRTH, J.: Verh. dtsch. Zool. Ges. 1974 (in press).
9. OGSTON, A.G.: Nature (Lond.) **162**, 963 (1948).
10. OGSTON, A.G.: Nature (Lond.) **181**, 1462 (1958).
11. PORTOGHESE, P.S.: Ann. Rev. Pharmacol. **10**, 51 (1970).
12. PRIESNER, E.: Fortschr. Zool. **22**, 49 (1973).
13. PRIESNER, E., JACOBSON, M., BESTMANN, H.J.: In press.
14. ARIENS, E.J.: Acad. Press. Inc. **1**, 197 (1964).
15. STEPHENSON, R.P.: Brit. J. Pharmacol. **11**, 379 (1956).
16. PATON, W.D.M.: Proc. Roy. Soc. London, **154**, 21 (1961).
17. SCHNEIDER, D.: Sci. Am. **231**, 28 (1974).

Cell Communication and Cyclic-AMP Regulation during Aggregation of the Slime Mold, *Dictyostelium discoideum*

G. Gerisch and D. Malchow

*Friedrich-Miescher-Laboratorium der Max-Planck-Gesellschaft,
74 Tübingen, Federal Republic of Germany*

and

B. Hess

*Max-Planck-Institut für Ernährungsphysiologie,
46 Dortmund, Federal Republic of Germany*

With 10 Figures

Introduction

The signal systems functioning in aggregation of *Dictyostelium* cells are being investigated with increasing intensity in the hope that this organism might function to some extent as a model for cell interactions in embryogenesis. The principal peculiarity of *Dictyostelium* resides in the formation of a multicellular organism by aggregation of single cells. During its growth-phase, the organism exists in the state of single, amoeboid cells. Several hours after end of growth these cells aggregate, forming a polar body along which they differentiale into either spores or stalk cells, the final cell types constituting the fruiting body [1]. As a microorganism, *D. discoideum* provides the advantages of growth in submerged mass culture, and of the ease to obtain and to cultivate mutants blocked in morphogenesis. In this paper we shall discuss cell communication by diffusible transmitters, and particularly the function of cyclic AMP in the aggregation phase of *D. discoideum*.

Chemotaxis and Signal Propagation

The orientation of aggregating cells towards aggregation centers is guided by concentration gradients of a chemotactic factor or possibly a series of factors. The chemotactic material is released from aggregation centers typically in pulses with a period of 2.5 to 5 min. The pulses of chemotactic activity are propagated from cell to cell as excitation waves (Fig. 1), which in an uniform cell layer

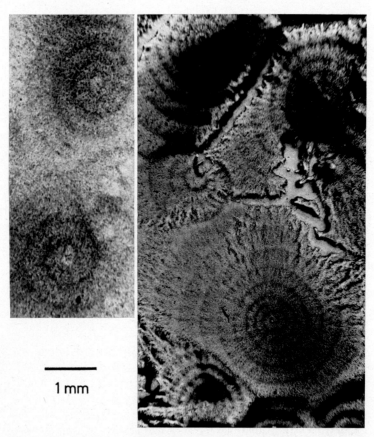

Fig. 1. Wave patterns of chemotactic activity in dense cell layers of *D. discoideum*. Left: Spiral-shaped waves in an early aggregation stage. Right: A later stage with aggregation territories already separated from each other by space which is depleted of cells as a result of their movement into the direction of a center. The chemotactic orientation towards a center is mediated by centrifugal relay of pulses. The visible waves coincide with zones of actual chemotactic response. (From [5] and [25])

spread with a constant speed of 40μ/min [2] to 120 [3] or up to 500 [4, 30] μ/min, depending on the number of cells per area. These values correspond to an input/output delay of > 15 sec. This means, when stimulated by transmitter, a sensitive cell responds after that time by transmitter release and thus continues the signal chain. A requirement for unidirectional signal propagation is a refractory phase, that is a phase of reduced sensitivity of a cell following its pulsing [2, 5, 6].

The wave patterns develop by self-organization from structureless populations of randomly distributed cells. The waves are either concentric or spiral-shaped. Formally the system could be treated as a group of diffusion-coupled oscillators [7, 8]. Noncellular analogues of these excitation waves are similarly shaped waves of reactivity in a chemical system, the Belousov-Zhabotinsky reaction [9].

Signal propagation extends the size of an aggregation territory beyond the range controlled by a center's direct chemotactic influence when any cell stimulated by transmitter is able to attract other cells chemotactically, and also to relay the signal that triggers the release of attractant. It is conceivable that the transmitter responsible for relaying of a signal is identical with the attractant, so that the cells respond to the same substance first by chemotactic orientation and, after a delay, by its release. KONIJIN et al. [10, 11] have shown that cAMP acts as an attractant. ROBERTSON et al. [12] have reported that cAMP when applied in pulses initiates propagated waves, thus acting as a transmitter.

Signalling and the response to intercellular signals is developmentally controlled. The ability to attract other cells increases two orders of magnitude when cells differentiate from the growth-phase to the aggregation state. Simultaneously, the sensitivity of the chemotactic response to aggregation centers as well as to cAMP increases to about the same extent [10]. The ability to propagate a wave develops likewise in the interphase between growth and full aggregation-competence [12]. Supposing that cAMP is the attractant as well as the transmitter, the molecular basis of the signal system would reside in the activity of adenylcyclase, the release mechanism for cAMP, the cAMP-receptor and the responses coupled to it, and in the cAMP phosphodiesterase activity.

Adenylcyclase and Phosphodiesterase Regulation

No data are available on the control of cAMP-transport through the plasma membrane. The possible contribution of the transport mechanism to the shape of the signal and to the periodicity of cAMP-release is unknown. The discussion on the control of cAMP in the intercellular space has to be focussed, therefore, on adenylcyclase and phosphodiesterase regulation.

According to ROSSOMANDO and SUSSMAN [13], adenylcyclase activity in cell homogenates does not significantly change when growth-phase cells differentiate into aggregating ones. However, an interesting interaction at the product level of the adenylcyclase and an ATP-pyrophosphohydrolase has been found (Fig. 10): 5'-AMP activates the adenylcyclase and cAMP the pyrophosphohydrolase, the responses to both effectors showing strong co-operativity [14]. As discussed below, the cross-activation of the two enzymes can result in oscillations of the cAMP level.

The life time of cAMP in the intercellular space is controlled both by soluble, extracellular phosphodiesterase and by cell-bound phosphodiesterase. The latter is also exposed to extracellular cAMP and is thus, presumably, a cell-surface constituent [15, 16]. The enzyme activities at these locations follow opposite time courses during development. The extracellular phosphodiesterase is inactivated by a specific, trypsin-sensitive inhibitor with a molecular weight of approx. 40000, which is released from the cells at the end of the growth-phase [17] (Fig. 2A). The enzyme activity reaches, therefore, a maximum at the end of cell growth. Under the conditions used by us, this regulation of the enzyme at the posttranslational level is drastic, the minima representing less than 5% of the peak activities (Fig. 2A). Although the phosphodiesterase activities may slowly increase again after the period of inhibitor release, they are still low when the cells reach full aggregation-competence. Formation of an extracellular inhibitor is restricted to those species of cellular slime molds which respond chemotactically to cAMP [18]. These results demonstrate a specific mechanism for the control of extracellular phosphodiesterase activity prior to aggregation, suggesting that the enzyme exhibits its main function during the growth-phase, where it suppresses cAMP-signals passing the extracellular space.

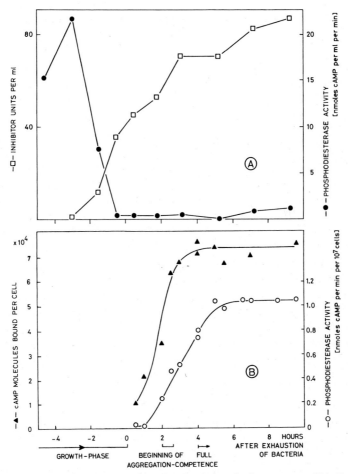

Fig. 2 A and B. Developmental regulation of phosphodiesterases and binding sites both interacting with extracellular cAMP. (A) Extracellular, soluble phosphodiesterase (●) is inactivated by an inhibitor which becomes detectable in the extracellular space at the end of the growth-phase (□). (B) Cell-bound phosphodiesterase activity (○) and cAMP-binding to cells (▲). The latter was tested by adding 7×10^{-8} M [³H] cAMP plus 5×10^{-4} M unlabeled cGMP and by measuring binding after 5 sec. (Data from [16] and [17])

The cell-bound phosphodiesterase is not affected by the inhibitor under *in vivo* conditions. This enzyme activity strongly increases between growth and aggregation-competence [15, 19] (Fig. 2B). The increase is controlled by a genetic system that simultaneously controls other developmentally regulated cell surface constituents, and controls also the inhibitor of extracellular phosphodiesterase [16, 17]. The enzyme limits the time window of a signal pulse, thus guaranteeing signal separation between consecutive periods. It fits to this function that the enzyme shows nonlinear kinetics, in contrast to the extracellular phosphodiesterase which shows Michaelis-Menten kinetics over the total range of cAMP-concentrations tested [20]. Either negative cooperativity or a set of enzymes with different K_m-values would sharpen the decay of a cAMP-pulse. It remains to be clarified if this is the only function of the cell-bound phosphodiesterase in the chemoreceptor system.

cAMP-Binding Sites

The investigation of cAMP-binding to possible receptor sites is complicated by the phosphodiesterase activity associated with aggregating cells. The phosphodiesterase can be preferentially inhibited by cGMP which shows a high affinity for the enzyme [21] and a low affinity for the receptor, as concluded from its weak chemotactic action [11]. When aggregation-competent cells were simultaneously incubated with [³H] cAMP and excess cGMP, binding was detected at 5 sec after nucleotide addition, and binding decayed almost completely within 5 min (Fig. 3A). At about the same rate, 5'-AMP appeared in the extracellular space (Fig. 3B). In the absence of cGMP the cell-bound phosphodiesterase hydrolyzed 95% of the added cAMP within a 5 sec period, and accordingly no binding was detected after that time (Fig. 3A and B). cAMP-binding to growth-phase cells was insignificant, despite of the low phosphodiesterase activity of these cells (Fig. 3A and B). These results indicate that binding of cAMP to receptor sites is transient and terminated by its hydrolysis, and that the cAMP-binding sites are under developmental control.

The dissociation constant of the cAMP-receptor complex is in the order of 1 to 2×10^{-7} M or lower [16]. This appears to be sufficient to explain the high sensitivity of the chemotactic response which is still detectable using a cAMP-concentration of 10^{-8} M [11]. From Scatchard plots a minimal number of 5×10^5 cAMP-binding sites per cell has been obtained for living, aggregation-competent cells. The potency for cAMP-binding increases up to that value after the end of growth in a similar time course as the activity of cell-bound phosphodiesterase increases (Fig. 2 B).

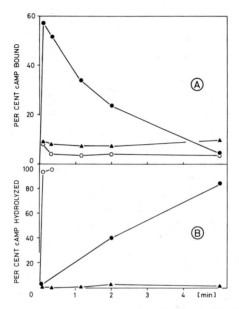

Fig. 3 A and B. Binding of cAMP to living cells (A), and its hydrolysis by cell-bound phosphodiesterase (B). Binding of 10^{-8} M [³H] cAMP to aggregation-competent cells was undetectable in the absence of cGMP ($\circ$, A), obviously because of the high rate of hydrolysis ($\circ$, B). Simultaneous addition of 5×10^{-4} M cGMP delayed hydrolysis ($\bullet$, B) and accordingly made the measurement of cAMP-binding possible ($\bullet$, A). No significant binding to growth-phase cells was detected in either presence ($\blacktriangle$, A) or absence (not shown) of cGMP, although the cell-bound phosphodiesterase activity of these cells was low ($\blacktriangle$, B). (Data from [16])

With respect to the association of transmitter-binding sites with a hydrolase, the receptor system by which the slime molds aggregate in response to periodic cAMP-pulses resembles the AcCh-receptor/cholinesterase system by which nerve impulses are transmitted through the synaptic cleft.

Optical Recording of Cellular Responses to cAMP

To relate the initial step of cAMP-interaction with receptor sites to the following cellular responses, a method providing sufficient time resolution is required for recording the latter in cell suspensions. Recording of light scattering (Fig. 4) is the method of

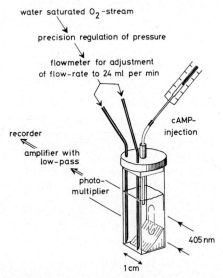

water saturated O_2-stream

precision regulation of pressure

flowmeter for adjustment of flow-rate to 24 ml per min

cAMP-injection

recorder

amplifier with low-pass

photo-multiplier

405 nm

1 cm

Fig. 4. Equipment used for measuring light scattering responses in cell suspensions. Suspensions of 2×10^8 cells/ml are aerated and simultaneously stirred through two needles by a carefully equilibrated O_2-stream. Noise produced by bubbling is supressed by a low pass filter in the recording pathway of optical density. A sloping surface of paraffin at the bottom of the optical cuvette prevents sedimentation of cells in the corners not directly seized by the oxygen bubbles. cAMP and other nucleotides are injected in a small volume of solute by a microsyringe

choice because all visible cAMP-induced responses of aggregating cells can be expected to influence light scattering: pseudopodial activity, cell elongation, and increased cell-to-cell adhesion [10]. The changes of light scattering in cell suspensions are characteristic of the developmental stage of the cells: growth-phase cells show only one predominant response peak, aggregation-competent cells additionally a slower response (Fig. 5). The heights of both peaks depend on the concentration of cAMP applied and both peaks reflect specific responses to cyclic nucleotides. 1000fold higher concentrations of cGMP and cIMP are required to get the same responses as to cAMP, but then the temporal response patterns are identical [22]. It is as

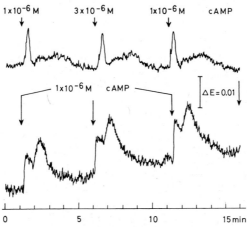

Fig. 5. Light scattering responses to cAMP in cell suspensions. Stirred suspensions of growth-phase cells (top) and of aggregation-competent cells (bottom) were stimulated by cAMP pulses. Responses of short duration were obtained, the temporal pattern of which depends on the developmental state: A fast, sharp response peak is characteristic for growth-phase cells, aggregation-competent cells showing an additional slower response. (Re-drawn from [22])

yet unclear to which type of cell behavior each peak is related. We suppose, however, that at least one peak is related to the chemotactic response of the cells.

The Cells Respond to Changes of cAMP-Concentration in Time

The light scattering method can be used to decide whether the cells respond to steady cAMP-concentrations or to the increase of concentrations in time. Both, the fast and the slow peaks are responses to a pulse-wise increase of cAMP-concentration. Both responses decay with time constants of one minute or less. In the case of the fast peak the time constant is about 10 sec, almost independent of the amplitude of the stimulus [22].

Because of the short life time of extracellular cAMP in suspensions of aggregation-competent cells. and because of the rapid liberation of cAMP from receptor sites, the decay of the responses might simply reflect the decrease of the number of cAMP-receptor complexes per cell. This explanation does not hold, however, when the lifetime of cAMP is extended by excess cGMP. Under these conditions binding is also extended (Fig. 3 A), but nevertheless the response pattern remains unchanged. The diagram of Fig. 6 illustrates that the shape of the response is determined at a step of signal processing later than the formation of the cAMP-receptor complex. Our results indicate that *Dictyostelium* cells show a typical "on-response" or, to re-phrase it, that they behave as fast adapting chemoreceptor cells.

A Possible Mechanism of Chemotactic Orientation

If the cells respond to changes of cAMP concentration in time, the chemoreceptor system of *D. discoideum* amoebae functions similar to the relaxation system of chemotactic bacteria [23, 24], as outlined by Adler and Koshland in this volume. The chemotactic orientation of the amoebae, however, is quite different from the alternating straight line/tumbling movement of the bacteria.

Fig. 6. Diagram showing the relation between extracellular cAMP concentrations (top), cAMP-binding to cells (middle), and light scattering responses (bottom). All possible combinations are listed and those found to be realized are shadowed. For reasons of simplicity, only one response peak is drawn. The scheme applies, however, for both the observed fast and slow responses. If the life-time of cAMP in the medium is short (A), binding to receptor sites would be also short in the case of rapid exchange between bound and free cAMP (Aa), or it would be long lasting in the case of slow exchange (Ab). If the lifetime of free cAMP is long (B), short-term binding (Ba) would be expected if the receptor exists in three states: (1) as free receptor, (2) as cAMP-receptor complex which is unstable and spontaneously deteriorates into (3) insensitive receptor without affinity to cAMP. If binding is short, initial binding could either cause a short-term response ($Aa\alpha$ and $Ba\alpha$), or it might trigger an extended response ($Aa\beta$ and $Ba\beta$), e.g., a response mediated by an enzyme which is activated *via* the cAMP-receptor complex, and then continues to function in the absence of bound cAMP. If binding is long lasting (Ab and Bb), the response could be nevertheless short ($Ab\alpha$ and $Bb\alpha$) if a fast adaptation step in signal processing exists; if not, the response would be as long as binding continues ($Ab\beta$ and $Bb\beta$)

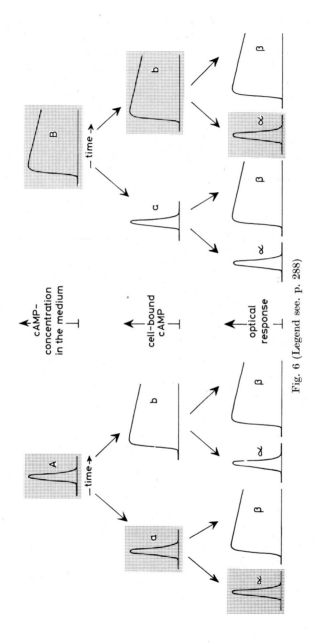

Fig. 6 (Legend see. p. 288)

The amoebae migrate with a front of pseudopods more or less precisely into the direction of a gradient.

As the bacteria, the amoebae are also attracted by non-pulsing sources of attractant, *e.g.* by the aggregation centers of an aper-

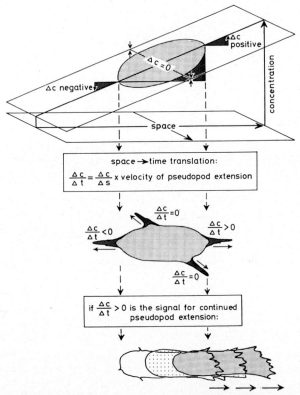

Fig. 7. A possible mechanism for the chemotactic response of an amoeboid cell. To detect the direction of a stationary concentration gradient (top), an amoeboid cell (shadowed area) has the possibilities of either measuring concentration differences over its total length, or along the length of individual pseudopods. If the latter is realized, it can be supposed that the response system functions on the basis of $\Delta c/\Delta t$ measurements during the extension of pseudopods in different directions (middle). If a positive $\Delta c/\Delta t$ would be a signal for the further extension of an elongating pseudopod, continued extension would be favored on the side of the amoeba directed towards the higher concentration, and would cause a movement into that direction (bottom)

iodically signalling mutant [25]. The obvious question is how a receptor system that responds to changes of concentration in time can guide a cell directly along a stationary spatial gradient. One possibility is illustrated in Fig. 7. The assumption is made that pilot pseudopods are protruded from any part of the cell surface, but that only those pseudopods which receive a positive input of $\Delta c/\Delta t$ are stimulated to continued extension. These pseudopods then constitute the front of the cells directed to the source of the gradient. Essential for the hypothesis is the assumption that pseudopod extension can be elicited by cAMP at any location of the cell surface. Experiments together with D. HÜLSER, Tübingen, using microcapillaries for local application of cAMP, have proven this assumption to be correct.

Spontaneous Periodic Activities in Cell Suspensions

Any cell that carries a propagated wave must function as a signal amplifier, because only a portion of the transmitter molecules released by a cell will reach and trigger other cells. Amplification expressed as number of transmitter molecules, means that the ratio of the molecules required for stimulation of a cell to those released in response to stimulation must be < 1. If cAMP is the transmitter, this amplification would be accesible to direct measurement in cell suspensions. Experiments of WICK [26] indicate an amplification factor of at least 10 in terms of extracellular cAMP-concentration when 2×10^8 cells/ml are triggered by 5×10^{-8} M cAMP. If the release of cAMP is autocatalytic as suggested by this experiment, it could function in cell suspensions as an intercellular coupling factor that synchronizes the activities of the individual cells. Small pulses of cAMP initially released by a few cells would trigger other cells to release cAMP, and thus would result in a burst of extracellular cAMP to which all sensitive cells contribute.

The light scattering responses demonstrate that cAMP-inputs to the chemoreceptor system can be easily recorded in cell suspensions. If the cells are able to generate cAMP-signals spontaneously and are able to synchronize their activities in stirred suspensions, similar responses should be detectable without experimental application of cAMP. In fact, periodic responses to autonomous signals have been recorded in suspensions of aggregation-competent cells,

the stage at which the cells are also able to propagate waves
(Fig. 8 bottom). Typically, these response have the shape of spikes
and are generated with a period of about 7 min. No spontaneous
periodic activity has been observed in suspensions of growth-phase
cells (Fig. 8, top), indicating developmental control of this activity.

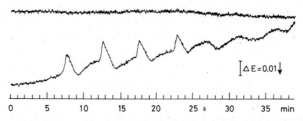

Fig. 8. Developmental control of spontaneous periodic activities in cell suspensions. In suspensions of cells harvested at the early interphase between
end of growth and the aggregation-competent state, no spontaneous changes
of light scattering have been recorded (upper curve). Synchronous oscillation
in aggregation-competent cells is indicated by periodic generation of spikes
and, later on, by continuation of sinusoidal oscillations of light scattering
(lower curve). The cells were harvested from suspension cultures, sedimented
and resuspended in fresh, cold buffer. Spike generation begins spontaneously
a few minutes after, transfer of these cells from an ice bath to 23° C (Re-
drawn from [22])

If the signal input-output delay is 15 sec as minimal value
calculated from the speed of wave propagation, a threefold cascade
of transmitter release would fit into a period of half a minute. In
spontaneously generated spikes this interval roughly corresponds
to the observed initiation period during which light scattering
slowly deviates from the base line prior to the final steep increase
of the response (Fig. 9).

Two results suggest that cAMP, in fact, controls the periodic
activity in cell suspensions. The first is a preliminary one and says
that the extracellular cAMP-level spontaneously oscillates synchronously with the changes of light scattering [26]. The second
result provides direct evidence that cAMP determines the phase of
the oscillating system: when a cAMP-pulse is applied within the
interphase between two spikes, a phase-shift is induced (Fig. 9).
This shows that the cAMP-receptor system is not only connected

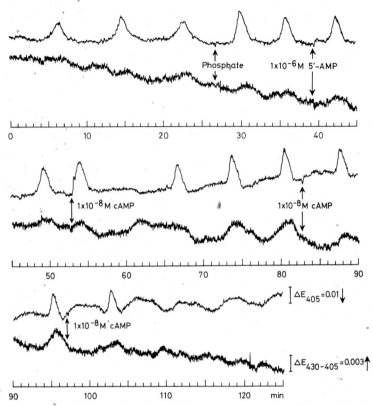

Fig. 9. Interaction of cAMP with the oscillating system, and the coupling of cytochrome b to this system. Upper curves ($\Delta E_{405\,nm}$): A continuous record of light scattering. Lower curves ($\Delta E_{430\,nm} - {}_{405\,nm}$): Simultaneous recording of the cytochrome b difference spectrum. Phosphate and 5'-AMP did not interfere with spontaneous spike generation in the cell suspension. However, a pulse of 10^{-8} M cAMP when applied in the second half of a period caused a phase shift of the oscillator underlying spike generation. In the period following the cAMP-pulse, no spike was formed. In the same cell suspension, cells did not respond to cAMP-pulses of the same amplitude when applied in the first half of a period. The redox state of cytochrome b oscillated in phase with spike generation, and showed the shift also in that period in which no spike was formed. When the system changed from spike generation to sinusoidal oscillations of light scattering, the periodic behavior of cytochrome b ceased.
(Re-drawn from [22])

to the chemotactic response apparatus, but is also linked to the
signal generator. It fits to the function of cAMP as a transmitter
that the cells are less sensitive to cAMP after than they are prior to
a spontaneous spike, indicating a phase of relative refractoriness
(Fig. 9) [22].

Towards an Understanding of the Oscillator Underlying Periodic Signalling

Several observations indicate that the generation of signal
pulses in *D. discoideum* is coupled to an oscillator the functioning
of which, however, does not, in turn, depend on pulse generation.
DURSTON [27] has shown that the pulse periods often are multiples
of a basic period of about 2.5 min, indicating that signal pulses may
be coupled either to each, or to any second or third etc. run of the
clock[1]. Similar observations have been made in cell suspensions.
Sinusoidal oscillations can continue after spike generation has
ceased, the only effect associated with this uncoupling being an
increase of frequency of about 20% [22]. In Fig. 9 the skipping of
a spike in one particular period is shown together with a record of
the cytochrome b difference spectrum. The redox state of cytochrome b oscillates in phase with spike generation, and does so even
in that period in which actually no spike is formed, which again
indicates continuing of intracellular oscillations in the absence of
spike generation.

GOLDBETER [28], using the data of ROSSOMANDO and SUSSMAN
[14], has demonstrated that the system shown in Fig. 10 is able to
oscillate. In principle, the model could explain the cytochrome
shifts accompanying spike generation. The shifts would follow from
coupling of the electron transport to ATP, the substrate of both
the adenylcyclase and the pyrophosphohydrolase. The triggering
of a pulse by cAMP could be explained by its action on the
pyrophosphohydrolase, which according to the scheme would be a
candidate for the cAMP-receptor. However, there remain several
observations which have to be fitted into this scheme. First, when
cells are triggered by small external cAMP pulses, their responses

---

[1] Indeed, the properties of entrainment and generation of subharmonics
have been demonstrated experimentally in case of the glycolytic oscillator
(see also Discussion remark by HESS, p. 296, this volume).

are not associated with a cytochrome b shift [22]. Second, cyto-chrome b shifts occur also in those periods in which no spike is formed. This suggests that the intracellular oscillator can be de-coupled from cAMP-release. Another complication is the dis-

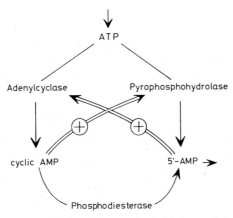

Fig. 10. Enzyme network for the control of the intracellular cAMP-level, which has been shown by GOLDBETER in a theoretical study [28] to be capable of oscillatory behavior. The scheme is based on cross-activation of adenyl-cyclase and pyrophosphohydrolase as reported by ROSSOMANDO and SUSS-MAN [14]

crepancy between the cAMP-concentration required for half-maxi-mal pyrophosphohydrolase-activation [14] and the apparent dis-sociation constant for cAMP-binding sites on intact cells [16]. These values differ by a factor of 10^4 or more.

The difference between the low external cAMP-concentrations which trigger a half-maximal response [11, 22] and the high intra-cellular cAMP level [29] is in the range of four orders of magnitude, and strongly suggests a signal transformation or amplification process at the plasma membrane. Interaction of cAMP with cell surface receptors is indicated by reversible, short-term binding of cAMP to living cells [16, 31]. These results render it improbable that external cAMP exerts its function by entering an intracellular cAMP pool. The question how binding of external cAMP to a mem-brane receptor is transformed into an intracellular signal guiding cell movement is still unsolved. Among the possible mechanisms of trans-membrane signal transformation, the functioning of the cAMP-receptor as a proteinkinase is a most attractive one. If asymmetrically orientated in the plasma membrane, with the regulatory subunit outside and the catalytic subunit inside, the enzyme could bind external cAMP and in response could phosphorylate a sub-membranous protein.

Own work reported in this paper has been supported by the Deutsche Forschungsgemeinschaft and the Stiftung Volkswagenwerk.

Addendum

B. Hess

The phenomena observed in *Dictyostelium* cells are the result of the molecular properties of the receptor and enzyme networks involved. As pointed out, the observed dynamics are analogs to a diffusion coupled sequence of oscillators. I would like to add that such phenomena are not only observed in biomolecular systems but also in pure chemical systems, such as the Belousov-Zhabotinsky reaction which describes the periodic catalytic oxidation of malonic acid by bromate in an acidic medium [for review see Nicolis, G., Portnow, J.: Chemical Oscillations in Chem. Rev. **73**, 364—384 (1973)]. The periodic time-course of this reaction, which can be recorded by the colour change of the catalysts (like cerium-ions or ferroin), can lead to a synchronization of the phase of oscillations in different locations and to the production of chemical waves closely resembling the oscillatory propagation pattern of *Dictyostelium discoideum*, which carries the information on the time and direction of movement leading to aggregation. Therefore, we asked the question whether diffusion coupled oscillatory chemical systems can also be used to transmit information over a longer distance. On the basis of a network description of the elementary chemical system, being extended to allow for diffusion processes, transmission properties were analysed mathematically, and it was found that triggered signals can be transferred almost undistorted and with nearly constant velocity. This model was confirmed experimentally and showed that a light pulse can well be carried over a few centimeters by the oscillating system. Not only physical but also chemical types of triggering could be used as information input. We pointed out that a combination of two or more signals in a specified way may be considered as modifying the information contained in the signals; such combinations may lead to a network made of "chemical wires". Thus, the analogy of the chemical system transmitting information to the *Dictyostelium* system or electronic analogs is obvious, and might lead to quite sophisticated questions on the biochemical nature of intercellular as well as intracellular cooperation [Busse, H., Hess, B.: Nature **244**, 203—205 (1973); Smoes, M.-L., Dreitlein, J.: J. Chem. Phys. **59**, 6277—6285 (1973); Bornmann, L., Busse, H., Hess, B., Riepe, R., Hesse, C.: Z. Naturforsch. **28** b, 824—827 (1973).

References

1. BONNER, J.T.: The cellular slime molds. Princeton (N.J.): University Press 1967.
2. GERISCH, G.: Wilhelm Roux' Arch. Entwickl.-Mech. Org. **156**, 127—144 (1965).
3. NANJUNDIAH, V.: Tübingen (personal communication).
4. MONK, M.: Edinburgh (personal communication).
5. GERISCH, G.: In: MOSCONA, A. A., MONROY, A. (Eds.): Current topics in development biology, Vol. 3, pp. 157—197. New York-London: Academic Press 1968.
6. COHEN, M. H., ROBERTSON, A.: J. theoret. Biol. **31**, 101—118 (1971).
7. SMOES, M.-L., DREITLEIN, J.: J. chem. Phys. **59**, 6277—6285 (1973).
8. WINFREE, A. T.: SIAM-AMS Proceedings 8 (1974).
9. WINFREE, A. T.: Science **175**, 634—636 (1972).
10. BONNER, J. T., BARKLEY, D. S., HALL, E. M., KONIJN, T. M., MANSON, J. W., O'KEEFE III, G., WOLFE, P. B.: Develop. Biol. **20**, 72—87 (1969).
11. KONIJN, T. M.: Advanc. Cyclic Nucleotide Res. **1**, 17—31 (1972).
12. ROBERTSON, A., DRAGE, D. J., COHEN, M. H.: Science **175**, 333—335 (1972).
13. ROSSOMANDO, E. F., SUSSMAN, M.: Biochem. Biophys. Res. Commun. **47**, 604—610 (1972).
14. ROSSOMANDO, E. F., SUSSMAN, M.: Proc. nat. Acad. Sci. (Wash.) **70**, 1254—1257 (1973).
15. MALCHOW, D., NÄGELE, B., SCHWARZ, H., GERISCH, G.: Europ. J. Biochem. **28**, 136—142 (1972).
16. MALCHOW, D., GERISCH, G.: Proc. nat. Acad. Sci. (Wash.) **71**, 2423—2427 (1974).
17. RIEDEL, V., GERISCH, G., MÜLLER, E., BEUG, H.: J. molec. Biol. **74**, 573—585 (1973).
18. GERISCH, G., MALCHOW, D., RIEDEL, V., MÜLLER, E., EVERY, M.: Nature (Lond.) New Biol. **235**, 90—92 (1972).
19. PANNBACKER, R. G., BRAVARD, L. J.: Science **175**, 1014—1015 (1972).
20. MALCHOW, D., NANJUNDIAH, V.: Biochem. Biophys. Acta, in press.
21. MALCHOW, D., FUCHILA, J.: FEBS Letters **34**, 5—9 (1973).
22. GERISCH, G., HESS, B.: Proc. nat. Acad. Sci. (Wash.) **71**, 2118—2122 (1974).
23. MACNAB, R. M., KOSHLAND, D. E., JR.: Proc. nat. Acad. Sci. (Wash.) **69**, 2509—2512 (1972).
24. BERG, H. C., BROWN, D. A.: Nature (Lond.) **239**, 500—504 (1972).
25. GERISCH, G.: Naturwissenschaften **58**, 430—438 (1971).
26. WICK, U.: Diplomarbeit, Universität Tübingen (1974).
27. DURSTON, A. J.: Develop. Biol. **37**, 225—235 (1974).
28. GOLDBETTER, A.: Rehovot (personal communication).
29. MALKINSON, A. M., ASHWORTH, J. M.: Biochem. J. **134**, 311—319 (1973).
30. SHAFFER, B. M.: Advances in Morphogenesis **2**, 109—182 (1962).
31. MALCHOW, D., GERISCH, G.: Biophys. Biophys. Res. Commun. **55**, 200—204 (1973).

Discussion

HEILMEYER (WÜRZBURG): Haben Sie gefunden, daß die cAMP-Wirkung in Gegenwart von ATP verändert ist ? Ich denke dabei an Literaturangaben, nach denen die Proteinkinase aus Muskel durch ATP/Mg^{2+} in der cAMP-Sensitivität um ungefähr den Faktor 10 herabgesetzt wird.

G. GERISCH: Wir haben nicht gefunden, daß extracelluläres ATP die Stimulierung durch cAMP in irgendeiner Weise beeinflußt, haben das aber nicht systematisch getestet. Man kann davon ausgehen, daß das ATP nicht in die Zelle hineingeht, ebensowenig wie das cAMP. Das cAMP bindet an die Zelloberfläche; die Hydrolyseprodukte erscheinen wieder im Medium. Ich möchte noch einmal betonen, daß die intracelluläre cAMP-Konzentration etwa 1000fach höher ist als das, was wir zur Stimulierung benötigen; d. h. es ist unwahrscheinlich, daß von außen zugegebenes cAMP dadurch wirkt, daß es den internen cAMP-pool auffüllt. Wir müssen für den cAMP-Stimulus ein Übersetzungssystem an der Membran fordern.

P. SUNDER-PLASSMANN (Münster): Herr Gerisch hat vorhin die frühe intercelluläre Signalbildung, bei der das cAMP im Mittelpunkt steht in Analogie zu ,,ganz primitiven synaptischen Systemen" gebracht. In der phylogenetischen Evolution treten nun die biogenen Amine noch differenzierender in diesen Regulationsmechanismus ein — dergestalt, daß jetzt engste Korrelaton zwischen β-receptor site der Zellmembran und dem Adenylat-Cyclase-System $\leftrightharpoons$ 3′, 5′-cAMP $\leftrightharpoons$ ATP $\leftrightharpoons$ Protein-Kinase entsteht. Hier bieten sich neuestens Korrespondenzen zum ,,antigen recognition mechanism" und der Heterogenität der Antikörper-Synthese in den B-Lymphozyten und der Θ-Antigen-Fixierung der T-Lymphocyten an [vgl. SUNDER-PLASSMANN et al.: Cybernetic Medicine 4, 15—23 (1973)].

Conjugation of the Ciliate *Blepharisma:* A Possible Model System for Biochemistry of Sensory Mechanisms

Akio Miyake

Max-Planck-Institut für Molekulare Genetik, D-1000 Berlin-Dahlem

With 2 Figures

Ciliate cells are separated from each other during most of their life cycle, but under certain conditions two cells temporarily unite to form a bicellular complex (conjugant pair) and undergo a series of developmental processes which are collectively called conjugation. Conjugant pairs are induced by interaction between cells of complementary mating types [1−3]. If two such mating types are separately cultured and mixed under appropriate conditions, they start interacting immediately and after 1−2 hrs of interaction cells unite in pairs. In many ciliates the specific substances which mediate this cell interaction (gamones) are cell-bound, but in *Blepharisma intermedium* gamones are excreted into the medium [3−5].

Cells of *B. intermedium* differentiate into mating types I and II. Their interaction consists of 7 steps [5], as shown in Fig. 1. Type I cells autonomously excrete Gamone I (Step 1). This gamone reacts with Type II cells (Step 2) and specifically transforms them so that they can form a cell union (Step 4) and at the same time induces them to produce and excrete Gamone II (Step 3). This gamone reacts with Type I cells (Step 5) and specifically transforms them so that they can form a cell union (Step 6). Transformed Types I and II cells unite to form conjugant pairs (Step 7). When Type I cells do not excrete Gamone I at the maximal rate, the production and excretion of this gamone can be enhanced by Gamone II. Therefore, the reaction chain consisting of Steps 1−3 and 5 is a positive feedback cycle.

Gamone I was purified and identified as a slightly basic glycoprotein of about 20000 molecular weight [6]. This gamone induces cell union in Type II cells (500−1000 cells/ml) at a concentration of 0.00006 µg/ml [6]. Gamone II is calcium-3-(2'-formylamino-5'-hydroxybenzoyl) lactate [7]. This gamone induces cell union in Type I cells (500–1000 cells/ml) at a concentration of 0.001 µg/ml [7]. Tryptophan appears to be a precursor of this gamone [3].

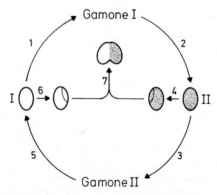

Fig. 1. Diagrammatic illustration of cell interaction in conjugation of *Blepharisma intermedium*. (Modified from [5])

Gamone-transformed cells can unite in all three possible combinations of mating types, but only heterotypic pairs (I–II) complete conjugation. Homotypic pairs (I–I, II–II) may remain united for days, but the process of conjugation appears to stop at the stage of pair formation. This provides an opportunity to investigate the two gamone-induced processes, namely 1) induction of gamone synthesis and 2) induction of cell union, under conditions that are effectively separated from other complicating processes of the conjugation.

Induction of homotypic union is inhibited by 10 µg/ml cycloheximide [8]. This also inhibits the incorporation of ^{14}C-L-leucine into 10% trichloroacetic acid-insoluble material, indicating that protein synthesis is needed for the induction of cell union. This assumption is supported by the finding that the leucine incorporation is greatly enhanced by gamone. The increased leucine incorporation is observed within 10 min after beginning the gamone treatment and continues for about 2 hr, when the cell union begins being formed. At this time the net leucine incorporation in gamone-treated cells may be 5 times as high as in untreated cells. Gamone of the same mating type has no such effect.

Induction of homotypic cell union takes about 2 hr. If cells are transferred to a gamone-free medium within one and a half hours, the cell union is never formed. If the transfer is made in the last 30 min of the induction, the cell union is formed although it lasts only for a brief period (up to 20 min). If the transfer is made after the cell union is formed the union persists longer, but cells eventually separate within a few hours. Thus, the cell union is induced after a continuous exposure to gamone and is maintained by a further continuous exposure to gamone. These results indicate that the formation and maintenance of cell union depend upon an accumulation of a certain amount of a hypothetical factor which is constantly produced during the gamone treatment but constantly disappears at the same time. The results of experiments on leucine incorporation and the effect of cycloheximide mentioned above suggest that this factor is a protein or proteins.

The Gamone II induction by Gamone I takes about 2 hr, suggesting that the Gamone II synthesizing machinery is built up anew after cells are treated with Gamone I. Contrary to the induction of cell union, a relatively brief exposure to gamone is effective for this induction. When cells are transferred to a gamone-free medium after 30 min of the treatment, Gamone II starts being produced 2 hr after beginning the treatment. However, the production is considerably less than in the control cells which are constantly exposed to Gamone I. When cells are transferred after 1 hr of the treatment, the Gamone II production is the same as the control, at least for a period of up to 4 hr. Thus, the building up of the Gamone II - producing system appears to continue after Gamone I is removed, and once built up, it functions normally, at least for several hours. Since tryptophan is a precursor of Gamone II, the Gamone II - producing system is likely to be an enzyme system which transforms tryptophan to Gamone II.

Based on these results, a molecular model of the cell interaction during the initiation of conjugation is constructed as a working model for future work (Fig. 2). Type I cells excrete Gamone I which is a glycoprotein. This molecule reacts with a hypothetical receptor (hatched area in Fig. 2) on Type II cells and induces protein synthesis. Some of these proteins are "cell-union-inducing proteins" and change the surface of the cell so that they can form a cell union (blackened area in Fig. 2). The others are enzymes which transform tryptophan to Gamone II, calcium-3-(2'-formylamino-5'-hydroxybenzoyl)-lactate. This molecule is excreted, reacts with a hypothetical receptor on Type I cells and induces protein synthesis. One of the induced proteins is Gamone I. The others are cell-union-inducing proteins, and Type I cells gain the capacity to unite.

Each step in this system is amenable to chemical analysis because, 1) the system is simple having only two types of cells, 2) each step can be experimentally induced in a relatively short, predictable time in a large amount of homogeneous cells, 3) both gamones have been purified, and 4) Gamone II has been synthesized [9].

In order to rationalize the use of this system as a model for the biochemistry of sensory functions, the processes in Figs. 1 and 2 may be translated as follows. An informational molecule, Gamone I, reacts with a receptor on Type II cells. This stimulus evokes a response in the form of the synthesis of cell-union-inducing proteins. The excited state of Type II cells induced by Gamone I is thus reflected by the synthesis of these proteins. The excited Type II

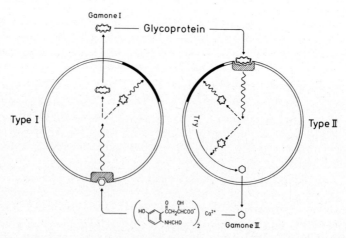

Fig. 2. Diagrammatic illustration of molecular mechanism of cell interaction in conjugation of *Blepharisma intermedium*

cells also produce and excrete a transmitter substance, Gamone II, which reacts with a receptor on Type I cells and stimulates them to synthesize proteins. Some of these proteins are the same cell-union-inducing proteins as induced in Type II cells. In this way, Type II cells transmit through Gamone II exactly the same excited state to Type I cells. It may be interesting to note that Gamone II is bio-chemically related to one of the neurotransmitters, serotonin. Once the accumulation of the cell-union-inducing protein reaches a certain threshold, cells gain the capacity to form a cell union, but in order to maintain the cell union, cells must be constantly stimu-lated. Thus, a prolonged excited state of cells results in the for-mation of a new pattern of cellular arrangement suggesting, though remotely, a relation to the embryonic development of nervous systems.

The attempt to regard the induction of conjugation in ciliates as a model for cell excitation may be further supported by the finding that ionic conditions which should bring about electrical depolarization in living cells, *i.e.*, KCl + Ca-poor conditions, induce in *Paramecium* the same effect as mating reaction and induce conjugation between cells of the same mating type [10, 11]. It is hoped that investigations on the molecular mechanism of these steps will contribute to the elucidation of the basic mechanism of sensory functions.

References

1. SONNEBORN, T. M.: Sex, sex inheritance and sex determination in *Para-mecium aurelia*. Proc. nat. Acad. Sci. (Wash.) **23**, 378 (1937).
2. METZ, C. B.: Mating substances and the physiology of fertilization in ciliates. In: WENRICH, D. H. (Ed.): Sex in microorganisms. Washington, D. C.: Amer. Ass. Advanc. Sci. 1954.
3. MIYAKE, A.: Cell interaction in conjugation of ciliates. Current Topics Microbiol. Immunol. **64**, 49 (1974).
4. MIYAKE, A.: Induction of conjugation by cell-free fluid in the ciliate *Blepharisma*. Proc. Japan Acad. **44**, 837 (1968).
5. MIYAKE, A., BEYER, J.: Cell interaction by means of soluble factors (gamones) in conjugation of *Blepharisma intermedium*. Exp. Cell Res. **76**, 15 (1973).
6. MIYAKE, A., BEYER, J.: Blepharmone: A conjugation-inducing glyco-protein in the ciliate *Blepharisma*. Science **185**, 621 (1974).
7. KUBOTA, T., TOKOROYAMA, T., TSUKUDA, Y., KOYAMA, H., MIYAKE, A.: Isolation and structure determination of Blepharismin, a conjugation initiating gamone in the ciliate *Blepharisma*. Science **179**, 400 (1973).

8. BEYER, J., MIYAKE, A.: On the molecular mechanism of gamone-induced conjugation in *Blepharisma intermedium*. Progress Protozool. Abstr. 4th Internat. Congr. Protozool. Clermont-Ferrand 1973, 280 (1973).

9. TOKOROYAMA, T., HORI, S., KUBOTA, T.: Synthesis of Blepharismone, a conjugation inducing gamone in ciliate *Blepharisma*. Proc. Japan Acad. **49**, 461 (1973).

10. MIYAKE, A.: Induction of conjugation by chemical agents in *Paramecium*. J. exp. Zool. **167**, 359 (1968).

11. MIYAKE, A.: Mechanism of initiation of sexual reproduction in *Paramecium multimicronucleatum*. Japan J. Genet. **44**, (Suppl. 1), 388 (1969).

Discussion

C. B. SHARMA (Regensburg): Dr. MIYAKE, at what level of protein biosynthesis does gamone I act ? Does this occur at transcriptional level or translational level ?

A. MIYAKE: Actinomycin D did not appreciably inhibit the induction of cell union [8] and this appeared to suggest that the control of protein biosynthesis might be at the level of translation. However, actinomycin D did not appreciably inhibit the uridine incorporation either under these conditions. It appears therefore that this antibiotic poorly enters these cells and cannot be used to answer such questions by simple experiments. In *Paramecium*, both puromycin and actinomycin S_3 inhibit the formation of cell union in conjugation. Therefore, it appears that the control is at the level of transcription in this case [11]. I think this problem must be investigated more thoroughly in *Blepharisma* at each step of cell union. There are at least two steps. First cells stick to each other by cilia and then they unite more intimately by the non-ciliated region of the cell surface. It is possible that the protein synthesis for the first step is controlled at the translational level, but the protein synthesis for the second step is controlled at the transcriptional level.

E. GROSS (Bethesda, Mdss.): You showed the gamone II as the Ca^{++}-salt. Is the Ca^{++}-ion necessary for the biological effect ? There are interesting structural features in gamone II, *e. g.* keto functions and two hydroxy groups. Since the compound is accessible synthetically, did you study the biological effect of chemically modified variants of gamone I ?

A. MIYAKE: This gamone was isolated as the Ca-salt, and the chemical structure was determined by X-ray crystallography with this Ca-salt. Because the suspension medium of the cells already contains 0.4 mM $CaCl_2$ [5], the Ca of gamone II should not give any significant change in the Ca-concentration. Whether the presence of Ca in the suspension medium is necessary for the effect of gamone II has not yet been seriously investigated. However, there are some indications that the dissociated ionic form of gamone II is more effective than the non-dissociated molecular form. That is, the lower the pH the more effective gamone II will be in the range pH

5.6—7.6. Such effect of pH was not observed for gamone I. Concerning the effect of structurally related compounds, only commercially available chemicals have so far been tested. Formylkynurenine, β-(indole-3) lactic acid and serotonin had no gamone II effect. 5-hydroxytryptophan and tryptophan competitively inhibited the effect of gamone II [3, 8]. Here the L-form was about four times more effective for the inhibition than the D-form, and this suggests that the L-configuration of the gamone is important. This may explain the fact that the synthetic gamone II is about half as active as the natural gamone II. This gamone had been synthesized only recently, and chemically modified variants have not yet been obtained.

B. HAMPRECHT (München): Dr. MIYAKE, do you have any indication that the cAMP system is involved in one or both of the gamones?

A. MIYAKE: This problem is being investigated by Dr. J. BEYER, my coworker in Berlin. He got some results which indicated that when gamones induce the cell union, the cAMP in the cell increases (unpublished). However, in some experiments the effect of gamone was not detected. He also found that theophylline, an inhibitor of phosphodiesterase, induced in some strains a weak cell attachment. Therefore to some extent this agent appears to mimic the effect of gamone. This result suggests that the cAMP is involved. However, when cAMP itself and mono- and dibutyryl cAMP were tested, no significant effect was detected. So at present there is only a slight indication that the cAMP system is directly involved in the induction of cell union by gamone.

Chemical Signal Transmission by Gamete Attractants in Brown Algae

LOTHAR JAENICKE

Institut für Biochemie der Universität zu Köln, 5000 Köln, An der Bottmühle 2, Federal Republic of Germany

With 2 Figures

I wish to present a system that might be useful in studying chemotaxis and transmission of chemical signals. It is the occurrence and action of highly specific, volatile and very lipophilic hydrocarbon sex attractants formed by the unicellular female gametes of some seaweeds to attract the unicellular motile males for conjugation [1].

Figure 1 shows the formulae of the four compounds known so far and their proposed biogenesis from poly-unsaturated fatty

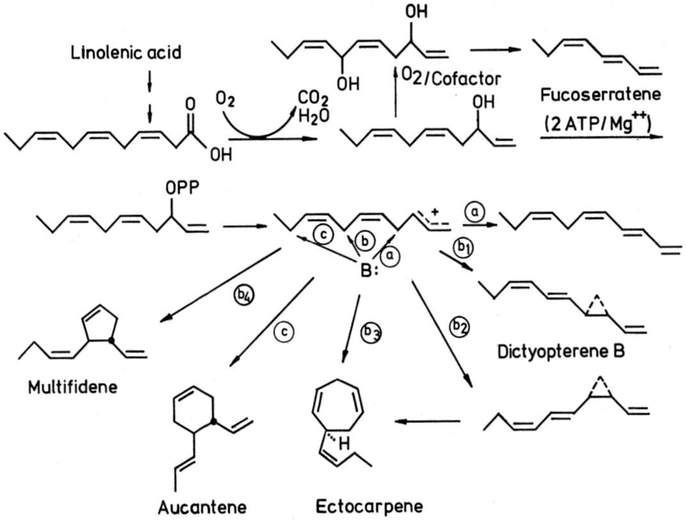

Fig. 1. Biogenetic connections of known gamones of seaweeds

acids. β-Oxidation and oxidative decarboxylation of *e.g.* linolenic acid yields a C_{11} triene-ol [2]. Supplied with an appropriate leaving group this gives a carbonium ion which can cyclize in different ways, giving the 7-membered ring $C_{11}H_{16}$ hydrocarbon ectocarpene in *Ectocarpus* [3], the di-substituted, prostaglandin-like $C_{11}H_{16}$ cyclopentene multifidene in *Cutleria* [2] with its accompanying inactive cyclohexene isomer aucantene [2], the $C_{11}H_{16}$ divinyl-cyclopropanes of *Dictyopteris* and, when further hydroxylated and degraded, fucoserratene in *Fucus* [4], now definitely established to be the *trans, cis*-1,3,5-octatriene. Syntheses of these compounds and biological studies on all of them are underway.

Our greatest gains have been made with ectocarpene, which was synthesized with strong tritium label in the side chain positions 1' and 2' by MARNER (see [5]). By exposing male gametes of *Ectocarpus* for different lengths of time to a gas phase containing the labeled gamone the kinetics of the uptake were studied. As shown in Fig. 2, short exposure times give high specific labeling. With increasing time, the labeling is diminished, apparently by some metabolic degradation of the side chain, the product of which is as yet

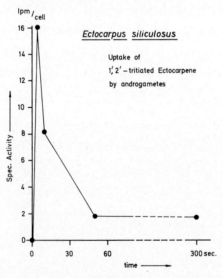

Fig. 2. Time course of uptake of label by *Ectocarpus* androgametes on exposure to tritiated ectocarpene

unidentified. A refractory phase of the receptors prevents further binding of the chemotactic substance. Finally, a steady state is reached.

This seems strongly indicative of a messenger/receptor mechanism with structural changes in the receiving protein of quite slow reversibility. According to recent, if also still preliminary radio-autographic evidence, obtained together with Prof. MÜLLER (Konstanz), the shortly exposed, highly labeled cells have most of the label over the large flagellum, none over the short flagellum which is supposedly a steering device, and relatively little over the cell body. After longer incubations the label over the flagellum is reduced dramatically, whereas most of the radioactivity is now over the cell. This, too, seems evidence for specific receiving sites (in the flagella ?), transport to the cell, and metabolic inactivation. It my be noted in passing that it is the large flagellum that is used by the male gametes to approach the female and to anker to her as a first step of cell-fusion. It might be that this simple, albeit quite subtle system will be useful in the elucidation of chemotaxis, chemical transmission and, as a model, for other sensory processes.

References

1. JAENICKE, L., MÜLLER, D. G.: Gametenlockstoffe bei niederen Pflanzen und Tieren. Fortschr. Chem. Org. Naturstoffe **30**, 62—100 (1973); — JAENICKE, L.: Sexuallockstoffe im Pflanzenreich. Festvortr. Rhein-Westf. Akademie der Wissensch. N 217. Opladen-Köln: Westdeutscher Verlag 1972.
2. JAENICKE, L., MÜLLER, D. G., MOORE, R. E.: Multifidene and Aucantene. C_{11} Hydrocarbons in the male attracting essential oil from the gyno-gametes of *Cutleria multifida* (Smith) Grev. (Phaeophyta). J. Amer. chem. Soc. **96**, 3324 (1974).
3. MÜLLER, D. G., JAENICKE, L., DONIKE, M., AKINTOBI, T.: Sex attractant in a brown alga: Chemical structure. Science **171**, 815—816 (1971).
4. MÜLLER, D. G., JAENICKE, L.: Fucoserraten, the female sex attractant of *Fucus serratus* L. (Phaeophyta). FEBS Letters **30**, 137—139 (1973).
5. JAENICKE, L., AKINTOBI, T., MARNER, F.-J.: Ein Beitrag zur Darstellung von Alkylcycloheptadienen: Synthese von Ectocarpen und seinen Homologen. Liebigs Ann. Chem. **1973**, 1252—1262.

Energy Transfer and Signal Conversion

On the Significance of Two-Dimensional Super-Structures in Biomembranes for Energy-Transfer and Signal Conversion

W. Kreutz, K.-P. Hofmann, and R. Uhl

Institut für Biophysik und Strahlenbiologie, Universität Freiburg im Breisgau, D-7800 Freiburg, Albertstraße 23, Federal Republic of Germany

With 9 Figures

The most evident two-dimensional super-structure so far determined in biomembranes is found in photosynthetic bacteria. Figure 1 shows an example of an electronmicroscopic picture of the

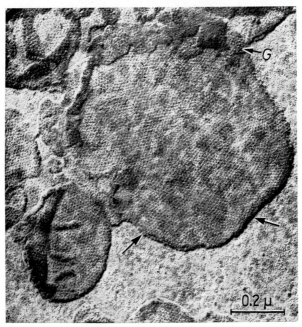

Fig. 1 a

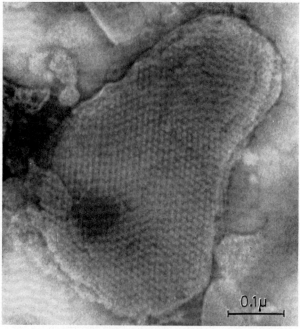

Fig 1 b

bacterium *Rhodopseudomonas viridis* by Giesbrecht and Drews
[1]. The whole membrane surface is covered with double chained
super-structures consisting of protein strands in a two-dimensional
association, forming several dislocation areas in the membrane
surface. Fig. 1 b gives a plane view of membranes of the same object
in a different state as obtained by Fritz, Göbel and Kreutz. In
this state corpuscular protein particles are attached onto the matrix in a hexagonal crystalline lattice arrangement. Apparently,
the matrix protein strands of Fig. 1 a define the coordination loci
(binding sites) for the protein particles seen in Fig. 1 b. The photosynthetic membrane of the higher plants also shows such combinations of linear super-structures and attached corpuscular
particles in orthogonal arrangements. In an earlier paper a detailed
discussion of these structural viewpoints was given [2]. The
quantitative evaluation of the X-ray diffraction diagrams of these
structures lead us to propose protein-chains for the matrix protein,

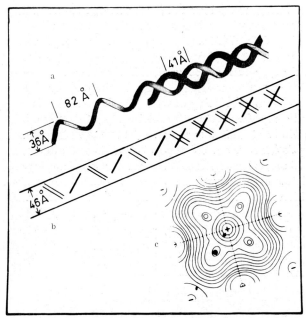

Fig. 2. (a) Single and double spiral. Diameter of the spiral backbone: 36—38 Å. Pitch height: single spiral 82 Å, double spiral 41 Å. (b) The schematic projection image corresponding to the single and double spiral. Diameter of the spiral backbone plus side chains: 46—48 Å. (c) The calculated electron density distribution giving one "overcrossing" in a double spiral

in which polypeptides are arranged in a zigzag-manner (Fig. 2 b) forming rings or loops [2]. In Fig. 2 b each zigzag line denotes the projection of the mass of one protein ring or loop. Probably this protein type represents a spiral-protein, either forming single or double spirals, as shown in Fig. 2 a.

This concept is derived from the electron density projection depicted in Fig. 2 c as well as from the ring-like electron density projection of the cross section of this protein [3]. The X-ray diffraction diagrams further demonstrate that the correlation of the individual membrane protein spirals are not to be regarded strictly crystalline but paracrystalline or liquid-crystalline. A detailed discussion on this structural situation in biomembranes is given elsewhere [4].

The biological significance of such defined two dimensional ($2d$-) superstructures will be demonstrated for two cases:

    1. for a defined efficient energy conduction *e.g.* photon transfer and

    2. for cooperative processes in biomembranes.

The photon transfer mechanism in the photosynthetic membrane offers a convincing example for Case 1. As this topic was treated comprehensively in an earlier paper [5], only a brief comment will be given in this report. For the establishment of distinct absorption levels, *e.g.* chlorophyll absorbing at 673 nm, 683 nm, and 695 nm, chlorophyll molecules must be kept in strict geometric correlation in order to achieve a strongly defined interaction of the transition moments, for instance in the form of dimers. Further-

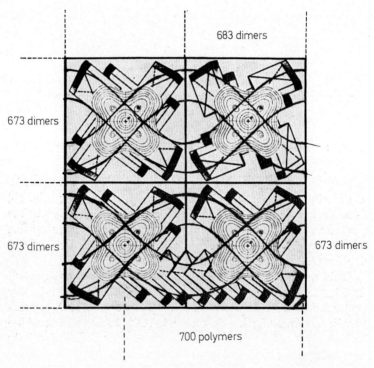

Fig. 3. View of spiral protein forming the backbone for underlying chloro-phyll-dimers

more, the geometric correlation of the dimers to one another must be guaranteed in order to obtain a defined exciton conduction or long-range Förster transfer mechanism. These conditions can be achieved only by a protein super-structure (Fig. 3).

In the case of cooperativity, for instance cooperative interaction between reaction partners, geometric arrangements with sufficiently long correlation periods are also demanded. As an example, cooperative membrane behavior can be demonstrated in the primary reactions of visual signal conversion in the rod outer segment (ROS)-disc-membrane. First, it should be added that the same or a very similar matrix-protein type as in the photosynthetic membrane can be detected also in the ROS-disc-membrane by X-ray diffraction, as Fig. 4a and b shows.

The distances between the diffraction rings in the X-ray pattern of Fig. 4a *per se* exclude a pure linear lattice. Furthermore, Fig. 4b directly demonstrates the separation into a linear lattice (stacking of the discs) in the "meridian" (vertical) and the planar lattice in the "equator" (horizontal). The $2d$-diffraction pattern can be explained with the same spiral structures of Fig. 2a and b. Compared with the photosynthetic membrane, the difference manifests itself essentially in the relative position of the spirals against each other. The conditions for cooperative behavior within the protein fraction of the membrane is, therefore, established in the disc membrane.

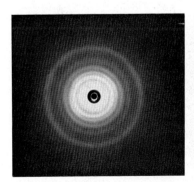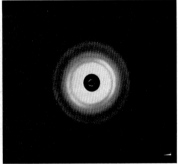

Fig. 4a and b. Diffraction pattern of isolated rod-outer-segments of bovine retina in humid state. (a) Unoriented, (b) oriented equatorial 93 Å-, 82 Å-, and 46.5 Å-reflections; meridian linear lattice reflections corresponding to a period of 246 Å (S. STANGE, unpublished)

Whether these possibilities are realized in nature can be outlined by investigations dealing with the bleaching behavior of rhodopsin and correlated processes. Rhodopsin molecules may be associated to the matrix protein in a corresponding way as demonstrated in Fig. 1a and 1b, *i.e.* the matrix protein strands should define the geometric coordination of the binding sites for the attachment of rhodopsins and the rhodopsins may fluctuate between the paracrystalline coordinated binding sites.

If a sequence of light flashes (3 min flash interval, 20 μsec flash duration) is applied on rod outer segments of bovine eyes in Ringer suspension in a light-flash photometer, a bleaching behavior of rhodopsin in dependence to the flash number is registered, as illustrated in Fig. 5a. The first applied narrow band flash of $\lambda_{max} = 512$ nm corresponds to a bleaching of about 2–3%. Since the amplitudes belonging to certain flash numbers are plotted logarithmically, the measurement shows that in the range of a bleaching rate of about 2–50% the amplitudes decrease faster than exponentially (sigmoidally). At more than 50% bleaching, the amplitudes behave exponentially. The absolute rate of the bleached

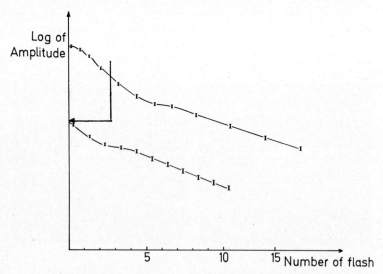

Fig. 5. Bleaching of the absorption change at 380 nm (metarhodopsin II) for two preparations of differently light adapted cattle eyes

rhodopsin prior to the experiments appears to depend on the seasonal dark adaptation of the animals before slaughtering. The amplitude series in Fig. 5b indicates this and shows a bleaching behavior corresponding to a higher light exposure prior to measurement (abscissa shifting). This interpretation is supported by DE GRIP et al. [6], who measured the season-dependent fraction of unbleached rhodopsin of cattle. The bleaching behavior of rhodopsin in dependence to the flash number has already been investigated by EMRICH [7]. Because of the lower sensitivity of his measuring equipment, 20 flashes were summed to reach one amplitude value. Each of his amplitude values corresponds to a bleaching rate of about 15%. Under these experimental conditions the superexponential initial phase was not detected by EMRICH. He found exponential behavior throughout the bleaching curve.

The signals obtained by single light flashes as shown in Fig. 5 were sufficiently intense so that application of flash groups could be avoided in our experiments. This is demonstrated in Fig. 6.

The measurements illustrated in Fig. 5a and b shows that the metarhodopsin I/II-reaction measured at 380 nm decreases superexponentially in the physiologically relevant range in dependence on the flash-number. This superexponential decay of the amplitudes cannot be due to experimental inhomogeneities in the preparation, light beam, etc., but may be interpreted as a cooperative effect: The rhodopsin molecules ought to be cooperatively coupled in the dark state and the coupling should be no longer efficient or exist no more at a bleaching degree of about 50%. The amplitude decay curve cannot be fully explained at this point. Taking into consideration

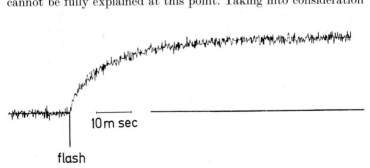

Fig. 6. Time course of the absorption change at 380 nm of a ROS-Suspension. Single flash. Excitation light: $\lambda_{max} = 512$ nm 20° C

Cone's experiments on lateral diffusion on rhodopsin [8], the ROS-disc-membrane should possess the following characteristics, in order to understand the cooperative bleaching behavior:

1. There are paracrystalline matrix structures ($2d$-lattice-protein, spiral-protein) which establish a sufficiently high order for the geometrical reaction coordination in short range regions performing direct or indirect (*via* lipids or protein) coupling of rhodopsins.

2. Rhodopsin possesses the ability to occupy these coordination sites for the duration of a certain correlation time by lateral diffusion.

3. The average range of the transfer mechanism is probably defined by three factors:

a) The average geometric extension of the paracrystalline matrix zones.

b) Interruption or decrease of the transfer coupling by bleached rhodopsin with increasing bleaching.

c) By correlation of the phase relation of the intrinsic rotation of rhodopsin as measured by Cone [9].

4. This mechanism guarantees an intrinsic regulation of the signals, in dependence on the light intensity, *i.e.* at low light intensity large amplification by bleaching of large cooperative units down to uncoupled monomers or oligomers.

5. The steepness of the curve in the region of cooperative coupling, as compared with the behavior in the end part of the curve, and also taking into consideration the height of the initial amplitudes, suggests that the coupling of rhodopsin is accomplished along linear chains.

It has been well established in a number of laboratories that a pH-change is coupled with the metarhodopsin I/II-transformation [10—13]. The behavior of the pH was therefore measured in dependence on the flash-number with a pH-indicator (bromocresol-purple, $\lambda_{max} = 595$ nm). Figure 7 gives a comparative measurement of the pH-decay (lower curve) as well as the M-I/II-reaction (upper curve) in the presence of the indicator under identical conditions. From Fig. 7 it is evident that the amplitudes of the pH-change and the M-I/II-signals run parallel up to a bleaching rate of about 50%. In the further course, however, the amplitude of the pH-change shows a faster decay than the M-I/II-transformation. This indicates that the lighttriggered release of binding sites for protons

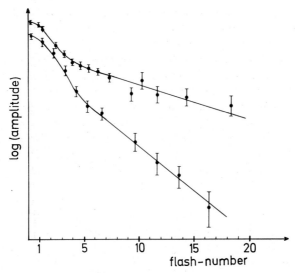

Fig. 7. Upper curve: Bleaching of rhodopsin in the presence of a pH-indicator. Lower curve: Decay of pH-change

comprises regions at least as large or larger than the cooperative coupled units of the M-I/II-reaction.

For the measurement of the pH-changes and their time course the following statement can be made: If the indicator is offered to the outer region of the outer-segments, the pH-signal shows a half decay time of about 100 msec at 20° C (Fig. 8b). If the indicator is added to the inner region of the outer segments, a 10 msec-signal is obtained (Fig. 8a). The protons, therefore, need a 90 msec permeation time in order to pass through the outer membrane. Furthermore, it can be demonstrated that the active indicator in the outside region is bound to the outer side of the outer membrane. To show this, the rods are bathed in indicator solution, centrifuged and resuspended in indicator-free solution. Thus, the pH-signal can be registered more easily than before. Both, the fast and slow pH-signal, can also be measured together in a superimposed form, if indicator is applied to the inside as well as to the outside of the outer segments.

Apart from the two signals described above, two further signals, unknown up to now, were found (Fig. 9 a—d). They differ in their bleaching behavior in a characteristic manner: one of these signals is negative in sign (Fig. 9d) with respect to the M-I/II-signal (Fig. 9a), while the other signal is positive (Fig. 9b). These signals were registered superimposed in the range between 600 and 800 nm (Fig. 9c), *i.e.* in a wavelength region in which the rhodopsin-metabolites show no absorption. The half-time decay of the positive signal is about 20 msec, that of the negative signal about 8 msec at a pH of 5.6 and 20° C. The amplitudes of these signals in dependence on the number of flashes is remarkable: the positive signal has already vanished after 5 flashes, whereas the negative signal behaves similarly to the M-I/II-reaction in bleaching.

This signal behavior suggests that within the outer segments a cooperative behavior exists apparently in different regions. This conclusion is strengthened by the fact that the time course of the signals changes inversely to the decay behavior of the amplitudes, *i.e.* the kinetically slowest signal bleaches fastest and therefore comprises the largest cooperative units. The spectral behavior of the negative signal indicates that this signal represents a scattering

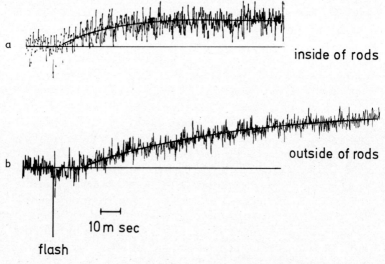

Fig. 8. Time course of the absorption change caused by pH-change, pH-Indicator: Bromocresolred; 595 nm excitation light: $\lambda_{max} = 512$ nm 20° C. Summation of 4 flashes

effect. The slow positive signal is very probably is not due to a scattering effect. Molecular interpretation is not yet possible. It might mean a further signal-dependent sensitivity step within the outer segments, which is self-regulating and effective only in a small range of low light intensity.

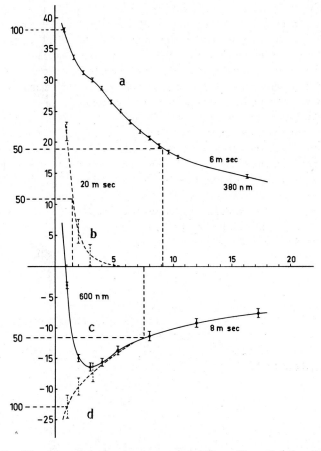

Fig. 9. *a* Bleaching of rhodopsin measured at 380 nm (6 msec). *b* Amplitude decay of a 20 msec-signal measured at 600 nm. *c* Superimposed amplitude decay curve of the 20 msec signal (*b*) and the 8 msec signal (*a*) measured at 600 nm. *d* Amplitude decay curve of a 8 msec signal measured at 600 nm

The cooperative bleaching of the amplitudes and the faster exhaustion of the H^+-binding sites, differing at least by the factor of 2, signify, that at least 2, but surely not more than 10 protons per photon absorbed, are bound. In the aqueous space between the discs, less than 10 protons are found at a pH = 6. This means that the light-triggered release of 2 to 10 proton-binding sites produces a vectorial proton suction in a radial direction towards the inner side of the outer membrane. The release of proton-binding sites also means a simultaneous release of at least 2 monovalent cations (K^+, Na^+) or one bivalent cation, for instance Ca^{++}. This proton suction and cation pressure will lead to an inverse exchange behavior on the inner surface of the outer membrane, namely to a proton release and Ca^{++}-binding. The disc-membrane would, therefore, represent a counteracting ion-exchanger pair.

An ion-exchange H^+ vs. Ca^{++} on the inner side of the outer membrane will cause a permeation decrease, especially if this exchange site is located at an Na^+-pore. Since there exist only about 10^3 pores in the outer-membrane of the outer segment, i.e. about 1 pore per disc, even a single ion-exchange already means a considerable hyperpolarization effect. The existence of a 1 : 1-exchanger, functioning as a reliable transmitter, guarantees the amplification by triggering the blocking of a small number of pores possessing a high permeation rate of 10^7 Na^+/sec per pore.

The light-triggered liberation of a fully deprotonated buffer-system out of the hydrophobic phase is supported by the following findings:

Firstly, flashlight photometric measurements on the pH-dependency of the pH-changes by Emrich [13] show a point of inflection at about pH 6.2 and exclusively positive signals, i.e. alkalinization over the whole pH-scale. The second experiment was carried out by McConnell, Rafferty, and Dilley [12], with pH-electrodes on intact discs and discs treated with Triton. With intact discs only positive signals were found, whereas with Triton-treated discs the signals become negative at pH 6.2. This implies that in the first case the buffer is fully loaded with metal cations, while in the other about one half of the buffer is loaded with protons and the other half with cations. As the aequeous inter-disc space will show a pH of about 6 or less, and because of the pK 6.2 of the buffer-system triggered by light, these experiments indicate that in the *in vivo* state the proton-binding sites are embedded in a hydrophobic region, and that they are exposed to the aqueous phase by the light action on rhodopsin.

The characteristics described provide the following general viewpoints for signal conversion in vision:

1. The initial direct or indirect cooperative coupling of rhodopsin offers an explanation for the high quantum efficiency of the visual system at very low light intensities.

2. The decrease in coupling at higher intensities regulates the input of the transmitter system in the further course of bleaching.

3. The transmitter system is established by a corresponding ion-exchange (proton/cation-exchange) at the disc and outer membrane.

4. The pore mechanism at the outer membrane triggered by the transmitter system effects the high amplification by regulation of the dark current.

References

1. GIESBRECHT, P., DREWS, G.: Arch. Mikrobiol. **54**, 297 (1966).
2. KREUTZ, W.: Angew. Chem. **84**, 597 (1972).
3. HOSEMANN, R., KREUTZ, W.: Naturwissenschaften **53**, 298 (1966).
4. KREUTZ, W. in: Summer School in Biophysics, COCHRAN, J., COLBOW, C. (ed.). Vancouver: Simon Frazer University Press (1974).
5. KREUTZ, W.: Naturforsch. **23** b. 520 (1968).
6. DE GRIP, W. J., DAEMEN, F. J. R., BONTING, S. L.: Vision Res. **12**, 1697 (1972).
7. EMRICH, H. M.: Pflügers Arch. Ges. Phys. **319**, 126 (1970).
8. POO, M. M., CONE, R. A.: Exp. Eye Res. **17**, 503 (1973).
9. CONE, R. A.: Nature (Lond.) New Biol. **236**, 39 (1972).
10. MATTHEWS, R. G., HUBBARD, R., BROWN, P. K., WALD, G.: J. gen. Physiol. **47**, 215 (1963).
11. FALK, G., FATT, P.: J. Physiol. (Lond.) **183**, 211 (1966).
12. McCONNELL, D. G., RAFFERTY, C., DILLEY, R. A.: J. biol. Chem. **243**, 5820 (1968).
13. EMRICH, H. M.: Habil.-Arbeit, Technische Universität Berlin 1972.

Discussion

H. M. EMRICH (München): Regarding the surplus proton-uptake at the beginning of photolysis, quantitative measurements have shown that initially 2—3 H^+ per formed M_{II} are bound. It therefore seems questionable whether the proton-uptake can function as a transmitter since this change of 2—3 H^+ can easily be eliminated by the buffer.

W. KREUTZ (Freiburg): First it must be said that up to now a quantitative determination of the number of bound protons has not been possible. All pertaining statements made up to now can only be regarded as estimations at best. Only one result can be considered reliable, namely, that for one bleached rhodopsin *at least* 2 protons are bound. In my report I based my considerations on this fact. Because of the coupling of the rhodopsins indicated by our measurements, about 10 protons could be bound per quantum absorbed in the initial phase of bleaching, which, because of the low H^+-concentration in the inter-disc space, produce a sufficiently strong H^+-abstraction. According to our concept, we even regard it a necessity that part of the protons are buffered away by the exchange system to facilitate the proposed transmitter mechanism. Moreover, the registration of a slow pH-change ($\approx$ 100 ms) in the outer phase of the ROS-discs demonstrates that the light-triggered H^+-binding causes a decrease of H^+ in the inter-disc space superceding the natural buffer capacity.

H. M. EMRICH: In my opinion, in taking up of a proton, an NH_2-group is transferred from the hydrophobic inner region of metarhodopsin into the aqueous phase. This would mean that no cation is liberated in exchange of a bound H^+.

W. KREUTZ: Your own investigations as well as those of McCONNEL et al. [11] in which the light-triggered proton binding, resp. proton release were measured, show that the pK-value of the proton-binding site amounts to about 6.2. Only your measurements indicate that a weak additional binding capacity with a pK 10.5 exists. This leads me to the conclusion that the major binding capacity for protons cannot be caused by a NH_2-group, but at best plays a secondary role. A comparison of the pH-amplitudes yielded by your measurements at pH 6.2 and 10.5 suggest an about tenfold higher binding capacity of the acceptor at pH 6.2 than the NH_2-acceptor at pH 10.5 coupled with rhodopsin 1:1.

B. HESS (Dortmund): A question regarding the cooperativity; first a technical question: What were the thicknesses of the preparations used for the flash-light experiments? Further, I did not understand how the cooperativity in the dimer range or in larger areas can be imagined. Does any hyperchromism occur? Can it be observed experimentally? In other words: If exposing a monomer, does the extinction-coefficient in the attached monomer partner rise? This should be detected experimentally.

W. KREUTZ: I take it that in your question concerning the preparation thickness you have in mind that there might exist an inhomogeneity of excitation, giving an explanation for the amplitude decay curve. The preparation thickness corresponds to an absorption of the excitation light of about 0.1 at 512 nm. Measurements with excitation light > 550 nm, i.e. with considerably lower absorption, exhibit the same decay curve. Also other aspects of inhomogeneity were carefully checked (*e.g.* by mixing the preparation after each flash, taking into account the geometry of the light beam *etc.*). These factors can be disregarded as cause for the amplitude decay curve.

Cooperativity in this connection as understood by us, means that in the initial range of bleaching 1 quantum, absorbed directly or indirectly, bleaches more than 1 rhodopsin, *i.e.* that there exists a rhodopsin-rhodopsin coupling on bleaching. The alternative is that always for 1 quantum absorbed only one rhodopsin is transformed to M_{II}, and that the overexponential amplitude decay curve of M_{II}-formation is due to secondary rhodopsin-M_{II} transformations caused by interactions between further rhodopsin and the surroundings (lipids, structural protein) in which a phase change was induced by the light-triggered primary rhodopsin-M_{II}-transformation.

Concerning the hyperchromism the following can be said: Our measurements are carried out at 380 nm, the maximum absorption of M_{II}. The analysis only reflects the course of bleaching. A continous change of the extinction coefficient of M_{II} in the course of bleaching would also offer an explanation for the measured bleaching curve. This interpretation would imply that the "surrounding phases" of the rhodopsins and, as a consequence, the interactions change in the membrane in the bleaching range from 0—50%, and that beyond 50% they become invariable. This interpretation of the M_{II}-amplitude decay must be kept in mind, but we consider it unlikely.

B. HESS: Is your concept on super-complexes in aggreement with the results obtained by CONE, [7] on the diffusion of rhodopsin?

W. KREUTZ: We must demand temporary complexes which become smaller or less effective by progressive bleaching. This is only possible if a rhodopsin exchange takes place between the complexes. This regrouping may appear as or signify a lateral diffusion.

B. HESS: How is the situation with artificial membranes, which are not stabilized by structural protein?

W. KREUTZ: The so-called artificial membranes generally consist of bimolecular lipid-vesicles to which proteins are attached. Such vesicles are smaller by about one order of magnitude in diameter than natural membranes. In these vesicles, van der Waals forces (reaching to about 1000 Å in lipids) suffice for stabilization. Apart from that, in such experiments the vesicles are only monofunctionally burdened in contrast to biomembranes which are poly-functional, introducing instability into the system.

L. JAENICKE (Köln): Could you make some additional comments on the "structural protein"?

W. KREUTZ: In connection with structural protein there is one special aspect of importance: recently the opinion has been forwarded that apart from the functional proteins no further essential protein could exist in biomembranes. In all biomembranes so far investigated there exists a protein part with no enzymatic activities which amounts to 10—30%. For instance, in the retina-disc about 80% rhodopsin, resp. opsin is found. There remains an undefined protein rest of 20%. Now, if a special protein exists in bio-membranes, which we call $2d$-lattice protein and which probably consists of super spirals in a $2d$-arrangement, contributing 20% of protein weight, it will play an important structural role because of its very fortunate ratio between plane (volume) requirement and molecular weight in the membrane. If spirals are arranged two-dimensionally, a membrane-plane section of about 80 Å × 40 Å can be covered by about 50 amino acids in the case of single spirals, respectively 100 amino acids in the case of double spirals. Thus, a maximal structural stability is obtained by a minimum demand of amino acids (M ≈ 10000). If this section were covered by an association of normal protein, a molecular weight greater than at least one order of magnitude than in the case of structural protein would be necessary. The existence of structural protein, therefore, cannot be questioned by the objection con-cerning the "rest-protein" only amounting to 20%. Such a small fraction of spiral protein suffices to constitute the matrix-structure of biomembranes.

B. HESS: I would like to discuss the structural protein in more detail, this being a rather controversial question. You might know that in the case of mitochondrial proteins the concept of the structural protein has been dis-carded. This is also strengthened by functional viewpoints. If isolated cyto-chrome oxidase is analysed, the same characteristics of this enzyme can be observed as in the membrane. The same applies to the purple membrane, *i.e.* from the functional standpoint the membrane proteins only have to be inser-ted into the membrane to obtain full activity. The structural protein is not necessary. Do rods represent an exceptional case, and can you offer further hints for the structure protein besides the structure analysis and the rest of about 20% in the protein composition of membranes?

W. KREUTZ: One of the most striking results in the field of biomembrane research since 20 years is that all biomembranes partly consist of a protein, possessing qualities which deviate from those of normal enzymatic protein. This protein was especially well characterized in the case of mitochondria. It possesses physico-chemical qualities (solubility, plane resp. space requirement, aggregation behavior etc.) which differ basically from those of normal enzymatic protein. It is hard luck for this protein that it is not fitted with enzymatic activities, *i.e.* with pure chemical functions. This may be the reason why biochemists regard it as non-existent. However, it is my con-viction that this protein is to fullfil a very important function, namely to establish the structural and, consequently, also the functional basis for bio-membranes. Its task is essentially of a physical nature, and its existence therefore cannot be discussed on the basis of chemical criteria.

H. STIEVE (Jülich): Can you give the approximate diameter of the super-spirals seen on the electronmicroscopic pictures you mentioned?

W. KREUTZ: On the electron microscopic pictures of J. H. MATHEJA, shown in the figure the lateral mean distance between the spiral axes amounts to about 50 Å.

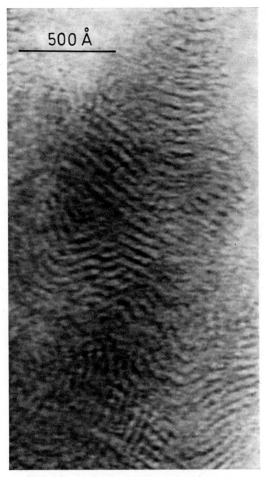

Figure. Electron micrograph of Folch-Lees protein from nerve myelin (phosphotungstic acid, negative contrast). Courtesy: J. H. MATHEJA

According to our earlier X-ray data (1961) and recent measurements (see Fig. 2, chapter 13) this distance should amount to 46—48 Å. The diameter of the actual spiral backbone, however, would be less by about 10 Å. Presumably about 5 Å long side-chains exist, keeping the spiral at distance. X-ray measurements further indicate that the pitch of the single spiral amounts to 82 Å, and that of the double spiral to 41 Å.

H. STIEVE: If there exists a long-range structure of amino acids, what factors then determine the helical structure, which apparently is rather periodic and also demands interaction between the chains?

W. KREUTZ: There are different possibilities for stabilization which — so it seems — may occur in the various biomembranes. First, there exists the possibility for the formation of double spirals (consisting of two left-hand or two right-hand spirals) representing a very stable configuration. Apparently, they are realized in the photosynthetic System II, in erythrocytes and in the Folch-Lees-protein of nerve myelin and are characterized by X-ray reflection corresponding to Bragg-spacing of 41 Å and 31 Å. A second possibility is offered by the defined association of a left-hand and a right-hand side by side spiral-aggregation, probably occuring in photosynthetic System I and in photosynthetic bacteria signified by 82 Å and 62 Å-X-ray reflections. A modification of this type of structure also seems to exist in the retina disc membranes producing 92—96 Å, 82 Å, and 62 ÅX-ray reflections. The third possibility is provided by a stabilization of the protein by interaction with lipids. I mainly have in mind hydrophobic interactions, indicated by the fact that this protein type can only be dissolved as a lipoprotein or loaded with detergents (replacing the lipids). If the lipids are taken off entirely from this protein, it is fully denatured.

H. STIEVE: May I put a further question on this topic? How do you imagine the incorporation of structural protein into the membrane? Looking at it figuratively, might it represent the bread with the lipid on top of it and above the lipid the floating rhodopsin? The structural protein must then not move at all?

W. KREUTZ: No, the structural protein can move, but restrictedly. It can form paracrystalline regions — fluid-like structures —; it can be mobile; however, essentially vertically to its long axis it will be relatively invariable and stable. Your picture of the protein lipid-disstribution, mentioned in your question, must not apply in this strict sense. According to my concept, the spiral protein can be incorporated into the lipid phase essentially producing lipid mono-layers and in between these regions bilayered lipid phases may exist, allowing linear shifting (movements) of other proteins in the lipid phase. Thus the spiral protein will guarantee a stable total super-structure, and at the same time will allow fluidic zones within the membrane.

On the Topography of Photoreceptor Membranes

F. J. M. Daemen, P. J. G. M. van Breugel, and S. L. Bonting

Department of Biochemistry, University of Nijmegen, Nijmegen, The Netherlands

Treatment with proteolytic enzymes has been shown to be a useful tool in elucidating structural details of biomembranes. We have obtained interesting data on the topography of bovine rod outer segment disk membranes (photoreceptor membranes), especially the localization of rhodopsin, by incubation with the proteolytic enzymes pronase, subtilisin, papain, chymotrypsin or trypsin. The results, which are rather similar for all these proteases, are collected in the table and show:

1. Rhodopsin, the principal photoreceptor membrane protein (85%) cannot be spectrally degraded by proteases at any enzyme concentration (6 hrs incubation at 30°) as long as the membrane structure is intact.

2. If, however, the arrangement of the membrane is disturbed by detergents, the typical rhodopsin absorption maximum at 500 nm is rapidly destroyed by proteases. Thus, either rhodopsin becomes accessible to the enzymes after interruption of lipid-protein interactions or the detergent unfolds the rhodopsin molecule itself.

3. In order to distinguish between these two possibilities, photoreceptor membranes were pretreated with phospholipase C, which destroys the membrane bilayer arrangement by removing the polar head groups from the phospholipids. Again, rhodopsin is no longer spectrally resistant against proteolytic attack, which suggests that, indeed, the lipid bilayer protects rhodopsin.

4. Another photoreceptor membrane protein, retinol oxidoreductase, is very sensitive to proteases, also in the intact membrane.

5. Peptide analysis by SDS-gel electrophoresis shows a progressive proteolytic breakdown of all membrane proteins in detergent. However, in the intact membrane, rhodopsin is apparently

only susceptible to a limited degree, which does not interfere with its absorption spectrum, while the other photoreceptor membrane proteins are largely degraded.

These results taken together clearly indicate that in bovine photoreceptor membranes rhodopsin is deeply embedded in the hydrophobic core of the phospholipid bilayer, and is only for a small part exposed to the aqueous phase.

Protease treatment of bovine photoreceptor membranes

Treatment	Rhodopsin absorbance	Oxido-reductase activity	Major peptides[a]
Untreated control	stable	stable	37000, minor higher M.W. bands
In suspension	stable	abolished	$\pm$25000; <15000; no higher M.W. band
In detergent[b]	rapid decay	abolished	>15000; no higher M.W. bands
In suspension after PL-ase C treatment	decay	abolished	—

[a] By SDS-gel-electrophoresis
[b] Digitonin; Triton X-100; Emulphogene BC-720; CTAB

Carrier and Pore Mechanisms in Lipid Membranes

E. Bamberg, R. Benz, P. Läuger, and G. Stark

*Universität Konstanz, Fachbereich Biologie, 7750 Konstanz,
Federal Republic of Germany*

With 13 Figures

One of the first steps in sensory excitation is a change in the ion permeability of a membrane. The elucidation of the transduction process is therefore closely related to our understanding of the mechanisms by which ions cross the cell membrane. As yet, most ion transport mechanisms in biological membranes are still obscure at the molecular level. On the other hand, in the last years some progress has been made in the investigation of lipid model membranes. We may expect that these studies may lead to a better insight into the possible ion transport mechanisms in the cell membrane.

The interior of a lipid membrane consists of the hydrocarbon chains of the lipid molecules, and therefore represents a medium of low dielectric constant. This means that the energy which is required to transfer an ion such as Na^+ or K^+ from the aqueous phase into the membrane is many times the mean thermal energy; *i.e.*, the membrane behaves like an extremely high barrier for the passage of these ions. But biological membranes are more or less permeable towards Na^+ or K^+, and therefore we have to assume that mechanisms exist within the membrane, by which the activation energy of ion transport is drastically reduced.

Two limiting cases for such transport mechanisms may be visualized: fixed pores and mobile carriers. A pore may be represented, for instance, by a large protein molecule which is built into the membrane structure and in which a special distribution of amino acids provides for a hydrophilic tunnel through the membrane. On the other hand, a carrier is a molecule which binds the transported ion on one membrane-solution interface, then moves to the opposite interface and releases the ion to the aqueous solution. The concept of carriers which facilitate the transport of ions through lipid membranes was a mere hypothesis for a long time, but in recent years a number of compounds like valinomycin, monactin, enniatin B (Fig. 1) have been characterized which act as ion carriers in the classical sense [1, 2].

These compounds share a common structural property: they are macrocyclic systems and contain both hydrophobic and hydrophilic groups. The six ester carbonyl groups of valinomycin may interact with a potassium ion. In this way a complex is formed in which the central ion is surrounded by a cage of six oxygen atoms.

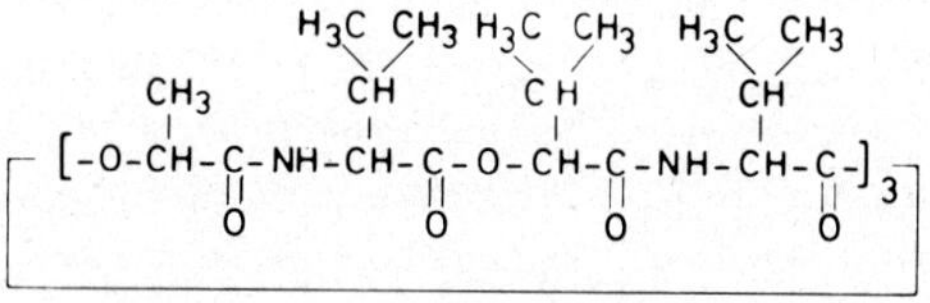

Valinomycin

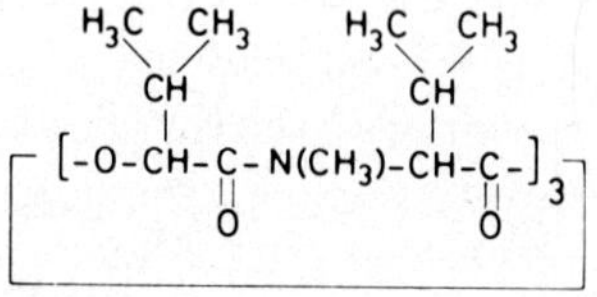

Enniatin B

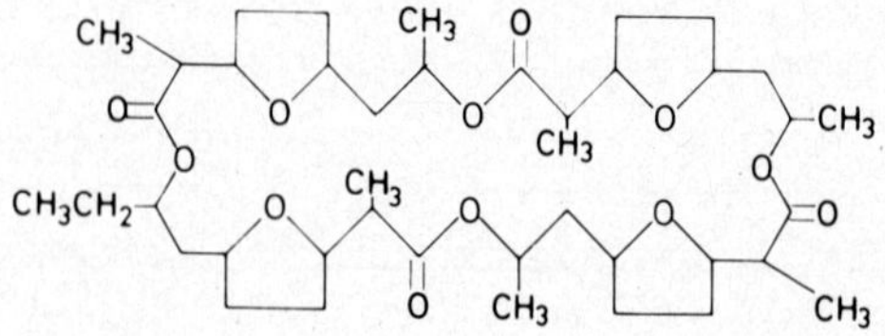

Monactin

Fig. 1. Structure of macrocyclic ion carriers

The interior of the complex offers to an ion an environment which is similar to the hydration shell of the ion in aqueous solution. The exterior surface of the complex is mainly hydrophobic. This picture is supported by X-ray data and spectroscopic measurements (Fig. 2).

The ability of valinomycin and other macrocyclic compounds to increase the potassium permeability of lipid membranes was first demonstrated with mitochondria [3]. For the interpretation of these results it has been proposed that these compounds act as carriers for potassium. But detailed information on the transport mechanism could not been obtained from these experiments, mainly as a consequence of the great complexity of biological membranes. In the past years, artificial model membranes have therefore been used extensively for the study of ion carriers.

Artificial lipid bilayer membranes with an area of several mm² may be obtained by a technique originally developed by MUELLER

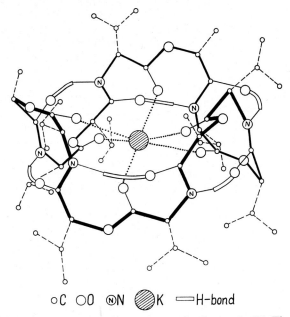

oC OO ⊗N ⊘K ⊏⊐H-bond

Fig. 2. Structure of the potassium complex of valinomycin [1]. The central cation is surrounded by six oxygen atoms of the ester carbonyl groups. The complex is stabilized by hydrogen bonds formed by the amide groups

and his associates [4]. These membranes are formed on a circular hole in a teflon wall in such a way that the membrane separates two aqueous electrolyte solutions (Fig. 3). The membrane thickness may be obtained from the electrical capacitance or from the optical

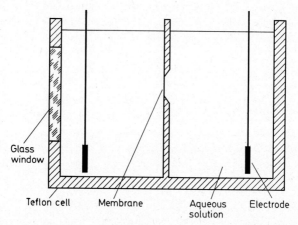

Fig. 3. Cell for electrochemical studies with artificial lipid membranes

reflectance of the film and has a value of about 60 Å (for dioleoyl-lecithin). The membrane contains small amounts of the solvent (usually n-decane), but otherwise has a structure similar to the structure of the bilayer regions of a biological membrane.

The electrical conductance λ_0 of an artificial bilayer membrane is extremely low; for instance, in a 1 M KCl solution values in the order $\lambda_0 = 10^{-7}\ \Omega^{-1}\ cm^{-2}$ are found. If small amounts of valino-mycin or monactin are added to the system, the membrane con-ductance increases by several orders of magnitude and the mem-brane becomes selectively potassium permeable [5]. It is seen from Fig. 4 that λ_0 is a linear function of valinomycin concentration over several decades. A similar result is obtained if valinomycin is added directly to the membrane forming solution. Likewise, if the valino-mycin concentration is held constant and the K^+ concentration c_M in the aqueous solution is varied, a linear relationship between λ_0 and c_M is found (only at c_M values in the vicinity of 1 M a saturating behavior is observed which is characteristic for carrier systems at high concentrations of the transported substrate where most of the carrier molecules are present in the complexed form). All these findings may be explained by the assumption that a distribution equilibrium exists for valinomycin between the aqueous phase and

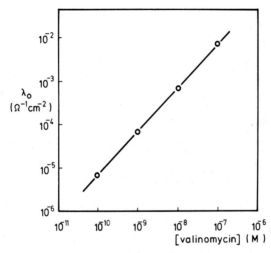

Fig. 4. Membrane conductance λ_0 as a function of valinomycin concentration in the aqueous phase at a fixed potassium concentration $c_M = 1$ M. Temperature $T = 25°$ C. The membrane has been formed from dioleoyllecithin in n-decane [5]

the membrane and, furthermore, that the electric current through the membrane is carried by a 1 : 1 complex of valinomycin with potassium.

The specificity by which valinomycin discriminates between different alkali ions is rather high. In Fig. 5 the membrane conductance λ_0 is plotted for different cations at a fixed valinomycin and ion concentration. It is seen, for instance, that the conductance in the presence of K^+ is higher by a factor of more than 10^3 than the conductance in the presence of Na^+. The origin of this high ion specificity is not fully understood [6, 7]; possibly, the specificity is a consequence of the steric constraints in the macrocyclic ring, which preclude an optimal electrostatic interaction between the relatively small Na^+ ion and the carbonyl oxygens of the ring.

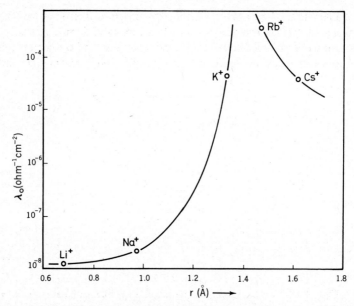

Fig. 5. Ion specificity of valinomycin [2]. The membrane conductance λ_0 is plotted at constant valinomycin concentration ($c = 10^{-7}$ M) and constant cation concentration ($c_M = 10^{-2}$ M). $T = 25°$ C. Membrane formed from dioleoyllecithin in n-decane

In the presence of a carrier, the ion transport through the membrane-solution interface may occur in either of two ways. The ion-carrier complex may form already in the aqueous phase and may then cross the interface. On the other hand, if complex formation in the water is negligible, a hydrated ion from the aqueous phase may react in the interface with a carrier molecule from the membrane. The complex then moves to the opposite interface where the ion is released by dissociation. If the first mechanism would be operative, diffusion polarisation should occur at high current densities, i.e., the carrier should be depleted at one interface and accumulated at the other. As such a diffusion polarisation is never observed in the valinomycin-potassium system, we may conclude that in this case complex formation occurs at the membrane solution interface [5]. The overall transport process (Fig. 6) may then be described by the rate constants for the formation (k_R) and dissociation (k_D) of the complex and by the rate constants for the translocation of the complex (k_{MS}) and of the free carrier (k_S) across the membrane. For instance, k_S indicates how many times per second a free carrier molecule jumps from one interface to the other.

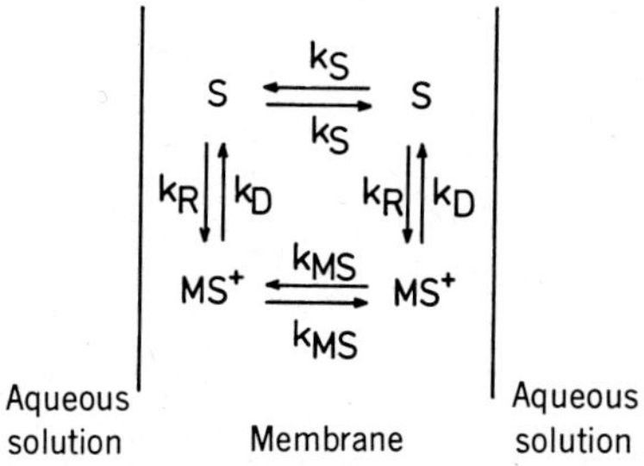

Fig. 6. Reaction scheme for the transport of an ion M^+ mediated by a carrier S

At this point it should be emphasized that the ion transport considered here (and also later in the section on pore mechanisms) is of a purely passive nature, *i.e.*, ions move down their electrochemical gradient which is given by the difference in the concentration and the difference in the electrical potential between both aqueous phases. Active transport leading to an accumulation of ions would be observed, however, if the carrier were chemically modified at one membrane-solution interface at the expense of metabolic energy, so that the affinity for the ion is different at the two sides of the membrane.

From the reaction scheme of Fig. 6 several questions arise. We want to know the time-scale of these processes, whether the translocation of the carrier occurs within milliseconds or within microseconds. Or we may ask whether there is a rate-limiting reaction in the overall transport process or whether all reactions take place at comparable rates. These questions are closely related to the problem of the origin of ion specificity which may be determined not only by thermodynamic factors (stability constants of the ion complexes) but also by kinetic parameters (rate constants). For an answer to these questions, one has to carry out a kinetic analysis of the carrier system. At first, this seems to be a rather difficult task because one has not only to determine the four rate constants (k_R, k_D, k_S, k_{MS})

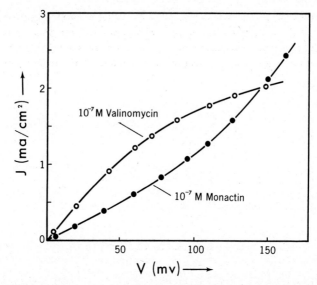

Fig. 7. Current density J as a function of the applied voltage V for monactin and valinomycin as carriers [5]. Phosphatidylserine membrane in 1 M KCl, 25° C. A superlinear behavior of J(V) is observed with monactin, whereas the current tends to saturate at high voltages in the case of valinomycin

but also the distribution coefficient of the carrier between water and the membrane. Such an analysis, however, becomes possible by a combination of steady-state conductance measurements with electrical relaxation experiments.

Very useful information is obtained simply by measuring the current J through the membrane as a function of the applied voltage V [5, 8]. Depending on the relative rates of the single transport steps, the J(V) curve may be either superlinear or saturating (Fig. 7). By measuring the shape of the J(V) characteristic at different ion concentrations, the numerical values of three different combinations of the rate constants and the partition coefficient γ_S of the carrier may be obtained (k_{MS}/k_D, k_R/k_S, and $\gamma_S k_S$). Evidently, steady-state conductance measurements are not sufficient for a complete kinetic analysis of the system. However, the additional information which is required may be obtained from electrical relaxation experiments [9].

Relaxation techniques have been widely used in chemical kinetics for the evaluation of rate constants. But this method is not restricted to chemical reactions, but may also be used for the kinetic analysis of transport processes in membranes. The principle of the

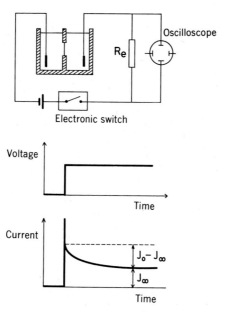

Fig. 8. Principle of the electric relaxation method [2]

method is well-known: The system is disturbed by the sudden displacement of an external parameter, and the time is measured which is required by the system to reach a new stationary state. In the case of a bilayer membrane it is convenient to choose as the variable external parameter the electric field strength in the membrane (Fig. 8). Immediately after a sudden displacement of the voltage, a capacitative current is observed which decays with a time constant equal to the product of the cell resistance and the membrane capacitance. This capacitative spike limits the time resolution of the method, which under favorable conditions is of the order of $1\,\mu s$. After the decay of the capacitative transient, the membrane current approaches with a characteristic time constant τ

a stationary value J_∞. The initial current J_0 is obtained by extrapolation to time zero. Such an experiment (Fig. 9) therefore yields
two additional independent informations; the relaxation time τ and
the relaxation amplitude $\alpha \equiv (J_0 - J_\infty/J_\infty)$. Both τ and α are related
in a straightforward way to the individual rate constants [9].

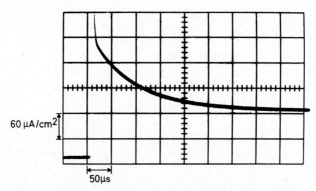

60 µA/cm²

50µs

Fig. 9. Relaxation of the membrane current after a sudden displacement of
the voltage from 0 to 60 mV. Phosphatidylserine membrane in 1 M KCl at
12° C. 10^{-3} M valinomycin has been added to the membrane-forming solution.
The capacitative spike is not completely visible

Together with the steady-state conductance data, the additional
information obtained from the relaxation experiment may be used
to calculate the single rate constants. For the system valinomycin/
K^+ and a phosphatidylinositol membrane the result reads [9]:

$$k_R \cong 5 \cdot 10^4 \, M^{-1} \, s^{-1}$$
$$k_D \cong 5 \cdot 10^4 \, sec^{-1}$$
$$k_S \cong 2 \cdot 10^4 \, sec^{-1}$$
$$k_{MS} \cong 2 \cdot 10^4 \, sec^{-1}.$$

From the numerical values of the rate constants a number of
interesting conclusions may be drawn. For instance, it is seen that
k_D, k_S, and k_{MS} are of the same order of magnitude, between 10^4
and $10^5 \, sec^{-1}$. At an ion concentration of $c_M = 1$ M also the product
$c_M k_R$ is of the same order ($5 \cdot 10^4 \, sec^{-1}$); under these conditions all
individual transport steps proceed at almost the same rate. The
jump time of the complex is given by the reciprocal of k_{MS} and is
equal to about 50 µsec. This value may be compared with the

diffusion time of a molecule of the size of valinomycin in water over a distance of the membrane thickness (~ 60 Å); this time is approximately $0.1 \, \mu$sec. The rate constant k_R for the formation of the ion-carrier complex in the membrane-solution interface is smaller by a factor of 10^3 than the corresponding rate constant for complex formation between valinomycin and potassium in methanolic solution [10]. The reason for the much slower rate in the membrane is not yet clear; a possible explanation may lie in the fact that the carrier molecule has to undergo a conformational change during complexation. Due to the high viscosity of the lipid environment of the carrier in the membrane, this conformational change may proceed with a much slower rate in the membrane as compared with the rate in an ordinary solution. This conclusion is in accordance with the finding that k_R strongly decreases with increasing chain length of the lipid and with decreasing temperature [11].

The function of a carrier may be compared with the function of an enzyme. An enzyme reduces the energy barrier which separates the reactants from the products of a chemical reaction. In an analogous way, the function of a valinomycin consists in reducing the extremely high activation barrier for the transport of an alkali ion across the hydrophobic interior of a lipid membrane. The activity of an enzyme may be characterized by two parameters: the half-saturation concentration and the turnover number. In the case of a carrier molecule, the half-saturation concentration may be defined as the ion concentration in the aqueous phase at which half of the membrane-bound carrier molecules are in the complexed form. Under the above conditions, this concentration is equal to $k_D/k_R \cong 1$ M. This means that valinomycin in the membrane has a rather low affinity for potassium.

The fact that valinomycin nevertheless is a very efficient potassium carrier results from the high turnover number of the molecule. In analogy to an enzyme, we may define a turnover number of an ion carrier as the maximum number of ions which can be transported per second by a single carrier molecule in the limit of high ion concentration. This turnover number f is related in a simple way to the rate constants [2]:

$$f = \left(\frac{1}{k_S} + \frac{1}{\mathrm{k}_{MS}} + \frac{2}{k_D} \right)^{-1}.$$

With the above values of the rate constants one obtains $f \cong 10^4 \text{ sec}^{-1}$, which means that a single valinomycin molecule is able to transport 10^4 potassium ions per second through the membrane.

At present we don't know to what extent Nature really uses carriers for ion transport. On the other hand, for certain biological transport systems it is rather certain that carriers are not involved. An example is the sodium channel of the nerve membrane, where different experiments lead to a number of about 10^8 Na^+ ions which pass per second through the open channel [12]. This number is by four orders of magnitude higher than the maximal transport rate of a single carrier molecule of the valinomycin type. It is therefore rather unlikely that the sodium channel is operated by a carrier mechanism. But, of course, the high transport rate could well be explained by a pore.

As yet, the functional characterization of membrane proteins which may act as pore molecules has not been very successful. But, fortunately, there exist a number of simpler molecules, such as gramicidin A, which are useful for studying the mechanism of ion transport through pores.

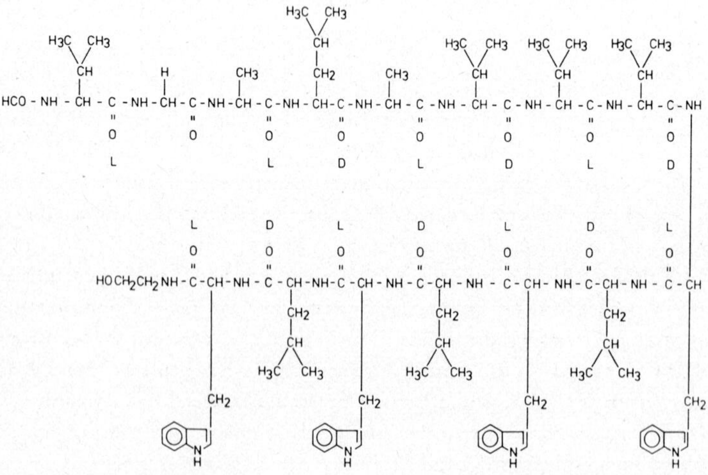

Valin-Gramicidin A

Fig. 10. Structure of Valine-gramicidin A

Gramicidin A is a linear peptide consisting of 15 amino acids (Fig. 10). This molecule has several characteristic properties. With the exception of glycin in position 2 it consists of strongly hydrophobic amino acids. As both end groups are blocked (by a formyl residue at the amino terminal and by an ethanolamino residue at the carboxyl terminal), the molecule is electrically neutral. Furthermore, there is a peculiar alternation in the optical configuration of the amino acids.

If gramidicin A is introduced into a biological or artificial membrane, the membrane becomes cation permeable. In this respect gramicidin is similar to the macrocyclic ion carriers. But it became soon clear that the action mechanism of gramicidin is quite different from the macrocyclic carriers, and that gramicidin presumably forms pores in a lipid membrane [17].

First, one may ask what conformation such a molecule could assume in a lipid membrane. An attractive possibility would be a helix. In order to act as a pore, the helix must have in its center a hydrophilic tunnel of the appropriate diameter and, besides this, the length must be sufficient to bridge the thickness of the membrane. As URRY has shown [13, 14], a helical conformation of gramicidin A is indeed feasible. The $\pi_{L,D}^{6}$-helix as proposed by URRY contains 6.3 amino acids per turn (Fig. 11). In the center of the helix a 4 Å wide hydrophilic channel is present which is lined by the oxygen atoms of the amide groups, whereas the hydrophobic residues are located at the periphery of the helix. Some evidence that gramicidin may assume an ordered, helical structure in certain organic solvents comes from circular dichroism measurements.

But here a difficulty arises: the length of the helix is only about 15 Å, much smaller than the hydrophobic thickness of a lipid bilayer (40—50 Å). URRY therefore proposed that the pore consists of a dimer of gramicidin A. The dimer has a length of about 30 Å and could be sufficient to span the hydrophobic core of the membrane, if a local thinning of the membrane is assumed. The dimer hypothesis is supported by the finding that the dimer formed by chemical linkage of two gramicidin monomers has a similar membrane activity as the monomer, but at much lower concentrations [14]. Furthermore, the kinetic experiments which are described below are in favor of the dimer model.

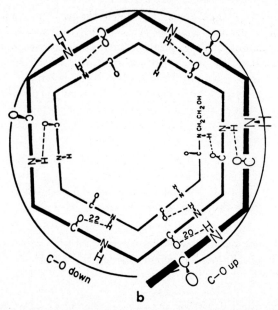

Fig. 11. Structure of the $\pi_{L,D}^6$ helix of gramicidin, as proposed by Urry [14]. The hydrophilic tunnel in the center of the helix is lined with the oxygen atoms of the amide groups, which alternately point up and down. The hydrophobic residues which are located at the periphery of the helix are not shown

It is interesting to investigate whether the observable transport properties of gramicidin A in a membrane agree with this picture. For this purpose it is again convenient to use artificial lipid membranes. A very instructive experiment consists in adding extremely small amounts of gramicidin A to the membrane and measuring the time course of the electric current at a constant voltage [15, 16]. Under these circumstances the current shows discrete fluctuations which have more or less the same amplitude (Fig. 12). If increasing amounts of gramicidin are added to the membrane, more and more fluctuations build up on top of each other until finally they fuse into an average macroscopic current. This experiment suggests that the single current fluctuation comes about by the formation and the disappearance of a single pore. One may then calculate the conductance Λ of a single pore: in 1 M NaCl at 25° C a value of $\Lambda = 1.1 \cdot 10^{-11}\ \Omega^{-1}$ is obtained [16]. This corresponds to a transport of 10^7 sodium ions per second through the single pore at a voltage of 100 mV. This value is larger by a factor of 10^3 than the turnover number of valinomycin, and would be difficult to reconcile with a carrier mechanism [15].

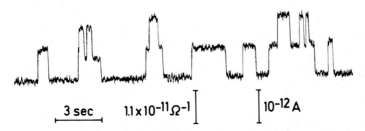

Fig. 12. Fluctuations of the membrane current in the presence of very small amounts of gramicidin A [16]. 1 M NaCl, 25° C, $V = 90$ mV. The membrane has been formed from dioleoyllecithin in n-decane. The base line corresponds to the membrane conductance without gramicidin

If the dimer hypothesis is correct, then the switching-on of the pore corresponds to the association of two gramicidin monomers, and the switching off to the dissociation of the dimer. This would mean that one could describe the pore-formation process in the same way as a bimolecular chemical reaction, which is characterized by the rate constants of association (k_R) and dissociation (k_D):

$$A + A \underset{k_D}{\overset{k_R}{\rightleftharpoons}} A_2.$$

This immediately leads us to the kinetics of pore formation, $i.e.$, to the question about the frequency of association and dissociation processes in the membrane.

Information about the pore kinetics may be obtained again by electrical relaxation experiments [18]. In order to understand why a voltage jump may displace the monomer-dimer equilibrium, one has to look once more at the geometrical situation in the membrane. The thickness of the hydrocarbon core of the membrane is about 50 Å, whereas the length of the dimer is only 30 Å. For the formation of the pore it would therefore be more favorable if the membrane were thinner. Indeed, it is found that pore formation is enhanced if the membrane thickness is reduced by changing the composition of the lipid [15]. If a voltage is applied to the membrane, charges of opposite sign build up at the two membrane surfaces. This gives rise to a pressure (in the same way as the plates of a charged plate-condenser attract each other) so that the membrane is elastically deformed. It can be shown by independent capacitance measurements that the membrane thickness decreases by a few percent within about one millisecond if a voltage of 100 mV is applied. This is a rather small effect which, however, is sufficient to displace the monomer-dimer equilibrium considerably.

For the application of the relaxation method one further needs an indicator for the concentration of the dimer in the membrane. This requirement is easy to fulfill: The unmodified lipid membrane is an almost perfect insulator, and the monomers are also likely to be non-conducting. The conductance is therefore proportional to the number of dimers in the membrane, *i.e.*, one may use the membrane current as an indicator for the dimer concentration. If a voltage is applied to the membrane at time zero, the membrane is quickly compressed. In this initial state there is a certain dimer concentration which determines the initial current. The dimer concentration and, correspondingly, the current then asymptotically increase towards new steady-state values.

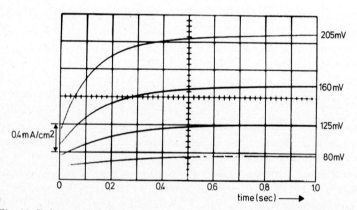

Fig. 13. Relaxation of the membrane current after a sudden displacement of the voltage [18]. 1 M NaCl, $2 \cdot 10^{-9}$M gramicidin, 25° C, dioleoyllecithin membrane. The amplitude of the voltage jump is indicated at the right side of the figure

This, indeed, is found experimentally (Fig. 13). Analysis of the time course $J(t)$ of the membrane current after the voltage jump shows that J is a purely exponential function of time t and therefore is described by a single relaxation time τ. On the other hand, theory tells us that for the dimer model, τ should be given by the expression

$$\frac{1}{\tau} = k_D + \text{const.} \sqrt{k_R \lambda_\infty}.$$

Thus, if τ is measured at different gramicidin concentrations and $1/\tau$ plotted as a function of the square root of the stationary membrane conductance λ_∞, a straight line should result. This expectation is verified by the experiment [18]. The observation that $1/\tau$ is a linear function of $\sqrt{\lambda_\infty}$ thus strongly supports the view that the pore is formed by a dimer of gramicidin A.

From the intercept and the slope of the $1/\tau$ versus $\sqrt{\lambda_\infty}$ plot, the values of k_R and k_D may be obtained. For a dioleoyllecithin membrane at $25°$ C one finds [16, 18]:

$$k_D \cong 1.6 \text{ sec}^{-1}$$
$$k_R \cong 1.8 \cdot 10^{14} \text{ cm}^2 \text{ mole}^{-1} \text{ sec}^{-1}.$$

$1/k_D \cong 0.6$ sec is the mean life-time if a dimer. This value agrees with the mean life-time of the conducting state which is directly obtained from the current fluctuations (Fig. 12). The value of k_R which describes the rate of association may be illustrated in the following way: If the monomers are present in the membrane in such a concentration that the mean distance is 1000 Å, then a given monomer will associate with another monomer with a frequency of 2 per sec. It is instructive to compare this reaction rate with the theoretical limit of a diffusion-controlled reaction. The diffusion of the monomers in the membrane may be visualized as a random walk in a two-dimensional space. The maximum possible association rate corresponds to the condition that every encounter would lead to the formation of a dimer. From an estimate of the diffusion coefficient, we would expect that the maximum association frequency in the above example would be between 10^3 and 10^4 per sec. The fact that the actually observed association rate is smaller by a factor of about 10^3 may be explained by the assumption that the two monomers have to be in a rather precise mutual orientation before the hydrogen bonds stabilizing the dimer may be formed.

In conclusion, we may say that the gramicidin system gives us an example of how the ion permeability of a lipid membrane may be controlled by the voltage. Under the influence of the electric field part of the inactive (monomeric) gramicidin is converted into the active form of a pore. It is feasible that also in other cases Nature uses the reversible association of peptide subunits for the control of ion permeability in membranes.

References

1. SHEMYAKIN, M.M., OVCHINNIKOV, YU. A., JVANOV, V.T., ANTONOV, V.K., VINOGRADOVA, E.J., SHKROB, A.M., MALENKOV, G.G., EVSTRATOV, A.V., LAINE, J.A., MELNIK, E.J., RYABOVA, J.D.: J. Membrane Biol. 1, 402 (1969).
2. LÄUGER, P.: Science 178, 24 (1972).
3. PRESSMAN, B.C., HARRIS, E.J., JAGGER, W.S., JOHNSON, J.: Proc. nat. Acad. Sci. (Wash.) 58, 1949 (1961).
4. MUELLER, P., RUDIN, D.O., TITIEN, H., WESCOTT, W.C.: Nature (Lond.) 194, 979 (1962).
5. STARK, G., BENZ, R.: J. Membrane Biol. 5, 133 (1971).
6. EISENMAN, G., SZABO, G., CIANI, S., McLAUGHLIN, S., KRASNE, S.: In: DANIELLI, J.F., ROSENBERG, M.D., CADENHEAD, D.A. (Eds.): In Progress in surface and membrane science: Vol. 6. NewYork 1973.
7. DIEBLER, H., EIGEN, M., ILGENFRITZ, G., MAASZ, G., WINKLER, R.: Pure appl. Chem. 20, 93 (1969).
8. LÄUGER, P., STARK, G.: Biocheim. biophys. Acta (Amster.) 211, 458 (1970).
9. STARK, G., KETTERER, B., BENZ, R., LÄUGER, P.: Biophys. J. 11, 981 (1971).
10. GRELL, E., FUNCK, TH.: J. Supramol. Structure 307 (1973).
11. BENZ, R., STARK, G., JANKO, K., LÄUGER, P.: J. Membrane Biol. 14, 339 (1973).
12. HILLE, B.: Progr. Biophys. molec. Biol. 21, 3 (1970).
13. URRY, D.W.: Proc. nat. Acad. Sci. (Wash.) 68, 672 (1971).
14. URRY, D.W., GOODALL, M.C., GLICKSON, J.S., MAYERS, D.F.: Proc. nat. Acad. Sci. (Wash.) 68, 1907 (1971).
15. HLADKY, S.B., HAYDON, D.A.: Biochim. biophys. Acta (Amst.) 274, 294 (1972).
16. BAMBERG, E., LÄUGER, P.: Biochim. biophys. Acta 367, 127 (1974).
17. KRASNE, S., EISENMAN, G., SZABO, G.: Science 174, 412 (1971).
18. BAMBERG, E., LÄUGER, P.: J. Membrane Biol. 11, 177 (1973).

Discussion

P. KARLSON (Marburg): The interesting model only accounts for increased permeability, *i.e.* a passive transport. It also lacks the vectorial aspect often observed in transport processes. Would it be possible to alter the model in such a way that it accounts also for vectorial (*i.e.* unidirectional) flow and active transport?

P. LÄUGER: An active transport mechanism may be realized by a carrier which becomes chemically modified at one membrane/solution interface at the expense of metabolic energy. If it is assumed that this chemical modification leads to a change in the affinity of the carrier for the ion, then the carrier may accumulate ions against an electrochemical gradient.

C. LIÉBECQ (Liège): You did not indicate the magnitude of the partition coefficients of these ionophore molecules between the water phase and the lecithin bilayer. Are they modified by the fixation of ions as in the valinomycin-K^+-complex?

P. LÄUGER: The partition coefficient γ_S of the carrier between the bilayer and water may be obtained from the kinetic analysis. For valinomycin, the values of γ_S for different lipids range between 10^4 and 10^5 at $25°$ C. The partition coefficient γ_{MS} of the ion carrier complex is not known with certainty, but some experiments indicate that λ_{MS} may be even larger than γ_S, in accordance with the expectation that the complex is more hydrophobic than the free carrier.

C. LIÉBECQ: You did not consider, in your kinetic analysis, the possible movements of the ionophore molecules, charged or not, from the water phase into the lecithin bilayer and *vice-versa*. Have you good reasons to neglect these additional reactions?

P. LÄUGER: The alternative mechanism that ion-carrier complexes which are already present in the aqueous phase move through the membrane/solution interface may be excluded experimentally from the absence of diffusion polarization during current flow.

E. GROSS (Bethesda): Is there an alternative to the carrier transport mechanism for valinomycin as you described it, for instance the association of valinomycin to a multimer to span the thickness of the membrane in a similar fashion as you indicate for gramicidin?

P. LÄUGER: The possibility that several valinomycin molecules cooperate in the transport of K^+ may be excluded by the finding that the membrane conductance generated by the carrier in the presence of K^+ is a strictly linear function of the carrier concentration.

E. GROSS: There are six analogues in the gramicidin series. Which of the analogues did you use in your work? Are there differences in the ion transport properties between the various analogues?

P. LÄUGER: For our gramicidin experiments we used two different samples. The one was commercial gramicidin which is a mixture of the A, B, and C analogues. Gramicidin B and C differ from A in that L-tryptophan in Position 11 is replaced by L-phenylalanine and L-tyrosine, respectively. The second sample was purified valine-gramicidin A. As may be expected, there was no significant difference between the results obtained with the two preparations.

Drugs to Explore the Ionic Channels in the Axon Membrane

W. ULBRICHT

Physiologisches Institut der Universität, D-2300 Kiel, Olshausenstraße 40—60, Federal Republic of Germany

With 9 Figures

The passive movement of ions along their electrochemical gradients that underlies the nerve action potential appears to be controlled by a finite number of discrete membrane sites that are now generally termed "channels". HILLE (1970) has summarized the compelling evidence in favour of this concept and of the existence of at least two distinctly different types of channels. The most telling argument is that each of the two types can be selectively blocked by drugs without affecting the other type of channel. One type mediates the transient sodium inward current during the upstroke of the action potential; it is hence called Na channel although other cations may, less readily, pass through it. By the same token the other type is termed K channel since it controls the delayed outward movement of K^+ ions during the falling phase of the action potential. Thus the two channels differ not only in their selectivity but also in their average kinetic behavior, as revealed by the macroscopic phenomenon of the ionic membrane current.

Block of Sodium Channels

The specific inhibitors of currents flowing through the Na channels are tetrodotoxin (TTX) and saxitoxin (STX). The two toxins have similar molecular weights (ca. 320 and 350, respectively), but their structures are quite different as seen in Fig. 1. Details on the chemistry and pharmacology of TTX and STX have recently been compiled by EVANS (1972). TTX is found in puffer fish and some kind of salamander, STX is produced by dinoflagellates on which certain shellfish feed that may considerably concentrate the toxin; therefore it has also become known as "paralytic shellfish poison". At equilibrium with only a few nM of either toxin half of the Na channels are blocked (Hille, 1968; Cuervo and Adelman, 1970; Schwarz et al., 1973), so that in 300 nM TTX no trace of Na current can be observed. In the families of current traces of Fig. 2, obtained in a voltage clamp experiment, the blocking effect is seen as loss of the inward (downward) component in Fig. 2B as compared to Fig. 2A. The figure also demonstrates that the late current (passing through the K channel) is entirely unaffected. This high specificity with respect to the "target" or "receptor" is paralleled

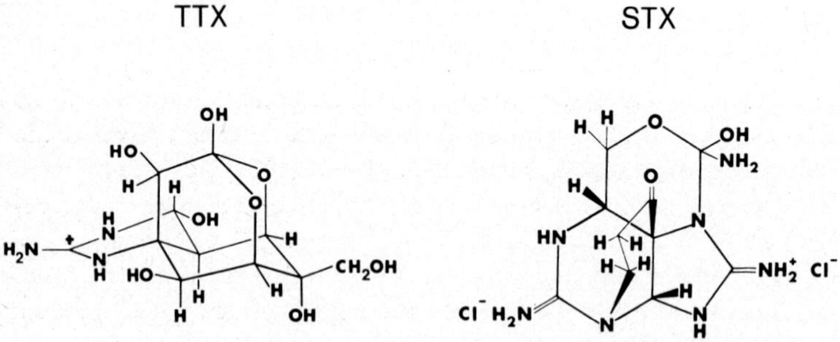

TTX   STX

Fig. 1. Structure of tetrodotoxin (TTX) and saxitoxin (STX). TTX is shown in one of the two active (cationic) forms

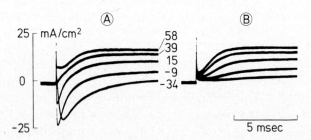

Fig. 2A and B. Effect of 300 nM tetrodotoxin (B) on the time course of membrane currents in a node of Ranvier as compared to the control in normal Ringer solution (A). Ordinate, current density in mA/cm², inward current negative; abscissa, time in msec. The numbers next to the traces give the membrane potential (inside with respect to outside), in mV, during the test pulses that were preceded by 50-msec conditioning prepulses to—110 mV. 15.5° C. (Unpublished record of Dr. H.-H. Wagner)

by the fact that slight changes in the structure of TTX render the molecule nearly ineffective in blocking the nerve membrane (see summary of NARAHASHI, 1972).

Interestingly, the toxin's sole effect is to reduce the amplitude of the sodium current while it does not affect its time course. An obvious explanation would be to assume that TTX simply reduces the number of operating channels by an all-or-none block with respect to the individual channel. Equilibrium experiments suggest the following reaction to underlie the block (HILLE, 1968):

$$\text{TTX} + R \underset{k_2}{\overset{k_1}{\rightleftharpoons}} \text{TTX} \cdot R$$

i.e. one TTX molecule binds to one receptor per channel to form a drug-receptor complex, $\text{TTX} \cdot R$, upon which the channel is promptly and completely occluded; k_1 and k_2 are the rate constants of association and dissociation, respectively. Their ratio, k_2/k_1, equals the equilibrium dissociation constant, K, that is about 3 nM in various nerve preparations as summarized by SCHWARZ et al. (1973).

Since the "receptor" must be part of the Na channel or at least closely linked to it, the highly specific reaction with TTX or STX is of particular interest to membrane physiologists. The first systematic attempt to determine the absolute reaction rates has been made by CUERVO and ADELMAN (1970) on squid giant axons. Unfortunately this axon is surrounded by a cell layer that impedes the diffusional access to the excitable membrane at which a stepwise change in TTX concentration would be required. In myelinated frog nerve fibres, however, the experimental situation is much more favourable (VIERHAUS and ULBRICHT, 1971 a) and it can be shown that TTX has ready access to the membrane that is located, in this preparation, in the nodes of Ranvier. SCHWARZ et al. (1973) studied the rates of TTX action in voltage clamp experiments on this preparation by recording the Na current during periodic depolarizing impulses of constant amplitude. A typical result is shown in Fig. 3, which gives the Na current relative to its control value after a sudden application of 3.1 (O) or 15.5 nM TTX (●). As can be seen, increasing the toxin concentration accelerates the block, and its exponential development quantitatively agrees with the kinetics following from the reaction scheme that also requires the offset to be independent of concentration. This is, indeed, observed during washout, as illustrated by the curve through the triangles. Agreement with simple kinetics, absence of apparent dif-

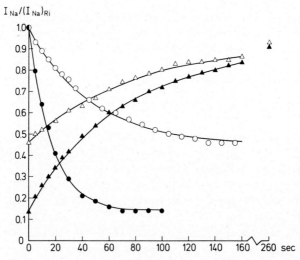

Fig. 3. Development of an recovery from tetrodotoxin-induced inhibition of Na currents, I_{Na}. Ordinate, I_{Na} relative to its value in normal Ringer solution, $(I_{Na})_{Ri}$. Abscissa, time after change of solution. Open symbols refer to the application of 3.1 nM-TTX, filled symbols to 15.5 nM-TTX. Circles and triangles give measurements during onset and offset, respectively. From
Schwarz et al. (1973)

fusion barriers and the marked dependence of the rates of TTX action on temperature suggest that the time course of block is, indeed, limited by the TTX-receptor reaction. Under this assumption, experiments of the kind shown in Fig. 3 yield mean values (at 20° C) of $3.3 \times 10^6 M^{-1} sec^{-1}$ for k_1 and $1.4 \times 10^{-2} sec^{-1}$ for k_2; the respective Arrhenius activation energies are 13.7 and 20.5 kcal/ mole (Schwarz et al., 1973). Interest in the reaction is continuing, especially since H^+ ions appear to compete with TTX for the same receptor (Wagner and Ulbricht, 1973, 1974; Ulbricht and Wagner, 1973).

Block of Potassium Channels

Potassium channels are reversibly blocked by tetraethylammonium (TEA) ions (TASAKI and HAGIWARA, 1957; ARMSTRONG and BINSTOCK, 1965; KOPPENHÖFER, 1967; HILLE, 1967). This effect is illustrated by Fig. 4 which also shows that the early sodium

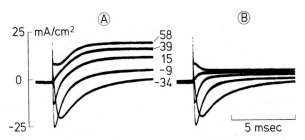

Fig. 4A and B. Effect of 5.8 mM tetraethylammonium chloride (B) on the time course of membrane currents in a node of Ranvier as compared to the control in normal Ringer solution (A). Ordinate, current density in mA/cm², inward current negative; abscissa, time in msec. Membrane potentials during the 5 test pulses are given in mV by the numbers next to the traces. Each pulse was preceded by a 50-msec conditioning pulse to —110 mV. 15.5° C. (Unpublished original record of Dr. H.-H. WAGNER; from the same fibre as for Fig. 2)

current is completely unchanged. As with TTX or STX only the amplitude (but not the time course) of the current through the channels in question is affected, and again a reaction scheme analogous to that for TTX suffices to explain the block at equilibrium with K of 0.4 mM for nodes of Ranvier (HILLE, 1967). All other alkylammonium ions are less effective or even ineffective; substitution of one ethyl group in TEA by a methyl group already raises K to 15 mM (HILLE, 1970).

As mentioned before, the falling phase of the action potential is, at least in part, brought about by the delayed K current. Therefore the repolarization of the membrane is hindered and hence the duration of the action potential is prolonged when the K channels are blocked by TEA. When this drug is suddenly applied during a train of action potentials, the rate of this lengthening action and hence the rate of TEA action can be determined. It was found that

the TEA-channel reaction was too fast to be resolved. Taking the
rate of change of the TEA *concentration* at the membrane into
consideration, k_2 of the reaction was estimated to be at least
$2 \times 10^2 \, \text{sec}^{-1}$ (VIERHAUS and ULBRICHT, 1971b). Obviously, the

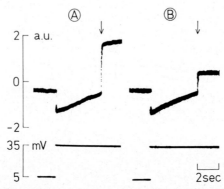

Fig. 5A and B. Current change (upper traces) on a sudden change in solution
during a depolarizing pulse (lower traces) in a voltage clamp experiment on
a node of Ranvier. Currents given in arbitrary units (a.u.), inward currents
negative. The membrane potential is given as deviation from the normal
resting potential, depolarization positive. In (A) and (B) the node was in
isotonic KCl (117 mM-KCl) which was changed, at the arrow, to Ringer
solution (2.5 mM-KCl) in (A) and to 117 mM-KCl + 1 mM-TEA in (B).
21.5° C. (Unpublished experiment)

TEA-receptor reaction is limited by the diffusional access of the
drug to the membrane, as can also be deduced from the voltage
clamp experiment in Fig. 5. Each of the two pictures shows the
membrane current during a long depolarizing impulse of small
amplitude. In Fig. 5A the pulse was applied to the node in 117 mM
KCl (isotonic KCl) that was changed at the arrow to normal
Ringer solution containing 2.5 mM-KCl. Since during sustained
depolarizations the membrane current is carried mostly by K^+
ions, an abrupt change in their concentration yields an equally fast
change in current. Figure 5B illustrates the situation with the K
concentration being kept constant at 117 mM, but when 1 mM TEA
was added at the arrow. Clearly, this pharmacologically induced
change in current was practically as fast as that in Fig. 5A and

obviously, several orders of magnitude faster than the TTX-induced changes of Fig. 3.

Drugs Affecting the Time Course of the Sodium Current

The blocking agents discussed in the preceding two sections are unique in that they are highly selective and without influence on the time course of the ionic currents. Most drugs affecting the excitable membrane, however, change the kinetics of the membrane permeabilities and usually act on both types of channels, although to a different extent. Of the agents with dominant effect on the Na current, the steroidal alkaloid veratridine may serve as a typical example. When a frog nerve fibre is treated with this alkaloid, a second considerably slower Na current component is observed in the voltage clamp. Figure 6 contains original current traces from such an experiment; the continuous trace shows the almost exponential inward current that develops with a time constant 10^4 times greater than in the unpoisoned nerve. Also, this inward current is flowing as long as the membrane is depolarized *i.e.* no inactivation is observed. At the end of the 12-sec impulse, a large inward current tail is seen that slowly subsides. This tail is caused by the sudden increase of the driving force acting on the Na^+ ions when the membrane is repolarized; the decay, then, reflects the

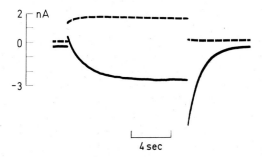

Fig. 6. Time course of membrane current of a node of Ranvier treated with 15 μM veratridine; voltage clamp experiment at 21.7° C. Ordinate, current (per nodal area) in nA, inward current negative; abscissa, time in sec. The continuous trace was observed in normal Na-containing Ringer solution, the interrupted trace in Na-free choline chloride solution. For either record the node was depolarized by 30 mV for 12 sec. [From ULBRICHT (1969b)]

much delayed shut-off due to this change in membrane potential. The interrupted trace in Fig. 6 was recorded in a Na-deficient medium in which no inward current was found, indicating that the slow current was indeed carried by Na^+ ions.

The effects of this alkaloid have been studied rather extensively (see summary of ULBRICHT, 1969a) and the results suggest that veratridine converts Na channels into "slow" channels in an all-or-none fashion (ULBRICHT, 1972a and b). This notion agrees with the observation that increasing the alkaloid concentration only augments the amplitude of the tail current without influencing its time constant, which was about 1 sec at room temperature for a step back to the resting potential (ULBRICHT, 1969b). Thus, the time constant characterizes the alkaloid veratridine and, interestingly, a wide range of typical time constants (approximately between 10 msec and 1 sec) have been observed with other ceveratrum alkaloids (HONERJÄGER, 1973). — In this context it appears necessary to point out that terms like "slow channel" refer to the average behavior as derived from the macroscopic ionic current. The real behavior of the individual channel is still completely unknown, and a channel may only be able to oscillate between two states: closed and fully permeable.

One of the reasons to believe that "slow" channels originate from normal Na channels is their susceptibility to TTX (ULBRICHT, 1966, 1969a). Even the kinetics of the TTX effect is unchanged in spite of the drastic modification of the channels. This is illustrated by Fig. 7, which stems from a node of Ranvier equilibrated in a veratridine solution and subjected about every 5 sec to a 3-sec depolarizing pulse by 30 mV. Although the pulse duration is not quite long enough for the slow inward current to reach its steady value, it can be shown that nevertheless the tails on repolarization are suited to measure changes in the alkaloid-induced permeability (ULBRICHT, 1972b). When TTX was added at the arrow, the decreasing amplitude of the tails quantitatively described the time course of the toxin effect. In the lower part of Fig. 7 the tail currents relative to the value in toxin-free solution are plotted as a function of time. Again the onset and offset could be nicely fitted by exponential functions leading to $k_1 = 3.4 \times 10^6 \, M^{-1} \, sec^{-1}$ and $k_2 = 1.14 \times 10^{-2} \, sec^{-1}$, i.e. quite comparable to the values obtained without veratridine (see p. 354). This clearly shows that the block by TTX is independent of the kinetic behavior of the Na channel usually ascribed to a mechanism or structure termed "gate". Most probably, TTX receptor and gate are separate entities, a notion that is supported by the recent discovery of a TTX-resistant minute "gating current" due to intramembrane movement of charge that, presumedly, accompanies the operation of the gate (details reviewed in ULBRICHT, 1974). In keeping with the gating concept, the veratridine experiments also suggest that Na inactivation may be connected to a gate separate from that responsi-

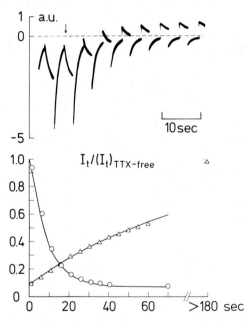

Fig. 7. Time course of tetrodotoxin action on a veratrinized node of Ranvier. Upper picture: Original current record; ordinate, membrane current in arbitrary units (a.u.), inward current negative. Abscissa, time in sec. The node had been equilibrated in $45\,\mu M$ veratridine and was subjected every 4.9 sec to a 2.8-sec depolarizing pulse by 40 mV; these pulses were followed by large inward current tails. At the arrow 31 nM-TTX was added, upon which the tails decreased. Lower diagram: Plot of the tail current, I_t, relative to the value in toxin-free veratridine solution, $(I_t)_{TTX\text{-}free}$ vs. time after the change of solution. Circles and triangles refer to the application and washout of TTX; the time constants of the fitted curves are 8.5 and 87.5 sec, respectively. 20.6° C. (Unpublished experiment)

ble for activation since the alkaloid does away with the former leaving the latter functioning, although at an enormously retarded speed. More evidence for separate gates will be presented later. Many agents that modify the Na channel are found in animals. For example, the skin secretions of a small Colombian frog that have been used for the preparation of arrow poisons by Indians contain batrachotoxin, a steroidal alkaloid (!) which has some structural resemblance with ceveratrum alkaloids. Batrachotoxin, like veratridine, leads to sustained membrane depolarizations by keeping the Na channels open (see short review of Albuquerque, 1972). Completely different agents viz. protein-like are the neurotoxins contained in the venoms of various scorpion species. Some of these compounds have a pronouncedly delaying effect on the inactivation of the Na permeability of frog nerve fibres (Koppenhöfer and Schmidt, 1968a and b) and squid axons (Narahashi et al., 1972). Recently a rather bizarre effect of a scorpion venom has been described, under whose influence Na channels reopen for several hundred msec after repolarization. Apparently the venom prevents the activation gate from closing promptly on repolarization so that the channel becomes permeable at rest as soon as the inactivation gate opens again in the course of recovery (Calahan, 1973). — It should be mentioned that these drugs, as veratridine, do not effect the TTX receptor of the modified Na channels.

The drug effects so far mentioned in this section suggest that the distinction between activation and inactivation is more than just a convenient way to describe the transient Na current normally observed in axons (Hodgkin and Huxley, 1952). A particularly telling clue to structurally separate gates is found in the experiments of Armstrong et al. (1973), who perfused squid axons with solutions containing pronase, a mixture of proteolytic enzymes. Figure 8 presents an example of their findings in an axon whose K channels have been blocked by internal TEA. Therefore only the Na component is seen that shows its normal time course in the early stage of pronase treatment (A) (see also Fig. 4B). After 12 min of this treatment the inactivation is completely abolished, and the current record C superficially resembles that of the veratrinized nodal membrane (Fig. 6), however on a completely different time scale. The important point is that pronase, in contrast to veratridine, has nearly no effect on activation (see super-

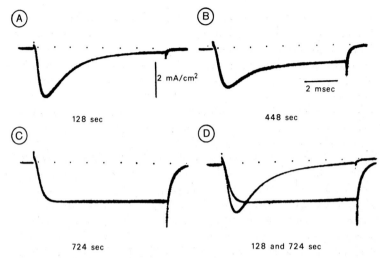

Fig. 8A—D. Effect of internally applied pronase on inward currents of the squid axon membrane. The axon was in sea water and filled with a K-rich solution containing, besides 1 mg pronase/ml, 15-mM-TEA to block the K channels. Voltage clamp records at 8° C during depolarizing pulses to zero absolute membrane potential following prepulses of −110 mV. (A) 128 sec after pronase perfusion when the inactivation of the Na current was still normal. (B) After 448 sec when the inactivation was intact in only part of the Na channels. (C) After 724 sec when the inactivation was completely abolished. (D) Superimposed traces of (A) and (C) to show that the activation was hardly affected. From ARMSTRONG et al. (1973)

imposed traces in D). Obviously, inactivation is linked to a protein structure that can be selectively destroyed. Since pronase acts in this way only when applied internally, one comes to the conclusion that the inactivation gate is located at or near the inside of the membrane from where the activation gate appears to be inaccessible to the enzyme.

Pharmacological Asymmetry of the Membrane

The example of pronase leads to an important aspect of drug effects on excitable membranes viz. that these effects depend on the surface of the membrane to which the drugs are applied. Thus in squid axons scorpion venom remains ineffective if applied to the axoplasmic side of the membrane (NARAHASHI et al., 1972). Like-

362 W. ULBRICHT

wise, TTX does not block, even at very high concentrations, from inside the squid axon (NARAHASHI et al., 1966) or the node of Ranvier (KOPPENHÖFER and VOGEL, 1969); STX shows a comparable preference for the outside of the squid axon membrane (NARAHASHI, 1971). Possibly the toxin receptor is near the external mouth of the Na channel; it appears to be inaccessable from inside the axon because TTX is insoluble in most organic solvents and probably cannot penetrate lipid membranes.

In squid axons TEA blocks only from inside (TASAKI and HAGIWARA, 1957; ARMSTRONG and BINSTOCK, 1965). In frog nerve fibres TEA acts from outside (see Figs 4 and 5) as well as from inside (KOPPENHÖFER and VOGEL, 1969). On internal application, however, the time course of the reduced K current is affected to some extent, a phenomenon that is considerably more pronounced with some TEA derivatives that contain a long chain, e.g. nonyltriethylammonium bromide, C_9 (ARMSTRONG and HILLE, 1972). Figure 9 gives an example of the effect of the internal C_9 as revealed in a voltage clamp experiment on a squid giant axon (ARMSTRONG, 1971). The experiment was done in the presence of TTX to suppress the Na currents and Fig. 9A shows that under the influence of C_9 the K outward current rises as in the control (B) but soon decreases again to a low final level. This phenomenon resembles the natural inactivation of the Na current, and Fig. 9A looks like the mirror image of Fig. 4B. ARMSTRONG (1969, 1971) has extensively studied this "inactivation" and concludes that C_9 enters (together with hydrated K^+ ions) the K channel when its "gate" opens on depolarization and exposes the relatively wide initial segment of

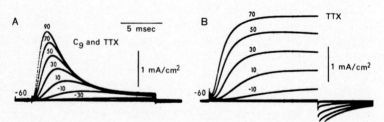

Fig. 9A and B. Squid membrane currents in sea water containing 100 nM-TTX. (A) From an axon into which nonyltriethylammonium (C_9) had been injected to final concentration of 0.11 mM. (B) From an uninjected axon; 9° C. From ARMSTRONG (1971)

the channel. There C_9 binds to a receptor whereby the passage to K^+ ions is blocked; the drug cannot move through the channel for its adjacent segment is too narrow. Closing the gate on repolarization is severely impeded or impossible until C_9 has eventually moved back to the axoplasm under the influence of the electrical field. Interestingly, C_9 is ineffective if applied externally to squid axons while in frog nerve fibres external application of C_9 blocks like TEA, *i.e.* irrespective of time and potential (see Fig. 4).

Another drug whose effect depends on the site of application is QX-314, a quaternary (triethyl) derivative of the local anaesthetic lidocaine. This drug blocks the Na channels of the nodal membrane and it is much more effective when applied internally, in which case it exerts an additional voltage-dependent effect (STRICHARTZ, 1973). This latter effect can be explained if QX-314 molecules enter Na channels whose gates are open and bind to sites that are halfway down the electrical gradient along the channel. In this respect, *i.e.* blocking only after opening, the drug effect resembles that of C_9 on the K channel and, interestingly, internal QX-314 shows some comparable effect on the K permeability.

The asymmetrical action of QX-314 is also observed in squid axons (FRAZIER et al., 1970) in which it has helped to identify the active form of local anesthetics. Most of these drugs are basic tertiary amines with a pK_a value between 7 and 9, so that they are partially dissociated at the physiological pH. The old question which form is active, the uncharged or the cationic form (see RITCHIE and GREENGARD, 1966), could be answered when the technique of the internally perfused squid axon permitted to apply the anesthetic to either membrane side and to vary, simultaneously, the pH of the internal and external medium. From extensive experiments of this kind, NARAHASHI (1971) concludes that local anesthetics act in their cationic form at the internal membrane surface, which they can reach from outside only in the uncharged configuration. These drugs then appear to be more effective at alkaline pH since this favours membrane penetration, after which the molecules may further dissociate because of the lower internal pH. The permanently charged quaternary local anesthetics (like QX-314) are practically unable to penetrate and are, hence, ineffective if applied to the outside. On internal application, however, they promptly block and this action is independent of pH. — Incidentally, veratridine, too, is more effective at increased pH (Ulbricht, 1969a), and it has been suggested that the veratrum alkaloids act at or near the internal membrane surface (Honerjäger, 1971). This could explain why good reversibility of the alkaloid effects is obtained only if the membrane can be washed from both sides, as in the perfused squid axon (Meves, 1966; Ohta et al., 1973).

Conclusion

The present, necessarily incomplete, review intended to show how drugs can help to form our ideas of the ionic channels through the membrane. The fact that the early Na current and the delayed K current can be selectively inhibited strongly support the notion of two distinctly different groups of channels. In each type, the gates appear to be located closer to the axoplasmic side of the membrane than the channel sites that discriminate between the ion species (for details on ionic selectivity, see review of Ulbricht, 1974). In the Na channel, activation and inactivation are shown to be linked to separate structures, and apparently the latter function is brought about by a channel component closest to the internal membrane surface. These conclusions from compelling pharmacological evidence may serve as an example for the effectiveness of drugs — at least those with highly selective actions — as tools in the study of the excitable membrane.

Acknowledgement

The author wishes to thank Miss E. Dieter for valuable technical help and Dr. H.-H. Wagner for reading the manuscript. The support by the Deutsche Forschungsgemeinschaft is gratefully acknowledged.

References

Albuquerque, E. X.: Fed. Proc. **31**, 1133 (1972).
Armstrong, C. M.: J. gen. Physiol. **54**, 553 (1969).
Armstrong, C. M.: J. gen. Physiol. **58**, 413 (1971).
Armstrong, C. M., Bezanilla, F., Rojas, E.: J. gen. Physiol. **62**, 375 (1973).
Armstrong, C. M., Binstock, L.: J. gen. Physiol. **48**, 859 (1965).
Armstrong, C. M., Hille, B.: J. gen. Physiol. **59**, 388 (1972).
Calahan, M.: Biophys. Soc. Abstr., 17th Ann. Meeting, 242a (1973).
Cuervo, L. A., Adelman, W. J.: J. gen. Physiol. **55**, 309 (1970).
Evans, M. H.: Int. Rev. Neurobiol. **15**, 83 (1972).

FRAZIER, D.T., NARAHASHI, T., YAMADA, M.: J. Pharmacol. exp. Ther. **171**, 45 (1970).
HILLE, B.: J. gen. Physiol. **50**, 1287 (1967).
HILLE, B.: J. gen. Physiol. **51**, 199 (1968).
HILLE, B.: Progr. Biophys. molec. Biol. **21**, 1 (1970).
HODGKIN, A.L., HUXLEY, A.F.: J. Physiol. (Lond.) **117**, 500 (1952).
HONERJÄGER, P.: Biophys. Soc. Abstr., 15th Ann. Meeting, 54a (1971).
HONERJÄGER, P.: Naunyn-Schmiedebergs Arch. Pharmakol. **280**, 391 (1973).
KOPPENHÖFER, E.: Pflügers Arch. ges. Physiol. **293**, 34 (1967).
KOPPENHÖFER, E., SCHMIDT, H.: Pflügers Arch. **303**, 133 (1968a).
KOPPENHÖFER, E., SCHMIDT, H.: Pflügers Arch. **303**, 150 (1968b).
KOPPENHÖFER, E., VOGEL, W.: Pflügers Arch. **313**, 361 (1969).
MEVES, H.: Pflügers Arch. ges. Physiol. **290**, 211 (1966).
NARAHASHI, T.: In: ADELMAN, W.J. (Ed.): Biophysics and physiology of excitable membranes. New York: van Nostrand Reinhold Co. 1971.
NARAHASHI, T.: Fed. Proc. **31**, 1124 (1972).
NARAHASHI, T., ANDERSON, N.C., MOORE, J.W.: Science **153**, 765 (1966).
NARAHASHI, T., SHAPIRO, B.I., DEGUCHI, T., SCUKA, M., WANG, C.M.: Amer. J. Physiol. **222**, 850 (1972).
OHTA, M., NARAHASHI, T., KEELER, R.F.: J. Pharmacol. exp. Ther. **184**, 143 (1973).
RITCHIE, J.M., GREENGARD, P.: Ann. Rev. Pharmacol. **6**, 405 (1966).
SCHWARZ, J.R., ULBRICHT, W., WAGNER, H.-H.: J. Physiol. (Lond.) **233**, 167 (1973).
STRICHARTZ, G.R.: J. gen. Physiol. **62**, 37 (1973).
TASAKI, I., HAGIWARA, S.: J. gen. Physiol. **40**, 859 (1957).
ULBRICHT, W.: Pflügers Arch. ges. Physiol. **289**, R 9 (1966).
ULBRICHT, W.: Ergebn. Physiol. **61**, 18 (1969a).
ULBRICHT, W.: Pflügers Arch. **311**, 73 (1969b).
ULBRICHT, W.: Pflügers Arch. **336**, 187 (1972a).
ULBRICHT, W.: Pflügers Arch. **336**, 201 (1972b).
ULBRICHT, W.: Biophys. Struct. Mech. (in press) (1974).
ULBRICHT, W., WAGNER, H.-H.: Phil. Trans. R. Soc. (in press) (1974).
VIERHAUS, J., ULBRICHT, W.: Pflügers Arch. **326**, 76 (1971a).
VIERHAUS, J., ULBRICHT, W.: Pflügers Arch. **326**, 88 (1971b).
WAGNER, H.-H., ULBRICHT, W.: Pflügers Arch. **339**, R 70 (1973).
WAGNER, H.-H., ULBRICHT, W.: Pflügers Arch. **347**, R 34 (1974).

Discussion

V.P. WHITTAKER (Göttingen): The very high affinity of the tetrodotoxin for the channels would seem to make it an ideal candidate for making an affinity column of, in an attempt to isolate the material which composes the channels. Can you tell me if any work on these lines has been done?

W. ULBRICHT: As far as I know TTX has no yet been successfully employed for affinity chromatography in the strict sense, but ³H-TTX has been helpful in identifying fractions of solubilized membrane proteins of high affinity for the toxin [BENZER, T. I., RAFTERY, M. A.: Proc. nat. Acad. Sci. (Wash.) **69**, 3634—3637 (1972); HENDERSON, R., WANG, J. H.: Biochemistry **11**, 4565—4569 (1972)].

V. P. WHITTAKER: Is there any physiological role of batrachotoxin in regulating sodium movement through the skin of the toad?

W. ULBRICHT: Batrachotoxin has no effect on the short-circuit current in the skin of *Rana pipiens* [ALBUQUERQUE, E. X., DALY, J. W., WITKOP, B.: Science **172**, 995—1002 (1972)].

U. THURM (Bochum): Some local anesthetics are said to displace calcium from the membrane. Could you link this to the observations you talked about?

K. ULBRICHT: Not convincingly, although competition between local anesthetics and calcium has, indeed, been assumed to underlie nerve block [see *e.g.* BLAUSTEIN, M. P., GOLDMAN, D. E.: Science **153**, 429—432 (1966)]. This particular explanation, however, implies a distinct role of calcium in the gating mechanism that, in my opinion, has not yet been proved. Moreover, since many local anesthetics appear to act at the axoplasmic side of the membrane the axon interior would probably have to serve as the pool of the competing Ca^{++} ions although this compartment contains very little or, in the case of the internally perfused axon, no calcium.

C. LIÉBECQ (Liège): I should like to know to what extent the resting potential is affected by those drugs that selectively block the sodium or potassium channels.

K. ULBRICHT: TTX (300 nM) has bee reported to lead to a slight hyperpolarization of the resting squid axon membrane and thus has the effect of a Na-free solution [FREEMAN, A. R.: Comp. Biochem. Physiol. **40**A, 71—82 (1971)]. TEA (about 5 mM) depolarizes the nodal membrane by a few mV [SCHMIDT, H., STÄMPFLI, R.: Pflügers Arch. ges. Physiol. **287**, 311—325 (1966)].

Mechanisms of Electrical Membrane Responses in Sensory Receptors, Illustrated by Mechanoreceptors[1]

Ulrich Thurm[2]

Arbeitsgruppe für Primärprozesse der Rezeptoren, Institut für Allgemeine Zoologie, Ruhr-Universität Bochum, D-4630 Bochum, Federal Republic of Germany

With 12 Figures

I. Introduction

Biochemical investigation of sensory transduction within receptor cells has to envisage the fact that these processes are performed by functional systems consisting of a number of submechanisms of quite different nature. This diversity corresponds to a highly differentiated structural organization of the transducing region of the cell. In a type of receptor cell in which the functional and structural organization had originally appeared rather "isotropic", *i.e.* in the Pacinian corpuscle, further investigation has also revealed a high level of structural complexity (Fig. 5A) [1]. The structural heterogeneity of the transducing regions need not handicap biochemical investigation but may actually be advantageous, since a spatial separation of the submechanisms facilitates a dissection of the functional complex so that the submechanisms can be studied separately. The following contribution is an attempt to outline principles of the functional organization of sensory receptor cells in order to give a framework of understanding for further investigation of the various functional elements and their interrelationship.

A sensory signal transmitted within a receptor cell is generally carried by an ionic current, called the receptor current. By chang-

---

[1] Dedicated to Professor Dr. B. Rensch on the occasion of his 75th birthday.

[2] Present address: Zoologisches Institut, Lehrstuhl f. Neurophysiologie d. Universität Münster, D-4400 Münster, Federal Republic of Germany.

ing the voltage across parts of the cell membrane this current elicits the next, different step of signal transmission, which is either the secretion of a synaptic transmitter substance carrying the signal to the next cell or the generation of nerve impulses appropriate to conduct the signal over a long distance still within the sensory cell (Fig. 1). The processes which transform the external stimulus into the receptor current comprise the sensory transduction. Only this stage of signal processing will be considered here.

Sensory transduction is a control process in which the energy for the cellular response is supplied by the metabolism of the organism. A threshold response of a sensory cell supplies up to $3 \cdot 10^{-9}$ A or about $1.5 \cdot 10^{-10}$ W [2]. A representative value of the stimulus energy controlling this current flow is $5 \cdot 10^{-19}$ Wsec, the energy delivered by a light quantum at about 500 nm wavelength. Mechanoreceptors indicate that the stimulus energy is necessary in order to *change* the strength of the receptor current; there is no need for a supply of stimulus energy during a constant current response. A mechanoreceptor kept constantly deformed may respond for at least several days. The input parameter which is in most unique relation to the energy flow of the response is obviously not the energy input of the stimulus but the conformation of some small, essential part of the cell. This is the input-output relation as it exists at a mechanical valve. The relative displacements effective in stimulating mechanoreceptor terminals are roughly in the order of Å units and below [3—5]. At this subcellular level of events the differences between sensory cells specialized for the different modalities of stimuli seem to become smaller than on the organ level: The stimulus-response relation is supposed, for photo- and chemoreceptors as well as for mechanoreceptors, to be a molecular deformation to current relationship (for photoreceptors, ref. [6]). In photo- and chemoreceptors, however, endogenous mechanisms exist which reverse the molecular result of the stimulus energy absorption, whereas in most mechanoreceptors the deformation is released only by a reversal of the original energy input. In every case the flow of external signals modulates an energy flow which is supplied by the receptor cell. Thus we have to deal with three main groups of problems (Fig. 1):

a) The molecular mechanisms receiving the stimuli which may be called the sensor mechanisms. These mechanisms determine the

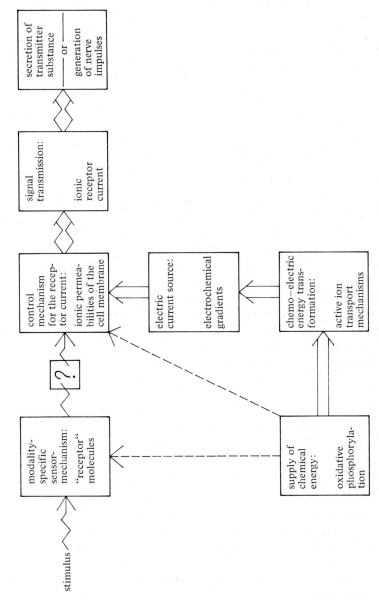

Fig. 1. Block-diagram of transduction and transmission of a signal within a receptor cell

specificity of a sensory cell for a certain modality and quality of stimuli.

b) The mechanisms supplying the energy and the ionic conditions for the receptor current.

c) The mechanisms controlling (modulating) the ionic current flow according to the state of stimulation of the sensor.

The sensor mechanism (a) and the control mechanism (c) have often been considered in the past to be part of the same macromolecule within the cell membrane. Indeed, one could think of pore molecules which possess a sensitive site (*e.g.*, a chromophore), thus directly controlling an ionic current through the membrane depending on the stimulus input. However, circumstantial evidence so far obtained for some photo- and mechanoreceptors rules against the common identity of the sensor and the current-control molecule (see Paragraph IV). This gives rise to the big question mark in Fig. 1 as to the means of coupling sensor and control mechanisms. I shall leave this question to stimulate discussion, rather than to discuss it within this survey (but see [7]).

II. The Spatial Distribution of Submechanisms

The physiology of sensory transduction is confronted with a marked "anisotropy" of the receptor cell terminals which contrasts the higher "isotropy" of the basic organization of nerve axons. This structural difference is associated with two essential differences in the functional basis of these cellular regions:

a) Since the receptor current is generated in a *terminal* structure, the current circuit is locally fixed, in contrast to the local circuits which move along an axon. Whereas in an unmyelinated axon every membrane area becomes the site of current inflow as well as of outflow successively, in a receptor terminal one area is subject only to the inflow, the other area only to the outflow of the net current. Moreover, the ionic composition of the inward and outward currents appear to be nonidentical in some receptors. Thus gradients of the ionic activities are to be expected along the receptor terminal between the sites of current inflow and outflow which can be matched only by local, metabolism dependent, transport processes.

b) The sensory cells of most types are part of epithelia which separate two liquid-filled spaces (Fig. 2). The "external" medium can differ very much from the intercellular medium, just as for instance fresh water does or the cochlear "endolymph" which has

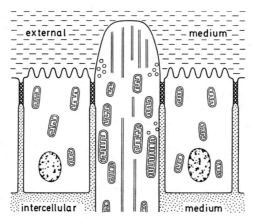

Fig. 2. Scheme of a receptor cell within a sensory epithelium. The apical segment of the receptor cell facing the external medium represents specialized terminal structures like microvilli or cilia. The crossed zones between the cells symbolize junctional complexes (*zonulae occludentes, adhaerentes* or *septatae*). Microtubules, mitochondria and vesicles are indicated in a distribution common to many types of epithelial receptor cells. (From [10])

a K^+/Na^+-ratio similar to the *intra*cellular K^+/Na^+-ratio. As Fig. 2 illustrates, the apical part of an epithelial receptor cell which is specialized for receiving the adequate stimuli is surrounded by this "external" medium, whereas the basal, larger part of the cell is in contact with the regular intercellular medium. Thus, it is known for several receptors that the ionic gradients across these different membrane areas differ (*e.g.* [8, 9]). It is a common property of epithelial cells that the membrane areas facing the different media are different in their permeabilities and in their possession of active transport mechanisms; this is the basis for the active roles of most epithelia. Together with the ionic concentration gradients, these differences can be sources for a transepithelial voltage gradient. Thus, we have to realize that sensory cells integrated into epithelia are, at least in several cases, subject to external electrochemical gradients, and that the working conditions for the membrane areas

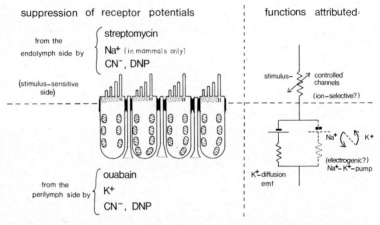

Fig. 3. Illustration of experimental results obtained by Matsuura et al. [11] at sacculus sensory epithelium of goldfish, demonstrating the functional separation and the differences in properties of the two sides of the epithelium.
Black connections between cells symbolize junctional complexes

separated by the epithelial boundary layer can be appreciably different [10].

The diversity of membrane properties at the apical versus the basal side of an epithelial sensory cell have clearly been shown by Matsuura et al. [11] for the stato-acoustic receptor in the sacculus of goldfish, as illustrated in Fig. 3. Their results demonstrate: (a) The media facing the two sides of the epithelium are separated by diffusion barriers; (b) the apical membrane differs from the basal membrane of the sensory epithelium with respect to the mechanisms involved; (c) the ionic requirement for the generation of receptor potentials is different for the apical and the basal membrane areas. As to the location of essential submechanisms it is concluded: A K^+-diffusion potential and a ouabain-sensitive Na^+-K^+-pump are located at the basal membrane area; the apical membrane possesses a streptomycin-sensitive function which may be associated with the stimulus-controlled K^+-permeability inferred for this membrane according to other authors; no K^+-diffusion source is needed at the apical side. Although "supporting" cells are present besides the receptor cells in the sensory epithelium, it is suggested, for other reasons, that these properties refer to the receptor cells.

The basic scheme of organization of the receptor region in epithelial sensory cells is remarkably similar throughout the animal kingdom e.g., from hydromedusae to man, and it is independent of the modality of the adequate stimuli (Fig. 4). Within the receptor region we generally find a sub-region which determines the modality of adequate stimuli — a modality-specific region, often called the outer segment. This segment is connected to a second subregion (inner segment), characterized by a high concentration of mitochondria and of vesicles of unknown function, both irrespective of the modality of adequate stimuli (see Section IV). The modality-specific subregion is often a modified ciliary shaft, in which cases the subregions are connected by the basal ciliary structures (Fig. 4). The stimulus-receiving, modality-specific subregion protrudes into the external medium, whereas in most cases the accumulation of mitochondria faces the basal membrane region which is surrounded by the intercellular medium. There are a few exceptions (e.g. the vertebrate photoreceptors) in which the subregion containing the accumulation of mitochondria — the inner segment — is also apical to the border line of intercellular membrane junctions (see Fig. 4 E).

The organization of the receptor region in epithelial primary receptor cells, as exemplified in Fig. 4, is analogous to the organization of the secondary receptor cells involved in the study of MATSUURA et al. [11] cited above (Fig. 3). We may therefore expect, that the spatial distribution of submechanisms as illustrated for the stato-acoustic receptors in Fig. 3 is not just a special case. Results on vertebrate photoreceptors and on insect mechanoreceptors substantiate this expectation (see Section V).

Since the accumulation of mitochondria is apparently essential for the generation of receptor potentials (see the following section), it has been a challenging problem to assign the kind of flow which bridges the considerable distances (up to 300 μm! [12]) between the site of primary stimulus action and the mitochondria: the flow either of chemical energy (e.g. ATP) or of ions or of an unknown

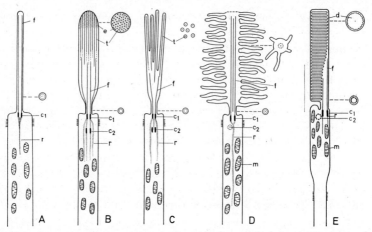

Fig. 4A—E. Diagrams of distal nerve processes of epithelial ciliary receptor cells for various modalities of adequate stimuli. (A) chemo- and/or mechano-receptor of the auriculum of a planarian [54]; (B) mechanoreceptor of insect hair or campaniform sensillum [39]; (C) chemoreceptor of insect hair sensillum [55]; (D) photoreceptor of a hydromedusan [56]; (E) rod-photoreceptor of vertebrates [57]. Hatched zones outside of the cells symbolize junctional complexes connecting to neighbouring cells. $c_{1,2}$, centrioles; e, intensely stained material associated with microtubules (tubular body); f, ciliary filaments; m, mitochondria; r, root filaments; t, microtubules

type of signal (*e.g.* transmitted as conformational changes of micro-tubules) [13, 14]. This question has now been decided rather convincingly in favour of an ionic current (see Section V).

III. The Supply of Chemical Energy

As is well known, the electrical energy which is used in the receptor current is supplied by electrochemical gradients across areas of plasma membrane. These gradients, in turn, are built up by ion transport mechanisms (pumps) which are driven by metabolic processes (Fig. 1). So far the Na^+-K^+-pump is the only ion transport mechanism which has been found in sensory cells to perform the chemo-electric energy transformation (see the effect of the inhibitor of this transport, ouabain, in the experiments of Fig. 3). Other types of ion pump, however, which are located in accessory cells contribute to the receptor current in some receptor organs (see below).

The oxidative metabolism has been found to be the main energy source for driving the ion pump of axon membranes as well as of receptors (*e.g.* [11, 15—17]). In insect eyes, where a large fraction of the volume consists of the receptive regions of the sensory cells, the O_2-consumption (per weight) in the unexcited state is higher than in nerve fibres, and it is further increased by adequate stimulation [15, 18, 19].

This high energy consumption per unit weight corresponds to the astoundingly high concentration of mitochondria in receptoric cell regions. We have found the ratio of the inner surface area of mitochondria per area of the surrounding neuron membrane to be about 10 times higher in receptive regions (outside the perikarion) than in axons of the same diameter (Fig. 5) [20]. This ratio is invariant with respect to the modality of the receptor or to the systematic position of the animal species. The same invariance is true for the *absolute amount* of the inner surface of mitochondria supplied within the receptive region. Within a frog muscle spindle (dendrites of only one sensory cell) this area amounts to 10 times the inner surface of the mitochondria of a liver cell ($4 \cdot 10^5 \mu m^2$ compared to $3 \cdot 10^4 \mu m^2$; [14, 21]).

The variance in the absolute amount of mitochondrial inner surface, however, spans a range of 1000 : 1, if one considers different types of receptors (with the muscle spindle being at the top of the scale). The absolute amount is only correlated with the morphological type of the receptor and not with the modality of the adequate stimuli [14].

That means, modality-specific energy requirements (*e.g.*, for regeneration of a photopigment) are probably small compared with the modality-unspecific energy needs of receptor regions. Similar accumulations of mitochondria are found in the transmitter-sensing postsynaptic regions. Questions dealing with the function of these accumulated mitochondria can be answered preliminarily by the comparison outlined below. It suggests that the fraction of these mitochondria needed to energize the receptor current is similar to that needed within axonal regions for the energy of spike currents.

In the comparison an inner mitochondrial area is calculated which, on the suppositions specified below, should correspond to a known receptor current strength. This value will then be compared with the measured values of the existing mitochondrial area. The calculation is done on the supposition

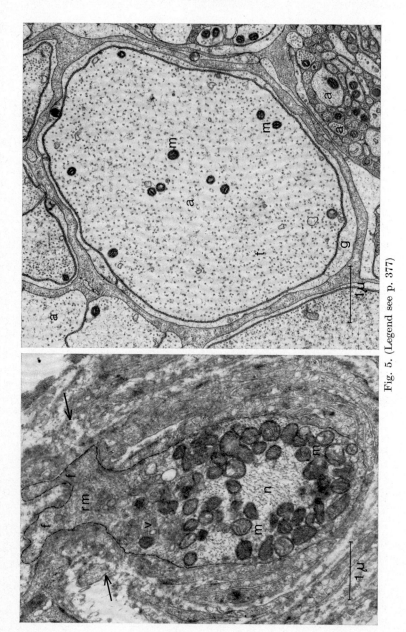

Fig. 5. (Legend see p. 377)

that in receptive regions, as in axons of identical diameter, equal areas of inner mitochondrial membrane are needed to reverse equal Na^+-influxes. This supposition does not include an assumption on the fraction of mitochondrial area active for energizing a special intensity of ion transport, but it assumes this fraction to be equal in axons and in receptive regions of equal diameter. The reason for referring to the cell diameter is the fact that in axons the ratio of inner mitochondrial surface to surrounding cell membrane considerably increases with the the axon diameter [20]. A mean value of Na^+-entry during an axon spike is $5 \cdot 10^{-7}$ A $\cdot$ sec $\cdot$ cm^{-2} [22]; i.e., during, for instance, 50 impulses/sec the Na^+-current has the mean of $2.5 \cdot 10^{-5}$ A$\cdot$cm^{-2} Within 10 μm-diameter axons of various animal species the ratio of inner mitochondrial area per unit axon surface is about 0.8. For these specifications about $3 \cdot 10^{-5}$ A of Na^+-influx are opposed by 1 cm^2 inner mitochondrial area.

In the ventral photoreceptor of *Limulus* [2, 23] the half maximal steady state receptor current is about $5 \cdot 10^{-9}$ A; this value might correspond again to the axonal frequency of 50 impulses/sec in spike generating receptors. Based on the aforementioned suppositions, the mitochondrial area corresponding to the receptor current is about $2 \cdot 10^4$ μm^2. This area is, indeed, as large as the mitochondrial area present within the inner segments of the big rods of frog's eye and is nearly 10 times above the mitochondrial area within the receptive region of squid photoreceptors; according to CLARK et al. [24] the value for the ventral photoreceptor of *Limulus* is expected to be within the same order of 10^4 μm^2.

The fact that mitochondria are packed more densely in most receptive regions than in axons may be related to the density of the receptor current: calculations relating measured receptor currents to corresponding membrane areas indicate that the receptor current density in the membrane of an inner receptor segment is higher than the mean current density in an axon membrane during an equivalent spike frequency.

The existence of a relatively small inner surface area of mitochondria (some 10^2 μm^2) is correlated in several types of receptors with a high concentration of mitochondria within certain accessory

---

Fig. 5. Cross sections of neurons within the receptive region (left) and the axonal region (right). Left: An encapsulated and lamellated receptor terminal (non-epithelial) from a sinus hair base of the mini-pig. In the upper half the surface membrane is outlined by dashes. Two fingerlike processes are obliquely cut in this cross-section of the otherwise cylindrical terminal. As demonstrated for the similarly organized Pacinian corpuscle, this receptor is probably stimulated by pressure in the direction of the arrows [59]. Courtesy of Dr. M. v. DÜRING. Right: Axons within the leg nerve of a whip spider. Courtesy of Dr. R. FOELIX. a, axon; f, fingerlike process; g, glial cell; m, mitochondria; n, neurofilaments; rm, receptor matrix consisting of 6 nm thick microfilaments [1, 43]; t, microtubules; v, vesicles

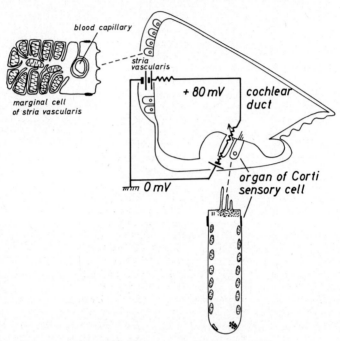

Fig. 6. Diagram of the mammalian cochlear duct showing the receptor current circuit (adapted from [25]), and the sensory and marginal cells having active functions within the circuit (adapted from [58])

cells. In two of these cases, *i.e.* the mammalian cochlea and insect epidermal receptors, it has been made very plausible that electrogenic ion transport mechanisms within these accessory cells (cells of the *stria vascularis* and the tormogen cells, respectively) contribute electrical energy to the generation of the receptor currents (Figs. 6 and 7) [10, 25—27]. These cells generate a transepithelial voltage of 50—100 mV (positive at the sensory cell apices) by intensive, acutely O_2-dependent, ion transport systems. These transport systems enrich the ionic milieu surrounding the apical receptor membrane with K^+ (*e.g.* [28, 9]). The pump mechanism performing these functions in insect sensory epithelia apparently belongs to the K^+-transport-type, known only in insects [29], which moves alkalications, preferentially K^+, only in the direction out of the cell [17, 30]. The highly folded membrane areas which are suggested to

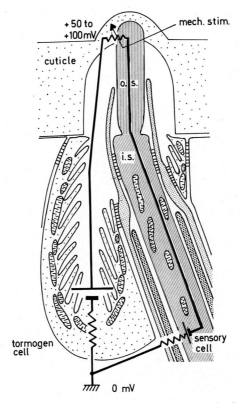

Fig. 7. Diagram of a campaniform mechanoreceptor unit of a fly showing the receptor current circuit (simplified) and accumulations of mitochondria (adapted from [10]). *i.s.*, inner segment; *o.s.*, outer segment of the receptor cell; *mech.stim.*, adequate mechanical stimulus

perform this transport are lined on the cytoplasmic side by particles of about 80 Å in diameter (Fig. 8) [10, 31] — one of the few cases in which a certain membrane activity is paralleled by some membrane structure visible in EM-sections.

IV. The Sensor and the Current Control Mechanism

As already mentioned, the sensor regions of many receptor cells are part of a more or less modified *cilium* (Fig. 4). Cells exist which have some sensitivity influencing the motor activity besides mo-

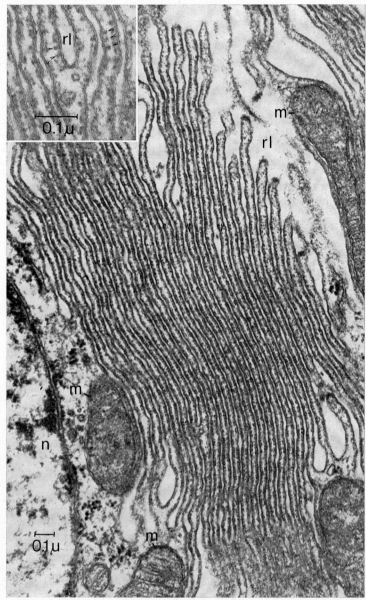

Fig. 8. (Legend see p. 381)

torically active cilia or flagella. I shall focus on the following questions within this brief survey: What is the nature of the functional relation between a sensor and a motor mechanism ? Could this relation be the reason for the development of specialized sensory mechanisms on the structural basis of a motor organelle ? Answering these questions might cast some light on the functional relationship between a molecular sensor and an effector or current-control mechanism.

We have looked for mechano-sensitivity in motile cilia, using the large abfrontal cilia on the gills of the mussel *Mytilus*, an object of classical studies in motor physiology of cilia. We found a sensitivity suprisingly similar in its characteristics to those of sensory hair cells of the vertebrate inner ear and of the lateral line system (Fig. 9) [32, 33]. The directional distribution of sensitivity has a unique relation to the plane and polarity of the ciliary movements, just like the relationship which exists in these sensory cells between sensitivity and the bilateral, polar ciliary structure. This suggests that the sensor mechanisms of both types of cells are of the same kind and are (more or less directly) associated with the cilia. The

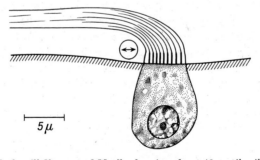

Fig. 9. Cell of a gill filament of *Mytilus* bearing about 40 motile cilia of 60μm length. The circle represents a glas needle in cross section which stimulates the cell by shearing displacements of the ciliary bases by $\geq$ 0.4μm. (From [32])

Fig. 8. Membrane lamellae of the tormogen cell of a campaniform receptor unit of the fly *Calliphora* (cf. Fig. 7). Note the particles (arrows) at the plasmic side of the membranes, as individually distinguishable in the inset. Courtesy of Dr. R. FOELIX. *m*, mitochondrion; *n*, nucleus; *rl*, receptor lymph cavity (external medium)

existence of this sensor mechanism does not seem to be a universal property of cilia, since we have found pronounced differences in the degree of sensitivity for different types of cells. The sensor might be similarly additional to the motor mechanism, as the photosensor, for instance, is in a flagellum of *Euglena*.

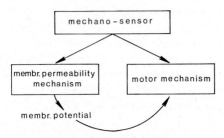

Fig. 10. Block-diagram of the inferred interrelation of sensor and response mechanisms in receptive and electrically responsive cells bearing motile cilia

Since a motor response is elicited in cilia following a stimulus, it is possible to use this response as an assay of sensitivity which is independent of the integrity of the membrane (other than a response in the membrane potential) comparable to the contractility of glycerol extracted or "skinned" muscle fibres. In this way the question of whether the sensor mechanism is identical with the current control mechanism within the cell membrane can be answered. We have found that the mechano-sensitivity remains unaffected in a medium which removes most ionic gradients across the cell membrane (activities of Na^+, K^+, Ca^{++}, and Mg^{++} in this medium similar to *intra*cellular activities) [33]. We are led to conclude that (a) the sensor mechanism is different from a permeability control mechanism and (b) that the motor mechanism can directly be activated without an interposed membrane depolarization. Since, on the other hand, the sensor mechanism appears to be of the same type as that controlling membrane permeabilities in sensory cells, we arrive at the scheme of interrelations shown in Fig. 10: The motor mechanism of the cilium and the membrane permeability control mechanisms are suggested to be parallel effectors activated by the sensor mechanism, independently of each other. Cells are known which are specialized, having only one of both effectors: cells which do not depolarize if stimulated mechanically but respond by ciliary motor activity, and conversely hair receptors of higher vertebrates which respond by a change in membrane potential without activating their cilium. In contrast, the homologous cells in lower vertebrates and similar sensory cells in molluscs display both kinds of response simultaneously (for references see [32, 34]). The comb-plate cells of ctenophores primarily have a motor function, but nevertheless respond by depolarizations (and motor activity) to passive bending of their cilia [35].

The concept, which has evolved from these results on ciliary mechanoreceptors and which has to be checked further, is that of the sensor as an autonomous mechanism which can be directly coupled to a motor mechanism as well as to a permeability control mechanism. This relationship would be the reason for the fact that many receptor cells have been specialized for their sensory function on the structural basis of a motor system. The validity of this concept also has to be checked for cells sensitive to stimuli of other modalities. In the ciliary vertebrate rod-photoreceptors the proof of a discontinuity between the membrane sacs (which contain the vast majority of the photopigment) and the surface membrane (which displays the permeability response) further the concept in the same direction: the separate identity of sensor and membrane-effector mechanisms is no longer doubted, and a major effort of research is directed towards elucidation of the process which functionally links both mechanisms (see [7, 38]). More circumstantial evidence suggests that also in *non*-ciliary photoreceptors the sensor mechanism is not identical with the molecules controlling membrane permeability (cf. [36]). A similar separate identity is suggested for the mechanisms in the chemosensitive subsynaptic membrane of cholinergic synapses [37].

In photoreceptors the sensor mechanism is easily recognized by the considerable amount of packed membranes containing the photosensitive pigment (Fig. 4 D and E) [cf. [6, 38]). Also, in ciliary mechanoreceptors of arthropods the modified shaft of the cilium develops a structural specialization, the tubular body (Figs. 4 B and 11) (*e.g.* [5, 39, 40]). (These receptors are to be distinguished from the sensory hair cells of *e.g.*, vertebrates, the cilia of which show the unmodified $9 \times 2 + 2$ configuration and which are mechanosensitive probably in the basal region of the cilia.) The tubular body

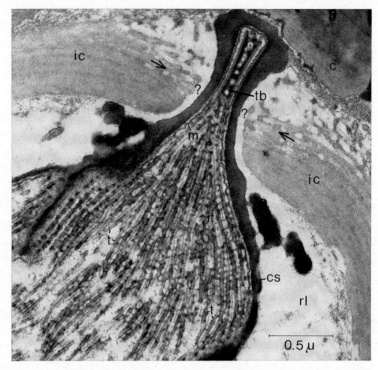

Fig. 11. Terminal of the outer segment of a campaniform mechanoreceptor of the fly *Calliphora*; longitudinal section. During an adequate stimulus, the inner cuticular layer (*ic*) probably compresses the terminal in direction of the arrows. The clefts at ? are probably caused by shrinkage. *c*, cuticle; *cs*, cuticular sheath; *it*, intertubular material; *m*, receptor membrane; *rl*, receptor lymph cavity; *t*, microtubules; *tb*, tubular body. Courtesy of Dr. R. Foelix

is a complex of plasmatic microtubules which along their length are interconnected and connected to the surface membrane by homogeneous material or defined bridges, which are distinguished by their intense osmium staining. The adequate stimulus is probably represented by a monoaxial diminution of the tip diameter by 30—1000 Å (0.5—15%) at the site of this tubular body [5, 41, 42]. It is not yet known whether the molecular mechanosensitive mechanism in these receptors is part of these plasmatic structures or of the surface membrane, or of the complex displayed by membrane plus the submembraneous material. Finger-like processes of the non-ciliary epidermal mechanoreceptors of vertebrates may be compared with this terminal region of modified cilia (see [43]) (Fig. 5A). These processes, which also are characterized by a special plasmatic configuration (similarly occurring in thermo-receptors), are presumably stimulated also by a deformation per-pendicular to their long axis [1].

In contrast to the latency of photoreceptors which is in the order of 10 msec, the latency in mechanoreceptors is generally less than 0.2 msec (e.g. [44]). This may suggest that the process which links sensor and current control mechanisms in photoreceptors is essentially different from that in mechanoreceptors.

V. Integration of Submechanisms

The fragmentary results obtained so far from epithelial mechano-receptors of vertebrates and insects and of vertebrate photo-receptors yield a common scheme (perhaps a preliminary one) which outlines the interrelation of the submechanisms within the circuits of ion and electrical charge flow (Fig. 12). Beyond their basic common features, the various receptor types differ in many details which in this scheme can be represented only by some "average" presentation. Indications exist that epithelial receptors for other modalities of stimuli and of other groups of animals also follow this scheme. Whether non-epithelial receptors differ from this scheme in more than the spatial distribution of the functional elements is a problem for further research. The scheme is based mainly on results worked out by CAVAGGIONI et al. [45], DAVIS [25], HAGINS et al. [47, 48], HONRUBIA and WARD [26], KAUFFMANN [49], KÜPPERS [9], MATSUURA et al. [11], NECKER [50], THURM [27], ZUCKERMANN [51].

The basic features of the scheme are as follows:

a) An electrical source which works on the basis of active Na^+-K^+-transport is present in the membrane of the basal segment of the receptoric region (inner segment of the distal nerve process of primary receptor cells). The source is mainly a K^+-diffusion electro-motive force (emf). The metabolic energy is supplied within this segment.

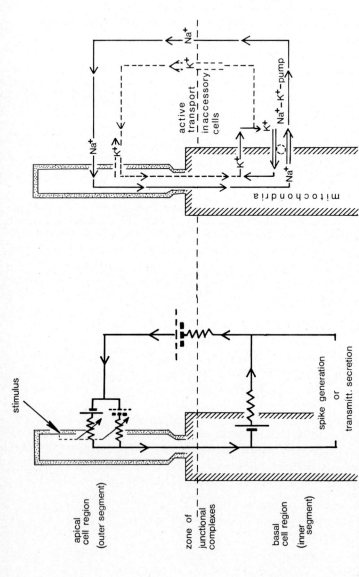

Fig. 12. Diagrams of receptor current circuits (left) and of cationic fluxes (right) in epithelial receptor cells. Summary of results for various receptor typs (see text). In vertebrate photoreceptors the zone of junctional complexes is located not at the distal but at the basal end of the inner segment

b) A depolarizing response of the sensory cell is caused by a stimulus-controlled increase in permeability of part of the apical membrane. The depolarizing current is carried by an inflow of cations. The emf underlying this current within the apical membrane is either positive inside (Na^+-gradient) or near to zero (small K^+-gradient due to high $[K^+]$ at the outside).

c) The site of the permeability change can be spatially separated from the site of the primary stimulus effect (sensor). For vertebrate photoreceptors this distance is in the order of 1 μm.

d) During depolarization, cations are flowing within the cell from the tip to the base of the receptoric region and *vice versa* outside the cell.

e) In some sensory epithelia, additional electrical sources located within the epithelial layer outside the sensory cells are included in the circuit of the receptor current. The polarity of these sources (apically positive) is such that it increases current flow within the receptor circuit.

Considerable differences apparently exist in the ionic composition of current influx into the apical membrane, corresponding to the various K^+/Na^+-ratios in the differing external media. For insect mechanoreceptors [27] and the sauropsid ear [49, 50] which have high $[K^+]$ in the external medium, data suggest two types of stimulus-controlled channels with different kinetic and dynamic behavior and different emfs, which may correspond to selective channels for Na^+ and K^+, respectively. In vertebrate photoreceptors, in contrast, during cell depolarization (occuring in darkness), the permeability of the apical membrane is much higher for Na^+ than for K^+ [45, 46].

At the end of this survey I would like to point to the instructive analogy which becomes apparent between this scheme of epithelial sensory cells and epithelial cells functioning in absorption and secretion of ions, like those of frog epidermis (cf. [52]) and of mammalian salivary duct [53] and of kidney distal tubules (cf. [52]). As in sensory cells, there is a passive influx of ions into these cells at their apical poles and an active transport out of the cells across the basal membrane. The epithelial sensory cells can be considered to be ion-transporting epithelial cells which are specialized for stimulus-dependent variability of their influx of ions.

References

1. Spencer, P.S., Schaumburg, H.H.: J. Neurocyt. **2**, 217 (1973).
2. Millecchia, R., Mauro, A.: J. gen. Physiol. **54**, 331 (1969).
3. Autrum, H.: Z. vergl. Physiol. **28**, 580 (1941).
4. Johnstone, B.M., Boyle, A.J.F.: Science **158**, 389 (1967).
5. Thurm, U.: Cold Spr. Harb. Symp. quant. Biol. **30**, 75 (1965).
6. Stieve, H.: Rhein.-Westf. Akad. Wissensch. N 239 (1974).
7. Stieve, H.: This volume.
8. Bosher, S.K., Warren, R.L.: Proc. roy. Soc. B **171**, 227 (1968).
9. Küppers, J.: In: Schwartzkopff, J. (Ed.): Mechanoreception. Symp. Bochum, Abhdlg. Rhein. Westf. Akad. Wissensch., Westd. Verl. Opladen (1974) (in press).
10. Thurm, U.: Verh. Dt. Zool. Ges., 64. Tagg. 79 (1970).
11. Matsuura, S., Ikeda, K., Furukawa, T.: Jap. J. Physiol. **21**, 563 and 579 (1971).
12. Kaissling, K.-E.: This volume.
13. Thurm, U.: Symp. Zool. Soc. Lond. **23**, 199 (1968).
14. Thurm, U.: In: Reichardt, W. (Ed.): Processing of optical data by organisms and by machines, 45. London: Academic Press 1969.
15. Ritchie, J.M.: J. Physiol. (Lond.) **188**, 383 (1967).
16. Langer, H.: Biol. Zbl. **81**, 691 (1962).
17. Stieve, H., Bollmann-Fischer, H., Braun, B.: Z. Naturforsch. **26 b**, 1311 (1971).
18. Autrum, H., Tscharntke, H.: Z. vergl. Physiol. **45**, 695 (1962).
19. Hamdorf, K., Kascheff, A.H.: Z. vergl. Physiol. **48**, 251 (1964).
20. Thurm, U.: In preparation.
21. Lehninger, A.L.: The mitochondrion. New York: W. A. Benjamin 1964.
22. Hodgkin, A.L.: The conduction of the nervous impulse. Liverpool Univ. Press 1964.
23. Millecchia, R., Bradbury, J., Mauro, A.: Science **154**, 1199 (1966).
24. Clark, A.W., Millecchia, R., Mauro, A.: J. gen. Physiol. **54**, 289 (1969).
25. Davis, H.: Cold Spr. Harb. Symp. quant. Biol. **30**, 181 (1965).
26. Honrubia, V., Ward, P.H.: J. acoust. Soc. Amer. **46**, 388 (1969).
27. Thurm, U.: In: Schwartzkopff, J. (Ed.): Mechanoreception. Symp. Bochum, Abhdlg. Rhein. Westf. Akad. Wissensch., Westd. Verl. Opladen (1974) (in press).
28. Bosher, S.K., Warren, R.L.: Proc. Roy. Soc. B. **171**, 227 (1968).
29. Harvey, W.R., Nedergaard, S.: Proc. nat. Acad. Sci. (Wash.) **51**, 757 (1964).
30. Küppers, J., Thurm, U.: Verh. dtsch. Zool. Ges., 67 Tagg. (in press) (1974).
31. Smith, D.S.: Tissue & Cell **1**, 443 (1969).
32. Thurm, U.: Verh. dtsch. Zool. Ges., 61. Tagg. 96 (1967).
33. Thurm, U.: Neurosci. Res. Progr. Bull. **8**, 496 (1970).
34. Dijkgraaf, S., Hessels, H.G.A.: Z. vergl. Physiol. **62**, 38 (1969).
35. Horridge, G.A.: Nature (Lond.) **205**, 602 (1965).

Discussion 389

36. CONE, R. A.: In: LANGER, H. (Ed.): Biochemistry and physiology of visual pigments, p. 275. Berlin-Heidelberg-New York: Springer 1973.
37. CHANGEUX, J.-P.: In: SCHNEIDER, D. (Ed.): Olfaction and taste. IV. Stuttgart: Wissensch. Verlagsges. 1972.
38. BONTING, S. L.: This volume.
39. THURM, U.: Science **145**, 1063 (1964).
40. GAFFAL, K. P., HANSEN, K.: Z. Zellforsch. **132**, 79 (1972).
41. BARTH, F. G.: J. comp. Physiol. **81**, 159 (1972).
42. THURM, U., STEDTLER, A., FOELIX, R.: Verh. Dt. Zool. Ges., 67. Tagg. (in press) (1974).
43. ANDRES, K. H.: In: SCHWARTZKOPFF, J. (Ed.): Mechanoreception. Symp. Bochum., Abhdlg. Rhein. Westf. Akad. Wissensch., Westd. Verl. Opladen (in press) (1974).
44. THURM, U.: Cold Spr. Harb. Symp. quant. Biol. **30**, 83 (1965b).
45. CAVAGGIONI, A., SORBI, R. T., TURINI, S.: J. Physiol. (Lond.) **232**, 609 (1973).
46. KORENBROT, J. I., CONE, R. A.: J. gen. Physiol. **60**, 20 (1972).
47. HAGINS, W. A., RÜPPEL, H.: Fed. Proc. **30**, 64 (1971).
48. YOSHIKAMI, S., HAGINS, W. A.: In: LANGER, H. (Ed.): Biochemistry and physiology of visual pigments. Berlin-Heidelberg-New York: Springer 1973.
49. KAUFFMANN, G.: J. comp. Physiol. **90**, 245 (1974).
50. NECKER, R.: Z. vergl. Physiol. **69**, 367 (1970).
51. ZUCKERMAN, R.: J. Physiol. (Lond.) **235**, 333 (1973).
52. KEYNES, R. D.: Quart. Rev. Biophys. **2**, 177 (1969).
53. KNAUF, H., FRÖMTER, E.: In: Electrophysiology of epithelial cells. Stuttgart: F. K. Schattauer Verl. 1971.
54. MACRAE, E. K.: Z. Zellforsch. **82**, 479 (1967).
55. ERNST, K. D.: Z. Zellforsch. **94**, 72 (1969).
56. EAKIN, R. M., WESTFALL, J. A.: Proc. nat. Acad. Sci. (Wash.) **48**, 826 (1962).
57. SJÖSTRAND, F. S.: J. cell comp. Physiol. **42**, 45 (1953b).
58. BERRIDGE, M. J., OSCHMANN, J. L.: In: Transporting epithelia. New York: Academic Press 1972.
59. ILYINSKY, O. B.: Nature (Lond.) **208**, 351 (1965).

Discussion

P. SUNDER-PLASSMANN (Münster): Die Mitochondrien-Ansammlung, wie sie von Herrn THURM in den Sinneszellen gezeigt wurde, findet sich auch im Bereich der Carotisgabel-Feldreceptoren, die teils baro- teils chemo-receptiver Art sind. Es ist nun von Interesse, daß sich ähnliche Beziehungen neuraler Korrespondenz (*N. vagus*) zwischen Mitochondrienfunktionen auch an bestimmten interstitiellen Zellen und solchen ektodermaler Natur des Thymusmarks feststellen ließen, besonders im Bereich perivasculärer Axone und an den Hassall-Körpern. Da sich markierte Antigen-Moleküle im Thymus hauptsächlich perivasculär finden, sehen wir hier Anhaltspunkte für den "antigen-recognition mechanism", dessen Substrat bekanntlich immer noch die schwächste Stelle der "clonal selection theory" darstellt.

U. THURM: Die Regel der Existenz von Mitochondrien-Anhäufungen in receptorischen Zellregionen gilt meines Wissens ganz allgemein; eine Ausnahme stellen nur einige Elektroreceptoren dar. Im Fall von Zellen, deren Erregbarkeit bekannt oder anzunehmen ist, kann eine entsprechende Mitochondrien-Anhäufung daher als Hinweis für eine receptorische Zellregion dienen.

Cell Cultures as Model Systems for Studying the Biochemistry of Differentiated Functions of Nerve Cells

B. Hamprecht

Max-Planck-Institut für Biochemie, D-8033 Martinsried, Federal Republic of Germany

With 21 Figures

1. Introduction

Nearly all the basic insights into the function of the nervous system were obtained by studying classical systems like the giant axons of molluscs and crustaceans, the neuromuscular junctions of invertebrates and vertebrates, the electric organs of the electric fish, the eyes of insects, crustaceans and vertebrates and the brains, spinal cords and ganglia of various vertebrates. Especially the organs of the central nervous system are extremely complex units composed of various classes of cells like neurons, astroglial, oligodendroglial and ependymal cells. The neurons of the brain form by no means a homogeneous population of cells. They can be classified further by the type of neurotransmitter they produce and by the types of receptors for neurotransmitters they carry on their cell surfaces. Thus, quite often it is difficult to assign certain biochemical effects observed with nervous tissue to one of its constituent cell types. In other words, we do not know the precise pattern of physiological, and therefore biochemical, functions a given cell type serves in the nervous system.

Despite the possibility of partial enrichment of certain cell types, primary cultures of cells from embryonic nervous tissue may still be a heterogeneous population of cells. In addition, such cultures are laborious to establish and for many purposes it is difficult to obtain sufficient quantities of cultured cells. While glial cells will proliferate in culture, neurons appear to undergo only a very limited number of cell divisions, if they divide at all.

Therefore, the advent of permanent clonal cell lines derived from tumors of the nervous system provided the possibility of working with "pure" cells much like using pure chemicals or pure strains of microorganisms. In addition, these cells can be grown in quantities sufficient for most investigations and there appear to be no limits to the number of generations which they can pass through.

The permanent cell lines most widely used are the neuroblastoma clones, derived from the spontaneous mouse tumor C 1300 [1—3]. Cell lines from a human neuroblastoma [4] and a human astrocytoma [5] have not yet been exploited appreciably,while a glioma clone isolated from a chemically induced tumor of the rat brain [6] is being studied intensively in many laboratories.

The first phase in the work with neuroblastoma and glioma cells, the establishment of the presence of characteristic neuronal and glial markers, is an indispensible procedure, if the cells are to be used as models for equivalent cells in the nervous system. Some mouse neuroblastoma clones contain choline acetyltransferase (E.C.2.3.1.6), the marker enzyme for cholinergic neurons, which catalyzes the formation of the neurotransmitter acetylcholine (ACh) [1—3]. In others, marker enzymes of adrenergic neurons are found, like tyrosine hydroxylase (E.C.1.14.3.a) [1—3] and dopamine-β-hydroxylase (E.C.1.14.2.1) [7, 8], which are engaged in the synthesis of the neurotransmitters dopamine and noradrenaline. Neuroblastoma cells have acetylcholinesterase (E.C.3.1.1.7) activity [9]; can be induced to extend processes [2, 10]; are excitable electrically [11] or by application of ACh to their cell surfaces [12, 13]. Besides receptors of ACh, neuroblastoma cells have receptors for prostaglandin E_1 [14, 15] and adenosine [16].

The rat glioma cells contain the brain specific S-100 protein [5], but not the enzymes necessary for the production of ACh or noradrenaline; they extend processes on treatment with N^6, $O^{2'}$-dibutyryl adenosine 3' : 5'-cyclic monophosphate (dibutyryl cyclic AMP [17]; they have noradrenaline receptors [18, 19]; they are unresponsive to electrical stimulation [20, 21]; their hyperpolarization response to ACh, which is antagonized by atropine, suggests the presence of muscarinic ACh receptors [21]. The presence of receptors for dopamine and histamine was suggested for human astrocytoma cells [22]. A neurinoma cell line derived from a Schwann cell tumor of a rat has been established recently [23].

2. Preparation of Rat Glioma × Mouse Neuroblastoma Hybrid Cells

Besides isolating clonal cell lines from tumors of neural origin, cell fusion appears to be a method for producing cell lines with interesting new combinations of neuronal properties. A first indication for such a possibility could be seen in the presence of choline acetyltransferase in hybrids obtained by fusion of 2 cell lines lacking the enzyme, i.e., by fusion of rat glioma line C6-BU-1 and mouse neuroblastoma line N4TG3 [20]. The phenomenon was explained as the activation of inactive genes during the formation of the hybrid cells [20]. High specific activity of choline acetyltransferase was the only remarkable feature of these hybrid cells, since their weak electrical activity and their lack of formation of processes were properties already characteristic of the parental neuroblastoma line [20].

However, when the line N4TG3 was substituted in the fusion process by another neuroblastoma line (N18TG2) derived from the same tumor [3, 24], hybrid cells of unusual properties were obtained, as will be demonstrated below. The formation of hybrid cells (Fig. 1C) by fusion of rat glioma line C6-BU-1 (Fig. 1A) and mouse neuroblastoma line N18TG2 (Fig. 1B) [26] was proved by the presence of marker chromosomes of both parent lines (Fig. 2C). The markers of the rat glioma line are small metacentric chromosomes (Fig. 2A), while large metacentric chromosomes are characteristic of the mouse neuroblastoma line (Fig. 2B). The mean number of chromosomes of the two C6-BU-1 × N18TG2 hybrids, 251 for clone 108CC5 and 155 for clone 108CC15, exceed the sum of 125 (C6-BU-1:40, N18TG2:85 chromosomes) and thus indicate that more than one cell of at least one of the parental lines participated in the fusion event.

3. Enzyme Activities of C6-BU-1 × N18TG2 Hybrid Cells. Choline Acetyltransferase

Using a newly developed assay [27] no trace of choline acetyltransferase can be detected in the parental glioma line (Fig. 3). On the other hand, low specific activity, which is essentially independent of the cell density, is clearly found in the neuroblastoma parent N18TG2 (Fig. 4). As in the case of the C6-BU-1 × N4TG3 hybrids,

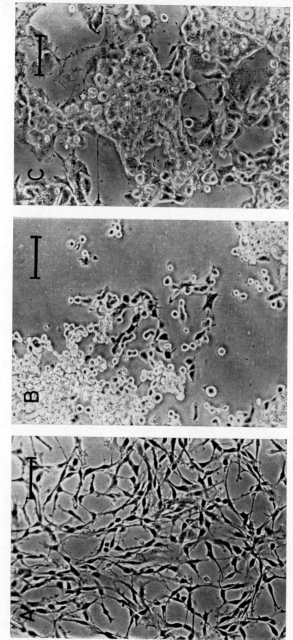

Fig. 1A—C. (A) Clonal glioma line C6-BU-1. (B) Clonal neuroblastoma line N18TG2. (C) C6-BU-1 × N18TG2 hybrid clone 108 CC5. The bar represents 0.1 mm. C6-BU-1 is a bromodeoxyuridine resistant mutant [20] of clonal line C6 [6], N18TG2 is a 6-thioguanine resistant mutant [24] of clonal line N18 [3]. In the hybrid the mutant parent cells complement each other to a wild-type cell, which can be selected for in HAT medium containing hypoxanthine, aminopterine and thymidine [25]

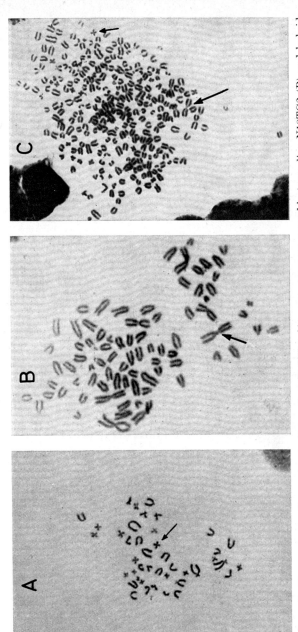

Fig. 2 A—C. Chromosomes of parent rat glioma line C6-BU-1 (A), parent mouse neuroblastoma line N18TG2 (B) and hybrid line 108CC5 (C). Short arrows indicate marker chromosomes of the parental rat cells, long arrows marker chromosomes of the parental mouse cells

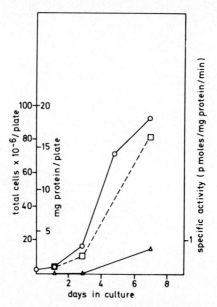

Fig. 3. Specific activity of choline acetyltransferase in rat glioma line C6-BU-1 as a function of the time in culture. Experimental details will be published elsewhere [26]. Specific activities at or below 1 pmole/mg protein/min are not clearly different from zero. ○ cells per plate, (100 mm in diameter), □ protein per plate, △ specific activity

also the C6-BU-1 × N18TG2 hybrid clones 108CC5 and 108CC15 show high specific activities (up to 200 pmoles/mg protein/min) of choline acetyltransferase. The specific activities are strongly dependent on the cell density, as shown for clone 108CC15 in Fig. 5A—D. When the hybrid cells are grown in the presence of 1 mM dibutyryl cyclic AMP, the specific activity of the enzyme is increased to 500 pmoles/mg protein/min (Fig. 5D), a value also found in homogenates of mouse brain [3].

Dopamine-β-Hydroxylase

On prolonged treatment of the C6-BU-1 × N18TG2 hybrids with dibutyryl cyclic AMP (for further details see Section 5) dense core vesicles, 1000—2000 Å in diameter can be detected by electron microscopy [28]. Vesicles of this kind from adrenergic nerves are

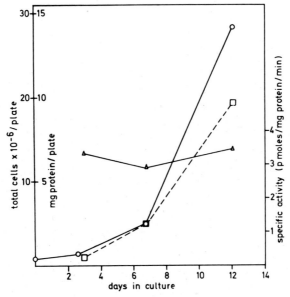

Fig. 4. Specific activity of choline acetyltransferase in mouse neuroblastoma line N18TG2 as a function of the time in culture. Details as in Fig. 3

known to contain noradrenaline, ATP, chromogranins and dopamine-β-hydroxylase, the enzyme responsible for the conversion of dopamine to noradrenaline. It is in line with this knowledge that the hybrid cells contain dopamine-β-hydroxylase activity [8]. The specific activity of the enzyme in the hybrids is 3—50 fold higher than in the parent neuroblastoma line N18TG2. The enzyme cannot be detected in the glioma cells [8]. Since the first enzyme of the pathway from tyrosine to noradrenaline, tyrosine hydroxylase, is missing in the hybrid cells, it is not surprising that catecholamines cannot be found in the hybrid cells [8]. It is probably for the first time that such clearcut evidence has been obtained for the presence of elements of two neurotransmitter systems in the same cell. The hybrid cells contain high activities of choline acetyltransferase a marker of the cholinergic cells. The clear vesicles of approximately 550 Å in diameter, which are found aside of the dense core vesicles in cells treated with dibutyryl cyclic AMP, resemble the acetylcholine storage vesicles of cholinergic nerve terminals. On the other

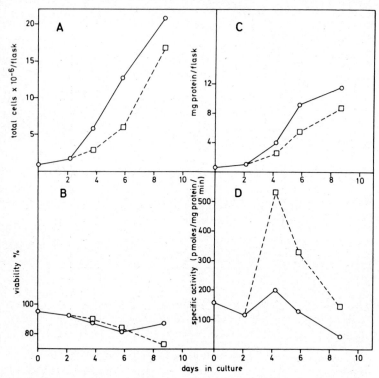

Fig. 5A—D. Specific activity of choline acetyltransferase in C6-BU-1 × N18TG2 hybrid cells clone 108CC15 as a function of the time in culture. (A) Cells per flask (75 cm²). (B) Viability of the cells. (C) Protein per flask. (D) Specific activity. ○ absence of, □ presence of dibutyryl cyclic AMP

hand, the list of adrenergic markers, albeit incomplete for the hybrid cells, comprises the dense core vesicles and dopamine-β-hydroxylase.

4. Receptors for Prostaglandin E_1 and Noradrenaline

The glioma cells, but not the neuroblastoma cells, can be stimulated by noradrenaline to strongly increase their intracellular levels of cyclic AMP [18, 19]. On the other hand, neuroblastoma cells show such a response only in the presence of prostaglandin E_1 [14, 15]. This compound exerts only a slight stimu-

Table 1. Levels of intracellular cyclic AMP in glioma and neuroblastoma cells and glioma × neuroblastoma hybrid clones in the presence of prostaglandin E_1 (PGE$_1$), noradrenalin (NA) and papaverine[a,b]

	Parent cells						Hybrid clone no.				
	C6-BU-1 Expt. no.			N18TG2 Expt. no.			108CC5 Expt. no.		108CC15 Expt. no.		
	1	2	3	1	2	3	1	2	1	2	3
Control	12	19	8	10	14	32	39	20	26	17	31
Paparverine	—	—	17	97	10	10	354	—	—	222	—
PGE$_1$	15	22	—	177	197	—	71	34	203	703	545
PGE$_1$ + papaverine	88	—	—	1863	—	—	3246	—	—	2554	3679
NA	—	—	713	—	—	8	25	9	8	6	—
NA + papaverine	—	—	1600	—	—	17	192	—	—	50	—
Total cells per flask × 10^{-6}	8	4[c]	17	18	24	48	8	9	7	19	21
Viability (%)	99	100	99	94	91	81	84	80	90	66	87

[a] Data from [29].

[b] The cells were incubated at 37° C for 10 min (in Krebs-Ringer-hydrogencarbonate buffer supplemented with 50 mM glucose) with prostaglandin E_1 (2.9 μM), noradrenalin (0.1 mM), papaverine (0.5 mM) and 3-isobutyl-1-methylxanthine (IBMX) (1 mM). For the determination of cyclic AMP and for other details see [29]. The dimension of the data is pmol/mg protein.

[c] Per 60 mm plate.

latory effect on C6-BU-1 cells. There is good evidence that hormonal responses of this kind are mediated by specific receptors on the cell surfaces. For theoretical as well as for practical reasons it is of great interest to know which of the parental receptors will be found in the glioma × neuroblastoma hybrid clones. Table 1 [29] demonstrates that in the hybrid cells the intracellular levels of cyclic AMP are increased by prostaglandin E_1 but depressed by noradrenaline. The results suggest that the prostaglandin receptors, which are markers of both parents, are expressed in the hybrids, and that

the stimulatory noradrenaline receptors (β-receptors) characteristic of the glioma parent are replaced by the inhibitory noradrenaline receptors of the neuroblastoma parent.

5. Action Potentials Elicited by Electrical Stimulation

When the hybrid cells (Fig. 1C) are seeded at low cell density
(400—2000 cells/cm²) and kept in complete growth medium [26]
supplemented with lmM dibutyryl cyclic AMP, the cells start send-
ing out processes. Eight to ten days after onset of the treatment the
extensions will have grown considerably and, after 2—6 weeks, may
have reached lengths of more than half a millimeter ("treated
cells") (Fig. 6).

After insertion of a microelectrode [30] into "treated cells",
membrane resting potentials in the range of —20 to —65 mV can
be measured.

In most nerve cells the membrane resting potential is relatively
close to the K^+ equilibrium potential [31], which can be calculated
from the exact data for the high K^+ concentration inside and the
low K^+ concentration outside the cell by using the Nernst equation:

$$E = \frac{RT}{F} \ln \frac{[K^+]_{outside}}{[K^+]_{inside}} \ .$$

Additions of K^+ ions to the medium outside the cells will
accordingly shift the membrane resting potential to more positive
values. This is, indeed, what is observed with the hybrid cells
(Fig. 7B). A similar addition of Na^+ ions to the same cell causes
only a comparatively slight effect (Fig. 7A). Although, from
technical reasons, exact data on the relationship between the K^+
concentration and the membrane resting potentials cannot be
obtained [26], the result suggests strongly that the transmembrane
gradient of K^+ and not of Na^+ ions is responsible for a large portion
of the membrane resting potential.

By depolarization, i.e. by passing current through the membrane
via the implanted electrode in such a way that the membrane
potential becomes less negative, active responses of the cell membranes in the form of action potentials are elicited, like in ordinary
nerve cells. Figure 8A and B show different forms of action potentials, which essentially differ in the strong hyperpolarizing after-

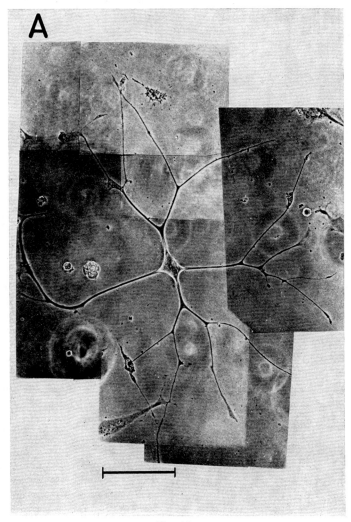

Fig. 6A.

Fig. 6A and B. C6-BU-1 × N18TG2 clonal hybrid cell line 108CC5 grown in
the presence [(A) 11 days, (B) 16 days] of dibutyryl cyclic AMP [(A) 4 mM;
(B) 1mM)]. The bars represent 0.1 mm. The pictures are taken from [8]

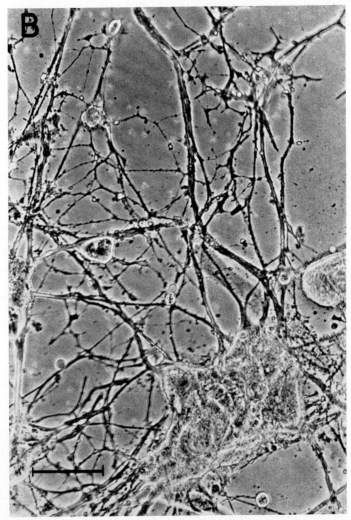

Fig. 6B. (Legend see p. 401)

potential of B. In some cases a long constant depolarizing current is accompanied by a train of action potentials, which lasts as long as the current is being passed through the membrane (Fig. 9A). When the current is increased, the height of the responses decreases and

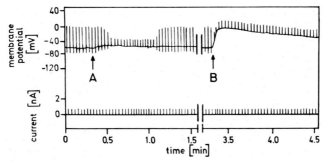

Fig. 7 A and B. Effect of alkali ions on the membrane resting potential of hybrid line 108CC5. The cells are attached to the bottom of the culture dish (60 mm in diameter) and are covered by 5 ml of culture medium. With a micropipette 1 μl of 2 M NaCl (A) or 3 M KCl (B), respectively, are added (time indicated by arrows) to the surface of the medium above the cell. The cell is impaled by a recording microelectrode. Whenever in the following figures substances other than ACh are tested for their influence on cells studied electrophysiologically, they are added in this way. Besides the effect of the ions on the membrane resting potential, the chart recorder diagram also demonstrates an effect on the action potentials (upper trace; long spikes directed upward), followed by a hyperpolarizing afterpotential, directed downward. The action potentials are elicited by square pulses of depolarizing current (lower trace) lasting for 100 msec

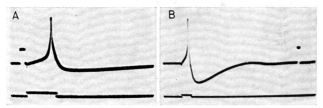

Fig. 8 A and B. Action potentials evoked by passing a depolarizing current through the cell membrane of hybrid cell 108CC5. (A) and (B) show oscilloscope pictures of different forms of action potentials from different cells. Upper trace: membrane potential. A calibration pulse of 20 mV, 20 msec appears before (A) or after (B) the action potential. Lower trace: Depolarizing current 1 nA; 100 msec (A), 50 msec (B)

their form changes (Fig. 9 B and C) until even the faint oscillatory activity (Fig. 9 D) subsides (Fig. 9 E). At this stage, the membrane has become depolarized constantly by about 30 mV. Similar phenomena have been described for lobster muscle fibres in the presence of Ba^{2+} ions [32] and for other systems [33].

In many nerve cells the action potential is composed of the
potential changes caused by an inward flow of Na^+ ions and a
delayed outward flow of K^+ ions [34]. With the exception of the
membranes of denervated muscle cells [35], an action potential of
this kind can be inhibited by blocking the sodium permeability
with tetrodotoxin [36]. Application of this poison, even in concentrations approximately 10^5 times higher than those effective in
other systems, did not affect the action potential (Fig. 10 A and B).
Although this result suggests that Na^+ ions play no part in the
action potential of the hybrid cells, the alternative of tetrodotoxin
insensitive Na^+ "channels" [35] cannot yet be ruled out. The
observation in mouse neuroblastoma cell lines that 86% of an

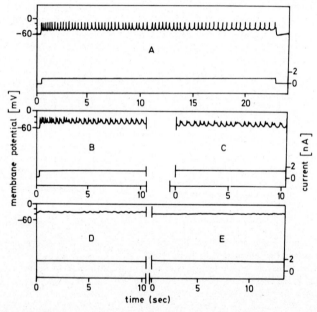

Fig. 9 A—E. Chart recorder diagrams of respective responses elicited by a
constant depolarizing current passing the plasma membrane of hybrid cell
108CC15. There appeared to be no limit as to the length of time the phenomenon could be observed. The experiment was ended after a total of approximately 30 min of recording. (A)—(E), different patterns of responses produced by increasing currents from 1.0—1.8 nA. Upper trace: membrane
potentials; lower trace: current

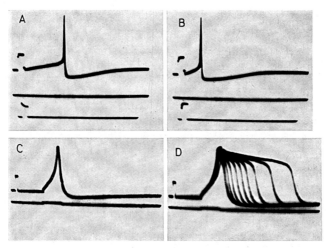

Fig. 10A—D. Effect of tetrodotoxin and tetraethylammonium ions on the action potential of the hybrid cells 108CC5. Oscilloscope recordings. (A) and (B) action potential before (A) and after (B) addition of $250\,\mu l$ 1 mM tetrodotoxin (in culture medium), to the medium (Ca^{2+} concentration approx. 12 mM) above the impaled cell. The action potentials (upper trace: membrane potential) are elicited by iontophoretic application of ACh (lowest trace: ACh current, 330 nA, 100 msec). A calibration pulse (20 mV, 100 msec) is preceding each action potential. (C) and (D) action potentials before (C) and after (D) addition (as above) of $20\,\mu l$ 0.1 M tratraethylammonium chloride (in culture medium). The cells are stimulated intracellularly by a pulse of depolarizing current (lower trace, 0.2 nA, 50 msec). Calibration pulse: 20 mV, 10 msec

action potential is sensitive to tetrodotoxin [37], however, lends little support to the latter explanation.

Tetraethylammonium ions block the K^+ permeability of the cell membranes [38—40] and thereby causes a prolongation of the action potentials [32, 41—43]. They also cause an increase in membrane resting potential [32]. Their action on the hybrid cells is very similar: they increase the membrane resting potential, they increase strongly the height and the duration of the action potential (Fig. 10C and D) and the magnitude of the hyperpolarizing after-potential. The prolongation of the action potential decreases steadily as the tetraethylammonium ions (applied locally) diffuse away from the cell into the surrounding medium (Fig. 10D). This result supports the view that K^+ ions participate in the action potential of the hybrid cells.

If we anticipate that the rising phase of the action potentials of the hybrid cells is not caused by sodium ions, calcium ions are good candidates to take their place, as known from studies of certain mammalian neurons [44] and smooth muscles [45—48], and of crustacean muscle [32, 49]. In fact, the increase of the Ca^{2+} concentration around the cells has a number of consequences. 1) The cells fire action potentials on depolarizations effected by much lower currents than before the increase of the Ca^{2+} concentration (Fig. 11 A and B). 2) The membrane resting potential increases. 3) The height of the action potential increases strongly (Fig. 11 A and B). 4) There is a dramatic increase in the hyperpolarizing "positive" afterpotential following the action potential (Fig. 11 A and B). Such an effect has already been described for the squid

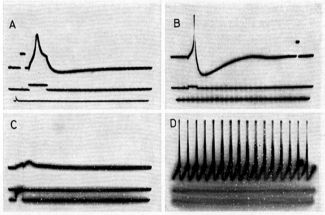

Fig. 11 A—D. Effect of the increase of the Ca^{2+} concentration in the external medium on the action potential of hybrid cells 108CC5. Oscilloscope recordings. Upper trace, membrane potential. Calibration pulse [(A), (B) and (D)] 20 mV, 20 msec. Middle trace, 50 msec pulse of depolarizing current: 1.5 nA (A), 0.5 nA (B). Lower trace, current of ACh applied iontophoretically: 230 nA, 100 msec [(C) and (D)]. A single pulse of ACh [not shown in (D)] elicited a train of more than 200 action potentials. A small section of the recording is reproduced in (D). (A) and (C): before; (B) and (D): after the addition of 10 µl (B) or 20 µl (D) 0.5 M $CaCl_2$ (dissolved in culture medium) to the medium above the impaled cell [hybrid clone 108CC15: (A) and (B); hybrid clone 108CC5: (C) and (D)]

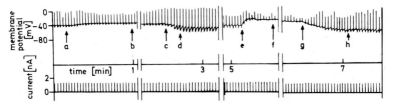

Fig. 12. Influence of Mg^{2+}, EGTA and Ca^{2+} on the resting membrane potential and the action potential of the hybrid cells 108CC5. Chart recorder diagrams. The duration of the depolarizing current pulses (spikes, lower trace) is 50 msec. The following additions to the culture dish were made: a, 1 μl 1 M $MgSO_4$; c and g, 2 μl 0.5 M $CaCl_2$;e, 1 μl 1 M Na-EGTA. Oscilloscope recordings taken at Points (a), (b), (d), (f), and (h) are shown in Fig. 13A—D, and C, respectively. The upward spikes in the upper trace represent depolarizations caused by the current pulses. Their nature (charging of the cell membrane or action potential) is only revealed by the recordings in Fig. 13. The downward spikes (voltage trace) are the hyperpolarizing afterpotentials

giant axon [50]. 5) A single stimulus may elicit as many as 200 action potentials (Fig. 11 C and D). 6) The sensitivity to ACh of the cells increases.

Antagonizing the Ca^{2+} by increasing the concentration of Mg^{2+} in the neighborhood of the impaled cell (Fig. 12a) or by decreasing the Ca^{2+} concentration by addition of the chelator ethyleneglycol- *bis* (β-aminoethylether) tetraacetic acid (EGTA) (Fig. 12e) shift the resting membrane potential to more positive values. These effects are always overcome by the new addition of Ca^{2+} ions (Fig. 12c and g). Parallel to this effect, Mg^{2+} strongly reduces the height of the action potential, as seen from the comparison of the oscilloscope recordings at Points a (Fig. 13A) and b (Fig. 13B). Also during the depolarization caused by EGTA the action potentials disappear as demonstrated by the recording taken in Fig. 12f (shown in Fig. 13D). In both cases the addition of Ca^{2+} (Fig. 12c and g) restores membrane resting potential and action potentials (Fig. 13C corresponds to Point d and also approximately to Point h, respectively, in Fig. 12). Especially the increase in the height of the action potentials due to the increase of the Ca^{2+} concentration in the medium is a good indication that Ca^{2+} ions are carrying the inward current during the action potential. However, the possibility that Ca^{2+} acts exclusively by facilitat-

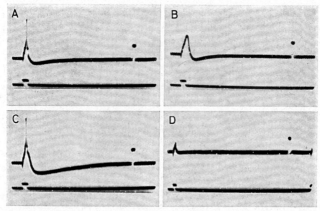

Fig. 13 A—D. Influence of Mg^{2+}, EGTA, and Ca^{2+} on the action potential of the hybrid cells 108CC5. Oscilloscope recordings. Upper trace, membrane potential; calibration pulse: 20 mV, 20 msec. Lower trace, depolarizing current: 1.3 nA, 50 msec. For details see Fig. 12

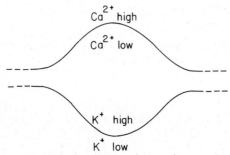

Fig. 14. Hypothetic ion gradients across the plasma membrane of the hybrid cells

ing the entry of Na^+ ions [51] remains to be ruled out. The ion gradients which are likely to be responsible for the electrical phenomena of the hybrid cells are illustrated in Fig. 14.

6. Action Potentials Elicited by ACh

Action potentials can be registered with an implanted microelectrode, when ACh from another micropipette is applied to the cell surface either iontophoretically (see Fig. 10A and B) or by

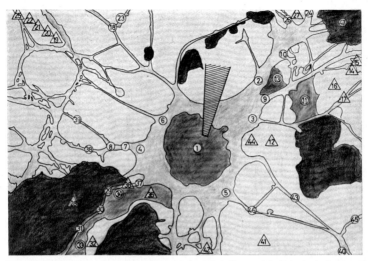

Fig. 15. Propagation of action potentials and ACh sensitivity of a hybrid cell (108CC5). The numbers in circles or double circles indicate spots on soma and neurites or on the lamellae, respectively that are sensitive to ACh. Application of ACh to sites that are marked by numbers in triangles did not elicit action potentials. A total of 47 sites was mapped. As this cell was the same as that in Fig. 17, the action potentials occurring during this experiment are practically identical to those in Fig. 17A and E

diffusion. When in a similar experiment (not shown here) choline is applied iontophoretically, no response is detected. This negative experiment is framed by two positive experiments with ACh, one preceding it and the other following it.

Action potentials elicited in one part of a hybrid cell are propagated to other parts of the cell. By iontophoretic application of ACh to its various parts, the cell depicted in Fig. 15 is stimulated to produce action potentials, which are sensed with the microelectrode impaled into the soma. Sensitivity to ACh is found practically on the entire cell surface, even on the very thin lamellae that extend from the sides of some cell processes (Fig. 15).

Repetitive doses of ACh cause a transient desensitization of the cell membrane, during which period the cells do not respond to ACh by firing action potentials. Only the first 2 pulses of ACh evoked action potentials in the hybrid cell. The depolarizations caused by the following ACh pulses were no longer large enough for triggering action potentials (Fig.16). However, already 1 min later an action potential (not shown) could again be elicited by a pulse of ACh

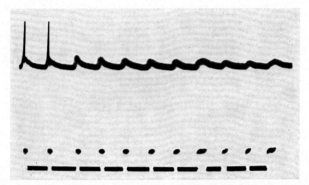

Fig. 16. Desensitization of the hybrid cell (clone 108CC5) membrane by repetitive doses of ACh applied iontophoretically. ACh pulses: 140 nA, 75 msec. Upper trace, membrane potential; lower trace, ACh current

applied at the same site. Desensitization of cells by high doses of ACh are known, *e.g.*, from studies of muscle [52, 53] or glioma cells [21].

In the presence of cholinergic antagonists like *d*-tubocurarine, atropine, hexamethonium, decamethonium, and phenyldimethylpiperazinium ions, ACh does not evoke action potentials. A typical experiment is depicted in Fig. 17. The application of ACh is followed by action potentials (Fig. 17 A). Now a solution of atropine is transferred to the surface of the medium above the impaled cell. After a brief lag phase, during which the drug diffuses down to the cell, the concentration of atropine at the cell surface is high enough to prevent ACh from eliciting action potentials (Fig. 17 B). During this period of insensitivity to ACh the cells are still capable of firing action potentials on electrical depolarization (Fig. 17 C). Subsequently, by finding still no response to ACh (Fig. 17 D) we assure ourselves that the cell, while it was being stimulated electrically, has not become sensitive to ACh. This indicates that the drug only inhibits the ACh receptors but not the system involved in the generation of the action potentials. The drug causes only a transi-

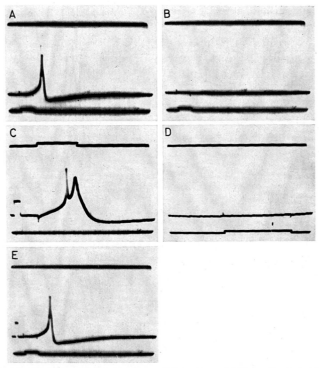

Fig. 17 A—E. Inhibition by atropine of the action of ACh on the hybrid cells 108CC5. Oscilloscope recording. Upper trace, depolarizing current for intracellular stimulation, 0.8 nA, 50 msec in (C); middle trace, membrane potential (calibration pulse 20 mV, 10 msec); lower trace, current for iontophoretic release of ACh [40 nA, 100 msec in (A), (B), (D), and (E)]. The cell is the same as that studied in Fig. 15. (A) Action potential elicited by ACh before the addition of atropine. (B) and (D) No action potentials in response to ACh directly after the addition of atropine (5 μl, 1 mM, in culture medium). (C) Action potential evoked by electrical stimulation during the period of inhibition by atropine. (E) Action potential in response to ACh after the atropine has diffused away from the cell surface

tory inhibition, since its concentration at the cell surface reaches a maximum and then decreases again, as the drug diffuses away. Thus about 1 min later, the cell responds to ACh again by firing an action potential (Fig. 17 E). Still studying the same cell, identical reversible inhibitions of the action of ACh are caused by 3 μl 1 mM

d-tubocurarine, 3—5 µl decamethonium and 5 µl 1 mM hexa-methonium. Lower amounts of these drugs do not inhibit the response to ACh. Atropine is a specific blocker of the muscarinic [54, 55] and d-tubocurarine of the nicotinic [56, 57] action of ACh, and hexamethonium [58] and decamethonium [58, 59] possess curare-like properties. In the hybrid cells the four substances are of similar potency in antagonizing the elicitation of action potentials by ACh. Thus, the ACh receptors which mediate the action potential response to ACh of the hybrid cells cannot be classified as nicotinic or muscarinic [54]. Besides its blocking properties, decamethonium may also act like ACh and depolarize membranes of muscle cells [60, 61]. With the hybrid cells this effect is not observed. However, 1,1-dimethyl-4-phenylpiperazinium ions, which act like acetyl-choline [62], show both types of the activities decamethonium is expected to possess. It lowers the membrane resting potential of the hybrid cells and antagonizes the action of ACh. The two effects are clearly separated, since the response to ACh is still inhibited when the membrane resting potential has already reached its original value. Inmidst this phase of insensitivity to ACh, action potentials can be elicited by electrical stimulation, demonstrating that only the ACh receptors are inhibited but not the system involved in the generation of the action potentials. Three minutes after the local addition of the drug to the culture dish, its concentration has already decreased sufficiently for ACh to evoke action potentials again. The experiment (not shown here) is performed on the cell used for the study in Fig. 17.

Although ACh causes action potentials with a large number of the hybrid cells, in a few cases its application is followed by a biphasic response consisting of a slow depolarization and a sub-sequent slow hyperpolarization (Fig. 18). d-Tubocurarine prevents both responses. However, the hyperpolarization response is the first one to reappear after the drug has diffused away to some extent. Atropine, on the other hand, preferentially blocks the hyperpolarization response. The hyperpolarization response re-appears partially as the atropine diffuses away from the cell surface. The inhibition is overcome completely by a 25% increase of the ACh current (last stimulation by ACh in Fig. 18). As already stated above for the other type of depolarization response (action potential), also this one is inhibited by both atropine and d-

tubocurarine and thus can neither be categorized as nicotinic nor as muscarinic. Deviations from the classical categories of ACh receptors [54] have also been reported for molluscan neurons [63]. The results presented here suggest three different types of ACh receptors in

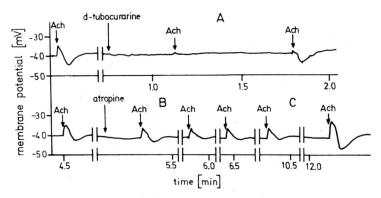

Fig. 18. Slow depolarizing and hyperpolarizing effects of ACh and their inhibition by d-tubocurarine or atropine in hybrid clone 108CC5. 3 μl of 1 mM solutions of the drugs in culture medium were applied to the medium above the cell studied. Chart recorder diagrams. At the arrows marked "ACh" an iontophoretic pulse of ACh was released onto the surface of the impaled cell. The pulses were 400 nA, 100 msec at all times indicated except the last one, where the pulse height was 500 nA

the population of hybrid cells, two of which may be found on the same cell. Binding of ACh to one of them causes the depolarization that precedes an action potential, binding to the other is followed by slow depolarization and binding to the third initiates the slow hyperpolarization response. Two types of cholinergic receptors on the same cell have been observed previously in other systems [63, and literature cited there].

α-Bungarotoxin, a constituent of the venom of the snake *Bungarus multicinctus*, binds specifically to ACh receptors and thus blocks the action of ACh on cells with cholinergic input [64, 65]. Figure 19 shows that a highly purified preparation of the toxin renders a previously sensitive cell (Fig. 19 A) insensitive to ACh (Fig. 19 B). However, it affects only the ACh receptors. The spike generating system is still functioning, as demonstrated by the

414 B. Hamprecht

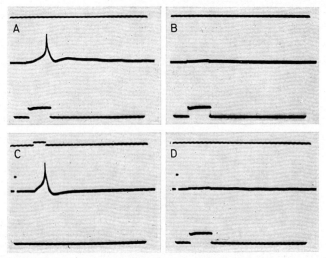

Fig. 19 A—D. Blockage by α-bungarotoxin of the response to ACh. Hybrid cell line 108CC5. Oscilloscope recordings. Upper trace, depolarizing current injected through the inserted microelectrode [(C): 0.4 nA, 50 msec]. Middle trace, membrane potential [(C) and (D): calibration pulse 20 mV, 10 msec]. Lower trace, ACh current [(A), (B), and (D): 140 nA, 75 msec]. (A) Action potential elicited by ACh before the addition of α-bungarotoxin, and (B) after the addition of α-bungarotoxin (10 μl of a solution containing 5 μg/μl in culture medium). No response to ACh. (C) Action potential on electrical stimulation. (D) Still no response to ACh

action potentials evoked by electrical stimulation (Fig. 19 C). The positive response to electrical depolarization is framed by two unsuccessful trials with ACh (Fig. 19 B and D). The inhibition by the toxin appears to be irreversible. The cell that was observed for the longest period did not regain sensitivity to ACh within 42 min after the addition of the toxin.

7. Importance of Thiol and Disulfide Groups for the Response to ACh

The intactness of disulfide bridges in the ACh receptor molecules of electroplax is essential for their function. After the reduction of disulfide bridges by dithiothreitol, electroplax do no longer respond to ACh [66]. Reoxidation, however, will restore their sensitivity to

ACh [66, 67]. If, after reduction, the receptor molecules are alkylated, no reactivation is possible [66, 67].

When active hybrid cells (Fig. 20 A) are treated with an agent that oxidizes thiol groups, 5,5'-dithiobis-(2-nitrobenzoic acid) (DTNB), they no longer fire an action potential in response to the original dose of ACh (Fig. 20 B), although they still do so when stimulated electrically (Fig. 20 C). A higher dose of ACh, however will evoke action potentials again. After addition of dithiothreitol, the original sensitivity to ACh returns (Fig. 20 D.). On addition of an even higher dose of dithiothreitol, the active response to ACh is lost again (Fig. 20 E), while electrical depolarization still evokes action potentials (Fig. 20 F). During the first 1.8 min after a new addition of DTNB the cell remains insensitive even to increased amounts of ACh. Approximately 1 min later the sensitivity to ACh returns transiently (Fig. 20 G) and then is lost again (Fig. 20 H).

The experiments demonstrate that both the oxidation of free sulfhydryl groups by DTNB and the reduction of disulfide bridges by dithiothreitol abolish the sensitivity to ACh. Oscillation between the inactive states of complete reduction and complete oxidation leads through an intermediate stage of sensitivity to ACh. Consequently, it is concluded that both thiol and disulfide groups are necessary for the cells to respond to the presence of ACh by firing action potentials.

This conclusion is supported by the results obtained with the thiol alkylating agent N-ethylmaleimide (NEM). After treatment with NEM, the cells are no longer responsive to the original dose of ACh (Fig. 21 A and B), although they still can be stimulated electrically (Fig. 21 C). Increasing the ACh current elicits action potentials (Fig. 21 D). New addition of NEM inhibits again (Fig. 21 E) and accordingly requires still higher doses of ACh for action potentials to be generated (Fig. 21 F), until finally even highest doses of ACh cause no more than a slight depolarization (Fig. 21 G), probably indicating a strongly reduced density of functioning receptor molecules at the surface of the cell. At this point, however, even the spike generating system must have been affected by NEM, as it can no longer be activated by electrical depolarization (Fig. 21 H).

These results are only partially analogous to those obtained with the electroplax system [66, 67]. Both systems are inhibited by treatment with dithiothreitol and by blocking of thiol groups.

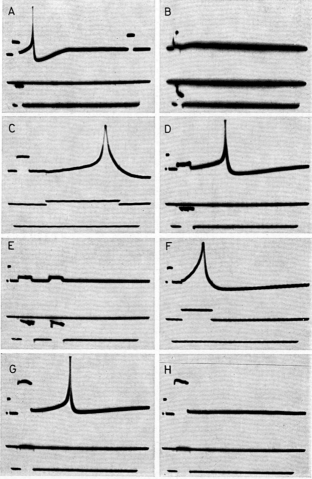

Fig. 20 A—H. Influence of DTNB and dithiothreitol on the response to ACh
of hybrid line 108CC5. Oscilloscope recordings. Upper trace, membrane
potential. Calibration pulse: 20 mV, 100 msec (A) or 20 msec (B)—(H).
Middle trace, depolarizing current 100 msec, 0.26 nA (C) or 0.6 nA (F).
Lower trace, ACh current 100 msec, 400 nA (A) and (B), 370 nA (D) and (E),
460 nA (G), 480 nA (H). (A) Before the addition of DTNB; action potential
elicited by ACh. (B) No response to ACh after the addition of 3 μl 1mM DTNB.
(C) Action potential on electrical stimulation. Subsequently, a trial with ACh
as in (B) proves that the cell is ACh insensitive during electrical stimulation.
As the response is identical to that in (B) it is not shown here. When the ACh

However, the response of the native electroplax can be inhibited only be a mercurial but not by NEM or DTNB [66]. In contrast, the hybrid cells are susceptible to both NEM and DTNB.

8. Conclusion

The C6-BU-1 glioma × N18TG2 neuroblastoma hybrid cells were shown to possess numerous properties characteristic of many types of neurons. They extend long processes, which contain two types of synaptic vesicles; they have enzymes necessary for the production of neurotransmitters. As electrically excitable cells they fire action potentials when depolarized by electric current or ACh. The action potentials are propagated over the whole cell surface. A constant depolarizing current evokes sequences of repetitive activity. There are indications for the resting membrane potential to be largely a K^+ potential and for Na^+ not to play an important role in the formation of the action potential. Ca^{2+} appears to be a good candidate for the ion carrying the inward current during the action potential. K^+ depolarizes, Ca^{2+} hyperpolarizes the plasma membrane. Increase of the Ca^{2+} concentration causes increases in the sensitivity of the cell to stimulation by electric current or ACh, long trains of action potentials as response to a single stimulus and strong hyperpolarizing afterpotentials following the action potential. Cholinergic antagonists like atropine or d-tubocurarine block the action of ACh at the cell surface in a reversible way. This contrasts to the well known irreversible action of the snake venom α-bungarotoxin. Some cells in the population of hybrid cells show a

---

current is increased from 400—500 nA, an action potential is generated (not shown). Immediately after the addition of 10 μl 0.1 M dithiothreitol, an ACh current of 380 nA is still not sufficient to trigger an action potential, although an action potential can be evoked electrically. During testing of electrical stimulation the cell does not become sensitive to ACh (400 nA; 5 min after the addition of dithiothreitol). However, 1 min later the cell can be stimulated by ACh (380 nA) (Fig. 20 D). (E) After the addition of 20 μl 0.1 M dithiothreitol no response to 2 pulses of ACh. (F) Action potential evoked electrically. The subsequent test for response to ACh (380 nA) is still negative. It precedes the addition of 100 μl 0.02 M DTNB; 1.8 min after this event an action potential is not even triggered by an ACh current of 460 nA, but it reappears 0.9 min later (G). (H) 4.1 min after the addition of DTNB the ACh sensitivity has disappeared again

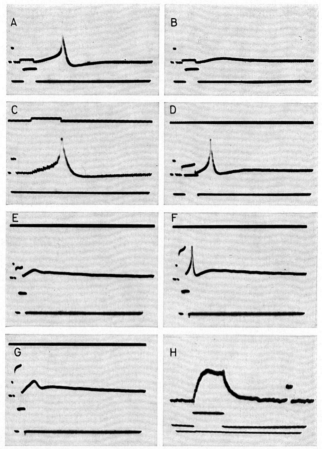

Fig. 21 A—H. Influence of NEM on the response to ACh of hybrid line 108CC5. All calibration pulses are 20 mV, 20 msec. The duration of all other pulses is 100 msec. (A) Response to ACh (270 nA) before the addition of NEM. (B) Inhibition of ACh action after addition of 5 μl 1 mM NEM. (C) Action potential stimulated electrically (0.7 nA) during the period of inhibition. After this trial the cell is still insensitive to an ACh current of 270 nA. (D) Reappearance of the action potential after increase of the ACh current (410 nA). (E) Another 5 μl of the NEM solution has no effect. Addition of 10 μl 1 mM NEM inhibits the ACh response. (F) After inreasing the ACh current once more (470 nA), an action potential reappears. (G) 10 μl 1 mM NEM added. ACh (460 nA) now evokes only a sub-threshold depolarization response. A further increase of the ACh current (510 nA) is without effect. (H) Nearly no activity seen on electrical stimulation (4.0 nA)

biphasic response to ACh, consisting of a slow depolarization following a slow hyperpolarization. These responses are inhibited differently by atropine or d-tubocurarine. High doses of ACh cause a desensitization effect. Both sulfhydryl and disulfide groups are necessary for the ACh receptors to function properly.

Thus, these hybrid cells are well established as models of nerve cells. As they can be grown as homogeneous populations in quantities sufficient for many biochemical investigations, a number of biochemical and pharmacological questions could be answered by studying these cells. Furthermore, hybridization of various cell types with at least one partner of neural origin may prove a powerful tool for the preparation of new cells with a welcome combination of properties.

Acknowledgements

A great deal of the experimental work described was performed during my stay at the National Institutes of Health, Bethesda, Maryland. I should like to thank Dr. M. NIRENBERG for the opportunity to work in his laboratory, Mr. W. KEMPER for the excellent collaboration during the electrophysiology experiments, Dr. T. AMANO for many stimulating discussions, Mrs. E. CHURCH for a few months of expert technical help, Drs. A. SYTKOWSKI and Z. VOGEL for a sample of α-bungarotoxin and the Max-Planck-Gesellschaft for a stipend that made my stay in the USA possible.

References

1. AUGUSTI-TOCCO, G., SATO, G.: Proc. nat. Acad. Sci. (Wash.) **64**, 311 (1969).
2. SCHUBERT, D., HUMPHREYS, S., BARONI, C., COHN, M.: Proc. nat. Acad. Sci. (Wash.) **64**, 316 (1969).
3. AMANO, T., RICHELSON, E., NIRENBERG, M.: Proc. nat. Acad. Sci. (Wash.) **69**, 258 (1972).
4. NICHOLLS, W. W., LEE, J., DWIGHT, S.: Cancer Res. **30**, 2110 (1970).
5. PERKINS, J. P., MACINTYRE, E. H., RILEY, W. D., CLARK, R. B.: Life Sci. **10**, 1069 (1971).
6. BENDA, P., LIGHTBODY, J., SATO, G., LEVINE, L., SWEET, W.: Science **161**, 370 (1968).
7. ANAGNOSTE, B., FREEDMAN, L. S., GOLDSTEIN, M., BROOME, J., FUXE, K.: Proc. nat. Acad. Sci. (Wash.) **69**, 1883 (1972).
8. HAMPRECHT, B., TRABER, J., LAMPRECHT, F.: FEBS Letters **42**, 221 (1974).
9. SEEDS, N. W., GILMAN, A. G., AMANO, T., NIRENBERG, M.: Proc. nat. Acad. Sci. (Wash.) **66**, 160 (1970).
10. BLUME, A., GILBERT, G., WILSON, S., FARBER, J., ROSENBERG, R., NIRENBERG, M.: Proc. nat. Acad. Sci. (Wash.) **67**, 786 (1970).

11. NELSON, P., RUFFNER, W., NIRENBERG, M.: Proc. nat. Acad. Sci. (Wash.) **64**, 1004 (1969).
12. HARRIS, A. J., DENNIS, M. J.: Science **167**, 1253 (1970).
13. NELSON, P. G., PEACOCK, J. H., AMANO, T.: J. cell. Physiol. **77**, 353 (1971).
14. GILMAN, A. G., NIRENBERG, M.: Nature (Lond.) **234**, 356 (1971).
15. HAMPRECHT, B., SCHULTZ, J.: FEBS Letters **34**, 85 (1973).
16. SCHULTZ, J., HAMPRECHT, B.: Naunyn-Schmiedeberg's Arch. Pharmacol. **278**, 215 (1973).
17. HAMPRECHT, B., JAFFE, B. M., PHILPOTT, G. W.: FEBS Letters **36**, 193 (1973).
18. GILMAN, A. G., NIRENBERG, M.: Proc. nat. Acad. Sci. (Wash.) **68**, 2165 (1971).
19. SCHULTZ, J., HAMPRECHT, B., DALY, J. W., : Proc. nat. Acad. Sci. (Wash.) **69**, 1266 (1972).
20. AMANO, T., HAMPRECHT, B., KEMPER, W.: Exp. Cell. Res **85**, 399 (1974).
21. HAMPRECHT, B., KEMPER, W., AMANO, T., NIRENBERG, M.: In preparation.
22. CLARK, R. D., PERKINS, J. P.: Proc. nat. Acad. Sci. (Wash.) **68**, 2757 (1971).
23. PFEIFFER, S. E., WECHSLER, W.: Proc. nat. Acad. Sci. (Wash.) **69**, 2885 (1972).
24. MINNA, J., GLAZER, D., NIRENBERG, M.: Nature (Lond.) New Biol. **235**, 225 (1972).
25. LITTLEFIELD, J. W.: Exp. Cell Res. **41**, 190 (1966).
26. HAMPRECHT, B.: In preparation.
27. HAMPRECHT, B., AMANO, T.: Anal. Biochem. **57**, 162 (1973).
28. DANIELS, M. P., HAMPRECHT, B.: J. Cell Biol. (in press).
29. HAMPRECHT, B., SCHULTZ, J.: Hoppe-Seyler's Z. physiol. Chem. **354**, 1633 (1973).
30. NELSON, P. G., PEACOCK, J. H., AMANO, T.: J. cell. Physiol. **77**, 353 (1971).
31. HODGKIN, A. L., HOROWICZ, P.: J. Physiol. (Lond.) **148**, 127 (1959).
32. WERMAN, R., GRUNDFEST, H.: J. gen. Physiol. **44**, 997 (1961).
33. SHANES, A. M.: Pharmacol. Revs. **10**, 165 (1958).
34. HODGKIN, A. L., HUXLEY, A. F.: J. Physiol. (Lond.) **116**, 449 (1952).
35. REDFERN, P., LUNDH, H., THESLEFF, S.: Europ. J. Pharmacol. **11**, 263 (1970).
36. NARAHASHI, T., MOORE, J. W., SCOTT, W. R.: J. gen. Physiol. **47**, 965 (1964).
37. SPECTOR, I., KIMHI, Y., NELSON, P. G.: Nature (Lond.) New Biol. **246**, 124 (1973).
38. ARMSTRONG, C. M., BINSTOCK, L.: J. gen. Physiol. **48**, 859 (1965).
39. SCHMIDT, H., STÄMPFLI, R.: Pflügers Archiv **287**, 311 (1966).
40. HILLE, B.: J. gen. Physiol. **50**, 1287 (1967).
41. LORENTE DE NÓ, R.: J. cell. comp. Physiol. (Suppl.) **33**, (1949).
42. BURKE, W., KATZ, B., MACHNE, X.: J. Physiol. (Lond.) **122**, 588 (1953).
43. TASAKI, I., HAGIWARA, S.: J. gen. Physiol. **40**, 859 (1957).
44. HIRST, G. D. S., SPENCE, I.: Nature (Lond.) New Biol. **243**, 54 (1973).

45. Nonomura,Y., Hotta,Y., Ohashi,H.: Science **152**, 97 (1966).
46. Kuriyama,H., Osa,T., Toida,N.: Brit. J. Pharmac. Chemother. **27**, 366 (1966).
47. Bennett,M.R.: J. Physiol. (Lond.) **190**, 465 (1967).
48. Hu,J., Prosser,C.L., Peterson,M.: Physiologist **13**, 228 (1970).
49. Fatt,P., Ginsborg,B.L.: J. Physiol. (Lond.) **142**, 516 (1958).
50. Shanes,A.M.: J. gen. Physiol. **33**, 57 (1949).
51. Weidmann,S.: J. Physiol. (Lond.) **129**, 568 (1955).
52. Thesleff,S.: Acta physiol. scand. **34**, 218 (1955).
53. Thesleff,S.: Acta anaest. scand. **2**, 69 (1958).
54. Dale,H.H.: J. Pharmacol. exp. Ther. **6**, 147 (1914).
55. Henderson,V.E., Roepke,M.H.: Physiol. Rev. **17**, 373 (1937).
56. Cowan,S.L.: J. Physiol. (Lond.) **88**, 3P (1936).
57. Kuffler,S.W.: J. Neurophysiol. **6**, 99 (1943).
58. Paton,W.D.M., Zaimis,E.J.: Brit. J. Pharmacol. **4**, 381 (1949).
59. Barlow,R.B., Ing,H.R.: Brit. J. Pharmacol. **3**, 298 (1948).
60. Paton,W.D.M., Zaimis,E.J.: J. Physiol. (Lond.) **112**, 311 (1951).
61. Burns,D., Paton,W.D.M.: J. Physiol. (Lond.) **115**, 41 (1952).
62. Chen,G., Partman,R., Wickel,A.: J. Pharmacol. exp. Ther. **103**, 330 (1951).
63. Levitan,H., Tauc,L.: J. Physiol. (Lond.) **222**, 537 (1972).
64. Chang,C.C., Lee,C.Y.: Arch. int. Pharmacodyn. **144**, 241 (1963).
65. Vogel,Z., Sytkowski,A.J., Nirenberg,M.W.: Proc. nat. Acad. Sci. (Wash.) **69**, 3180 (1972).
66. Karlin,A., Bartels,E.: Biochim. biophys. Acta Amsterdam **126**, 525 (1966).
67. Bartels,E., Deal,W., Karlin,A., Mautner,H.G.: Biochim. biophys. Acta Amsterdam **203**, 568 (1970).

Discussion

H. Stieve (Jülich): I have one question to Dr. Hamprecht's very interesting paper. What is the exact biological function that you are going to tackle and which you are going to solve more easily with your cell cultures than with classical nervous systems?

B. Hamprecht: First of all, we are trying to produce synapses with the cells. As I mentioned, they produce acetylcholine and they have acetylcholine receptors — so it is tempting to try to make synapses in a purely homogeneous cell population and to find out how synapses are being made, and I think this provides an opportunity to apply drugs right to a given cell without interfering with other cells. And, of course, you could also think of heterologous systems by using as target cells muscle cell cultures. This is point number one. But there are a number of morphological studies we have in mind. Maybe I should mention that we have found (Traber and Hamprecht, in preparation) that these hybrid cells are sensitive to morphine and that we can study the action of morphine on these cells, and we know what we are dealing with, whereas when you are using a brain — you never know which type of cell is really responding to morphine. These are just some examples. Other examples would be to study the uptake of neurotransmitters in those cells. And again, you don't have glial cells around; but you could take glial cells as well and then find out what the uptake studies in brain slices have meant. And you could study the effect of ions on the interplay of cells. For example, at present we are studying the production of prostaglandins by glioma cells (TRABER and HAMPRECHT, in preparation) and the idea is that prostaglandins might stimulate nerve cells. So the glioma cells would produce prostaglandin; the nerve cells — the neuroblastoma or the hybrid cells as a model — would make cAMP — in response to this, more noradrenaline would be produced and this would stimulate the glial cells and you would have a sort of an oscillation cycle which would be damped by the increase of the phosphodiesterase activity in response to the elevation of the cAMP.

B. HESS (Dortmund): I would like to ask one question — perhaps to my ignorance. Do you need glucose or oxygen to show all these phenomena, spikes and so on?

B. HAMPRECHT: These cells are generally grown in the presence of glucose and of oxygen. But we have not taken any measures to find out whether we could starve the cells and still obtain these responses, or we could exclude oxygen. We haven't done that, yet.

B. HESS: Are the responses which you observe responses to pulses, to concentration gradients, or responses to concentrations?

B. HAMPRECHT: They are not pulses. We add the drugs in a volume of a few microliters of a relatively concentrated solution to the surface of the medium above the cell impaled with a microelectrode. The cell is attached to the bottom of the culture dish. The drug will diffuse down to the surface of the cell, and after some time, of course, it will have diffused away into the environment.

B. HESS: You couldn't do it by a steady concentration?

B. HAMPRECHT: That we haven't checked. It is very difficult in this system at the moment, because when we change the medium totally, the cells become inactive, and we have not found out, yet, what the reason is.

E. GROSS (Bethesda, Md.): Sind die Sulfhydrylgruppen, von denen Sie sprachen und auf die Sie verschiedene SH-Reagentien einwirken lassen, am Acetylcholin-Receptor zu plazieren?

B. HAMPRECHT: Well, that is a guess. At least they are not involved in the spike-generating mechanism. But we do not know whether they are really exactly at the acetyl choline receptor. They might as well be at a step between the choline receptor and the spike-generating mechanism—if there is any intermediate step! That we cannot localize.

P. KARLSON (Marburg): Has the nerve growth factor any action on your cell cultures ?

B. HAMPRECHT: We haven't tried it on the hybrid cells, but LLOYD GREENE in NIRENBERG's laboratory (GREENE, personal communication) has tried it on some neuroblastoma cells — and there was no response whatsoever.

P. KARLSON: If you give dopamine, would these cells produce adrenaline ?

B. HAMPRECHT: We haven't done that experiment yet.

Immunogenetic Studies on Cell Surface Components of the Mammalian Nervous System

MELITTA SCHACHNER

Department of Neuropathology, Harvard Medical School and Department of Neuroscience, Children's Hospital Medical Center, 300 Longwood Avenue, Boston, MA 02115/USA

With 1 Figure

Interest in the composition of the outer membrane surface of nerve cells stems from its possible significance for morphogenesis and differentiation. The ontogenetic specification of tissue organization has been elaborated to a very elegant extreme in the nervous system, since most of its functional properties derive from the particular ways in which nerve cell contacts are organized. In terms of cytoarchitecture, the outstanding feature of the nervous system is that each neuron receives information from many other neurons and in turn transmits to many target cells, the extent of this convergence and divergence varying among regions and among classes of cells. Evidence from morphological and biochemical studies suggests that this functional specialization involves the development of topographically distinct sites on the surface membrane of a given nerve cell [1—3]. It is commonly assumed that these mosaic surface properties, which seem to mediate the specificity of surface contacts, become established in the mammal during embryonic and early postnatal development [3]. Direct molecular data on these organizational features at any stage of development, under any normal or pathological conditions are, however, very scarce.

An approach to identification, localization and, we hope, functional analysis of surface components is available through immunological methods. Encouraged by the success of immunogeneticists in the serological characterization of surface properties of the mouse lymphoid system [4], I have started a search for cell surface components, not only unique to nervous tissue, but also specific for a particular cell class and a particular developmental event. One problem with this approach, and a problem which underlies any characterization of nervous tissue at the molecular level, is the heterogeneity of the cell population under study. To raise specific antibodies one has to start with a cell population which has to meet at least the morphological and biochemical criteria of purity, let alone the immunological ones. Methods for dissociation and enrichment of nerve cell classes are available [5—8]; but the homogeneity and, in the case of the mouse, quantities obtained by the described techniques seemed to be an obstacle for our purposes. It is, indeed, with the help of cell surface specific antibodies that we would want to contribute to the presently available methods for isolation of particular cell classes [9]. To break into this vicious circle we have turned to the use of tumours as sources of antigen. This approach was made under two assumptions: (i) Tumours can be obtained as a relatively homogeneous and defined cell type. (ii) Tumours retain some properties characteristic of the normal counterpart that they are derived from. Furthermore, tumours may express developmental features which are thought to result from derepression of genes active during embryonal life.

A variety of nervous system tumours of inbred mouse strains have now been used by us to induce and characterize antibodies, not only unique to nervous tissue, but specific for a particular cell type within the nervous system. NS-1 (nervous system antigen-1) [10] is the first specific cell surface component to be discovered with an exclusive representation not only on nervous tissue, but confined to the subclass of glial cells by the presently accessible criteria. Antibodies to NS-1 were induced in C57BL/6 inbred mice and (C57BL/6 × DBA/2)F_1 hybrids with the methylcholanthrene induced glial cell tumour of probably oligodendrocytic origin, glioblastoma G26 of the C57BL/6 strain. The cytotoxicity test, a serological test designed for the exclusive and quantitative detection of antigenic components on the cell surface, was used to analyze these antibodies on glioblastoma G26 as the target indicator cell. As shown by absorption of anti-NS-1 antiserum with different tissues (Fig. 1), NS-1 is found solely on brain tissue of all mouse strains tested and of several other mammalian species, including man. It is present on cells of three of the four mouse glial cell tumours tested, but not the C1300 neuroblastoma, a tumour of neuronal origin. NS-1 occurs in higher concentration in regions of the nervous system richer in white than in gray matter, and in lower than normal concentrations in brains of myelin deficient neurological mutant mice. The concentration of NS-1 gradually increases postnatally

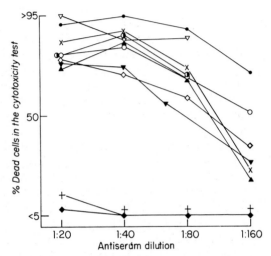

Fig. 1. Representation of NS-1 on various mouse tissues as determined by absorption of cytotoxic antibody. ● unabsorbed antiserum (C57BL/6 X DBA/2)F$_1$ anti-G26; antiserum absorbed with: × C57BL/6 liver; ○ K36 spontaneous leukemia of (C57BL/6 X AKR)F$_1$ hybrid; + C57BL/6 brain; ◆ glioblastoma G26; ◇ C57BL/6 spleen; ▲ C57BL/6 thymocytes; ▼ C57BL/6 kidney; ◑ C57BL/6 epidermal cells; ▽ C57BL/6 testicular cells

and reaches the adult level between the third and fourth week. The existence of more than one allele or genetic locus controlling NS-1 activity is suggested by the occurrence of higher amounts of NS-1 in brains of the A and C57BL/6 than of the Balb/c and DBA/2 mouse strains.

The availability of NS-1 antiserum enables a variety of investigations regarding the molecular structure of NS-1 and the genetics of the apparent allelic nature of its expression. Antibodies are being used as modifiers of physiological functions on living cells both *in vitro* and *in vivo*. With the refinement of immunohistological techniques, it should be possible to determine the distribution of

NS-1 among particular classes of glial cells and its topographical distribution on the cell surface within a particular cell at various developmental stages. It is hoped that the availability of neurological mouse mutants [11] with morphogenetic defects will offer a way to dissect by means of neuroimmunogenetic methods the developmental organization of a mammalian brain into critical individual steps.

References

1. JACOBSON, M.: Developmental neurobiology, p. 465. New York: Holt, Rinehart, and Winston (1970).
2. GAZE, R. M.: The formation of nerve connections, p. 299. New York: Academic Press (1970).
3. SIDMAN, R. L.: Contact interaction among developing mammalian brain cells. In: MOSCONA, A. (Ed.): Symposium on cell surface development. Proceedings of the Seventh International Congress of Developmental Biology. New York: John Wiley and Sons, Inc., 1974 (in press).
4. BOYSE, E. A., OLD, L. J.: Some aspects of normal and abnormal cell surface genetics. Ann. Rev. Gent. 3, 269—290 (1969).
5. HAMBERGER, A., HYDEN, H.: Inverse enzymatic changes in neurons and glia during increased function and hypoxia. J. Cell Biol. 16, 521—525 (1963).
6. ROSE, S. P. R.: Preparation of enriched fractions from cerebral cortex containing isolated metabolically active neuronal and glial cells. Biochem. J. 102, 33—43 (1967).
7. NORTON, W. T., PODUSLO, S. E.: Neuronal soma and whole neuroglia of rat brain: A new isolation technique. Science 167, 1144—1146 (1970).
8. BARKLEY, D. S., RAKIC, L. L., CHAFFEE, J. K., WONG, D. L.: Cell separation by velocity sedimentation of postnatal mouse cerebellum. J. Cell Physiol. 28, 271—280 (1973).
9. SCHACHNER, M., HÄMMERLING, U.: The postnatal development of antigens on mouse brain cell surfaces. Brain Res. 73, 362—371 (1974).
10. SCHACHNER, M.: NS-1 (nervous system antigen-1), a glial-cell specific antigenic component of the surface membrane. Proc. nat. Acad. Sci., USA. 71, 1795—1799 (1974).
11. SIDMAN, R. L., GREEN, M. C., APPEL, S. H.: Catalog of the neurological mutants of the Mouse, pp. 1—82. Cambridge, Mass.: Harvard Univ. (1965).

Neurotransmission

Einleitung zu den Vorträgen NACHMANSOHN und NEUMANN

W. HASSELBACH

*Max-Planck-Institut für medizinische Forschung, 69 Heidelberg, Jahnstr. 29,
Federal Republic of Germany*

Als ich 1949 als Hilfsassistent auf Probe zu H. H. WEBER ins
Physiologische Institut der Universität des Landes Württemberg-
Hohenzollern, nach Tübingen kam, erzählte er voll Begeisterung
von den Vorbereitungen zum 1. Mosbacher Kolloquium. Nach der
Wiederbelebung der nationalen Kongresse sollte wieder ein Tor zur
internationalen Wissenschaft geöffnet werden. Auch ein Physiologe
— einer, der allerdings als junger Ordinarius noch die physiologische
Chemie mitvertrat — gehörte also zu den Vätern der Mosbacher
Tagungen. Aus vielen Gründen hat sich dann in den folgenden
Jahren die Physiologie der Biochemie oder die Biochemie der
Physiologie entfremdet. Um so größer ist die Freude des Physiolo-
gen, der mit Bedauern die Trennung und die Wege der Wieder-
annäherung über die physikalisch-chemische Biologie etc. mit
Schmunzeln beobachtet hat, daß mit dem diesjährigen Thema die
biologische Chemie der Physiologie Reverenz erweist. Wie eng die
Beziehungen zwischen diesen beiden großen Teildisziplinen der
Biologie trotz äußerlicher Trennung immer waren, daran hat uns
GEORGE WALD erinnert. Seine Heimkehr war eine Heimkehr zur
Stätte des Wirkens von KÜHNE und MEYERHOF. Als Physiologen
haben sie an den Fundamenten der Biochemie gearbeitet. Wie weit
die Brücken in unserer Wissenschaft gespannt sind, wurde mir auch
klar, als GEORGE WALD die Arbeiten des Gießener Zoologen
W. J. SCHMIDT würdigte. Seine bahnbrechenden Arbeiten, in denen
er mit optischen Methoden zur Aufklärung der molekularen Architektur biologischer Strukturen beigetragen hat, sollten auch in
einer Zeit, in der sich der Fortschritt zu überschlagen droht, nicht
vergessen werden. W. J. SCHMIDT ist vor wenigen Wochen (14. 2.
1974) im Alter von fast 90 Jahren, von der wissenschaftlichen
Öffentlichkeit kaum bemerkt, in Frankfurt gestorben.

Ein Versuch eines Brückenschlages sind auch die Beiträge des heutigen Vormittags. Die physikalische Neurobiochemie will die Ergebnisse der Neurophysiologie interpretieren und verständlich machen. Der Meyerhof-Schüler und Biochemiker David Nachmansohn ist nie müde geworden, mit der ihm eigenen Beharrlichkeit die elektrische Manifestation der Nervenerregung zu hinterfragen. Die Physiologen dagegen sind diesen elektrischen Manifestationen verhaftet. Einmal, weil nur sie eine räumliche und zeitliche Analyse ermöglichen und zum anderen, weil sich ein weitgehend geschlossenes System entwickelt hat, das den Fortschritt der Physiologie in den letzten 30 Jahren repräsentiert. Es ist vor allem der formale Charakter der Analyse, wie er z. B. in den Beziehungen der Leitfähigkeit für die Natrium- und Kaliumionen zum Ausdruck kommt, der den Biochemiker mit Unbehagen erfüllt.

$$g_{K^+} = g^o_{K^+} \cdot n^4 \qquad \frac{dn}{dt} = \alpha_n \, (1 - n) - \beta_n \cdot (n)$$

$$g_{Na^+} = g^o_{Na^+} m^3 \cdot h \, \frac{dm}{dt} = \alpha_m \, (1 - m) - \beta_m \cdot (m)$$

$$\frac{dh}{dt} = \alpha_h \, (1 - h) - \beta_h \cdot (h) \, .$$

Mit den g_{K^+}, g_{Na^+}, den Leitfähigkeiten der Membran für die Kalium- und Natriumionen, und der Kabel-Gleichung

$$\frac{1}{R V^2} \cdot \frac{\delta \psi}{\delta t} = C \cdot \frac{\delta \psi}{\delta t} + g_{K^+} \, (\psi - E_{K^+}) + g_{Na^+} \, (\psi - E_{Na^+})$$

$R = $ Widerstand des Axoplasma $\psi = $ Membranpotential
$V = $ Fortleitungsgeschwindigkeit $C = $ Membrankapazität
                                      $E = $ Gleichgewichtspotentiale

können die elektrischen Phänomene der Nervenleitung hinreichend gut beschrieben werden. Der Biochemiker möchte die m, n und h's mit physiologisch relevanten Substanzen und ihren Umsetzungen identifizieren können und die Exponenten der Gleichung verstehen. Eine gleichzeitige Beobachtung der chemischen und elektrischen Prozesse ist aus naheliegenden Gründen nicht möglich. Wir sind also auf Indizien angewiesen, die vermehrt und miteinander verknüpft werden müssen. David Nachmansohn hat auf diese Weise ein großes Gebäude errichtet, über dessen Architektur er uns zusammen mit Herrn Neumann berichten will.

Biochemical Foundation of an Integral Model of Nerve Excitability[1]

DAVID NACHMANSOHN

Departments of Neurology and Biochemistry, Columbia University, New York, N.Y., USA

With 9 Figures

A. Introduction

Cell Membranes. During recent years cell membranes have moved to the center of biological research: (1) They are the site of some of the most vital cellular functions, such as, *e.g.*, energy supply, photosynthesis, vision, nerve impulse conduction and others. (2) It has been realized that there is a strong impact of structure and organization on chemical reactions. Whereas classical biochemistry generally analyzed chemical reactions in solution, it has become apparent that structural factors such as microenvironment, cooperativity, allosteric effects, allotopy, regulatory effects, protein-protein, protein-lipid interactions and many others may modify and drastically change the reactions observed in solution. A vast amount of information about the chemical events in membranes has accumulated. Perhaps the most important result has been a conceptual change. Since the turn of the century lipids were considered as the essential component acting as barriers and preventing the exchange of compounds between the inside of the cell and its outer environment. Today it is well established that proteins are the essential components responsible for the function of membranes. Many cell membranes are formed by two-thirds of proteins, and only one-third of phospholipids. From some membranes 30 dif-

[1] This lecture is based on a more extended presentation to appear in a special volume of Biomembranes [MANSON, L. (Ed.)], dedicated to the memory of AHARON KATCHALSKY.

The work was financially supported by the U.S. Public Health Service Grant NS-03304-12, National Science Foundation Grant NSF-GB-31122X, and the New York Heart Association.

ferent proteins (or more) have been extracted and identified. Membranes are highly dynamic structures, the site of many chemical reactions. Proteins account more readily for the specificity, the efficiency and the diversity of membrane functions than phospholipids (see *e.g.* [1—4]).

In contrast to the large amount of information on the chemical composition of membranes, we are still very far from a real knowledge of the molecular organization of the various constituents in the intact membrane. Indeed, in the last years more than ten different membrane models have been proposed. Without discussing their merits, we would like to bring two models as an illustration of the development during the last decade: the model of ROBERTSON [5] of the "unit membrane", and the model of SJOESTRAND and BARAJAS [6] representing the inner membrane of mitochondria (Fig. 1). The latter model incorporates the many enzymes showing their subunits and coenzymes well established to be present in this membrane; it also accounts for the proper relationship between the amount of proteins and phospholipids. This model is rather attractive because it integrates a great number of the known membrane constituents.

Recognizing the central importance of the proteins and the necessity of preserving them in their native conformation, SJOESTRAND and BARAJAS have introduced new techniques for the preparation and fixation of the specimen for electron microscopy; they avoided the usual standard techniques which almost certainly denature the proteins. With the new techniques the membranes have a thickness of 150—200 Å as compared to the 80—100 Å obtained with the standard procedures. A striking feature of their electron micrographs is the indication of many globular formations within the membrane (SJOESTRAND and BARAJAS [7]).

Excitable Membranes. Excitable membranes have the special ability of transiently changing their permeability in a controlled way to those ions which are the carriers of the electrical exchange currents accompanying membrane potential changes such as the nerve impulses. As was emphasized by A. V. HILL (1960), there appears to be no alternative to the assumption that *"the early production and absorption of heat after a stimulus are largely due to chemical reactions associated with, and following, the permeability cycle"*. Furthermore, various biochemical and electrophysiological

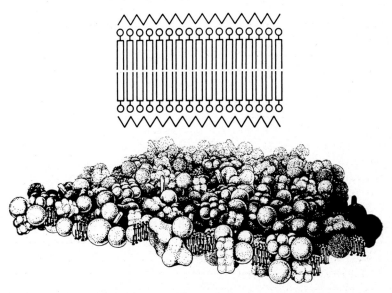

Fig. 1. Top: Model of ROBERTSON [5] of the "unit membrane", proposed to be 80 Å thick and formed by a bimolecular layer of phospholipids surrounded on the inside and outside by proteins attached to the phospholipids by Coulombic forces. Bottom: Model of SJOESTRAND and BARAJAS [6] of the inner mitochondrial membrane. The model tries to integrate the enzymes and coenzymes with their subunits biochemically established to be located in this membrane. The phospholipids of this membrane are known to form only a relatively small fraction of this membrane, as indicated in the picture. Thickness about 150—200 Å

observations (see for instance TASAKI [8]) are incompatible with assumption of simple electrodiffusion processes as an explanation for the generation of the action potential (see also COLE [9]). It should be realized that the increased ion fluxes during electrical activity appear, indeed, to result from complex intramembrane processes. It is obvious that an elucidation of the mechanism requires the analysis of these membrane processes.

B. Chemical Foundation of the Integral Model of Nerve Excitability

A chemical theory of the events associated with the conduction of nerve and muscle fibres has been elaborated during the last three

decades. It is based essentially on the properties and function of
the proteins processing acetylcholine (AcCh): (i) the enzyme AcCh-
esterase which hydrolyses the ester, (ii) the AcCh-receptor, the
target protein of AcCh, (iii) the enzyme choline-O-acetyltransferase
(choline acetylase) that synthesizes AcCh, and (iv) a storage site
(presumably a protein) to which AcCh is probably bound. The
storage protein is still a postulate, whereas the other three have
been isolated, purified and characterized. The early results are summarized in reviews [10, also 10a] and in a monograph [11], the later
developments in a series of presentations [12—19].

Instrumental for the progress was, since 1937, the use of electric
organs of electric fish. These organs are specialized for their function, the generation of electricity, to a degree which is virtually
without parallel in living organisms. DU BOIS-REYMOND, who
had worked for 20 years with these organs, predicted in 1877 that
this material would permit us one day to explain the mechanism of
the electrical activity in nerve and muscle fibres. For the biochemist
interested in proteins processing AcCh, these organs offer unique
material: 92% of this tissue is water and only 3% is proteins;
their paramount importance became apparent when it was
found, in 1937, that the tissue contains fantastic amounts of
AcCh-esterase. Obviously, other factors were essential for the
advances such as, *e.g.*, the spectacular progress of protein chemistry
in the last two decades, the development of instruments of an
amazing degree of precision, the aforementioned advances of our
knowledge of cell membranes and others.

I. Role of Acetylcholine in the Excitable Membrane

(a) The Acetylcholine Cycle. In the 1939's it was assumed that
AcCh acts as a "neurohumoral" transmitter, which is released
from nerve endings and, after crossing the non-conducting gap,
stimulates the effector cell, nerve or muscle. The results of the biochemical analyses of the proteins processing AcCh, indicated very
soon that this hypothesis is untenable. Twenty years ago the
following hypothesis was proposed for the role of AcCh in the
permeability changes of excitable membranes: (see Fig. 2; the
picture is taken from my Harvey Lecture in 1953 [10]). In this view
AcCh is released by stimulation from the storage protein and acts

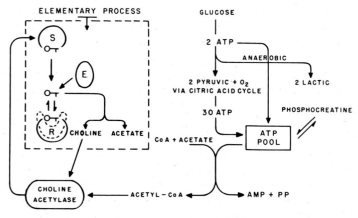

Fig. 2. Sequence of energy transformations associated with conduction, and integration of the acetylcholine system into the metabolic pathways of the nerve cell. The elementary process of conduction had been, in 1953, tentatively pictured as follows: (1) In resting condition acetylcholine ($\multimap$) is bound, presumably to a storage protein (S). The membrane is polarized. (2) AcCh is released by current flow (possibly hydrogen ion movements) or any other excitatory agent. The free ester combines with the receptor (R), presumably a protein. (3) The receptor changes its configuration (dotted line). This process increases the Na ion permeability and permits rapid Na influx. This is the trigger action by which the potential primary source of EMF, the ionic concentration gradient, becomes effective and by which the action current is generated. (4) The ester-receptor complex is in dynamic equilibrium with the free ester and the receptor; the free ester is hydrolysed by acetylcholinesterase (E). (5) The hydrolysis of the ester permits the receptor to return to its original shape. The permeability decreases, and the membrane is again in its original polarized condition [10]

on the AcCh receptor protein (*both* proteins were at that time a postulate). AcCh induces a conformational change of the receptor, initiating thereby a series of processes leading to an increased permeability to ions. AcCh is hydrolysed (in micro-seconds) by AcCh-esterase, permitting the receptor to return to its resting condition; the barrier for ions is reestablished. All those processes were assumed to take place within the membrane in a structurally well organized form. During recovery AcCh is resynthesized by choline acetylase (choline-O-acetyltransferase) using ATP hydrolysis as source of energy; ATP is provided by the glycolytic or citric acid cycles.

It is unnecessary to describe all the modifications of the cycle during the last 20 years induced by the advances of our information. Figure 3 shows the present view of the control function of AcCh in the membrane: the AcCh cycle worked out by E. NEUMANN and myself during the last year in connection with the integral model of nerve excitability [90]. The physicochemical foundation of this integral model will be presented in the lecture of E. NEUMANN.

In the framework of the integral model it is assumed that a decrease of the resting potential, $\Delta \psi_r$ by 15—20 mV (corresponding to a change of the electric field strength by 15—20 kV/cm) induces a conformational change in the storage site. This assumption is based on experiments of NEUMANN and KATCHALSKY [20] and NEUMANN and ROSENHECK [21] on the behavior of polyelectrolytic macromolecular organizations in electric fields. The field-induced conformational change in the storage site is assumed to release bound AcCh which is translocated to the AcCh receptor, changing its conformation upon association; thereby Ca^{++} ions are released from the receptor in its resting form. The Ca^{++} ions are involved in gateway processes which permit the passage of ions, possibly again by conformational changes of gateway proteins and/or phospholipids (or lipo- or glycoproteins).

Simultaneously AcCh is translocated to AcCh-esterase, which hydrolyses the ester to choline, acetate and protons. This is one of the apparently irreversible reactions in the cycle. For the resynthesis of AcCh energy is required, provided by ATP-hydrolysis. Choline-O-acetyltransferase acetylates choline and translocates it to the storage protein. The result of all these processes is the passage of 15000—30000 ions per molecule of AcCh activated across the membrane in both directions. The cycle reflects a stationary state of continuous activity. As with all events in living cells the processes take place continuosly, but during activity their rate is greatly increased.

(b) Macromolecular Conformation and Ca^{++} Ions. It may be useful to recall a few physicochemical aspects of macromolecular conformational changes in connection with Ca^{++} ions [90]. Structural changes of proteins and macromolecular organizations such as membranes are often cooperative in nature. One of the consequences of cooperativity is the possibility of far-reaching conformational

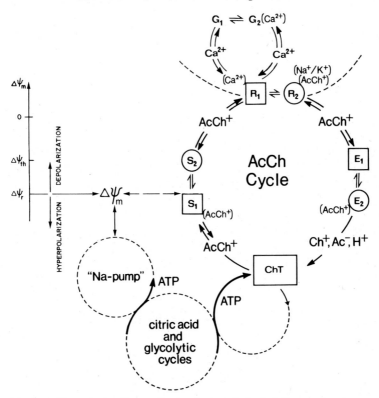

Fig. 3. AcCh cycle, for the cyclic chemical control of stationary membrane potentials $\Delta\psi$ and transient potential changes. The binding capacity of the storage site for AcCh is assumed to be dependent on the membrane potential, $\Delta\psi_m$, and is thereby coupled to the "Na^+/K^+ exchange-pump" (and the citric acid and glycolytic cycles). The control cycle for the gateway G_1 (Ca^{2+} binding and closed) and G_2 (open) comprises the SRE assemblies and the choline-O-acetyltransferase (Ch-T); Ch-T couples the AcCh synthesis cycle to the translocation pathway of AcCh through the SRE-assemblies. The continuous subthreshold flux of AcCh through such a subunit is maintained by the virtually irreversible hydrolysis of AcCh to choline (Ch^+), acetate (Ac^-) and protons (H^+) and by steady supply flux of AcCh to the storage from the synthesis cycle. In the resting stationary state, the membrane potential ($\Delta\psi_r$) reflects dynamic balance between active transport (and AcCh synthesis) and the flux of AcCh (through the control cycles surrounding the gateway) and of the various ions asymmetrically distributed across the membrane. Fluctuations in membrane potential (and exchange currents) are presumably amplified by fluctuations in the local AcCh concentrations maintained at a stationary level during the continuous translocation of AcCh through the cycle

changes by small local changes of environmental conditions. Moreover, conformational changes induced by binding of a ligand at one site may change the reactivity of other, possibly even far more remote, sites of a macromolecular system (allosteric effects). Ca^{++} ions are particularly effective in inducing large conformational changes as for instance in muscular contractions, and are particularly efficient in systems that contain regions of a relatively high negative surface charge. In such polyelectrolytic regions the osmotic coefficient for Ca^{++} is in the order of 0.01, *i.e.* about 99% of Ca^{++} counterions are bound [22]. The high binding capacity is one of the reasons for the assumption that Ca^{++} ions play an essential role in maintaining structural and functional integrity of protein and lipoprotein organization. For almost a century the need for Ca^{++} ions in nerve excitability was proposed [23]. More recently, TASAKI [8], in particular, has emphasized that Ca^{++} ions are absolutely necessary for nerve excitability.

II. The Proteins Processing Acetylcholine

(a) AcCh-esterase. The enzyme AcCh-esterase was for the first time isolated from electric tissue of *Torpedo marmorata* in 1938 [24]. Until then horse serum esterase was generally used, which is a mixture of several esterases, but does not contain AcCh-esterase. AcCh-esterase is not absolutely specific, but may be distinguished from other esterases by several special features such as, *e.g.*, the bell-shaped activity-substrate concentration curve. The enzyme was purified in the early forties virtually to homogeneity of the protein [25]. The availability of a highly active preparation permitted the analysis of important properties. The turnover number of the enzyme is about 8×10^5 AcCh molecules/sec, its turnover time about 70 μsec. This high rate of the enzyme activity is a prerequisite for the assumption of the chemical control of the electrical activity by the AcCh cycle, since the speed of the two activities must be similar. The molecular groups in the active site were analysed and the reaction mechanisms of many compounds explained, which play an important role in biology and medicine [11, 26]. Of particular interest was the elucidation of the mechanism of organophosphates, compounds widely used as insecticides; some of them are the famous "nerve gases", potential chemical warfare agents. These

compounds form a phosphorylated enzyme with a rather stable
P-O bond (with the O of the serine of the active site). The phosphoryl group may be removed, in an S_N2 reaction, by nucleophilic
compounds; one of the most potent compounds is pyridine-aldoxine
methiodide, synthesized by WILSON and GINSBURG [27]. It was
shown in animal experiments that this compound is a potent anti-
dote against organophosphate insecticide poisoning, especially in
combination with atropine [28] and is used today successfully all
over the world.

Later AcCh-esterase was purified with improved methods and it
was crystallized in 1967 [29]. Today, there exist several purification
methods, using affinity chromatography. ROSENBERRY et al. [30]
succeeded with such a method to obtain homogeneous protein in a
single step with a rather high yield.

(b) AcCh Receptor. The assumption that the AcCh receptor
is a protein (see Fig. 2) has been a postulate. The development of a
monocellular electroplax preparation by SCHOFFENIELS [31, 32]
and the refined method worked out by HIGMAN and coworkers
[33—36] made it possible to analyse the properties of the receptor.
Evidence was obtained, by a series of different types of experiments,
that the receptor is, indeed, a protein [37—41]. However, in experiments on the intact membrane it was impossible to decide whether
the different molecular groups in the active sites of enzyme and
receptor are part of one protein or whether enzyme and receptor are
two different proteins. CHANGEUX and his associates [42] succeeded
in separating the two proteins using a snake venom, the α-toxin of
Naja naja (MEUNIER et al., 1971). In the last few years the receptor
protein has been isolated, purified and characterized in many
laboratories all over the world, *e.g.* [43—47]. You will hear about
the receptor in the lecture of Dr. RAFTERY.

(c) Choline-O-Acetyltransferase. The enzymatic formation of
AcCh in a soluble system was discovered in 1942 [48]. The AcCh
synthesis requires the energy of ATP hydrolysis. The enzymatic
synthesis of AcCh *in vitro* was the *first* experimental demonstration
of an ATP-dependent acetylation. The observations were so unexpected that — as happens frequently in such cases — several
journals refused to accept them for publication [49]. The synthesizing enzyme was first referred to as choline acetylase and is

now called choline-O-acetyltransferase. This enzyme has been purified extensively by standard procedures from squid head ganglia. Recently, a very efficient procedure using affinity chromatography, led to a preparation with a high degree of purity, as was described by HUSAIN and MAUTNER [50].

(d) Storage Site. The storage site for AcCh in the excitable membrane is most likely a protein. Only a protein would account for the specificity of binding; a relatively high binding constant is suggested by the great difficulty of removing AcCh from the membrane. The protein nature of the storage site has been postulated in 1953 [10].

III. The Localization of AcCh-esterase

AcCh-esterase and choline-O-acetyltransferase are present in all types of excitable membranes from the lowest to the highest species in living organisms, as has been established by chemical analysis: in motor and sensory, in "cholinergic" and "adrenergic" fibres, in peripheral and central nervous system, in vertebrates and in invertebrates, and in muscle fibers. Not a single exception has been found [11, 12].

On the basis of biochemical data it was assumed for more than 30 years that AcCh-esterase is localized at or near the membranes. This evidence was of necessity only indirect. Electron microscopy in combination with staining techniques has established unequivocally that the enzyme is localized in excitable membranes. With myelinated nerve fibres the findings were in the beginning irregular. BRZIN and DETTBARN [51] had shown, using the magnetic diver, that in the myelinated axons of frog sciatic nerve AcCh-esterase is present at the Ranvier nodes as well as in the intermediate sections. Assuming that the myelinated axons are so rich in lipids that the lipid insoluble AcCh does not reach the membrane even in slices only 500 Å thick, BRZIN [52] incubated the slices in Triton X-100 before adding the reagents necessary for the test of AcCh-esterase activity (acetylthiocholine and copper sulfate). With this pretreatment the enzyme appeared regularly in the membrane of the myelinated axons (Fig. 4).

The enzyme is not only present in all excitable membranes, but also no difference has been found in conducting and synaptic parts.

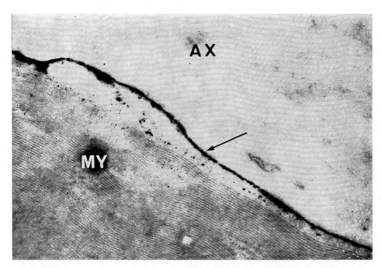

Fig. 4. Large myelinated (MY) ventral root axon (AX) taken from a frog sciatic nerve. The slice was treated with Triton X-100 before the incubation for testing acetylcholinesterase activity with the standard procedure for histochemical staining of the enzyme (adding acetylthiocholine and copper sulfate). The hydrolytic product, thiocholine, forms a precipitate with copper sulfate. The dense end product is present in the axolemmal (plasma) membrane (arrow) [52]

Figure 5 shows an isolated excitable membrane of the electroplax of *Electrophorus* treated with the usual staining techniques for testing the enzyme [53]. Although 99% of this membrane are formed by the conducting and only 1—2% of synaptic parts, the electron micrograph shows the uniform distribution along the entire membrane. The uniformity of the distribution is still more distinctly shown in electron micrographs of the excitable membrane of the electroplax prepared by N. THOMAS, R. DAVIS, and G. KOELLE with a new staining method, using gold thiolacetic acid and leading to a gold-sulfide precipitate (paper still in preparation). The elegance of this new method is seen in Fig. 6, which shows the motor end plate of an intercostal muscle of mouse. The picture shows unequivocally the presence of the enzyme in the membrane of the nerve terminal and in the strongly folded postsynaptic membrane [53a].

In the excitable membrane of a single electroplax there are 10^{11} molecules of AcCh-esterase. One gram membrane may hydrolyse more than 30 kg of AcCh per hour. This is a truly amazing concentration. The number of AcCh receptors in this membrane is of the same order of magnitude.

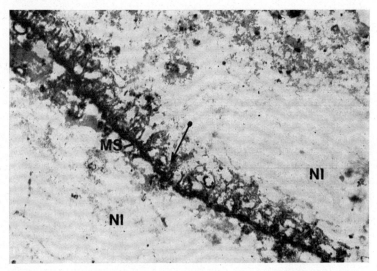

Fig. 5. Electron micrograph of an isolated fragment of excitable membrane from the electroplax of *Electrophorus*, tested for AcCh-esterase activity by standard procedures. The picture shows the uniformity of distribution of AcCh-esterase at the innervated membrane surface (MS). No staining was found in the non-innervated (NI) membrane [53]

IV. Experimental Basis for the Direct Link or the Proteins with Electrical Activity

(a) Effects of Specific Inhibitors of Either Enzyme of Receptor on the Electrical Activity. Neither the localization of AcCh-esterase in excitable membranes nor the high concentration are an indication for the direct role of the AcCh cycle in the electrical activity. It must be emphasized that the chemical theory is based on an entirely different type of experimental facts. During the last

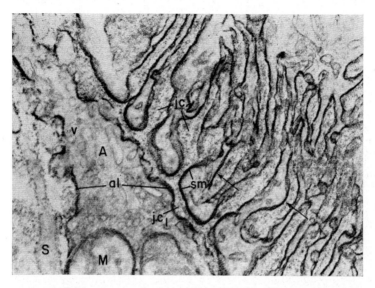

Fig. 6. Electron microscopic histochemical localization of acetylcholinesterase at the motor end plate of mouse intercostal muscle. A high magnification (× 63 000) view of the junctional complex, showing the axon terminal (A)
containing mitochondria (M) and numerous synaptic vesicles (v), the junctional cleft (jc), and junctional folds of the sarcolemma (sm). The electron-
dense granules, 40—50 Å in diameter, represent gold sulfide, the reaction
product of the goldthiolacetic acid method for the detection of acetylcholinesterase and nonspecific cholinesterase. The axolemma (al) exhibits marked
enzymic activity both on the surface facing the primary junctional cleft (jc_1)
and at the surface facing the teloglial Schwann cell sheath (S) (the axonal
terminal is somewhat separated from the Schwann cell in this micrograph).
Where the plane of section is perpendicular to the sarcolemma (arrows), the
particles form a dense line about 120—140 Å thick [53a]

30 years it has been shown in a vast number of experiments using
different types of preparations, compounds and methods, that
potent and specific inhibitors of the enzyme or of the receptor have
strong effects on the different electrical parameters of excitable
membranes. Obviously, not all preparations are equally suitable to
offer this type of evidence in view of the complexity of the structures
by which excitable membranes are insulated and surrounded by
protective barriers. This problem will be discussed in more detail

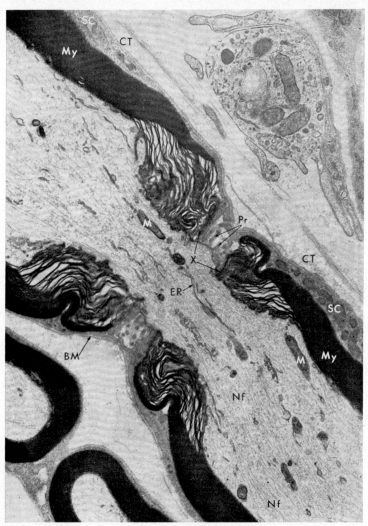

Fig. 7. Electron micrograph showing a Ranvier node of a single fibre from the sciatic nerve of mouse. The sheath of myelin forms a compact tube (My) over most of the internodal area. In the region of the node, finger-like processes (Pr) of neighboring Schwann cells (SC) interdigitate and cover the nodal area. A basement membrane (BM) and connective tissue fibres (CT) of the endoneurium complete the wrappings of the fibre. At the node, the membrane of the axon is free of myelin and is exposed to the interstitial fluids which diffuse through the basement membrane and between the Schwann cell processes. Axoplasm is rich in neurofilaments (Nf) and contains slender elements of the endoplasmic reticulum (ER) and small numbers of mitochondria (M). [97]

in Section V. But a few examples may be given as an illustration. When curare (d-tubocurarine), a potent inhibitor of the AcCh receptor, is added to an isolated axon of the frog sciatic nerve and the electrical activity is recorded at a single Ranvier node (Fig. 7), the electrical response is rapidly and reversibly blocked [53 b—d]. Physostignine, a potent and competitive inhibitor of AcCh-esterase ($K_I = 10^{-7}$ M) added to the same preparation, increases within seconds the electrical response, in concentrations of 10^{-5} to 10^{-6} M, then the activity is slowly decreased and in a few minutes it is blocked [53 c].

A particularly interesting demonstration of the block of electrical activity by the inhibition of the AcCh receptors presents a series of experiments carried out with local anesthetics on the monocellular electroplax preparation by E. BARTELS [54, 55]. These compounds are structural analogs of AcCh. By systematic stepwise substitution of AcCh (see Table 1) BARTELS has shown how AcCh, a receptor activator acting on synaptic junctions only, is transformed into a typical local anesthetic which is a receptor inhibitor and acts on both synaptic and conducting parts of the membrane. Benzoylcholine is structurally and in its activity a typical transitory form, which may exhibit both types of action according to experimental conditions. Under appropriate experimental conditions it is possible to demonstrate the typical competitive nature between the action of AcCh and that of local anesthetics.

(b) Parallelism between Chemical Stimulation of Isolated Membranes of the Electroplax of Electrophorus and Electrical Stimulation of the Intact Membrane. CHANGEUX and his associates [53] have prepared isolated fragments from the excitable membranes of electroplax of *Electrophorus*. These fragments are part of the *conducting and not of the synaptic* membrane. They form microsacs which permit the analysis of some properties and function of the membrane proteins. The microsacs may be filled with radioactive Na^+ or other ions. This preparation permits us to study the effects of AcCh receptor activators or inhibitors on the efflux of the ions. An interesting result of these experiments with the microsacs is the effect on the efflux of Na^+ ions [56]. A remarkable parallelism was found between the effect of chemical stimulation (or inhibition) on the Na^+ efflux and the effects of the same compounds on the electri-

Table 1. Local anesthetics as "antimetabolites" of acetylcholine

Compound	Synaptic Junctions		Conducting Membrane
	Activator	Inhibitor	
	M concentration		
$CH_3-\overset{\underset{\|}{CH_3}}{\overset{\|}{N}}-CH_2-CH_2-O-\overset{\underset{\|}{CH_3}}{C}-O^{(-)}$ (+) Acetylcholine	2.5×10^{-6}	O	O
$CH_3-\overset{\underset{\|}{CH_3}}{\overset{\oplus\|}{N}}-CH_2-CH_2-O-C-O^{(-)}$ (cyclohexyl) Hexahydrobenzoylcholine	5×10^{-4}	O	O
$CH_3-\overset{\underset{\|}{CH_3}}{\overset{\oplus\|}{N}}-CH_2-CH_2-O-C-O^{(-)}$ (phenyl) Benzoylcholine	5×10^{-4}	5×10^{-4}	1×10^{-3}
$CH_3-\overset{\underset{\|}{CH_3}}{\overset{\oplus\|}{N}}-CH_2-CH_2-O-C-O^{(-)}$ (phenyl–NH_2) p–Aminobenzoylcholine	O	1×10^{-3}	2.5×10^{-3}
$C_2H_5-\overset{\underset{\|}{H}}{\overset{\oplus\|}{N}}-CH_2-CH_2-O-C-O^{(-)}$ (phenyl–NH_2) with C_2H_5 Procaine	O	2.5×10^{-4}	5×10^{-4}
$CH_3-\overset{\underset{\|}{CH_3}}{\overset{\oplus\|}{N}}-CH_2-CH_2-O-C-O^{(-)}$ (phenyl–$NH-C_4H_9$) Tetracainemethiodide	O	2×10^{-5}	1×10^{-5}

Table 1: (Legend see p. 447)

cal response of the intact electroplax, measured two years earlier by CHANGEUX and PODLESKI [57] (Fig. 8).

The flux of Na^+ ions across the membrane of the microsacs, Φ_{Na}, expressed in moles/cm²/sec, has been calculated by KASAI and CHANGEUX [56]. This value is surprisingly similar to that calculated by HODGKIN and HUXLEY [58] for the influx of Na^+ ions into the interior of the squid giant axon as a result of electrical stimulation. The two values were obtained on the basis of the same equation. It seems difficult to interpret this surprising similarity of the effects of chemical and electrical stimulation upon the Na^+ ion fluxes across the membrane, except by the assumption that the electrical stimulation has activated the same molecular control mechanism in both membranes. As will be discussed in Section V, this chemical mechanism has been demonstrated not only in the membrane of the squid axon, but it is also linked directly to its electrical activity.

(c) **Basic Excitation Units.** A concept of fundamental importance for the understanding of nerve excitability and the integral model has been suggested by E. NEUMANN: the notion of a Basic

---

The Table shows that local anesthetics are typical derivatives of AcCh. All data are derived from experiments performed on the monocellular electroplax preparation of *Electrophorus*. At the concentrations given the compounds have comparable effects. Whereas AcCh is an activator of the receptor, local anesthetics are inhibitors. The effects of activators may be recognized by their depolarizing action; they act on synaptic junctions only. The inhibitors block electrical activity without depolarization; they act on conducting as well as synaptic parts of the membrane. The stepwise substitutions show the transition from one type of the effect on the receptor to the other. The substitution of the methyl group at the carbon of the carbonyl group by a saturated ring strongly decreases the depolarizing action (about 100 fold), but the compound still remains an activator, acting on the synapse only. The substitution by an unsaturated ring already transforms the properties of the molecule: benzoylcholine is not only structurally but also functionally a typical transitory form between AcCh and the local anesthetics: depending on the experimental conditions it may produce either of two effects, and it already has the ability to penetrate the structural barriers surrounding the conducting parts of the membrane. Therefore it affects both parts. The addition of a single amino group to the phenyl ring of benzoylcholine in para position transforms the molecule into a typical local anesthetic: this compound is a receptor inhibitor and acts on synaptic and on conducting parts of the membrane. By small additional substitutions either at the carbonyl group or at the ammonium group, one may obtain very effective local anesthetics [54, 55].

Excitation Unit (BEU). In this concept the gateway is a permeation zone through which normally Na^+ ions pass during the action potential; this gateway is surrounded by several complexes

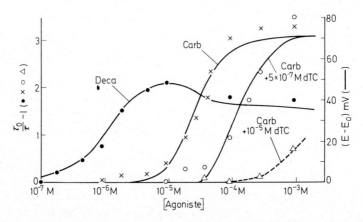

Fig. 8. Parellelism between chemical stimulation of isolated membranes ("microsacs") and electrical stimulation of the intact isolated electroplax of *Electrophorus*. The dose-response curves of the chemical stimulation of the microsacs were evaluated by measuring the rate of ^{22}Na efflux from the microsacs. τ is the period of time required for the 50% loss of ^{22}Na of the vesicles in the presence of carbamylcholine, $\tau = \tau_0$ in its absence. The dose-response curves on the electroplax of activators: carbamylcholine (carb), decamethonium (deca) — or inhibitors: d-tubocurarine (dTC) — have been taken from [57]; they were evaluated as usual by electrical parameters (voltage changes are given on the right side). The data show the striking similarity of the affinities to the AcCh receptor tested on the cellular level (isolated electroplax) and of those tested on the subcellular level (isolated membranes, "microsacs")

of S (storage), R (receptor), and E (enzyme) proteins, (see Fig. 4 in the following article and NEUMANN et al. [90]). This concept is of decisive value for the interpretation of many electrophysiological observations such as threshold, graded or all-or-none response, accommodation and many others. The concept is only briefly mentioned here; it is essential for the understanding of the following section discussing the role of AcCh in synaptic junctions.

V. Role of AcCh at Motor Endplates and at Synaptic Junctions

(a) **Problem of the Role of AcCh at Junctions.** The well known hypothesis of neurohumoral transmission attributes to AcCh function only at synaptic junctions. It is postulated that AcCh is released from the nerve terminal and acts, after crossing the non-conducting gap, as a mediator of the impulse between nerve and nerve or nerve and muscle. This view explicitly postulates a fundamentally different mechanism: chemical transmission of AcCh across junctions and purely electrical propagation of nerve impulses along fibres. It is the assumption of such a basic difference which appeared unacceptable to many prominent neurobiologists. On the basis of electrical signs, conducting and synaptic parts of excitable membranes share many similar properties; therefore, these facts were considered to be hardly compatible with the view of an entirely different mechanism. Not the facts but only the interpretations were questioned and rejected (see *e.g.* [59, 60]).

Since the role of AcCh as a neurohumoral transmitter across junctions is still a widely accepted view, it appears imperative to analyse, at least briefly, the main data on which the original hypothesis was based, to review some more recent data contradicting the original hypothesis and requiring drastic modifications, and finally to discuss how in the light of the information presently available one may explain and reconcile the early observations with the integral model of nerve excitability presented here. Without a detailed discussion of the peculiar properties of synaptic transmission in general, only those aspects will be stressed which refer to the specific function of AcCh at junctions. This question cannot be omitted or ignored without making it extremely difficult for the reader to understand and evaluate how the two seemingly contrasting views as to the function of AcCh can be reconciled and form part of the integral model. An alternative interpretation of the function of AcCh at the junction will be discussed. It is compatible with the integral model attributing to AcCh the same role in conducting and synaptic parts of excitable membranes.

(b) **Early Observations that Suggested a Special Function of AcCh at Synaptic Junctions**

1. External Application of AcCh. One of the most fundamental facts supporting a transmitter role of AcCh appeared to be the powerful action of externally applied AcCh on junctions, in contrast to the total failure of AcCh to affect conduction of fibres even in high concentrations. As in the famous experiments of CLAUDE BERNARD on curare, frog sciatic nerve fibres were used to test the effect of AcCh on conduction. These fibres are composed of several thousand axons in which the conducting membranes are surrounded by a myelin sheath 30000—50000 Å thick; in addition, the entire fiber is surrounded by a sheath of connective tissue. Thus, the excitable membrane is well protected against many compounds and particularly against lipid insoluble quaternary ammonium derivatives such as AcCh and curare. Only at the Ranvier node myelin is absent, although even there one finds a base membrane and some tissue covering the excitable membrane (see Fig. 7). As mentioned before, when compounds acting on the AcCh-receptor or on AcCh-esterase are applied to a single axon preparation and the electrical activity is measured on a single Ranvier node, the effects are similar to those observed on motor endplates. Thus, the limitation of the actions of curare and AcCh are fully explained by the structural barriers, protecting and insulating the conducting parts of the membrane; these barriers are usually less efficient or absent at the junctional parts.

Even the so-called unmyelinated axons are surrounded by Schwann cells rich in lipids; for instance, in the isolated giant axon of *Loligo*, the Schwann cell is about 4000 Å thick. Neither AcCh nor curare are able to penetrate into the interior of these axons, as has been repeatedly demonstrated with radioactive and stable isotopes [61—63]. They obviously do not reach the conducting membrane and cannot affect its activity. However, after exposure of the squid giant axon to a few µg of phospholipase A for a few minutes, both AcCh and d-tubocurarine do affect electrical activity; experiments with radioactively labeled compounds have shown that under these conditions they are found in the axoplasm [63, 64]. Electron micrographs of axons exposed to phospholipase A showed a slight disintegration of the outer layer of the Schwann cell; in agreement with electrophysiological evidence the excitable membrane was *not* affected [65].

In contrast, tertiary analogs of AcCh which are lipid soluble reach the conducting membrane without any pretreatment; they are also found inside the axoplasm. Specific inhibitors of either enzyme or the receptor affect reversibly the electrical activity of the squid giant axon. Table 2 illustrates the difference between the action of tertiary and quaternary ammonium derivatives on axonal and synaptic parts of the membrane, without or with pretreatment with phospholipase A. The effects of local anesthetics and the similarity of their action on conducting and synaptic parts of the membrane has been discussed in Section IV.

Table 2. Similarities and differences between tertiary and quaternary nitrogen derivatives in their actions on axonal and synaptic parts of excitable membranes

Compound	Axon (squid)		Synapse
	Untreated	After phospholipase A	(electroplax)
a) Atropine	2×10^{-3}	3×10^{-4}	3×10^{-4}
Physostigmine	7×10^{-3}	1×10^{-3}	0.7×10^{-3}
Procaine[a]	3×10^{-3}		1×10^{-3}
Dibucaine[a]	3×10^{-5}		3×10^{-5}
b) Acetylcholine	$(\geqq 10^{-1})$	2×10^{-4}	3×10^{-6}
d-Tubocurarine	$(\geqq 10^{-2})$	3×10^{-5}	3×10^{-6}
Benzoylcholine	2×10^{-2}		1×10^{-3}

[a] Local anesthetics (analogs of acetylcholine).

Permeability barriers protecting conducting (axonal) parts of excitable membranes against the action of quaternary analogs of ammonium derivatives (but less or not at all of tertiary ones). Exposure of axons to Phospholipase A (in a few μg for a few minutes) strongly reduces the protection by the barriers. Apparently no such barriers exist at synaptic parts of many excitable membranes. The squid giant axons has been used to test the barrier-reducing effect of Phospholipase A in conducting (axonal) parts. This axon is unmyelinated; however, it is covered, as are all axons, by a layer of Schwann cells, which is in this particular axon 4000 Å thick. Schwann cells are rich in phospholipids. Reliable values for testing the effects of compounds on the synaptic parts can be obtained from the monocellular electroplax preparation. The molar concentrations of a few representative tertiary compounds are given at which impulse conduction is blocked (without depolarization) in the axons, before and after exposure to Phospholipase A. Many quaternary ammonium derivatives such as AcCh and d-tubocurarine (in the concentrations given in brackets) did not affect conduction at all. However, after exposure of the axon to phospholipase A, the concentrations of AcCh and d-tubocurarine are close to the concentration values required to block impulse transmission across the synaptic junction. (a) tertiary, (b) quaternary compounds. (Data taken from [64].)

There are a few axons where the conducting parts of the membrane are poorly protected and react directly to AcCh without any previous pretreatment: for instance, the lobster walking leg [66], and the rabbit vagus (after its connective tissue sheath has been removed) [67]. Recently a hybrid type of neuroblastoma fibres has been found in which an action potential may be produced either by electrical stimulation or by electrophoretic application of AcCh [68].

2. *The Artificially Induced Appearance of AcCh Outside Nerve Fibres.* Under physiological conditions there is no release of AcCh from the nerve terminals. The appearance in the perfusion fluid of junctions has only been demonstrated under unphysiological conditions. The observations of OTTO LOEWI [69] on the ,,*Vagusstoff*" described in the textbooks as the classical foundation of the neuro-humoral transmitter role of AcCh are only reproducible in severely deteriorated heart preparations, as was shown by ASCHER [70]. AcCh is found outside nerve fibres in many other nerve preparations, including for instance the *ganglion nodosum*, which has no synapses, when they are severely damaged [71]. It is known that OTTO LOEWI tried for more than ten years in the United States to repeat his experiments originally performed in Europe and finally abandoned his efforts. He attributed his failure to a species difference (*Rana pipiens* in the United States)[2]. But even if we disregard LOEWI's experiments, DALE and his coworkers [79] emphasized that they were unable to find any trace of AcCh in the junctional perfusion fluid *unless eserine*, a potent inhibitor of AcCh-esterase, was present. Obviously, in the presence of an inhibitor of the rapid and powerful removal mechanism of AcCh released, AcCh will escape from the membrane and appear in the surrounding gap. It should be recognized that the experiments of DALE [79] are in direct contradiction to LOEWI's interpretation of an actual release of the *Vagusstoff* (AcCh) in the absence of an inhibitor. Nevertheless, the release of AcCh from damaged nerve is still today considered as one of the basic evidence for its neurohumoral transmitter role.

In view of the insulating barriers surrounding all conducting membrane parts, AcCh appears even in the presence of eserine only

---

[2] BRUECKE in Vienna and his associates unsuccessfully tried to reproduce LOEWI's experiments using *Rana esculenta* (personal communication to D.N. in 1958).

in the perfusion fluid of junctions. However, in preparations in which AcCh may reach the conducting membrane because of incomplete protection [72], such as the axons of the walking leg of lobster, AcCh is released even in resting condition when they are kept in saline solution containing eserine [73]. This is in full agreement with the observations of LORENTE DE NÓ [71] mentioned before, who demonstrated the appearance of AcCh on several sites outside synaptic junctions. Moreover, it was shown in the 1930's that AcCh is released from the cut surfaces of axons into the surrounding fluid when they are stimulated [74—77] because at the cut axon surface there is no barrier. These findings were repeatedly confirmed and even extended to several types of nerves (see e.g., [78]).

A further experiment may be mentioned which seemed to suggest that AcCh is released on stimulation exclusively from the nerve terminals. DALE and his associates [79] reported that they were unable to find AcCh in the perfusion fluid after the motor nerve had been cut. However, McINTYRE and his associates [80] have demonstrated in very extensive and careful investigations that AcCh appears in the perfusion fluid of muscle which has been stimulated directly, even after complete degeneration of the motor nerve endings; thus there is a release of AcCh from the post- as well as the presynaptic membrane. In these studies an explanation was found for the negative results of the earlier findings: occasional failure of AcCh appearance in the perfusion fluid was found to be due to the obliteration of small blood vessels following complete denervation; therefore, the appearance of AcCh in the perfusion fluid of these muscles was sometimes prevented.

In summary, the interpretation of the original observations on which the role of AcCh as a neurohumoral transmitter were based has become untenable in the light of the facts presented.

(c) Data Supporting a Similar Role of the AcCh Cycle in Pre- and Postsynaptic Membranes. In contrast to the difficulties facing the assumption that AcCh is a neurohumoral transmitter across junctions, the evidence for a similar role of the compound in both conducting and synaptic parts of the membrane has found increasingly strong experimental support. In the 1930's knowledge of the structural aspects of synaptic junctions was extremely limited. This situation changed only in the 1960's, mainly due to the rise of electron microscopy. BARRNETT [81] was the first to demonstrate by electron microscopy combined with histochemical straining techniques that AcCh-esterase is located in *both* junctional membranes, *i.e.*, the nerve terminal and the postsynaptic membrane. This result was consistent with the conclusions based on a series of indirect biochemical data (for a summary see [11]). In the last decade both the methods of electron microscopy and of staining techniques were remarkably improved. A particularly elegant picture of the neuromuscular junction and the localization of AcCh-esterase in pre- and postsynaptic membranes is shown in Fig. 6, taken from KOELLE [53a]. Besides demonstrating the presence of AcCh-esterase in both junctional membranes, this figure illustrates the complexity of shape and structure of a junction.

The presence of an AcCh receptor and its function in the nerve terminals was first indicated by the results of MASLAND and WIGTON [82]: they found that AcCh, neostigmine and curare act in a similar way on pre- and postsynaptic membranes of the neuromuscular junction and that AcCh produces antidromic impulses. Since these experiments did not fit the current notions of neurohumoral transmission, they were completely ignored for more than a decade. But in the 1950's these observations were confirmed and greatly extended by many investigators. Today it is well recognized that nerve terminals are just as sensitive as the postsynaptic membrane to AcCh and its structural analogs (for details see *e.g.* [83, 84]). Antidromic impulses in motor nerve produced by AcCh and analogs injected into the neuromuscular junctions were recorded at the ventral roots. Thus, both AcCh-esterase and -receptor are not only present at both junctional membranes, but they function in the same way in both membranes.

K^+ Ion Efflux from Nerve Endings. COWAN [85] demonstrated a strong efflux of K^+ ions from stimulated axons. Similarly, FELDBERG and VARTIAINEN [86] found an efflux at synaptic junctions following stimulation. ECCLES [87] considered at that time these findings as evidence that K^+ ions are the transmitters carrying the impulse from the nerve terminal to the postsynaptic membrane. The question of the mechanism by which the K^+ ions are released from the nerve terminal has not been raised and could not have been answered. For many years no electrical activity could be

detected at nerve terminals. This failure was considered as strong evidence for the assumption that, in contrast to axons, transmission of impulses across junctions requires chemical transmitters. But in 1963, action potentials in nerve terminals were demonstrated by HUBBARD and SCHMIDT [88]; these findings were confirmed by KATZ and MILEDI [89]. Thus, another objection has been removed which was used as support for a fundamentally different role of AcCh in conducting and junctional parts of the membrane.

(d) Alternative Interpretation of the Function of AcCh at Junctions

1. Similarity of the Role of the AcCh Cycle in All Excitable Membranes. In view of the remarkable advances of the information about cell membranes in general and the information about the presence and function of the proteins processing AcCh in excitable membranes both in their conducting and synaptic parts in particular, a re-evaluation of the role of AcCh at synaptic junctions appears necessary. The observations on which the original hypothesis of AcCh as neurohumoral transmitter was based have found an entirely different explanation, and have made the early interpretation untenable. On the other hand, the data in the preceding paragraphs strongly support a similar role of AcCh in synaptic as well as in conducting membrane parts.

Thus, the alternative interpretation, postulated for many years, appears more satisfactory than the original hypothesis proposed: the AcCh cycle controls the ion movements across the terminal membrane in a way similar to that proposed for the conducting membrane. The signal given by the release of AcCh is greatly amplified: for 1000 molecules of AcCh released in a nerve terminal, many millions of Na^+ ions will enter the axon and an equivalent amount of K^+ ions will flow into the non-conducting gap. The amount of K^+ ions in the non-conducting gap of about 200—400 Å may easily reach the concentration required to produce the change of potential, $\Delta(\Delta\psi)$, across the postsynaptic membrane [90]. The K^+ concentration in the synaptic cleft will become high enough to induce the conformational change of the storage protein in the postsynaptic membrane leading to a release of AcCh, and thus initiate the same sequence of events as in the conducting and terminal membranes. The basic excitation units proposed for the axonal membrane are assumed to be present in the nerve terminal as well as in the post-synaptic membrane (Fig. 9).

In summary, the view presented postulates that the AcCh cycle, the basic elementary process controlling the permeability changes

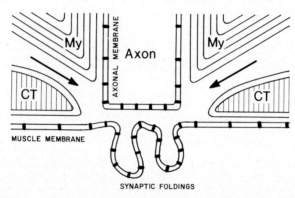

Fig. 9. Scheme of a cross section through a synaptic junction between a neuron and a muscle cell. The bars across the excitable membranes represent cross sections of the suggested basic excitation units (BEU); the density of BEU is assumed to be higher in the synaptic region than in the axonal parts. MY, membrane layers of myelin protecting the axonal membrane; CT, protective layers (*e.g.* connective tissue) of the muscle membrane. The arrows indicate the sites of relatively easy access for external application of chemicals to the excitable membranes of nerve and muscle

required for ion fluxes, is the same in the entire excitable membrane. This concept applies on the basis of experimental evidence to excitable membranes throughout the animal kingdom; it is a universal characteristic of excitability. In contrast, there is no evidence that AcCh at junctions becomes a neurohumoral transmitter across the synaptic cleft.

2. *Differences between Conduction and Transmission.* However, it must be emphasized that the view of the universal role of the AcCh cycle in nerve excitability in no way contradicts the existence of marked and important differences between conduction along axons and transmission across junctions. There are striking differences of structure, shape, organization and environment. Many of the differences in electrical parameters such as, *e.g.*, the duration of

the action potential may be attributed to such factors. Inspecting the complex shape of a neuromuscular junction (see Fig. 6), we may imagine that geometrical factors alone influence the time interval in which the different parts of the postsynaptic membrane are affected, *e.g.* by presynaptically released K^+ ions. Due to the lack of insulating barriers at most junctions, the pharmacological action of externally applied AcCh and curare is usually restricted to junctions. This apparent limitation of action may apply to most drugs.

Finally, it must be recalled that we do not know the molecular organization of cell membranes. This factor, however, may well play an important role in the differences between conduction and transmission. In the framework of our model, the Basic Excitation Unit (BEU) may not be evenly distributed; the BEU density may be greater at junctions than at axons, but at present no unequivocal quantitative data on esterase and receptor densities are available. In addition, neuroeffectors such as for instance catecholamines, developed at a later stage of evolution, may influence the elementary processes taking place at junctions. These amines may act, for instance, as modulators of the cholinergic control or on the processes in the gateways directly or indirectly. The control of the permeability changes in axonal and synaptic parts of the membrane by the AcCh cycle has been occasionally referred to as the "unified concept of transmission and conduction". This interpretation is an oversimplification and may cause serious misinterpretation. The notion of a unified role concerns exclusively the specific intramembranous control action of AcCh in junctional and axonal membrane parts. This concept is the main difference between the integral model and the hypothesis of neurohumoral transmission.

Attributing to ATP, myosin and actin a central role in the molecular events during muscular contraction does not exclude marked differences between many parameters in the contractile processes of rabbit striated and smooth muscle, or the muscles of holothuria and worms; a great variety of additional factors are involved which will strongly influence and modify the parameters observed, even if the underlying elementary process is the same.

3. Excitatory and Inhibitory Effects of Nerve Stimulation. Nerve stimulation may have excitatory and inhibitory effects. This difference is widely attributed to excitatory and inhibitory transmitters. AcCh usually initiates a series of reactions leading to increased membrane permeability causing depolarization and excitation. But in some preparations such as, for instance, in the heart, *vagus* stimulation or artificial external application of AcCh have inhibitory effects: the membrane is hyperpolarized, presumably by decreasing K^+ permeability. It has been speculated that these opposite results of stimulation, *i.e.* depolarizations and hyperpolarizations, may be attributable to different types of neurohumoral transmitters in spite of the evidence that a compound such as AcCh may have both excitatory and inhibitory effects.

However, an understanding of these seemingly opposite effects requires an understanding of the precise molecular events. We are at present very far from having this information. We do not know why AcCh usually increases, but in some cases apparently decreases Na^+ permeability or increases the permeability to Cl^- ions. Various factors such as structural organization, small changes in environment, reactions involving S-S or S-H groups of membrane proteins surrounding the gateways, may readily account for the apparently opposite effects of the same control mechanism. It should be recalled that ATP is required both for muscular contraction and for relaxation. For many years this phenomenon escaped a satisfactory interpretation until it was found that the effect is controlled by Ca^{++} ions (see *e.g.*, [91, 92]). In the case of the AcCh receptor there are S-S groups near the anionic group of the active site [93]. Reducing these S-S groups by dithiothreitol (DTT) drastically changes or modifies the effect of compounds acting on the receptor. It was found, for instance, that trimethylbenzene diazonium fluoroborate (TDF) applied to an electroplax forms a covalent bond with the receptor at or near the active site and blocks irreversibly the response to receptor activators. After exposure of the electroplax to DTT, which reduces the S-S groups in the neighborhood of the active site, TDF in 10^{-6} M becomes a potent reversible receptor activator depolarizing the membrane [94]. Similarly, hexamethonium, a curare-like reversible inhibitor of the receptor of the electroplax, becomes an activator of the receptor after exposure to DTT [95]. Thus, such a minor change as the reduction of S-S groups in the receptor protein may transform an inhibitory into an excitatory action. Before we know more about the specific molecular processes taking place in the membrane and in its proteins, the assumption of excitatory and inhibitory transmitters based simply on changes of electrical parameters or release or external application of metabolites such as amino acids, hormones etc. seems premature. On the basis of the present knowledge, there appears to be little justification for the proposal of various transmitters acting independently of the specific AcCh control mechanism (in the pre- and postsynaptic membranes).

It may be briefly mentioned in this connection that the action of some compounds such as e.g. veratridine, and of certain neurotoxins such as tetrodotoxin or batrachotoxin used in recent years to affect ion permeabilities is also still not understood in molecular terms.

VI. Concluding Remarks

One of the fundamental notions of biochemical thinking is the biochemical unity of life, a notion which has played an essential role in the development of biochemistry since the time of PASTEUR. Nature has shown little imagination in modifying chemical mechanisms associated with a given function. The specific chemical processes associated with various cellular mechanisms are remarkably similar from the most primitive cells to those in the most highly developed organisms. Thus, it appears pertinent to assume that such a specific system as the AcCh cycle is associated with the ion permeability changes during electrical activity is ubiquitous and required for all forms of bioexcitability; one of the universal and most vital characteristics of living organisms. The adaptation of the same specific system to the great diversity of the needs of a variety of organisms may be achieved by many additional factors such as changes of form and shape, structure and organization, and additional chemical factors: altogether they may modify the effects of specific chemical reactions in any way required.

Typical for chemical processes in cells is their cyclic character. This important principle was first recognized by OTTO MEYERHOF half a century ago. He found that only about one sixth of the lactic acid formed anaerobically from glycogen during muscular contraction by a series of intermediary steps is oxidized, as we know today via the citric acid cycle, but five sixths of the lactic acid formed is resynthesized during recovery to glycogen by the energy derived from the oxidation. His observations provided the basis for the explanation of the well known Pasteur effect. MEYERHOF was the first to recognize the far-reaching general implications of these findings. The series of cycles associated with most cellular functions apparently prevent unnecessary waste by minimum energy dissipation, using the excess energy for reversing most of the processes and thereby restoring the initial state with maximum efficiency. The series of cyclic processes (AcCh cycle) suggested to be associated with the control of transient changes of electrical properties and the maintenance of nerve excitability may well have a similarly essential bioenergetic function.

The integral model of excitability (see also the next article) does not claim to provide final answers; the model suggests new experiments but also leaves many questions open. J. J. Thompson once said "a theory is a tool and not a creed". A hypothesis derives its value from its ability to stimulate new experiments. The results in turn may be used for correcting, modifying or even discarding a working hypothesis. The elements on which the integral model is based may be subdivided into three categories: (i) well established biophysical and biochemical data; (ii) indirect evidence which requires further experimental support; and (iii) postulates which, however sound the reasoning may be, present a challenge for experimental tests.

But in contrast to a theory there are certain axioms, basic notions without which no field of science can develop, be it biology or physics. At the foundation of all sciences there are fundamental assumptions which cannot be further reduced but have to be accepted by an act of faith [96]. One axiom in biochemistry is that expressed by Justus von Liebig in 1846 in his ,,*Einführung in die Thierchemie*", that no manifestation of life is conceivable without molecular changes, *i.e.*, without chemical processes. A second axiom is the basic similarity of the elementary processes underlying a specific cellular mechanism. A third axiom is the paramount role of proteins, including enzymes, in all mechanisms of living cells.

References

1. Loewenstein, W. R. (Ed.): In: Biological membranes: recent progress. Ann. N. Y. Acad. Sci. **137**, 403—1048 (1966).
2. Racker, E. (Ed.): In: Membranes of mitochondria and chloroplasts, Vol. I, pp. 127—171. New York: Van Nostrand, Reinhold Co. 1970.
3. Manson, L. A. (Ed.): In: Biomembranes, Vol. I, p. 293. New York: Plenum Press 1971.

4. ROTHFIELD, L. I. (Ed.): In: Structure and function of biological membranes, p. 486. New York: Academic Press 1971.
5. ROBERTSON, J. D.: In: KATZ, B., BUTLER, J. V. A. (Eds.): Progress in biophysics, pp. 343—418. New York: Pergamon Press 1960.
6. SJOESTRAND, F. S., BARAJAS, L.: J. ultrastruct. Res. **32**, 293—306 (1970).
7. SJOESTRAND, F. S., BARAJAS, L.: J. ultrastruct. Res. **25**, 121—155 (1968).
8. TASAKI, I.: Nerve excitation. Springfield., Ill: Charles C. Thomas 1968.
9. COLE, K. S.: Physiol. Rev. **45**, 340—379 (1965).
10. NACHMANSOHN, D.: Harvey lectures 1953, 1954, pp. 57—99. New York: Academic Press 1955.
10a. NACHMANSOHN, D.: Erg. Physiol. **48**, 575—683. Berlin-Heidelberg-New York: Springer 1955.
11. NACHMANSOHN, D.: Chemical and molecular basis of nerve activity, pp. 235. New York: Academic Press 1959.
12. NACHMANSOHN, D.: Cholinesterases and anticholesterinase agents. In: KOELLE, G. B. (Ed.): Handbuch d. exp. Pharmakologie, Ergw. XV/1, pp. 701—740; Ergeb. XV/2, pp. 40—45. Berlin-Heidelberg-New York: Springer 1963.
13. NACHMANSOHN, D.: In: KAPLAN, N. O., KENNEDY, E. P. (Eds.): Current aspects of biochemical energetics: Lipmann dedicatory volume, pp. 145—172. New York: Academic Press 1966a.
14. NACHMANSOHN, D.: In: LOEWENSTEIN, W. R. (Ed.): Biological membranes: recent progress. Ann. N. Y. Acad. Sci. **137**, 877—900 (1966b).
15. NACHMANSOHN, D.: Proc. nat. Acad. Sci. (Wash.) **61**, 1034—1041 (1968).
16. NACHMANSOHN, D.: Science **168**, 1059—1066 (1970).
17. NACHMANSOHN, D.: Handbook of sensory physiology. In: LOEWENSTEIN, W. R. (Ed.): Principles of receptor physiology, Vol. I, pp. 18—102. Berlin-Heidelberg-New York: Springer 1971a.
18. NACHMANSOHN, D.: Proc. nat. Acad. Sci. (Wash.) **68**, 3170—3174 (1971b).
19. NACHMANSOHN, D.: The structure and function of muscle. In: BOURNE, G. H. (Ed.): Physiology and biochemistry, Vol. III, pp. 32—117. New York: Academic Press 1973.
20. NEUMANN, E., KATCHALSKY, A.: Proc. nat. Acad. Sci. (Wash.) **69**, 993—997 (1972).
21. NEUMANN, E., ROSENHECK, K.: J. Membrane Biol. **10**, 279—290 (1972).
22. KATCHALSKY, A. (Ed.): In: Connective tissue: intercellular macromolecules, pp. 9—41. Boston: Little, Brown and Co. 1964.
23. BRINK, F.: Pharmacol. Rev. **6**, 243—298 (1954).
24. NACHMANSOHN, D., LEDERER, E.: Bull. Soc. chim. Biol. (Paris) **21**, 797—808 (1939).
25. ROTHENBERG, M. A., NACHMANSOHN, D.: J. biol. Chem. **168**, 223—231 (1946).
26. NACHMANSOHN, D., WILSON, I. B.: Advances in enzymology. Vol. XII, pp. 259—339. New York: Interscience 1951.
27. WILSON, I. B., GINSBURG, S.: Arch. Biochem. Biophys. **54**, 569—571 (1955).

28. KEWITZ, H., WILSON, I. B., NACHMANSOHN, D.: Arch. Biochem. Biophys. **64**, 456—465 (1956).
29. LEUZINGER, W., BAKER, A. L., CAUVIN, E.: Proc. Nat. Acad. Sci. USA **59**, 620—623 (1968).
30. ROSENBERRY, T. L., CHANG, H. W., CHEN, Y. T.: J. Biol. Chem. **247**, 1555—1565 (1972).
31. SCHOFFENIELS, E., NACHMANSOHN, D.: Biochim. Biophys. Acta **26**, 1—15 (1957).
32. SCHOFFENIELS, E.: Biochim. Biophys. Acta **26**, 585—596 (1957).
33. HIGMAN, H. B., BARTELS, E.: Biochim. Biophys. Acta **54**, 543—554 (1961).
34. HIGMAN, H. B., BARTELS, E.: Biochim. Biophys. Acta **57**, 77—82 (1962).
35. HIGMAN, H. B., PODLESKI, T. R., BARTELS, E.: Biochim. Biophys. Acta **75**, 187—193 (1963).
36. HIGMAN, H. B., PODLESKI, T. R., BARTELS, E.: Biochim. Biophys. Acta **79**, 138—150 (1964).
37. WEBB, G. D.: Biochim. Biophys. Acta **102**, 172—184 (1965).
38. PODLESKI, T. R.: Doctoral Thesis, Columbia University, New York (1966).
39. PODLESKI, T. R.: Biochem. Pharmacol. **18**, 211—226 (1969).
40. PODLESKI, T. R., NACHMANSOHN, D.: Proc. Nat. Acad. Sci. USA **56**, 1034—1039 (1966).
41. PODLESKI, T. R.: Proc. Nat. Acad. Sci. USA **58**, 268—273 (1967).
42. MEUNIER, J.-C., HUCHET, M., BOQUET, P., CHANGEUX, J.-P.: C. R. Acad. Sci. Paris, Serie D **272**, 117—120 (1971).
43. OLSEN, R. W., MEUNIER, J.-C., CHANGEUX, J.-P.: FEBS Letts. **28**, 96—100 (1972).
44. SCHMIDT, J., RAFTERY, M. A.: Biochemistry **12**, 852—856 (1973).
45. KARLIN, A., COWBURN, D.: Proc. Nat. Acad. Sci. USA **70**, 3636—3640 (1973).
46. ELDEFRAWI, M. E., ELDEFRAWI, A. T.: Arch. Biochem. Biophys. **159**, 362—373 (1973).
47. CHANG, H. W.: Proc. Nat. Acad. Sci. USA **71**, 2113—2117 (1974).
48. NACHMANSOHN, D., MACHADO, A. L.: J. Neurophysiol. **6**, 397—404 (1943).
49. NACHMANSOHN, D.: Annual review of biochemistry **41**, 1—28 (1972).
50. HUSAIN, S. S., MAUTNER, H. G.: Proc. Nat. Acad. Sci. USA **70**, 3749—3753 (1973).
51. BRZIN, M., DETTBARN, W.-D.: J. Cell Biol. **32**, 577—583 (1967).
52. BRZIN, M.: Proc. Nat. Acad. Sci. USA **56**, 1560—1563 (1966).
53. CHANGEUX, J.-P., GAUTRON, J., ISRAEL, M., PODLESKI, T.: C. R. Acad. Sci. Paris, Serie D **269**, 1788—1791 (1969).
53a. KOELLE, G. B.: Ann. N. Y. Acad. Sci. **183**, 5—20 (1971).
53b. DETTBARN, W.-D.: Nature, Lond. **186**, 891—892 (1960).
53c. DETTBARN, W.-D.: Biochim. Biophys. Acta **41**, 377—386 (1960).
53d. DETTBARN, W.-D. In: Proceed. Symp. Compar. Bioelectrogenesis. C. Chagas and Paes de Carvalho, eds. Elsevier Publ. Co., p. 262—287 (1961).
54. BARTELS, E.: Biochim. Biophys. Acta **109**, 194—203 (1965).
55. BARTELS, E., NACHMANSOHN, D.: Biochem. Zeitschr. **342**, 359—374 (1965).

56. KASAI, M., CHANGEUX, J.-P.: C. R. Acad. Sci. Paris **270**, 1400—1403 (1970).
57. CHANGEUX, J.-P., PODLESKI, T. R.: Proc. Nat. Acad. Sci. USA **59**, 944—950 (1968).
58. HODGKIN, A. L., HUXLEY, A. F.: J. Physiol. **116**, 449, 473, 497, and **117**, 500 (1952).
59. ERLANGER, J.: J. Neurophysiol. **2**, 370—379 (1939).
60. FULTON, J. F.: Physiology of the nervous system. Oxford Univ. Press, New York (1938, 1943).
61. BULLOCK, T. H., NACHMANSOHN, D., ROTHENBERG, M. A.: J. Neurophysiol. **9**, 9—22 (1946).
62. ROTHENBERG, M. A., SPRINSON, D. B., NACHMANSOHN, D.: J. Neurophysiol. **11**, 111—116 (1948).
63. HOSKIN, F. C. G., ROSENBERG, P.: J. Gen. Physiol. **46**, 1117—1127 (1964).
64. ROSENBERG, P.: Mem. Inst. Butantan Simp. Internac. **33**, 477—508 (1966).
65. MARTIN, R., ROSENBERG, P.: J. Cell. Biol. **36**, 341—353 (1968).
66. DETTBARN, W-D., DAVIS, F. A.: Biochim. Biophys. Acta **66**, 397—405 (1963).
67. ARMETT, J., RITCHIE, J. M.: J. Physiol. **152**, 141—158 (1960).
68. HAMPRECHT, B.: Hoppe-Seyler's Z. Physiol. Chem. **355**, 109—110 (1974).
69. LOEWI, O.: Arch. ges. Physiol. (Pflueger's) **189**, 239—242 (1921).
70. ASCHER, L.: Arch. ges. Physiol. (Pflueger's) **210**, 689—696 (1925).
71. LORENTE DE NÓ, R.: Am. J. Physiol. **121**, 331—349 (1938).
72. DE LORENZO, A. J. D., DETTBARN, W-D., BRZIN, M.: J. Ultrastruc. Res. **24**, 367—384 (1968).
73. DETTBARN, W.-D., ROSENBERG, P.: J. Gen. Physiol. **50**, 447—460 (1966).
74. CALABRO, W.: Riv. biol. **15**, 299—320 (1933).
75. BERGAMI, G.: Atti. acad. naz Lincei, VI: **23**, 518—521 (1936a).
76. BERGAMI, G.: Boll. soc. ital. biol. sper. **11**, 275—277 (1936b).
77. BERGAMI, G., CANTONI, G., GUALTIEROTTI, T.: Arch. Ist. Biochim. ital. **8**, 267—298 (1936).
78. BRECHT, K., CORSTEN, M.: Pflügers Arch. ges. Physiol. **245**, 160—169 (1941).
79. DALE, H. H., FELDBERG, W., VOGT, M.: J. Physiol. (Lond.) **86**, 353—380 (1936).
80. McINTYRE, A. R.: In: BOVET, D., BOVET-NITTI, F., MARINI-BETTOLO, G. B. (Eds.): Curare and curare-like agents, pp. 211—218. Amsterdam: Elsevier 1959.
81. BARRNETT, R. J.: J. Cell Biol. **12**, 247—262 (1962).
82. MASLAND, R. L., WIGTON, R. S.: J. Neurophysiol. **3**, 269—275 (1940).
83. RIKER, W. F., JR., WERNER, G., ROBERTS, J., KUPERMAN, A.: Ann. N. Y. Acad. Sci. **81**, 328—344 (1959).
84. WERNER, G., KUPERMAN, A. S.: Cholinesterase and anticholinesterase agents. In: KOELLE, G. B. (Ed.): Handbuch d. exp. Pharmakologie, Ergw. XV, pp. 570—678. Berlin-Heidelberg-New York: Springer 1963.
85. COWAN, S. L.: Proc. roy. Soc. B **115**, 216—260 (1934).

86. Feldberg, W., Vartiainen, A.: J. Physiol. (Lond.) **83**, 103—128 (1934).
87. Eccles, J. C.: J. Physiol. **84**, 50—52 (1935).
88. Hubbard, J. I., Schmidt, R. F.: J. Physiol. **166**, 145—167 (1963).
89. Katz, B., Miledi, R.: Proc. Roy. Soc. B **161**, 453—482 (1965).
90. Neumann, E., Nachmansohn, D., Katchalsky, A.: Proc. nat. Acad. Sci. (Wash.) **70**, 727—731 (1973).
91. Ebashi, E., Lipmann, F.: J. Cell Biol. **14**, 389—400 (1962).
92. Hasselbach, W., Makinose, M.: Biochem. Z. **339**, 96—111 (1963).
93. Karlin, A., Winnik, M.: Proc. nat. Acad. Sci. (Wash.) **60**, 668—674 (1968).
94. Podleski, T., Meunier, J.-C., Changeux, J.-P.: Proc. nat. Acad. Sci. (Wash.) **63**, 1239—1246 (1969).
95. Karlin, A.: J. gen. Physiol. **54**, 245—264 (1969).
96. Born, M.: Natural philosophy of cause and chance. London-New York: Oxford University Press 1949.
97. Porter, K. R., Bonneville, M. A.: An Introduction to the Fine structure of cells and tissues. Philadelphia: Lea and Febiger 1964.

Towards a Molecular Model of Nerve Excitability*

EBERHARD NEUMANN**

Max-Planck-Institut für Biophysikalische Chemie, 3400 Göttingen-Nikolausberg, Postfach 968, Federal Republic of Germany

With 7 Figures

1. Introduction

Bioelectricity and excitability, universal properties of all higher organisms, are already encountered in algae and lower animals. It is, however, most convenient to study bioelectrical phenomena in specialized neuronal tissue evolved for the absorption, processing and transmission of environmental information and for the coordination and regulation of higher organismic function. Such specialized nerve tissue, particulary suited for electrophysiological studies, are the giant axons of certain squids. The coupling of biochemical events and electrical parameters in excitable membranes are readily demonstrable at most neuromuscular junctions or with the isolated electroplax of the electric eel *Electrophorus electricus*.

Although numerous experimental data have been accumulated in the various disciplines working on bioelectricity, the mechanism of nerve excitability and synaptic transmission is still an unsolved problem. Many mechanistic interpretations of nerve behavior and the various molecular and mathematical models cover only a part of the known facts, are thus selective and of only limited value. According to AGIN [1], there is no need for further (physically) unspecific mathematical models (such as for instance the Hodgkin-Huxley scheme for squid giant axons). "What is needed is a quantitative theory based on elementary physicochemical assumptions, and which is detailed enough to produce calculated membrane

---

* Financial support of the ALFRED P. SLOAN Foundation and the Stiftung Volkswagenwerk is gratefully acknowledged.

** Dedicated to the memory AHARON KATZIR-KATCHALSKY (1913—1972).

behavior identical with that observed experimentally. At the present time such a theory does not exist. Its construction will be an important advance, for like all theories its lifetime will be short, and in the process of destroying it we will learn things which are new and exciting".

The first proposal of a *physically specific* mechanism for the control of bioelectricity is due to NACHMANSOHN [2, 3]. The chemical hypothesis of NACHMANSOHN remained on a qualitative level, and until recently there was no detailed link between the numerous biochemical data on excitability and the various electrophysiological observations. A first attempt at integrating some basic data of biochemical and pharmaco-electrophysiological studies has been initiated by the late AHARON KATCHALSKY, and a first report has been recently given [4].

The present account is a further step towards a specific quantitative physico-chemical model for the control of ion flows during excitation. After an introductory survey on fundamental electrophysiological and biochemical observations, our integral model is developed and some basic electrophysiological excitation parameters are formulated in terms of specific membrane processes.

2. Problems in Biomembrane Electrochemistry

It is well known that bioelectricity and nerve excitability are electrically manifested in stationary membrane potentials and the various forms of transient potential changes such as, *e.g.*, the action potential [5, 6]. Although these electrical properties reflect membrane processes, bioelectricity and excitability are intrinsically coupled to the metabolic activity of the excitable cells. Now, inherent to all living cells is a high degree of coupling between energy and material flows. But already on the subcellular level of membranes intensive chemo-diffusional flow coupling occurs, and apparently time-independent properties reflect balance between active and passive flows of cell components.

The specific function of the excitable membrane requires the maintenance of nonequilibrium states [7]. The intrinsic nonequilibrium nature of membrane excitability is most obviously reflected in the asymmetric ion distributions across excitable membranes. These nonequilibrium distributions are metabolically mediated and maintained by "active transport" (*e.g.*, Na^+/K^+ exchange-pump). A fundamental requirement for such an active chemo-diffusional flow coupling is spatial anisotropy of the coupling medium [8], including the membrane structure [7].

Anisotropy is apparently a characteristic property of biological membranes. Furthermore, cellular membranes including nerve membranes may be physico-chemically described in terms of a layer structure. For instance, it was found that the internal layer of the axonal membrane contains proteins required for excitability. Proteolytic action on this layer causes irreversible loss of this property [9].

The membrane components of excitable membranes include ionic constituents: fixed charges (some of them may serve to facilitate locally permselective ion diffusion), mono- and divalent metal ions, especially Ca^{2+}-ions, and in particular ionic side groups of membrane proteins directly involved in the control of electric properties. Local differences in the distribution of fixed charges may create membrane regions with different permeability characteristics, and (externally induced) ionic currents may amplify either accumulation or the depletion of ions within the membrane. Structural inhomogeneity of excitable membranes may thus lead to the observed nonlinear dependencies between certain physical parameters, *e.g.* between current intensity and potential [10]. A well known example of this nonlinearity is the current rectification in resting stationary states of excitable membranes. Correspondent to current rectification, there is a straightforward dependence of the membrane potential on the logarithm of ion activities only in limited concentration ranges [11, 12]. Thus, various chemical and physical membrane parameters show the intrinsic structural and functional anisotropy of excitable membranes. This recognition reveals the approximate nature of any classical equilibrium and nonequilibrium approach to electrochemical membrane parameters on the basis of linearity, and involving the assumption of a homogeneous isotropic membrane. Since, however, details of the membrane anisotropy are not known, any exact quantitative nonequilibrium analysis of membrane processes and ion exchange currents across excitable membranes faces great difficulties for the time being.

3. Stationary Membrane Potentials

It is only in the frame of a number of partially unrealistic, simplifying assumptions that we may approximately describe the electro-chemical behavior of excitable membranes, within a limited range of physico-chemical state variables [13]. Explicitly, we use the formalism of classical irreversible thermodynamics restricted to linearity between flows and driving forces. The application of the Nernst-Planck equation to the ion flows across excitable membranes represents such a linear approximation, widely used to calculate stationary membrane potentials.

There is experimental evidence that large contributions to the resting stationary membrane potential, $\Delta \psi_r$, are attributable to ion selectivities. Indeed, it appears that excitable membranes have developed dynamic structures which are characterized by perm-selectivity for certain ion types and ion radii. This property may be described by "Nernst" terms which, however, are strictly valid only for electrochemical equilibria. These Nernst terms may be calculated by application of the Nernst-Planck equation relating the ion flow J_i to the gradient of the electrochemical potential $V \tilde{\mu}_i$ of the ion type i,

$$J_i = U_i \cdot C_i V(-\tilde{\mu}_i) \tag{1}$$

where U_i is the ionic mobility and C_i is the molar concentration. The electrochemical potential of ion i of valency Z_i is defined by

$$\tilde{\mu}_i = \mu_i^0 + RT \ln a_i + Z_i \cdot F \cdot \psi . \tag{2}$$

In Eq. (2), μ_i^0 is the standard chemical potential and a_i the thermodynamic activity which in dilute solution may be approximated by $a_i \cong C_i$; RT is the (molar) thermal energy, F is the Faraday constant, and ψ is the electrical potential.

In the frame of the linear model, the flux component $J_i(x)$ perpendicular to the membrane surfaces, at the point x within the membrane is given by

$$J_i(x) = U_i(x) \cdot C_i(x) \cdot \frac{d}{dx}(-\tilde{\mu}_i) . \tag{3}$$

Integration of Eq. (3) within the membrane boundaries ($x = 0$ and $x = d$, the membrane "thickness") in a closed form requires restrictive assumptions. Despite the experimentally suggested inhomogeneity of excitable membranes, the following approximations are used: (1) the ion mobilities are the same throughout the membrane and (2) space charge effects are negligible, so that we may assume approximate microscopic electroneutrality. Thus, $\nabla^2 \psi \cong 0$ within the membrane. The Laplace equation $\nabla^2 \psi = 0$ is equivalent to the constant field condition that usually is not an appropriate physical assumption [13, 14].

For the condition of stationarity, *i.e.* at zero net membrane current ($I_m = 0$), the uniform model treatment yields the Nernst contributions

$$(\Delta \psi_N)_{I_m = 0} = \frac{RT}{F} \sum_i \frac{t_i}{Z_i} \ln \frac{a_i^{(o)}}{a_i^{(i)}} \tag{4}$$

where t_i is the transference number representing the fraction of membrane current carried by ion type i. (The fraction t_i may vary between 0 and 1.)

Although stationary states of excitable membranes always reflect balances between active transport processes and passive "leakage" fluxes, we may safely neglect flow contributions associated with active transport as long as the time scale considered does not exceed the millisecond range.

The electrical potential difference of an excitable membrane under "resting" conditions (stationary case of $I_m = 0$) may thus be approximated

$$\Delta \psi_r = (\Delta \psi_N)_{I_m = 0}. \tag{5}$$

This relationship is useful for a limited number of practical cases.

It should be realized that the measured potential difference (measured for instance with calomel electrodes in connection with salt bridges) cannot be used to calculate the exact value for the average electric field, $\overline{E}$ across the permeation barrier of thickness d. $\overline{E}$ may be defined by

$$\overline{E} = -\frac{1}{d} \Delta \psi'. \tag{6}$$

The electrical potential difference $\Delta \psi'$ associated with the permeation barrier results from different sources. Although these sources are mutually coupled, we may formally separate the various contributions. Due to the presence of fixed charges at membrane surfaces [15] there are Donnan potentials $\Delta \psi_D^{(o)}$ and $\Delta \psi_D^{(i)}$ from the inside (i) and outside (o) interfaces between membrane and environment. Furthermore, there are interdiffusion potentials $\Delta\psi_U$ arising from differences in ionic mobilities within ion exchange domains of intramembraneous fixed charges (TASAKI, 1968). We may sum up these terms to $\Delta\psi_{DU} = \Delta\psi_D^{(o)} + \Delta\psi_D^{(i)} + \Delta\psi_U$. Thus,

$$\Delta\psi' = (\Delta\psi_N)_{I_m = 0} + \Delta\psi_{DU}. \tag{7}$$

Compared to $\Delta\psi_{DU}$, the "Nernst" contributions to $\Delta\psi'$ appear relatively large. Inserting Eqs. (4) and (7) in Eq. (6), we obtain for the average electric field in the resting stationary state:

$$(\overline{E})_{I_m = 0} = -\frac{1}{d}\left(\Delta\psi_{DU} + \frac{RT}{F}\sum_i \frac{t_i}{Z_i}\ln\frac{a_i^{(o)}}{a_i^{(i)}}\right) \tag{8}$$

Among the various ions known to contribute to $\Delta\psi$ *(in vivo)* are the metal ions Ca^{2+}, Na^+, K^+, protons, and Cl^- ions. In the resting state the value of the stationary membrane potential, $\Delta\psi_r$, is different for different cells and tissues. Distribution and density of fixed charges, ion gradients and the extent to which they contribute to $\Delta\psi_r$ differ for different excitable membranes.

Variations of the natural ionic environment lead also to alterations in the Donnan and interdiffusion terms. Since ions are an integral part of the membrane structure, for instance as counterions of fixed charges, any change in ion type and salt concentration but also variations in temperature and pressure may cause changes in the lipid phase [16] and in the conformation of membrane proteins. As a consequence of such structural changes, membrane "fluidity" and permeability properties may be considerably altered. It is known that, for instance, an increase in the external Ca^{2+} ion concentration increases the electrical resistance of excitable membranes [10].

4. Transient Changes of Membrane Properties

A central problem in bioelectricity is the question: what is the mechanism of the various transient changes of membrane parameters associated with nerve activity? Before discussing a specific physico-chemical model for the control of electrical activity, it appears necessary to recall a few fundamental electrophysiological and chemical observations on excitable membranes.

4.1 Transient Changes in $\Delta\psi$

The various transient expressions of nerve activity, such as depolarizations and hyperpolarizations of the resting stationary potential level, reflect changes of dielectric-capacitive nature, inter-diffusional ion redistributions and "activations" or "inactivations" of different gradients or changes of the extent with which these gradients contribute to the measured parameters. At constant pressure and temperature, the ion gradient contributions to $\Delta\psi$ may be modelled as variations of the t_i parameters.

(It should be realized that, in general, the actually measured parameters such as potential differences, ionic conductivity or membrane resistance may contain larger contributions from cell membranes — of glia or Schwann cells — between the excitable membrane and the measuring electrodes.)

a) Threshold Behavior. Transient changes in $\Delta\psi$ may be caused by various physical and chemical perturbations orginating from adjacent membrane regions, from adjacent excitable cells, or from external stimuli. Phenomenologically we differentiate sub- and suprathreshold responses of the excitable membrane to stimulation. Subthreshold changes are, for instance, potential changes which attenuate with time and distance from the site of perturbation; this phenomenon has been called electrotonic spread. If, however, the intensity of depolarizing stimulation exceeds a certain threshold value, a potential change is triggered that does not attenuate, but propagates as such along the entire excitable membrane. This suprathreshold response is called *regenerative* and has been termed *action potential* or *nerve impulse.*

b) Stimulus Characteristics. In order to evoke an action potential, the intensity of the stimulation has to reach the threshold with a certain minimum velocity [10]. If the external stimulus for instance is a current of gradually increasing intensity, I, the minimum slope condition for the action potential may be written

$$dI/dt \geqq (dI/dt)^{\min}. \tag{9}$$

The observation of a minimum slope condition for the generation of action potentials is of crucial importance for any mechanistic approach to excitability.

On the other hand, when rectangular current pulses are applied, there is an (absolute) minimum intensity, I_{th}, called rheobase, and a minimum time interval, Δt, of current application. It is found that the product of suprathreshold intensity and minimum duration is approximately constant. Thus, for $I \geq I_{th}$,

$$I \cdot \Delta t \simeq \text{constant.} \tag{10}$$

Equation (10) describes the well known strength-duration curve. Whereas the strength-duration product does not depend on temperature, the temperature coefficient of the rheobase ($d I_{th}/d T$ related to a temperature increase of $10°$ C) Q_{10} is generally about 2 (see e.g., [10]).

It is recalled that the value of I_{th} is history dependent. The threshold changes as a function of previous stimulus intensity and duration. Hyperpolarizing and depolarizing subthreshold prepulses also change the threshold intensity of the stimulating current. See Section 3d).

It appears that, in general, the induction of the action potential requires the *reduction* of the intrinsic membrane potential $\Delta \psi_r$ below a certain threshold value, $\Delta \psi_{th}$. This potential decrease $\Delta (\Delta \psi) = \Delta \psi_r - \Delta \psi_{th}$ is usually about 15—20 mV and has to occur in the *form of an impulse*, $\int \Delta (\psi) dt$, in which a minimum condition between membrane potential and time must be fulfilled:

$$\frac{d \Delta \psi}{dt} \geq \left(\frac{d \Delta \psi}{dt} \right)^{\min} . \tag{11}$$

The condition for the initiation of an action potential may be written

$$\Delta \psi_r - \int \left(\frac{d \Delta \psi}{dt} \right)^{\min} dt = \Delta \psi_{th}$$

or in the more general form:

$$\Delta \psi_r - \frac{1}{\Delta t} \int \Delta (\Delta \psi) \, dt \leq \Delta \psi_{th} . \tag{12}$$

The potential change $\Delta (\Delta \psi)$ is equivalent to a change in the intrinsic field, E, across the membrane of the thickness d. Thus $\Delta E = -\Delta (\Delta \psi)/d$, and with Ohm's law we have $d \cdot \Delta E = -R_m \cdot I$, where R_m is the membrane resistance.

Including Eq. (4) we may write

$$\int \Delta(\Delta \psi)\, dt = -d \int \Delta E\, dt = \int R_m \cdot I\, dt$$

$$= \frac{RT}{Z_i F} \int \Delta \ln \frac{a_i^{(o)}}{a_i^{(i)}}\, dt \,. \tag{13}$$

With Eq. (13) we see how the intrinsic membrane potential may be changed: by an (external) field (voltage or current) pulse or by an ion pulse involving those ions that determine the membrane potential [cf. Eq. (4)]. Such an ion pulse may be produced if the concentration of K^+ ions on the outside of excitable membranes is sufficiently increased within a sufficiently short time interval (impulse condition). Similarly, a pH change can cause action potentials [17].

As seen in Eq. (4), the membrane potential is dependent on temperature. Therefore, temperature (and also pressure) changes alter the stationary membrane potential in excitable membranes. Moreover, action potentials can be evoked by thermal and mechanical shocks (see, *e.g.*, [18]).

It is furthermore remarked that under natural conditions electrical depolarization produces an action potential only if the excitable membrane was kept above a certain (negative) level of polarization; in squid giant axons the minimum membrane potential is about —30 to —40 mV. This directionality of membrane polarization and the requirement of field reduction for regenerative excitation are a further manifestation of the intrinsic anisotropy of excitable membranes.

c) Propagation of Local Activity. In many excitable cells, $\Delta \psi_r$ is about —60 mV to —90 mV, where the potential of the cell interior is negative. Assuming an average membrane thickness, $d = 100$ Å, we calculate with Eq. (2) an average field intensity of approximately 60—90 kV/cm (cf., however, [19].) The field vector in the resting stationary state is directed from the outside to the inside across the membrane of the excitable cell. (It is this electric field which partially compensates the chemical potential gradient of the K^+ ions.) Any perturbation which is able to change locally the intrinsic membrane potential, *i.e.* the membrane field, will also affect adjacent parts of the membrane or even adjacent cells. If the field change remains below threshold or does not fulfil the minimum slope condition, there will be only subthreshold attenuation of this field change. A nerve impulse in its rising phase may, however, reduce the membrane field in adjacent parts to such an extent and within the required minimum time interval, that suprathreshold responses are triggered. It is recalled that electric fields represent long-range forces (decaying with distance).

d) Refractory Phases. Another important observation suggestive for the nature of bioelectricity is the refractory phenomenon. If a nerve fibre is stimulated a second time shortly after a first impulse was induced, there is either an impulse that propagates much slower or only a subthreshold change. Immediately after stimulation a fibre is *absolutely refractory*, no further impulse can be evoked. This period is followed by a *relatively refractory phase* during which the threshold potential is more positive and only a slowly propagated impulse can be induced. The various forms of history dependent behavior are also called *accomodation* or *adaption* of the fibre to preceding manipulations.

4.2 Time Constants of $\Delta \psi$ Changes

If rectangular current pulses of fixed duration but of variable amplitude and amplitude directions are locally applied to an excitable membrane, a series of local responses are obtained. Figure 1 shows schematically the time course of these local responses upon hyper- and depolarizing stimulations: subthreshold potential changes and action potential [20].

It appears that the threshold level reflects a kind of instability. When the stimulus is switched off, fluctuations either result in the action potential (path $c \rightarrow c'$) or in a return to the resting level (path $c \rightarrow c''$). If, for phase c, the stimulus of the same intensity would last longer, an action potential would develop immediately from the hump visible in the late phase of stimulation.

In view of a rather continuous transition from a subthreshold response to the action potential, the notion of a threshold in the context of an all-or-none law for the action potential becomes less rigorous.

It has been found that a large section of the time course of sub- and suprathreshold responses can be described with linear differential equations of first order. Furthermore, the time constants τ_m associated with these sections are very similar for subthreshold potential changes as well as for the initial rising phase (also called *latency;* see Fig. 1) of the action potential.

The actual values for τ_m are different for different excitable membranes and are dependent on temperature. In squid giant axons the value of τ_m at about 20° C is about 1 msec, the corre-

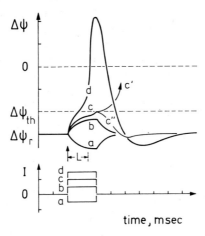

Fig. 1. Sub- and suprathreshold responses of the membrane potential, $\Delta\psi$, to stimulating rectangular current pulses of fixed duration but variable intensity, I. *a* inward current pulse causing hyperpolarization, *b* subthreshold outward current ($I < I_{\mathrm{th}}$) causing depolarization, *c* threshold outward current (I_{th}) causing either an action potential (path *c'*) or return to resting stationary potential $\Delta\psi_r$ (path *c''*), *d* suprathreshold outward pulse ($I > I_{\mathrm{th}}$) causing action potential. *L*, latency phase of the action potential; $\Delta\psi_{\mathrm{th}}$, threshold potential

sponding value for lobster giant axons is about 3 msec. The temperature coefficient ($d\tau_m^{-1}/dT$ related to a temperature increase of 10° C) Q_{10} is about 2 [10].

As outlined by COLE, a time constant in the order of milliseconds can hardly be modelled by simple electrodiffusion: an ion redistribution time of 1 msec requires the assumption of an extremely low ion mobility of 10^{-8} cm sec^{-1}/Vcm^{-1}. However, even in "sticky" ion exchange membranes, ionic mobilities are not below 10^{-6} cm sec^{-1}/V cm^{-1}. Furthermore, the temperature coefficients of simple electrodiffusion are only about 1.2—1.5.

Thus, magnitude and temperature coefficient of τ_m suggest that electrodiffusion is not rate-limiting for a large part of the ion redistributions following perturbations of the membrane field.

This conclusion is supported by various other observations. The time course of the action potential can be formally associated with a series of time constants, all of which have temperature coefficients of about 2—3 (see, e.g., [10]). The various phases of the action potential are prolonged with decreasing temperature. In the framework of the classical Hodgkin-Husley phenomenology, prolonged action potentials should correspond to larger ion movements. However, it has been recently found that in contrast to this prediction, the amount of ions actually transported during excitation decreases with decreasing temperature [21].

It thus appears that ion movements (caused by perturbations of stationary membrane states) are largely rate-limited by membrane processes. Such processes may comprise phase changes of lipid domains or conformational changes of membrane proteins. Changes of these types are usually cooperative, and temperature dependencies are particularly pronounced within the cooperative transition ranges.

Prolonged potential changes and smaller ion transport at decreased temperatures may be readily modelled, if at lower temperature configurational rearrangements of membrane components involve smaller fractions of the membrane than at higher temperature.

There is a formal resemblance between the time constant τ of a phase change or a chemical equilibrium and the RC term of an electrical circuit with resistance R and capacity C [22]. If a membrane process is associated with the thermodynamic affinity A and a rate $J_r = d\xi/dt$, where ξ is the fractional advancement of this process, we may formally define a reaction resistance $R_r = (\partial A/\partial J_r)$ and an average reaction capacity $\overline{C}_r = -(\partial A/\partial \xi)^{-1}$. The time constant is then given by $\tau = R_r \cdot \overline{C}_r$.

The time course of electrical parameters may thus be formally modelled in terms of reaction time constants for membrane processes of the type discussed above. For the chemical contribution of the observed subthreshold change in the membrane potential

$$\Delta \psi = I_m R_m \left(1 - \exp\left[-t/\tau_m\right]\right) \tag{14}$$

caused by the rectangular current pulse of the intensity I_m across the membrane resistance R_m, we have $\tau_m = R_r C_r$.

As already mentioned, the time constants for subthreshold changes and for the first rising phase of the action potential are almost the same. Furthermore, the so-called "Na$^+$-ion activation-inactivation curves (in voltage clamp experiments) for both sub-and suprathreshold conditions are similar in shape, although much different in amplitude" (PLONSEY [23]). These data strongly suggest that sub- and suprathreshold responses are essentially based on the same control mechanism; it is then most likely the molecular organization of the control system that accounts for the various types of response.

4.3 Proteins Involved in Excitation

Evidence is accumulating that proteins and protein reactions are involved in transient changes of electrical parameters during excitation. As briefly mentioned, the action of proteases finally leads to inexcitability. Many membrane parameters such as ionic permeabilities are pH-dependent. In many examples, this dependency is associated with a pK value of about 5.5 suggestive for the participation of carboxylate groups of proteins.

Sulfhydryl reagents and oxidizing agents interfere with the excitation mechanism, e.g. prolonging the duration and finally blocking the action potential [24]. The membrane of squid giant axons stain for SH groups provided the fibres had been stimulated [25]. These findings strongly suggest the participation of protein specific redox reactions in the excitation process.

Of particular interest appear the effects of ultraviolet radiation on Ranvier nodes. The spectral radiation sensitivity of the rheobase and of the fast transient inward current (normally due to Na$^+$ ions) in voltage clamp is very similar to the ultraviolet absorbance spectrum for proteins [26, 27]. The results of Fox [27] also indicate that the fast transient inward component of the action current is associated with only a small fraction of the node membrane.

The conclusions on locally limited excitation sites are supported by the results obtained with certain nerve poisons. Extremely low concentrations of tetrodotoxin reduce and finally abolish the fast inward component of voltage clamp currents (for review see [28]).

The block action of this toxin is pH dependent and is associated with a pK value of about 5.3.

It thus appears that the ionic gateways responsible for the transient inward current involve protein organizations comprising only a small membrane fraction.

4.4 Impedance and Heat Changes

a) Impedance Change. The impedance change accompanying the action potential is one of the basic observations in electro-physiological studies on excitability [10]. It is generally assumed that the impedance change reflects changes in ionic conductivities (ionic permeabilities). Figure 2 shows schematically that the conductance first rises steeply and in a second phase decays gradually towards the stationary level. In contrast to the pronounced resistance change, the membrane capacity apparently does not change during excitation [29]. This result, too, suggests that only a small fraction of the membrane is involved in the rather drastic permeability changes during excitation.

b) Heat Exchange Cycle. The action potential is accompanied by relatively large heat changes [30]. These heat changes may be

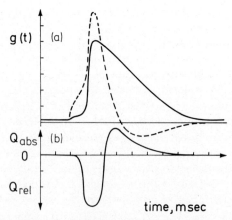

Fig. 2a and b. Schematic representation of (a) conductivity change, $g(t)$, accompanying the action potential (dashed line) and (b) heat exchange cycle. $Q_{rel'}$, heat released during rising phase and $Q_{abs'}$, heat absorbed during falling phase of the action potential

thermodynamically modelled in terms of a cyclic variation of membrane states. The complex chain of molecular events during a spike may be simplified by the sequence of state changes $A \to B \to A$, where A represents the resting stationary state and B symbolizes the transiently excited state of higher ionic permeability.

The heat changes occur under practically isothermal-isobaric conditions. If we now associate the Gibbs free energy change, ΔG, with the (overall) excitation process $A \rightleftharpoons B$, we may write

$$\Delta G = \Delta H - T \Delta S \,, \tag{15}$$

where ΔH is the reaction enthalpy (as heat exchangeable with the environment), and ΔS the reaction entropy.

More recently, it has been confirmed that the rising phase of the action potential is accompanied by heat release, Q_{rel}, while during the falling phase the heat Q_{abs} is reabsorbed [31]; see Fig. 2. In our simple A-B model, the first phase is associated with

$$\Delta G_{A \to B} = \Delta H_{A \to B} - T \Delta S_{A \to B}$$

and the second one with

$$\Delta G_{B \to A} = \Delta H_{B \to A} - T \Delta S_{B \to A} \,.$$

In general, for a cyclic process (where the original state is restored), $\oint dG = 0$ or

$$\Delta G_{A \to B} + \Delta G_{B \to A} = 0 \,.$$

In the hypothetical case of ideality (reversibility), $\Delta H = Q$ and $Q_{rel} + Q_{abs} = 0$.

Since no *natural* process occurs ideally (*i.e.* completely reversible), there are always irreversible contributions. This means a part of $\Delta G_{A \to B}$ and of $\Delta G_{B \to A}$ will dissipate into heat. We may formally split ΔG in a reversible (exchangeable) contribution ΔG^{rev} and an irreversible contribution ΔG^{irr} [32]. Thus,

$$\Delta G_{A \to B} = \Delta G^{rev}_{A \to B} + \Delta G^{irr}_{A \to B}$$

$$\Delta G_{B \to A} = \Delta G^{rev}_{B \to A} + \Delta G^{irr}_{B \to A} \,.$$

By definition $\Delta G^{irr} = - T \Delta S^{irr} \leq 0$, since the change in the inner entropy ΔS^{irr} is always larger or equal to zero (see, *e.g.*, [8]).

The measured heats are then given by

$$Q_{\text{rel}} = \Delta H_{\text{A} \to \text{B}}^{\text{rev}} + \Delta G_{\text{A} \to \text{B}}^{\text{irr}}$$
$$Q_{\text{abs}} = \Delta H_{\text{B} \to \text{A}}^{\text{rev}} + \Delta G_{\text{B} \to \text{A}}^{\text{irr}} \ .$$

Since in a cycle $\Delta H_{\text{A} \to \text{B}}^{\text{rev}} + \Delta H_{\text{B} \to \text{A}}^{\text{rev}} = 0$, we find for the "difference" between heat released and heat absorbed,

$$\Delta Q = Q_{\text{rel}} + Q_{\text{abs}} = (\Delta G_{\text{A} \to \text{B}}^{\text{irr}} + \Delta G_{\text{B} \to \text{A}}^{\text{irr}}) = -T \Delta S^{\text{irr}} \leqq 0 \ .$$

Due to irreversible contributions we have for the absolute values $|Q_{\text{rel}}| > |Q_{\text{abs}}|$ (Q_{rel} counting negative!). It is found experimentally that $|Q_{\text{abs}}| \cong 0.9 |Q_{\text{rel}}|$. As stressed by Guggenheim [33], $\Delta G^{\text{irr}} < 0$ or $\Delta S^{\text{irr}} > 0$, *only if phase changes and/or chemical reactions are involved*. Then, for our case we may write

$$\Delta Q = \Delta G^{\text{irr}} = - \sum_j A_j \xi_j < 0 \ ,$$

where A is the affinity and ξ is the extent of membrane processes j involved [32].

Since the action potential most likely involves only a small fraction of the excitable membrane, the measured heat changes Q_{rel} and Q_{abs} appear to be very large. Since, on the other hand, the mutual transition $A \to B \to A$ "readily" occurs, the value of $\Delta G (= \Delta G_{A \to B} = -\Delta G_{B \to A})$ cannot be very large. In order to compensate a large ΔH (here $\cong Q$), there must be a large value for ΔS; see Eq. (15). This means that the *entropy change associated with the membrane permeability change during excitation is also very large*.

It is, in principle, not possible to deduce from heat changes the nature of the processes involved. However, large configurational changes — equivalent to a large overall ΔS — in biological systems frequently arise from conformational changes of macromolecules or macromolecular organizations such as membranes or from chemical reactions. In certain polyelectrolytic systems, such changes even involve metastable states and irreversible transitions of domain structures [32].

The large absolute values of Q and the irreversible contribution ΔQ suggest structural changes and/or chemical reactions to be associated with the action potential. Furthermore, there are observations indicating the occurrence of metastable states and non-equilibrium transitions in excitable membranes, at least for certain perfusion conditions [6].

Summary of This Section. (1) Due to various similarities, sub- and suprathreshold responses appear to reflect a common basic mechanism (more complex than simple electro-diffusion). (2) Proteins and, in some examples, redox reactions are involved in excitation. (3) Large changes in heat and membrane resistance accompanying the action potential point to configurational re-arrangements of membrane components: phase changes, conformational transitions or chemical reactions. (4) Evidence is accumulating suggesting that excitability comprises only a small membrane fraction. (5) Many features of subthreshold responses may be analyzed as membrane relaxations to small perturbations of stationary states (tractable with linear differential equations of first oder). Suprathreshold responses are basically nonlinear and may be seen as relaxations to (locally) large perturbations of the excitable membrane.

5. The Cholinergic System and Excitability

Among the oldest known macromolecules associated with excitable membranes are some proteins of the cholinergic system. The cholinergic apparatus comprises acetylcholine (AcCh), the synthesis enzyme choline-O-acetyltransferase (ChT), acetylcholine-esterase (AcCh-E), acetylcholine-receptor (AcCh-R) and a storage site (S) for AcCh. Since details of this system are outlined by NACHMANSOHN in the previous chapter, here only a few aspects essential for our integral model of excitability are discussed.

5.1 Localization of the AcCh System

Chemical analysis has revealed that the concentration of the cholinergic system is very different for various excitable cells. For instance, squid giant axons contain much less AcCh-E (and ChT) than axons of lobster walking legs (see, *e.g.*, [34]); motor nerves are generally richer in cholinergic enzymes than sensory fibres [35].

The search for cholinergic enzymes in nerves was greatly stimulated by the observation that AcCh is released from isolated axons of various excitable cells, provided inhibitors of AcCh-E such as physostigmine (eserine) are present. This release is appreciably increased upon electric stimulation [36, 37] or when axons are exposed to higher external K^+ ion concentrations [38]. Since larger increases of external K^+ concentration depolarize excitable membranes, reduction of membrane potential appears to be a prerequisite for AcCh liberation from the storage site.

Evidence for the presence of axonal AcCh storage sites and receptors are still mainly indirect. However, direct evidence more and more accumulates for extrajunctional AcCh receptors [39]; binding studies with α-bungarotoxin (a nerve poison with a high affinity to AcCh-R) indicate the presence of receptor-like proteins in axonal membrane fragments [40].

Recently, another protein which also binds AcCh, α-bungarotoxin (and other cholinergic ligands) has been isolated by CHANG from the electric organ of *Electrophorus electricus* [75]. We recall that the receptor protein (R) may be operationally defined as the membrane component which upon binding of AcCh and other agonists causes a membrane permeability change and which upon binding of α-bungarotoxin and other antagonists prevents AcCh- (or electrically) induced permeability changes. To account for specificity and efficiency, the receptor protein should bind AcCh with a high binding constant and with a binding stoichiometry of not more than one or a few AcCh molecules per receptor protein. The other protein (called by CHANG AcCh-R II) would not match this operational definition, because it has a high binding capacity for AcCh associated with a relatively low binding constant. This protein would, however, meet the properties required for a membrane storage site for AcCh and may thus be called S-protein.

There are still discrepancies as to the presence and localization of the cholinergic system. However, the differences in the interpretations of chemico-analytical data and the results of histochemical light- and electron microscopy investigations gradually begin to resolve; there appears progressive confirmation for the early chemical data of an ubiquituous cholinergic system. For instance, AcCh-E reaction products can be made visible in the excitable membranes of more and more nerves formerly called noncholinergic (see, *e.g.*, [41]). Catalysis products of AcCh-E are demonstrated in pre- and postsynaptic parts of excitable membranes (see, *e.g.*, [41] and [42]). In a recent study, stain for the α-bungarotoxin receptor complex is visible also in presynaptic parts of axonal membranes (see Fig. 1 in [39]). These findings suggest the presence of the cholinergic system in both junctional membranes and thus render morphological support for the results of previous studies on the pre- and postsynaptic actions of AcCh and inhibitors and activators of the cholinergic system [43, 44].

5.2 The Barrier Problem

Histochemical, biophysical and biochemical and, particularly, pharmacological studies on nerve tissue face the great difficulty of an enormous morphological and chemical complexity. It is now recognized that due to various structural features not all types of nerve tissue are equally suited for certain investigations.

The excitable membranes are generally not easily accessible. The great majority of nerve membranes is covered with protective tissue layers of myelin, of Schwann- or glia cells. These protective layers insulating the excitable membrane frequently comprise structural and chemical barriers that impede the access of test compounds to the excitable membrane. In particular, the lipid-rich myelin sheaths are impervious to many quarternary ammonium compounds such as AcCh and *d*-tubocurarine (curare).

In some examples such as the frog neuro-muscular junction, externally applied AcCh or the receptor inhibitor curare have relatively easy access to the synaptic gap, whereas the excitable membranes of the motor nerve and the muscle fibre appear to be largely inaccessible. On the other hand, the cholinergic system of neuromuscular junctions of lobsters are protected against external action of these compounds, whereas the axons of the walking legs of lobster react to AcCh and curare (cf., *e.g.*, [45]).

Penetration barriers also comprise absorption of test compounds within the protective layers. Furthermore, chemical barriers in the form of hydrolytic enzymes frequently cause decomposition of test compounds before they can reach the nerve membrane. For instance, phosphoryl phosphatases in the Schwann cell layer of squid giant axons cause hydrolysis of organophosphates such as the AcCh-esterase inhibitor diisopropylfluorophosphate (DFP), and impulse conduction is blocked only at very high concentrations of DFP [46].

A very serious source of error in concentration estimates and in interpretations of pharmacological data resides in procedures that involve homogenization of lipid-rich nerve tissue (see, *e.g.*, [47]). For instance, homogenization liberates traces of inhibitors (previously applied) which despite intensive washing still adhered to the tissue. Even when the excitable membrane was not reached by the inhibitor, membrane components react with the inhibitor during homogenization [48]. Thus, block of enzyme activity observed after homogenization is not necessarily an indicator for block during electrical activity (cf. e.g., [20], p. 90).

As demonstrated in radiotracer studies, failure to interfere with bioelectricity is often concomitant with the failure of test compounds to reach the excitable membrane. Compounds like AcCh or *d*-tubocurarine (curare) act on squid giant axons only after (enzymatic) reduction of structural barriers [49]. Diffusion barriers even after partial reduction are often the reason for longer incubation times and higher concentration of test compounds as compared to less protected membrane sites.

In this context it should be mentioned that the enzyme choline-*O*-acetyltransferase, sometimes considered to be a more specific indicator of the cholinergic system, is frequently difficult to identify in tissue and is *in vitro* extremely unstable [50].

In the light of barrier and homogenization problems, it appears obvious that any statements on the absence of the cholinergic system or on the failure of blocking compounds to interfere with excitability are *only useful*, if they are based on evidence that the test compound had actually reached the nerve membrane.

5.3 Electrogenic Aspects of the AcCh System

Particularly suggestive for the bioelectric function of the cholinergic system in axons are electrical changes resulting from eserine and curare application to Ranvier nodes, where permeability barriers are less pronounced [51, 52]. Similar to the responses of certain neuromuscular junctions, eserine prolongs potential changes also at nodes; curare first reduces the amplitude of the nodal action potential and then also decreases the intensity of subthreshold potential changes in a similar way as known for frog junctions.

In all nerves the generation of action potentials is readily blocked by (easily permeating) local anesthetics such as procaine or tetracaine. Due to structural and certain functional resemblance to AcCh which is particularly pronounced for tetracaine (see Fig. 3),

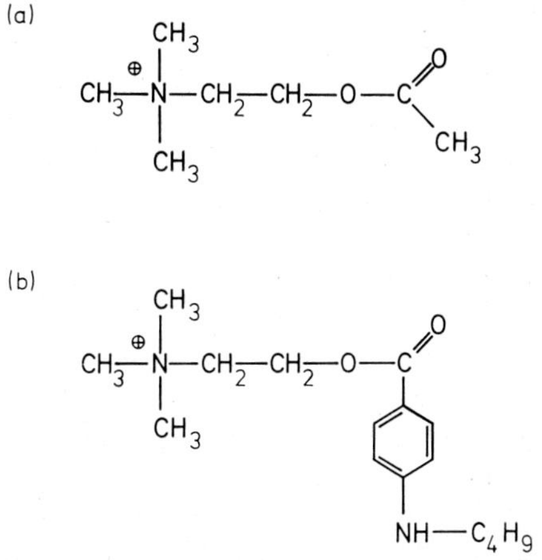

(a)

(b)

Fig. 3a and b. Chemical structure of the acetylcholine ion (a) and of the tetracaine ion (b). Note that the structural difference is restricted to the acid residue: (a) CH_3 and (b) the amino-benzoic acid residue rendering tetracaine lipid-permeable

these compounds may be considered as analogs of AcCh. In a recent study it is convincingly demonstrated how (by chemical substitution at the ester group) AcCh is successively transformed from a receptor activator (reaching junctional parts only) to the receptor inhibitor tetracaine reaching readily junctional and axonal parts of excitable membranes [53]. Local anesthetics are also readily absorbed in lipid bilayer domains of biomembranes (see for review [54]).

External application of AcCh without esterase inhibitors faces not only diffusion barriers, but esterase activity increases the local proton concentration [45]; the resulting changes in pH may contribute to changes in membrane potential.

Only very few nerve preparations appear to be suited to demonstrate a direct electrogenic action of externally applied AcCh. Diffusion barriers and differences in local concentrations of the cholinergic system may be the reason that the impulse condition for the generation of action potentials cannot be fulfilled everywhere (see Section 4.1 b). Some neuroblastoma cells produce subthreshold potential changes and action potentials upon electrical stimulation as well as upon AcCh application [55—57, see also p. 391 ff.].

There are thus, without any doubt, many pharmacological and chemical similarities between synaptic and axonal parts of excitable membranes *as far as the cholinergic system is concerned*. On the other hand, there are various differences. But it seems that these differences can be accounted for by structural and chemical factors.

As to this problem, two extreme positions of interpretation may be distinguished. On the one side more emphasis is put to the differences between axonal and junctional membranes. An extreme view considers the responses of axons to AcCh and structural analogs as a pharmacological curiosity [58, 59]; and, in general, the cholinergic nature of excitable membrane is not recognized and acknowledged. However, the presence of the cholinergic system in axons and the various similarities to synaptic behavior suggest the same basic mechanism for the cholinergic system in axonal and synaptic parts of excitable membranes.

Since until now there has been *no direct experimental evidence for* AcCh *to cross the synaptic gap*, the action of AcCh may be alternatively assumed to be restricted to the interior of the excitable membrane of junctions and axons. This assumption is based on the fact that no trace of AcCh is detectable outside the nerve unless AcCh-esterase inhibitors are present. According to this alternative hypothesis, *intramembraneous* AcCh combines with the receptor and causes permeability changes mediated by conformational changes of the AcCh receptor.

This is the basic postulate of the chemical theory of bioelectricity (NACHMANSOHN, this issue), attributing the primary events of all forms of excitability in biological organisms to the cholinergic system: in axonal conduction, for subthreshold changes (electronic spread) in axons and pre- and postsynaptic parts of excitable membranes.

In the framework of the chemical model the various types of responses, excitatory and inhibitory synaptic properties are associated with structural and chemical modifications of the *same basic mechanism involving the cholinergic system.* Participation of neuroeffectors like the catecholamines or γ-aminobutyric acid and other additional reactions within the synapse possibly give rise to the various forms of depolarizing and hyperpolarizing potential changes in postsynaptic parts of excitable membranes. The question of coupling between pre- and postsynaptic events during signal transmission cannot be answered for the time being. It is, however, suggestive to incorporate in transmission models the transient increase of the K^+ ion concentration in the synaptic gap after a presynaptic impulse.

5.4 Control Function of AcCh

It is recalled that transient potential changes such as the action potential result from permeability changes caused by proper stimulation. However, a (normally proper) stimulus does not cause an action potential if (among others) certain inhibitory analogs of the cholinergic agents such as, *e.g.*, tetracaine are present. Tetracaine also reduces the amplitudes of subthreshold potential changes; in the presence of local anesthetics, for instance procaine, mechanical compression does not evoke action potentials [18]. It thus appears that the (electrical and mechanical) stimulus does *not directly* effect sub- and suprathreshold permeability changes, suggesting preceding events involving the cholinergic system.

If the AcCh-esterase is inhibited or the amount of this enzyme is reduced by protease action, subthreshold potential changes and (postsynaptic) current flows as well as the action potential are prolonged (see, *e.g.*, [51, 52, 60]). Thus AcCh-E activity appears to play an essential role in terminating the transient permeability changes. The extremely high turnover number of this enzyme (about 1.4×10^4 AcCh molecules per sec, *i.e.*, a turnover time of 70 μsec) is compatible with a rapid removal of AcCh [61].

In summary, the various studies using activators and inhibitors of the cholinergic system indicate that both initiation and termination of the permeability changes during nerve activity are (active) processes associated with AcCh. It seems. however, possible to decouple the cholinergic control system from the ionic permeation sites or gateways. Reduction of the external Ca^{2+} ion concentration appears to cause such a decoupling; the result is an increase in potential fluctuations or even random, *i.e.* uncontrolled firing of action potentials (see, *e.g.*, [10]).

6. The Integral Model

In the previous sections, some basic electrophysiological observations and biochemical data are discussed that any adequate model for bioelectricity has to integrate. It is stressed that among the features excitability models have to reproduce are the threshold behavior, the various similarities of sub- and suprathreshold responses, stimulus characteristics and the various forms of conditioning and history-dependent behavior.

In the present account we explore some previously introduced concepts for the control of electrical membrane properties by the cholinergic system [4]. Among these fundamental concepts are (i) the notion of a basic excitation unit (BEU); (ii) the assumption of an AcCh storage site particularly sensitive to the electric field of the excitable membrane; (iii) the idea of a continuous sequential translocation of AcCh through the cholinergic proteins (AcCh-cycle). Finally, we proceed towards a formulation of various excitation parameters in terms of nonequilibrium thermodynamics.

6.1 Key Processes

In order to account for the various interdependencies between electrical and chemical parameters, it is necessary to distinguish between a minimum number of single reactions associated with excitation.

A possible formulation of some of these processes in terms of chemical reactions has been previously given [4]. The reaction scheme is briefly summarized.

1) Supply of AcCh to the membrane storage site (S), following synthesis (formally from the hydrolysis products choline and acetate)

$$S + AcCh = S(AcCh) . \qquad (16)$$

For the uptake reaction two assumptions are made: (i) the degree of AcCh association with the binding configuration S increases with increasing membrane potential (cell interior negative), (ii) the uptake rate is limited by the conformational transition from state S to $S(AcCh)$, and is slow as compared to the following translocation steps.

Vesicular storage of AcCh as indicated by WHITTAKER and coworkers [62 see also p. 515 ff.] is considered as additional storage for membrane sites of high AcCh turnover, for instance at synapses.

2) Release of AcCh from the storage from $S(AcCh)$, for instance by depolarizing stimulation

$$S(AcCh) = S' + AcCh . \tag{17}$$

Whereas $S(AcCh)$ is stabilized at large (negative) membrane fields, S' is more stable at small intensities of the membrane fields. The field-dependent onformational changes of S are assumed to gate the path of AcCh to the AcCh-receptors.

The assumptions for the dynamic behaviour of the storage translocation sequence

$$S + AcCh \underset{k_{-1}}{\overset{k_1}{\rightleftharpoons}} S(AcCh) \underset{k_{-2}}{\overset{k_2}{\rightleftharpoons}} S' + AcCh \tag{18}$$

may be summarized as follows: the rate constant, k_2, for the release step is larger than the rate constant, k_1, for the uptake, and also $k_2 \gg k_{-2}$. (See also Section 6.5.)

3) Translocation of released AcCh to the AcCh-receptor (R) and association with the Ca^{2+}-binding conformation $R(Ca^{2+})$. This association is assumed to induce a conformational change to R' that, in turn, releases Ca^{2+} ions

$$R(Ca^{2+}) + AcCh = R'(AcCh) + Ca^{2+} . \tag{19}$$

4) Release of Ca^{2+} *ions* is assumed to change structure and organization of gateway components, G. The structural change from a closed configuration, G, to an open state, G', increases the permeability for passive ion fluxes.

5) AcCh *Hydrolysis.* Translocation of AcCh from $R'(AcCh)$ to the AcCh-esterase, E, involving a conformational transition from E to E'

$$R'(AcCh) + E = E'(Ch^+, Ac^-, H^+) + R' . \tag{20}$$

The hydrolysis reaction causes the termination of the permeability change by re-uptake of Ca^{2+} ions,

$$R' + Ca^{2+} = R(Ca^{2+}) \tag{21}$$

concomitant with the relaxation of the gateway to the closed configuration, G.

Thus, the reactions (20) and (21) "close" a reaction cycle which is formally "opened" with reactions (16) and (18).

Since under physiological conditions (i.e. without esterase inhibitor) no trace of AcCh is detectable outside the excitable membrane (axonal and synaptic parts), the sequence of events modelled in the above reaction scheme is suggested to occur in a specifically organized structure of the cholinergic proteins; a structure that is intimately associated with the excitable membrane.

6.2 Basic Excitation Unit

Before proceeding towards a model for the organization of the cholinergic system, it is instructive to consider the following well known electrophysiological observations.

In a great variety of excitable cells the threshold potential change to trigger the action potential is about 20 mV. This voltage change corresponds to an energy input per charge or charged group within the membrane field of only about one kT unit of thermal energy (k Boltzmann constant; T absolute temperature) at body temperature. If only one charge or charged group would be involved, thermal motion should be able to initiate the impulse. Since random "firing" is very seldom, we have to conclude that several ions and ionic groups have to "cooperate" in a concerted way in order to cause a suprathreshold permeability change.

Furthermore, there are various electrophysiological data which suggest at least two types of gateways for ion permeation in excitable membranes (for summary see [10]): a rapidly operating ion passage normally gating passive flow of Na^+ ions (into the cell interior) and permeation sites that normally limit passive K^+ ion flow.

There are various indications such as the direction of potential change and of current flow, suggesting that the rising phase of the action potential has predominantly contributions from the "rapid gateway"; the falling phase of the overall permeability change involves larger contributions of the K^+ ion gateways (see also [63]). There is certainly coupling between the two gateway types: electrically through field changes and possibly also through Ca^{2+} ions transiently liberated from the "rapid gateways". As explicitly indicated in Eqs. (19) and (21), Ca^{2+} ion movement precedes and follows the gateway transitions. Recent electrophysiological studies on neuroblastoma cells confirm the essential role of Ca^{2+} ions in subthreshold potential changes and in the gating phase of the action potential [54].

At the present stage of our model development we associate the direct cholinergic control of permeability changes only to the rapidly operating gateway, G. As seen in Fig. 2, the rising phase of the conductance change caused by the permeability increase is rather steep. This observation, too, supports a cooperative model for the mechanism of the action potential.

The experimentally indicated functional cooperativity, together with the (experimentally suggested) locally limited excitation sites, suggest a structural anchorage in a cooperatively stabilized membrane domain.

In order to account for the various boundary conditions discussed above we have introduced the *notion of a basic excitation unit* (BEU). Such a unit is suggested to consist of a gateway G that is surrounded by the cholinergic control system. The control elements are interlocked complexes of storage (S), receptor (R) and esterase (E), and are called SRE-assemblies. These assemblies may be organized in different ways and, for various membrane types, the BEUs may comprise different numbers of SRE assemblies. As an example, the BEU schematically represented in Fig. 4 contains 6 SRE units controlling the permeation site, G.

The core of the BEU is a region of dynamically coupled membrane components with fixed charges and counter ions such as Ca^{2+} ions. Figure 4 shows that the receptors of the SRE assemblies form a ring-like array. We assume that this structure is cooperatively stabilized and, through Ca^{2+} ions, intimately associated with the gateway components. In this way the Ca^{2+}-dependent conformational dynamics of the receptors is coupled to the transition behavior of the gateway.

The receptor ring of a BEU is surrounded by the "ring" of the storage sites and (spatially separated) by the "ring" of the AcCh esterases. The interfaces between the different rings define local reaction spaces through which AcCh is exchanged and translocated.

The BEUs are assumed to be distributed over the entire excitable membrane, axonal, pre- and postsynaptic and dendritic parts; the BEU density may vary for different membrane parts. The high density of cholinergic proteins found in some examples may be due to clustering of BEUs.

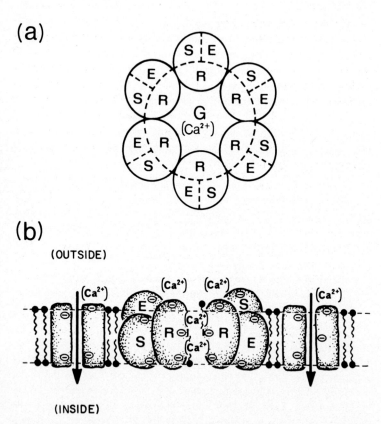

Fig. 4a and b. Scheme of the AcCh-controlled gateway, G. (a) Basic excitation unit (BEU) containing in this example 6 *SRE*-assemblies, viewed perpendicular to the membrane surface. S, AcCh storage site; R, AcCh receptor protein; E, AcCh-esterase. (b) Cross section through a BEU flanked by two units which model ion passages for K^+ ions; the arrows represent the local electrical field vectors due to partial permselectivity to K^+ ions in the resting stationary state. The minus signs, $\ominus$, symbolize negatively charged groups of membrane components

Different membrane types may not only vary in the number of *SRE* assemblies per BEU but also in the type and organization of the gateway components, thus assuring permselectivities for various ion types, particularly in synaptic parts of excitable membranes. It is only the cholinergic control system, the *SRE*-element which is assumed to be the same for all types of rapidly controlled gateways for passive ion flows.

a) Action Potential. In the framework of the integral model, the induction of an action potential is based on cooperativity between several *SRE* assemblies per BEU. In order to initiate an action potential a certain critical number of receptors, $\overline{m}^c$ per BEU, has on average to be activated within a certain critical time interval, Δt^c, (impulse condition). During this time interval at least, say 4 out of 6 *SRE* assemblies have to process AcCh in a concerted manner. Under physiological conditions only a small fraction of BEUs is required to generate and propagate the nerve impulse.

b) Subthreshold Responses. Subthreshold changes of the membrane are seen to involve only a few single *SRE* assemblies of a BEU. On the average not more than one or two *SRE* elements per BEU are assumed to contribute to the measured responses (within time intervals of the duration of Δt^c).

The (small) permeability change caused by Ca^{2+} release from the receptor thus results from only a small part of the interface between receptor and gateway components of a BEU: the ion exchanges $AcCh^+/Ca^{2+}$ and Na^+ are locally limited.

In the framework of this model, spatially and temporally attenuating electrical activity such as subthreshold axonal, postsynaptic, and dendritic potentials are the sum of spatially and temporally additive contributions resulting from the local subthreshold activity of many BEUs.

Although the permeability changes accompanying local activity are very small (as compared to those causing the action potentials), the summation over many contributions may result in large overall conductivity changes. Such changes may even occur (to a perhaps smaller extent) when the core of the gateway is blocked. It is suggested that compounds like tetrodotoxin and saxitoxin interact with the gateway core only, thus essentially not impeding subthreshold changes at the interface between receptor ring and gateway.

Influx of Ca^{2+} ions particularly through pre- and postsynaptic membranes may affect various intracellular processes leading, *e.g.*, to release of hormones, catecholamines, etc.

6.3 Translocation Flux of AcCh

As discussed before, the excitable membrane as a part of a living cell is a nonequilibrium system characterized by complex chemo-diffusional flow coupling. Although modern theoretical biology tends to regard living organisms only as quasi-stationary, with oscillations around a steady average, our integral model for the subthreshold behavior of excitable membranes is restricted to stationarity. We assume that the "living" excitable membrane (even under resting conditions) is in a state of continuous subthreshold activity (maintained either aerobically or anaerobically). However, the nonequilibrium formalism developed later on in this section can also be extended to cover non-linear behavior such as oscillations in membrane parameters.

In the frame of the integral model, continuous subthreshold activity is also reflected in a continuous sequential translocation of AcCh through the cholinergic system. The *SRE* elements comprise reaction spaces with continuous input by synthesis (ChT) and output by the virtually irreversible hydrolysis of AcCh. Input and output of the control system are thus controlled by enzyme catalysis.

a) Reaction Scheme. Since AcCh is a cation, translocation may most readily occur along negatively fixed charges, may involve concomitant anion transport or cation exchange. The reaction scheme formulated in Section 6.1 gives therefore only a rough picture. Storage, receptor and esterase represent macromolecular subunit complexes with probably several binding sites and the exact stoichiometry of the AcCh reactions is not known.

The conformationally mediated translocation of the AcCh-ion, A^+, may then be reformulated by the following sequence:

1) Storage Reaction

$$S(A^+) + C^+ = S'(C^+) + A^+ \tag{22}$$

(C^+ symbolizes a cation, $2C^+$ may be replaced by Ca^{2+}).

2) Receptor Reaction

$$A^+ + R(\text{Ca}^{2+}) = R'(A^+) + \text{Ca}^{2+}. \tag{23}$$

3) Hydrolysis Reaction

$$R'(A^+) + E = R' + E'(A^+) \rightarrow (\text{Ch}^+, \text{Ac}^-, \text{H}^+). \tag{24}$$

As already mentioned, the nucleation of the gateway transition (causing the action potential) requires the association of a critical number of A^+, $\bar{n}^c$, with the cooperative number of receptors, $\bar{m}^c$, in the Ca^{2+} binding form $R(\text{Ca}^{2+})$, within a critical time interval Δt^c. This time interval is determined by the life time of a single receptor-acetylcholine association.

Using formally $\bar{n}^c$ and m^c as stoichiometric coefficients the concerted reaction inducing gateway transition may be written:

$$\bar{n}^c A^+ + \bar{m}^c R(\text{Ca}^{2+}) = \bar{m}^c R'(\bar{n}^c A^+) + \bar{m}^c \text{Ca}^{2+}. \tag{25}$$

Storage and receptor reactions, Eqs. (22) and (23), represent gating processes preceding gateway opening ("Na^+-activation") and causing the latency phase of the action potential. The hydrolysis process causes closure of the cholinergically controlled gateway ("Na^+-inactivation"). In the course of these processes the electric field across the membrane changes, affecting all charged, dipolar, and polarizable components within the field. These field changes particularly influence the storage site and the membrane components controlling the K^+ permeation regions (see [65]). Figure 5 shows a scheme modelling the "resting" stationary state and a transient phase of the excited membrane.

The complexity of the nonlinear flow coupling underlying suprathreshold potential changes may be tractable in terms of the recently developed network thermodynamics covering inhomogeneity of the reaction space and nonlinearity [22]. An attempt at such an approach, which formally includes conformational metastability and hysteretic flow characteristics [66, 67] is in preparation [68].

b) Reaction Fluxes. For the nonequilibrium description of the translocation dynamics we may associate reaction fluxes with the translocation sequence, Eqs. (22—24).

(a) Resting stationary state

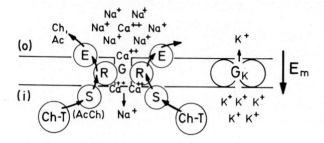

(b) Excited state

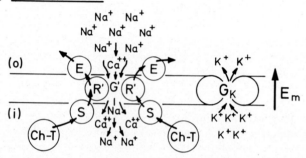

Fig. 5a and b. Schematic representation of a membrane section (a) in the "resting" stationary state and (b) in a transient phase of excitation. In (a), the majority of the acetylcholine receptors is in the Ca^{2+} ion-binding conformation R; the cholinergically controlled rapidly operating gateway is in the closed state G, and the permeability for Na^+ (and Ca^{2+}) ions is very small as compared to the permeability for K^+ ions through the slow gateway G_K. The electric field vector, E_m, pointing from the outside boundary (o) to the inside boundary (i) of the membrane is largely due to the K^+ ion gradient. In (b), most of the receptors are in the acetylcholine-binding conformation R', and the rapid gateway is in its open configuration G' (Na^+-activation phase). The change in the electric field (directed outward during the peak phase of the action potential) accompanying the transient Na^+ (and Ca^{2+}) influx causes a transient (slower) increase in the permeability of G_K, thus inducing a (delayed) transient efflux of K^+ ions. Hydrolysis of acetylcholine (AcCh) leads to relaxation of R' and G' to R and G, restoring the resting stationary state. Translocation of AcCh, occasionally in the resting stationary state and in a cooperatively increased manner after suprathreshold stimulation, through a storage site (S) of relatively large capacity, receptor and AcCh-esterase is indicated by the curved arrows. The hydrolysis products choline (Ch) and acetate (Ac) are transported through the membrane where intracellular choline-O-acetyltransferase (ChT) may resynthesize AcCh (with increased rate in the refractory phase)

1) The release flux is defined by

$$J(S) = \frac{d[\bar{n}_r]}{dt} \qquad (26)$$

where $\bar{n}_r$ is the average number of A^+ released into the reaction space between storage- and receptor ring.

2) The receptor flux including association of A^+ and conformation change of R is given by

$$J(R) = \frac{d[\bar{n}]}{dt} \qquad (27)$$

where $\bar{n}$ is the average number of A^+ associated with R.

3) The esterase (or decomposition flux) is defined by

$$J(E) = \frac{d[\bar{n}_e]}{dt} \qquad (28)$$

where $\bar{n}_e$ is the average number of A^+ processed through AcCh-esterase.

Stationary states of the cholinergic activity are characterized by constant overall flow of AcCh; neither accumulations nor depletions of locally processed AcCh occur outside the limit of fluctuations. Thus, for stationary states,

$$J(S) = J(R) = J(E) = \text{constant}. \qquad (29$$

Statistically occurring small changes in membrane properties such as the so-called *miniature end plate potentials* are interpreted to reflect amplified fluctuations in the subthreshold activity of the cholinergic system.

Oscillatory excitation behavior observed under certain conditions (see, *e.g.*, [10]) may be modelled by periodic accumulation and depletion of AcCh in the reaction spaces of the BEUs.

6.4 Field Dependence of AcCh Storage

In the simplest case, a change of the membrane potential affects the chain of translocation events already at the beginning, *i.e.* at the storage site. Indeed, the observation of AcCh release by electrical stimulation or in response to K^+-ion induced depolarization support the assumption of a field-dependent storage site for AcCh.

Denoting by $\bar{n}_b$ the amount of AcCh bound on an average to S, we may define a distribution constant for the stationary state of the storage translocation by $K = \bar{n}_b/\bar{n}_r$. This constant (similar to an equilibrium constant) is a function of temperature T, pressure p, ionic strength, I, and of the electric field, E. A field dependence of K requires that the storage translocation reaction involves ionic, dipolar, or polarizable groups.

The isothermal-isobaric field dependence of K at constant ionic strength may be expressed by the familiar relation:

$$\left(\frac{\partial \ln K}{\partial E}\right)_{p,T,I} = \frac{\Delta M}{RT} \tag{30}$$

where ΔM is the reaction moment; ΔM is (proportional to) the difference in the permanent (or induced) dipole moments of reaction products and reactants. If a polarization process is associated with a finite value of ΔM, K should be proportional to E^2 (for relatively small field intensities up to $100\ \text{kV/cm}$). Furthermore, a small perturbation of the field causes major changes in K only on the level of higher fields (see, e.g., [69]). It is therefore of interest to recall that, under physiological conditions, excitable membranes generate action potentials only above a certain (negative) potential difference.

The suggestion of a field-induced conformational change in a storage protein to release AcCh derives from recent studies on field effects in macromolecular complexes and biomembranes. It has been found that electric impulses in the intensity similar to the depolarization voltage changes for the induction of action potentials are able to cause structural changes in biopolyelectrolytes [70, 71] and permeability changes in vesicular membranes [72]. In order to explain the results, a polarization mechanism has been proposed that is based on the displacement of the counterion atmosphere of polyelectrolytes or of oligo-electrolytic domains in membrane organizations.

If the conformational dynamics of the storage site does indeed involve a polarization mechanism, we may represent the dependence of bound AcCh, $\bar{n}_b$, on the electric field of the membrane as shown in Fig. 6. Increasing membrane potential increases the amount of bound AcCh and thus also the number of AcCh ions that, after fast reduction of the membrane potential, are translocatable to the receptor.

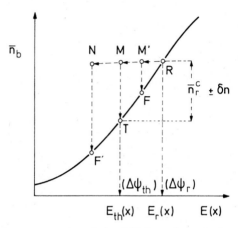

Fig. 6. Model representation of the field-dependent stationary states for AcCh storage. The mean number, $\bar{n}_b$, of AcCh ions bound to the storage site at the membrane site, x, of the release reaction, as a function of the electric field, $E(x)$, (at constant pressure, temperature and ionic strength). The intervals $M'F$, MT, and NF' correspond to the maximum number of AcCh ions released, n_r, for 3 different depolarization steps: (a) a subthreshold change from the resting state R to F, (b) a threshold step R to T, releasing the threshold or critical number n_r^c ($\pm\,\delta n$, fluctuation), and (c) a suprathreshold step R to F' with $n_r > n_r^c$

6.5 Relaxations of AcCh Translocation Fluxes

It is recalled that the receptor reaction [cf. Eqs. (23) and (25)] plays a key role in coupling the control function of AcCh with the permeability change of the gateway. Uptake of AcCh from the storage ring, conformational transition and Ca^{2+} ion release comprise a sequence of three single events. It is therefore assumed that the processing of AcCh through the receptor is slower than the preceding step of AcCh release from the storage. The receptor reaction is thus considered to be rate-limiting. Therefore, any (fast) change in the membrane field will lead to either a transient accumulation or a depletion of AcCh in the reaction space between S-ring and R-ring of a BEU.

In the case of a fast depolarization, there is first a transient increase in the storage flux $J(S)$ causing transient accumulation of AcCh in the S-R reaction space. The accumulation rate $J(A^+)$ is defined by

$$J(A^+) = \frac{d[\bar{n}_a]}{dt} = J(S) - J(R) \tag{31}$$

where the receptor flux is also considered as rate-limiting for the (fast) esterase flux $J(E)$. The number $\bar{n}_a$ of transiently accumulated AcCh is calculated by integration of Eq. (31). Recalling the definitions of the single fluxes, Eqs. (26) and (27) ,$\bar{n}_a = \bar{n}_r - \bar{n}$; after adjustment of the flux system to stationarity $\bar{n}_a = 0$.

Since flux intensities increase with increasing driving forces (see, e.g., Katchalsky [7]), $J(S)$ will increase with increasing perturbation intensity, thus causing an increase in the rate of all following processes.

It is recalled that in the framework of our integral model, the time course of changes in electrical membrane parameters such as the membrane potential is controlled by the cholinergic system and the gateway dynamics.

a) Subthreshold Relaxations. Subthreshold perturbations do not induce the gateway transitions and are considered to cause membrane changes of small extent only. The time constant, τ_m, for subthreshold relaxations of chemical contributions to membrane potential changes [see Eq. (14)] is thus equal to the time constant, τ_R, of the rate limiting receptor flux. For squid giant axons $\tau_R = \tau_m = 1$ msec, at $20°$ C.

The relaxation of $J(R)$ to a lasting subthreshold perturbation (e.g. current stimulation) is given by

$$\frac{dJ(R)}{dt} = -\frac{1}{\tau_R} (J(R) - J'(R)) \tag{32}$$

where $J'(R)$ is the stationary value of the new flux. Equivalent to Eq. (32), we have for $\bar{n}$,

$$\frac{d[\bar{n}]}{dt} = -\frac{1}{\tau_R} ([\bar{n}] - [\bar{n}]') \tag{33}$$

describing an exponential "annealing" to a new level of AcCh, $\bar{n}'$, processed through the receptor-ring.

It is evident from the reaction scheme, Eqs. (22)—(33), that the time constant τ_R is the relaxation time of a coupled reaction system. In order to demonstrate the dependencies of τ_R on various system parameters such as the local concentrations of the reaction partners, we may calculate τ_R using a few simplifying assumptions.

We recall that the release step is fast as compared to the receptor reaction. Furthermore, for subthreshold perturbations the changes in the local concentration of the metal ions is certainly small in comparison to the concentration changes of the cholinergic reaction partners (buffer-condition). We denote by s and r the single binding sites of S and R, and use the simplified reaction scheme

(1)
$$s_1(A^+) + C^+ \underset{k'_{21}}{\overset{k'_{12}}{\rightleftarrows}} s_2(C^+) + A^+,$$

(2)
$$A^+ + r_1(Ca^{2+}) \underset{k'_{32}}{\overset{k'_{23}}{\rightleftarrows}} r_2(A^+) + Ca^{2+}.$$

Due to the buffer condition, we may approximate

$$k''_{12} \cong k'_{12}[C^+] \quad \text{und} \quad k''_{32} = k'_{32}[Ca^{2+}].$$

With
$$s_1(A^+) = \bar{n}_b, \, r_2(A^+) = \bar{n} \, , \, [A^+] = [\bar{n}_r] \cong [s_2(C^+)],$$

the two reaction fluxes are:

(1)
$$j(s) = -\frac{d[\bar{n}_b]}{dt} = k''_{12}[\bar{n}_b] - k'_{21}[\bar{n}_r]^2,$$

(2)
$$j(r) = \frac{d[\bar{n}]}{dt} = k'_{23}[\bar{n}_r] [r_1(Ca^{2+})] - k''_{32}[\bar{n}].$$

Applying normal mode analysis [73], we obtain the relaxation times $\tau(s)$ and $\tau(r)$:

$$1/\tau(s) = 4k'_{21}[\bar{n}_r]' + k'_{12}[C^+]$$

$$1/\tau(r) = k'_{23}\left\{[\bar{n}_r]' + \frac{[r_1(Ca^{2+})]' \cdot (k'_{12} + k'_{23}[\bar{n}_r]')}{k'_{12} + 4k'_{21}[\bar{n}_r)'}\right\} + k'_{32}[Ca^{2+}][\bar{n}]'.$$

It is noted that the rate coefficients k' contain conformational contributions; the concentration terms are primed and represent the stationary values of the new flux conditions.

In case of strongly concerted interactions, we may approximate $\tau(s) = \tau_S$ associated with $J(S)$, and $\tau(r) = \tau_R$ associated with $J(R)$.

b) Parameters of Suprathreshold Changes. It is recalled that the induction of an action potential is associated with three critical parameters:

$$\bar{n}^c, \; \bar{m}^c, \; \Delta t^c = \tau_R .$$

For a perturbation, the intensity of which increases gradually with time, the condition $\bar{n} \geqq \bar{n}^c$ corresponding $\bar{n}_r \geqq \bar{n}_r^c$ (within a BEU) can only be realized, if the minimum slope condition leading to

$$\frac{dJ(S)}{dt} \geqq \frac{dJ(S)^{\min}}{dt}$$

and to [the equivalent expression for $J(R)$]

$$\frac{dJ(R)}{dt} \geqq \frac{dJ(R)^{\min}}{dt} \tag{34}$$

is fulfilled (see Section 4.1 b; Eqs. (9) and (11)].

For rectangular (step) perturbations the threshold conditions are:

$$J(S) = \frac{[\bar{n}_r]}{\tau_R} \geqq \frac{[\bar{n}_r^c]}{\tau_R} ,$$

$$J(R) = \frac{[\bar{n}]}{\tau_R} \geqq \frac{[\bar{n}^c]}{\tau_R} .$$

Since $J(S)$ increases with the intensity of the (step) perturbation, the time intervals $\Delta t \; (< \tau_R)$ in which $\bar{n}^c$ AcCh ions start to associate with the receptor become smaller with larger stimulus intensities. We may write this "strength-duration" relationship for suprathreshold perturbations in the form

$$J(S) \cdot \Delta t = [\bar{n}_r^c] \quad \text{and} \quad J(R) \cdot \Delta t = [\bar{n}^c] . \tag{35}$$

[Compare Eq. (10).] The time intervals Δt of the receptor activation correspond to the observed latency phases.

The expressions corresponding to the rheobase (see Section 4.1) are

$$J(S)_{\text{th}} = \frac{[\bar{n}_r^c]}{\tau_R} \quad \text{and} \quad J(R)_{\text{th}} = \frac{[\bar{n}^c]}{\tau_R} . \tag{36}$$

These equations clearly demonstrate the impulse condition [release of $\bar{n}_r \gtreqless \bar{n}_r^c$ within Δt^c, cf. Eq. (12)] for the induction of action potentials.

Since $\bar{n}_r^c$ and $\bar{n}^c$ are numbers describing functional cooperativity, the strength-duration products Eq. (35) do not depend on temperature. The fluctuations $\pm \delta n$ for $\bar{n}_r$, however, increase with increasing temperature (and may finally lead to thermal triggering of action potentials). The flux equivalents of the rheobase, Eq. (36) are reaction rates which in general are temperature dependent (having a Q_{10} coefficient of about 2).

There are further aspects of electrophysiological observations which the integral model at the present stage of development may (at least qualitatively) reproduce.

If the membrane potential is slowly reduced, subthreshold flux relaxation of the ratio $\bar{n}_b/\bar{n}_r$ may keep $\bar{n}_r$ always smaller than $\bar{n}_r^c$. Thus, corresponding to experience, slow depolarization does not (or only occasionally) evoke action potentials.

In order to match the condition $\bar{n}_r > \bar{n}_r^c$ starting from the resting potential, the depolarization has in any case to go beyond the threshold potential, where

$$\bar{n}_b(M) - \bar{n}_b(T) = \bar{n}_r^c \quad \text{(see Fig. 6)}.$$

For stationary membrane potentials $\Delta \psi < \Delta \psi_{\text{th}}$, the maximum number of AcCh-ions that can be released by fast depolarization within Δt^c is smaller than $\bar{n}_r^c$. Thus, corresponding to experience, below a certain membrane potential, near below $\Delta \psi_{\text{th}}$, no nerve impulse can be generated.

c) **Refractory Phenomena.** After the gateway transition to the open state, the receptors of the BEUs have to return to the Ca^{2+}-binding conformation $R(Ca^{2+})$ before a second impulse can be evoked [cf. Eq. (25)]. Even if $\bar{n}^c$ AcCh ions were already available, the time interval for the transition of $\bar{m}^c$ receptors is finite and causes the observed absolutely refractory phase.

Hyperpolarizing prepulses shift the stationary concentration of $\bar{n}_b$ to higher values (see Fig. 6). Due to increased "filling degree", the storage site appears to be more sensitive to potential changes (leading, among others, to the so-called "off-responses"). On the other hand, depolarizing prepulses and preceding action potentials temporarily decrease the actual value of $\bar{n}_b$, thus requiring increased stimulus intensities for the induction of action potentials.

The assumptions for the kinetic properties of the storage site mentioned in the discussion of Eq. (18) are motivated by the accommodation behavior of excitable membranes. The observation of a relatively refractory phase suggests that the uptake of AcCh into the storage form $S(A^+)$ is slow compared to the release reaction. Therefore, after several impulses there is partial "exhaustion" of the storage site. If during the (slow) refilling phase there is a new stimulation, $\bar{n}_b$ may still be lower than the stationary level. Therefore, the membrane has to be depolarized to a larger extent in order to fulfil the action potential condition $\bar{n}_r \geqq \bar{n}_r^c$.

6.6 The AcCh Control Cycle

The cyclic nature of a cholinergic permeability control in excitable membranes by processing AcCh through storage, receptor, esterase and synthetase is already indicated in a reaction scheme developed 20 years ago (see Fig. 11 of [2]). The complexity of mutual coupling between the various cycles directly or indirectly involved in the permeability control of the cholinergic gateway is schematically represented in Fig. 7. In this representation it may be readily seen that manipulations such as external application of AcCh and its inhibitory or activating analogs may interfere at *several sites* of the AcCh cycle. In particular, the analysis of pharmacological and chemical experiments faces the difficulty of this complexity.

In the previous sections it has been shown that basic parameters of electrophysiological phenomenology may be modelled in the framework of a nonequilibrium treatment of the cholinergic reaction system. The various assumptions and their motivations by experimental observations are discussed and the cholinergic reaction cycle is formulated in a chemical reaction scheme.

In conclusion, the integral model at the present level of development appears to cover all essential pharmaco-electrophysiological and biochemical data on excitable membranes. The model is expressed in specific reactions subject to further experimental investigations involving the reaction behavior of isolated membrane components as well as of membrane fragments containing these components in structure and organization.

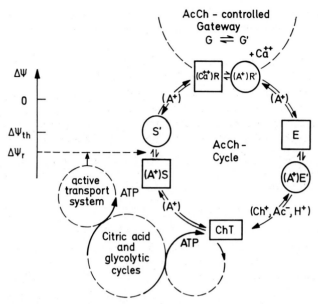

Fig. 7. Acetylcholine (AcCh)cycle, for the cyclic chemical control of stationary membrane potentials $\Delta\psi$ and transient potential changes. The binding capacity of the storage site (S) for AcCh is assumed to be dependent on the membrane potential, $\Delta\psi$, and is thereby coupled to the active transport system (and the citric acid and glycolytic cycles). The control cycle for the gateway G (Ca^{2+}-binding and closed) and G' (open) comprises the SRE assemblies (see Fig. 4) and the choline-O-acetyltransferase (ChT); ChT couples the AcCh synthesis cycle to the translocation pathway of AcCh through the SRE-assemblies. The continuous subthreshold flux of AcCh through such a subunit is maintained by the virtually irreversible hydrolysis of AcCh to choline (Ch^+), acetate (Ac^-) and protons (H^+) and by steady supply flux of AcCh to the storage from the synthesis cycle. In the resting stationary state, the membrane potential ($\Delta\psi$) reflects dynamic balance between active transport (and AcCh synthesis) and the flux of AcCh (through the control cycles surrounding the gateway) and of the various ions asymmetrically distributed across the membrane. Fluctuations in membrane potential (and exchange currents) are presumably amplified by fluctuations in the local AcCh concentrations maintained at a stationary level during the continuous translocation of AcCh through the cycle [74]

Acknowledgements

This study is based on numerous discussions with Prof. DAVID NACHMANSOHN whom I thank for the many efforts to reduce my ignorance in the biochemistry of excitable membranes. Thanks are also due to Prof. Manfred Eigen for his critical interest and generous support of this work. Finally, I would like to thank the Stiftung Volkswagenwerk for a grant.

Note Added in Proof

Recently it has been found that acetylcholine induces a conformational change in the isolated acetylcholine-receptor protein (from *Electrophorus electricus*). This configurational change controls the binding of calcium ions to the polyelectrolytic macromolecule. The kinetic analysis of this fundamentally important biochemical reaction [see Eq. (19)] results in number values for apparent rate constants and equilibrium parameters of the participating elementary processes, but also reveals the stoichiometry of the interactions between receptor, acetylcholine, and calcium ions. [Chang, H. W., Neumann, E.: Proc. Natl. Acad. Sci. USA, (in press).]

References

1. Agin, D.: Excitability phenomena in membranes. In: Rosen, R. (Ed.): Foundations of mathematical biology, pp. 253—277. New York: Academic Press 1972.
2. Nachmansohn, D.: Metabolism and function of the nerve cell. In: Harvey Lectures 1953/1954, pp. 57—99. New York: Academic Press 1955.
3. Nachmansohn, D.: Proteins in bioelectricity. Acetylcholineesterase and -receptor. In: Loewenstein, W. R. (Ed.): Handbook of sensory physiology, Vol. 1, pp. 18—102. Berlin-Heidelberg-New York: Springer 1971.
4. Neumann, E., Nachmansohn, D., Katchalsky, A.: An attempt at an integral interpretation of nerve excitability. Proc. nat. Acad. Sci. (Wash.) **70**, 727—731 (1973).
5. Hodgkin, A. L.: The conduction of the nervous impulse, Springfield, Ill.: C. C. Thomas 1964.
6. Tasaki, I.: Nerve excitation. Springfield, Ill.: C. C. Thomas 1968.
7. Katchalsky, A.: Membrane thermodynamics. In: Quarton, G. C., Melnechuk, T., Schmitt, F. O. (Eds.): The neurosciences, pp. 326—343. New York: The Rockefeller University Press 1967.
8. Prigogine, I.: Thermodynamics of irreversible processes, 3rd ed. Springfield, Ill.: Thomas Publ. 1968.
9. Tasaki, I., Singer, I.: Membrane macromolecules and nerve excitability: a physico-chemical interpretation of excitation in squid giant axons. Ann. N. Y. Acad. Sci. **137**, 793—806 (1966).
10. Cole, K. S.: In: Tobias, C. A. (Ed.): Membranes, ions, and impulses. Berkeley, Calit.: University of California Press 1968.
11. Hodgkin, A. L., Keynes, R. D.: The potassium permeability of a giant nerve fibre. J. Physiol. (Lond.) **128**, 61—88 (1955).
12. Tasaki, I., Takenada, T.: Ion fluxes and excitability in squid giant axon. In: Hoffman, J. F. (Ed.): The cellular functions of membrane transport. Englewood Cliffs, N. J.: Prentice-Hall Inc. 1964.

13. AGIN, D.: Electroneutrality and electrondiffusion in the squid axon. Proc. nat. Acad. Sci. (Wash.) **57**, 1232—1238 (1967).

14. SEGAL, J. R.: Surface charge of giant axons of squid and lobster. Biophys. J. **8**, 470—489 (1968).

15. ZELMAN, A., SHIH, H. H.: The constant field approximation: numerical evaluation for monovalent ions migrating across a homogeneous membrane. J. theor. Biol. **37**, 373—383 (1972).

16. TRÄUBLE, H., EIBL, H.: Electrostatic effects on lipid phase transitions: membrane structure and ionic environment. Proc. nat. Acad. Sci. (Wash.) **71**, 214—219 (1974).

17. TASAKI, I., SINGER, I., TAKENAKA, T.: Effects of internal and external ionic environment on excitability of squid giant axon. J. gen. Physiol. **48**, 1095—1123 (1965).

18. JULIAN, F. J., GOLDMAN, D. E.: The effects of mechanical stimulation on some electrical properties of axons. J. gen. Physiol. **46**, 197—313 (1962).

19. CARNAY, L. D., TASAKI, I.: Ion exchange properties and excitability of the squid giant axon. In: ADELMAN, W. J., JR. (Ed.): Biophysics and physiology of excitable membranes, pp. 379—422. New York: Van Nostrand Reinhold Co. 1971.

20. KATZ, B.: Nerve, muscle, and synapse. New York: McGraw-Hill 1966.

21. LANDOWNE, D.: Movement of sodium ions associated with the nerve impulse. Nature (Lond.) New Biol. **242**, 457—459 (1973).

22. OSTER, G. F., PERELSON, A. S., KATCHALSKY, A.: Network thermodynamics: dynamic modelling of biophysical systems. Quart. Rev. Biophys. **6**, 1—134 (1973).

23. PLONSEY, R.: Bioelectric phenomena. New York: McGraw-Hill 1969.

24. HUNEEUS-COX, F., FERNANDEZ, H. L., SMITH, B. H.: Effects of redox and sulfhydryl reagents on the bioelectric properties of the giant axon of the squid. Biophys. J. **6**, 675—689 (1966).

25. ROBERTSON, J. D.: The ultrastructure of synapses. In: SCHMITT, F. O. (Ed.): The neurosciences, Vol. 2, pp. 715—728. New York: The Rockefeller University Press 1970.

26. MURALT, A. V., STÄMPFLI, R.: Die photochemische Wirkung von Ultraviolettlicht auf die erregten Ranvierschen Knoten der einzelnen Nervenfaser. Helv. physiol. Acta **11**, 182—193 (1953).

27. FOX, J. M.: Veränderungen der spezifischen Ionenleitfähigkeiten der Nervenmembran durch ultraviolette Strahlung. Dissertation. Homburg-Saarbrücken: 1972.

28. EVANS, M. H.: Tetrodotoxin and saxitoxin in neurobiology. Int. Rev. Neurobiol. **15**, 83—166 (1972).

29. COLE, K. S.: Dielectric properties of living membranes. In: SNELL, F. et al. (Eds.): Physical principles of biological membranes, pp. 1—15. New York: Gordon and Breach 1970.

30. ABBOT, B. C., HILL, A. V., HOWARTH, J. V.: The positive and negative heat production associated with a single impulse. Proc. Roy. Soc. B **148**, 149—187 (1958).

31. HOWARTH, J.V., KEYNES, R.D., RITCHIE, J.M.: The origin of the initial heat associated with a single impulse in mammalian non-myelinated nerve fibres. J. Physiol. (Lond.) **194**, 745—793 (1968).
32. NEUMANN, E.: Molecular hysteresis and its cybernetic significance. Angew. Chem. (int. Edit.) **12**, 356—369 (1973).
33. GUGGENHEIM, E.A.: Thermodynamics. New York: Interscience 1949.
34. BRZIN, M., DETTBARN, W.-D., ROSENBERG, PH., NACHMANSOHN, D.: Cholinesterase activity per unit surface area of conducting membranes. J. Cell Biol. **26**, 353—364 (1965).
35. GRUBER, H., ZENKER, W.: Acetylcholinesterase: histochemical differentiation between motor and sensory nerve fibres. Brain Res. **51**, 207—214 (1973).
36. CALABRO, W.: Sulla regolazione neuro-umorale cardiaca. Riv. biol. **15**, 299—320 (1933).
37. LISSÁK, K.: Liberation of acetylcholine and adrenaline by stimulating isolated nerves. Amer. J. Physiol. **127**, 263—271 (1939).
38. DETTBARN, W.-D., ROSENBERG, PH.: Effects of ions on the efflux of acetylcholine from peripheral nerve. J. gen. Physiol. **50**, 447—460 (1966).
39. PORTER, C.W., CHIU, T.H., WIECKOWSKI, J., BARNARD, E.A.: Types and locations of cholinergic receptor-like molecules in muscle fibres. Nature (Lond.) New Biol. **241**, 3—7 (1973).
40. DENBURG, J.L., ELDEFRAWI, M.E., O'BRIEN, R.D.: Macromolecules from lobster axon membranes that bind cholinergic ligands and local anesthetics. Proc. nat. Acad. Sci. (Wash.) **69**, 177—181 (1972).
41. KOELLE, G.B.: Current concepts of synaptic structure and function. Ann. N. Y. Acad. Sci. **183**, 5—20 (1971).
42. LEWIS, P.R., SHUTE, C.C.D.: The distribution of cholinesterase in cholinergic neurons demonstrated with the electron microscope. J. Cell Sci. **1**, 381—390 (1966).
43. MASLAND, R.L., WIGTON, R.S.: Nerve activity accompanying fasciculation produced by Prostigmine. J. Neurophysiol. **3**, 269—275 (1940).
44. RIKER, W.F., JR., WERNER, G., ROBERTS, J., KUPERMAN, A.: The presynaptic element in neuromuscular transmission. Ann. N.Y. Acad. Sci. **81**, 328—344 (1959).
45. DETTBARN, W.-D.: The acetylcholine system in peripheral nerve. Ann. N.Y. Acad. Sci. **144**, 483—503 (1967).
46. HOSKIN, F.C.G., ROSENBERG, PH., BRZIN, M.: Re-examination of the effect of D.FP on electrical and cholinesterase activity of squid giant axon. Proc. nat. Acad. Sci. (Wash.) **55**, 1231—1235 (1966).
47. NACHMANSOHN, D.: Proteins of excitable membranes. J. gen. Physiol. **54**, 187—224 (1969).
48. HOSKIN, F.C.G., KREMZNER, L.T., ROSENBERG, PH.: Effects of some cholinesterase inhibitors on the squid giant axon. Biochem. Pharmacol. **18**, 1727—1737 (1969).
49. ROSENBERG, P., HOSKIN, F.C.G.: Demonstration of increased permeability as a factor in the effect of acetylcholine on the electrical activity of venomtreated axons. J. gen. Physiol. **46**, 1065—1073 (1963).

50. NACHMANSOHN, D.: Actions on axons and the evidence for the role of acetylcholine in axonal conduction. In: KOELLE, G.B. (Ed.): Cholinesterases and anticholinesterase agents. Handb. d. exp. Pharmakologie, Erg. XV, pp. 701—740. Berlin-Heidelberg-New York: Springer 1963.

51. DETTBARN, W.-D.: The effect of curare on conduction in myelinated, isolated nerve fibres of the frog. Nature (Lond.) 186, 891—892 (1960).

52. DETTBARN, W.-D.: New evidence for the role of acetylcholine in conduction. Biochim. biophys. Acta (Amst.) 41, 377—386 (1960).

53. BARTELS, E.: Relationship between acetylcholine and local anesthetics. Biochim. biophys. Acta (Amst.) 109, 194—203 (1965).

54. SEEMAN, P.: The membrane actions of anesthetics and tranquilizers. Pharmacol. Rev. 24, 583—655 (1972).

55. HARRIS, A.J., DENNIS, M.J.: Acetylcholine sensitivity and distribution on mouse neuroblastoma cells. Science 167, 1253—1255 (1970).

56. NELSON, P.G., PEACOCK, J.H., AMANO, T.: Responses of neuroblastoma cells to iontophoretically applied acetylcholine. J. Cell Physiol. 77, 353—362 (1971).

57. HAMPRECHT, B.: Cell cultures as model systems for studying the biochemistry of differentiated functions of nerve cells. Hoppe-Seylers Z. physiol. Chem. 355, 109—110 (1974).

58. ARMETT, C.J., RITCHIE, J.M.: The action of acetylcholine on conduction in mammalian non-myelinated fibres and its prevention by anti-cholinesterase. J. Physiol. (Lond.) 152, 141—158 (1960).

59. RITCHIE, J.M.: The action of acetylcholine and related drugs on mammalian non-myelinated nerve fibres. Biochem. Pharmacol. 12 (S), 3 (1963).

60. TAKEUCHI, A., TAKEUCHI, N.: Actions of transmitter substances on the neuromuscular junctions of vertebrates and invertebrates. In: KOTANI, M. (Ed.): Advan. in Biophys. 3, 45—95. Baltimore: University Park Press 1972.

61. NACHMANSOHN, D.: Chemical and molecular basis of nerve activity. New York: Academic Press 1959.

62. WHITTAKER, V.P.: The biochemistry of synaptic transmission. Naturwissenschaften 60, 281—289 (1973).

63. NEHER, E., LUX, H.D.: Rapid changes of potassium concentration at the outer surface of exposed single neurons during membrane current flow. J. gen. Physiol. 61, 385—399 (1973).

64. SPECTOR, I., KIMHI, Y., NELSON, P.G.: Tetrodotoxin and cobalt blockage of Neuroblastoma action potentials. Nature (Lond.) New Biol. 246, 124—126 (1973).

65. ADAM, G.: Theory of nerve excitation as a cooperative cation exchange in a two-dimensional lattice. In: SNELL, F., et al. (Eds.): Physical principles of biological membranes, pp. 35—64. New York: Gordon and Breach 1970.

66. KATCHALSKY, A., SPANGLER, R.: Dynamics of membrane processes. Quart. Rev. Biophys. 1, 127—175 (1968).

67. BLUMENTHAL, R., CHANGEUX, J.-P., LEFÈVRE, R.: Membrane excitability and dissipative instabilities. J. Membrane Biol. 2, 351—374 (1970).

68. RAWLINGS, P.K., NEUMANN, E.: In preparation.
69. EIGEN, M.: Dynamic aspects of information transfer and reaction control in biomolecular systems. In: QUARTON, G.C., MELNECHUK, T., SCHMITT, F.O. (Eds.): The neurosciences, pp. 130—142. New York: The Rockefeller University Press 1967.
70. NEUMANN, E., KATCHALSKY, A.: Long-lived conformation changes induced by electric impulses in biopolymers. Proc. nat. Acad. Sci. (Wash.) 69, 993—997 (1972).
71. REVZIN, A., NEUMANN, E.: Conformational changes in rRNA induced by electric impulses. Biophys. Chem. 2, 144—150 (1974).
72. NEUMANN, E., ROSENHECK, K.: Permeability changes induced by electric impulses in vesicular membranes. J. Membrane Biol. 10, 279—290 (1972).
73. EIGEN, M., DeMAEYER, L.: Relaxation methods. In: FRIESS, S.L., LEWIS, E.S., WEISSBERGER, A. (Eds.): Technique of organic chemistry, Vol. 8, p. 895. New York: Interscience Publ. Inc. 1963.
74. NEUMANN, E., NACHMANSOHN, D.: In: MANSON, L. (Ed.): Biomembranes, Vol. 7. London. New York: Academic Press 1974.
75. CHANG, HAI WON: Purification and characterization of acetylcholine receptor-I from electrophorus electricus. Proc. nat. Acad. Sci. (Wash.) 71, 2113—2117 (1974).

Discussion

H. STIEVE (Jülich): This is a very potent model — which reminds me in some respects of ADAM's model — but I was unable to grasp so many details in the short time. Therefore I would like to ask you: Can you derive from your model critical experiments which can verify or disprove essential parts of the model?

E. NEUMANN: ADAM's molecular model for excitation does not specify the protein matrix on which ion exchange is assumed to take place upon depolarization; furthermore, the experimental data on the various inhibitors such as curare or physostigmine that interfere with electrical activity not only of synaptic junctions but also of axons (provided these structural analogs of AcCh can reach the excitable membrane) are not taken into account. Thus the elegant model of ADAM covers only part of experimental observations on axonal excitation.

I recall that our integral model is suggested by experimental facts, direct and partially indirect biochemical and pharmaco-electrophysiological data. These experimental results have been correlated and modelled in a specific reaction scheme for the initiation and termination of the excitation process. If it turns out that the *in vitro* measured thermodynamic and kinetic parameters associated with the reaction scheme are beyond reasonable values (*e.g.* compared to the rate of increase and decrease of the ion flows during excitation), then our model has to be modified. Thus the specific reaction scheme itself suggests critical experiments.

V. P. WHITTAKER (Göttingen): How essential is it that the coupling provided by the acetylcholine cycle in your scheme should in fact involve acetylcholine ? It seems to me that it could just as easily involve some other substance, for example ATP, that is a ubiquitous neuronal constituent, or be a hypothetical substance X. I am sure you must be aware of the vast amount of work, showing that some neurons contain the compounds of the cholinergic system and others do not. This has been shown very elegantly, for example, in the lobster by KRAVITZ [HALL, Z. W., BOWNDS, M. O., KRAVITZ, E. A.: J. Cell. Biol. **46**, 290—299 (1970)] where individual neurons can be indentified as having excitatory or inhibitory motor function or sensory function.

E. NEUMANN: The specific reaction scheme and the flux expressions are formulated using symbols; symbols, of course, may represent anything, also ATP or even a hypothetical substance X. There are, however, at present no experimental data suggesting an ATP-control for the transiently increased ion flows during excitation. Secondly, the field of excitation theories would not need any further unspecific model involving an unspecific substance X (see AGIN, 1972).

I would like to recall again that the specific reaction scheme of our integral model is suggested by direct and partially indirect experimental observations: for instance, AcCh release from axonal and other non-synaptic parts of excitable membranes upon depolarization in the presence of eserine, interference of inhibitory structural analogs of AcCh with electrical *etc.*, as discussed in my paper.

The question of the absence of cholinergic compounds in some nerves is a controversial problem which is not finally decided. There is, however, growing evidence confirming early analytical-chemical data on an ubiquitous presence of cholinergic compounds in nervous tissue. In the light of refined techniques, more and more nerves and synapses formally called non-cholinergic (an interpretation mainly derived from histochemical attempts using light microscopy) "unexpectedly contain cholinergic compounds".

See, *e.g.* KOELLE, G. B.: Ann. N. Y. Acad. Sci. **183**, 5—20 (1971); KASA, P., MANN, S. P., HEBB, C.: Nature (Lond.) **226**, 812 (1970); GRUBER, H., ZENKER, W.: Brain Res. **51**, 207—214 (1973).

Recent developments show that some old methods were not suited to detect, for instance, low concentrations of the enzyme choline-O-acetyltransferade [see, *e.g.*, KASA et al.: Nature (Lond.) **226**, 812 (1970); HAMPRECHT, B., AMANO, T.: Analyt. Biochem. **57**, 162—172 (1974)]. Furthermore, analytical methods involving lipid-rich tissue frequently suffer from homogenization artefacts [see *e.g.*, NACHMANSOHN, D.: Handbook of sensory physiology, Vol. 1, pp. 18—102. Berlin-Heidelberg-New York: Springer 1971, and references cited therein]. Of particular importance is that choline-O-acetyltransferase isolated in solution and in tissue slices is very unstable. The analytical chemistry and histochemistry of this enzyme (the *in vivo* concentration of which is sometimes very low) requires extremely sensitive detection methods and careful experimental skill.

D. NACHMANSOHN: Dr. WHITTAKER, may I first comment on your second remark. Chemical-analytical investigations, performed over a period of four decades, using tissue from the lowest phyla up to the highest of neurons, demonstrate the presence of two cholinergic proteins: a special type of esterase referred to as AcCh-esterase and choline-*O*-acetyltransferase. It is remarkable that so far no exception was found (for summaries see NACHMAN-SOHN, 1959, 1963). Moreover, indirect biochemical evidence suggested that AcCh-esterase is localized at or near the surface of axons (see, *e.g.* NACHMAN-SOHN and MEYERHOF, 1940); at that time membranes were not yet visualized by electron microscopy. Numerous reports appeared particularly in the 1950's, which claimed that AcCh-esterase is absent in many excitable cells (see, *e.g.*, KOELLE, 1963). These statements were based on staining techniques with the use of the light microscope. In the specimen slices used in these techniques, the thickness of nerve covering tissue layers may prevent the access of the added substrate (acetylthiocholine) to the enzyme. The absence of staining outside the junction was for more than a decade the only evidence for the assumption that in muscle fibres the enzyme is located exclusively at the motor end plate. In some tissues, in which the enzyme concentration was extremely high when chemical methods were used, the enzyme appeared to be hardly visible or even absent when staining techniques were applied. Even in certain electric organs, no AcCh-esterase was detected. All these reports were in sharp contrast to the results obtained with chemical methods demonstrating the presence of AcCh-esterase in all types of excitable fibres from the lowest to the highest forms of life.

When later in the 1960's staining techniques were applied in combination with electron microscopy, the situation changed drastically. The enzyme was found to be closely associated with the excitable membranes in the conducting parts as well as in the two junctional membranes, those of the nerve terminal and of the postsynaptic membrane. [For further details see also the text of my lecture.]

Now, your first question. I may remind you that ATP has a turnover time several orders of magnitude too small for a rapid control of electrical activity. AcCh-esterase, however, is an enzyme with one of highest known turnover numbers. The chemical theory proposing a cholinergic control of bioelectricity is *not* based purely on the ubiquitous presence of AcCh-esterase, but rather on the inseparability of electrical activity and proper function of AcCh-receptor and AcCh-esterase.

I. OSTROWSKI (Frankfurt/M.): Kann eine sehr rasch erfolgende Ester-hydrolyse als Stimulus für die Erzeugung eines Aktionspotentials fungieren ?

E. NEUMANN: Es gibt meines Wissens noch keine experimentelle Evidenz für diesen Vorschlag. Es ist jedoch bekannt, daß eine geringfügige *Verkleine-rung* der Protonenkonzentration in der Perfusionsflüssigkeit perfundierter Tintenfisch-Axonen zur Auslösung von Aktionspotentialen führen kann [TASAKI, I., SINGER, I., TAKENADA, T.: J. gen. Physiol. 48, 1095—1123 (1965)]. Andererseits depolarisieren gewisse Axonen des Hummers langsam bei etwa pH 2, erzeugt durch Hydrolyse von AcCh, das in hohen Konzentrationen (etwa 0.01 M) in Abwesenheit von Esteraseinhibitoren von außen appliziert wurde [DETTBARN, W.-D., BARTELS, E.: Biochem. Pharm. **17**, 1833 (1968)]. Bisher gibt es noch keinen Beweis für das *in vivo*-Auftreten derart hoher Konzentrationen von freiem AcCh.

W. GUDER (München): Since I have no information about nerves, I would like to ask a question with regard to the cycle in axons. You have shown that AcCh-esterase is there, but how do you think AcCh is resynthesized in that membrane, because I haven't seen any mitochondria. Where do you think that the ATP comes from in the membrane of the nerves?

E. NEUMANN: I would like to draw your attention to ultrastructural studies of squid giant fibers by G.M. and R.VILLEGAS, J. gen. Physiol., **51**, 44s—60s (1968). Electronmicrographs of sections of giant axons (*e.g.* stellar nerve of the squid *Dosidicus gigas*) not only demonstrate thick Schwann cell layers covered by a basement membrane (impervious to many chemical compounds), but also show large cistern of the endoplasmatic reticulum and many mitochondria. The authors explicitly state that the peripheral axoplasma (close to the excitable membrane) shows about 40 mitochondria per 100 μm^2. In this context it is of interest that electrical activity of squid giant axons can be maintained aerobically or anaerobically for several hours, even if about 90% of the axoplasma is extruded. It has been shown that the envelope of 10% axoplasma adjacent to the excitable membrane is associated with high glycolytic activity, providing about 80% of the total axoplasmic ATP production [HOSKIN, F.C.G.: Nature (Lond.) **210**, 856—857 (1966)].

W. HASSELBACH (Heidelberg): Can you explain the observed heat changes during excitation quantitatively with your model? How large is the contribution of the heat of hydrolysis?

E. NEUMANN: The heat changes accompanying the action potential reflect contributions of very many single events, among them the heat of AcCh-hydrolysis. An answer to your question would require the measurement of heat for all single reactions occurring in a specific structure and membrane organization. This is a task that, at the present stage of technology, is not solvable. The integral model does, however, give a (qualitative) explanation for the cyclic release and uptake of heat during the action potential, as well as for the (small) fraction of heat not reabsorbed. [See the text of the lecture.]

D. NACHMANSOHN: Dr. HASSELBACH, I am surprised about your question whether the integral model is able to explain *quantitatively* the observed heat changes during excitation. You are working on problems of muscular contraction on which I, too, worked in MEYERHOF's laboratory. In discussing the heat changes observed during muscular contraction and relaxation, HILL has stressed for many decades that the heat changes are the result of many chemical reactions, and that thermodynamics cannot supply explanations about any specific chemical mechanism. It is even impossible, as was pointed out by ROSSI-FANELLI, ANTONINI and WYMAN a few years ago when they measured heat changes of a single component in solution (hemoglobin), to provide a precise answer for the contributions of enthalpy and entropy changes. All the more it is impossible to analyse the heat changes observed in a complex structure and to contribute them to specific chemical reactions, since there are a great number of reactions going on simultaneously.

As to the heat of hydrolysis of AcCh-esterase, this is a reaction which definitely has nothing to do with the supply of energy for electrical activity, since the action of the enzyme is a recovery process permitting the AcCh-receptor to return to its resting condition and thus reestablish the barrier for ion movements, taking place during activity. The question of the results of the heat changes during electrical activity is just as complex as that during muscular activity: the process is associated with a whole series of reactions going on simultaneously. The question has been repeatedly discussed, most recently in an article of mine in a Handbook on muscle [NACHMANSOHN, D.: In: BOURNE, G. H. (Ed.): The structure and function of muscle, Vol. III, pp. 32—117. New York: Academic Press 1973].

Aspects of the Biochemistry of Cholinergic Transmission in *Torpedo* and *Loligo*

V. P. WHITTAKER

Abteilung für Neurochemie, Max-Planck-Institut für biophysikalische Chemie, 34 Göttingen, Postfach 968, Federal Republic of Germany

With 7 Figures

Introduction

Our knowledge of the biochemistry of adrenergic transmission has been greatly aided by the study of the mammalian adrenal medulla. The cells of this tissue are embryologically derived from nervous tissue and contain numerous granules, $0.2-0.5$ μm diameter, which may be regarded as hypertrophied noradrenergic synaptic vesicles. These granules are readily isolated by subcellular fractionation and their composition has been studied in some detail [1]. They are known to contain large amounts of adrenaline and some noradrenaline, sequestered within a lipoprotein membrane along with a number of soluble acidic proteins (the main component of which is known as chromogranin A) and appreciable amounts of ATP. The stoichiometry has been worked out in some detail: the molar ratios chromogranin: catecholamine: ATP are about $1:200:50$. A detailed description of the structure of the granule core and a knowledge of the physical forces involved is, however, still lacking. Synaptic vesicles isolated from noradrenergic nerves have a generally similar composition and their main core protein is immunochemically identical with chromogranin.

By contrast, no such convenient model of the cholinergic neuron exists among mammalian tissues. In spite of the functional importance of cholinergic neurons in the mammalian nervous system, in all mammalian tissues cholinergic neurons are either heavily outnumbered by non-cholinergic or constitute only a very small proportion by weight of the total tissue, so that biochemical

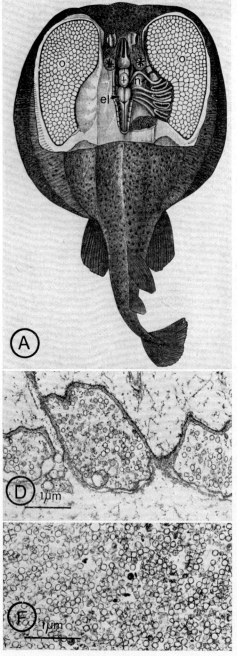

Fig. 1 A, D, F

Fig. 1. (A) Drawing of *Torpedo marmorata* showing (el) electric lobes containing the cells of origin of cholinergic electromotor neurons, (n) electromotor nerve trunks, (o) electric organ. (B and C) Light microscopic cross-section of electric lobes showing (cb) cell bodies and (a) axons of the electromotor neurons: in (C) the somata of these neurons have shrunk revealing the absence of axosomatic contacts; note also the numerous small glial nuclei (arrows). (D) Electron-microscopic cross-section of an electrocyte showing nerve terminals. (E) Fraction enriched in cell bodies of electromotor nerves isolated by tissue fractionation techniques. (F) Fraction enriched in synaptic vesicles prepared by centrifugation in a zonal rotor as shown in Fig. 2. (G) Isolated glial nuclei of similar type to those marked by arrows in (C). Electron micrographs are by H. ZIMMERMANN; histology is by K. WÄCHTLER; (A) and (B) are from FRITSCH [13] retouched

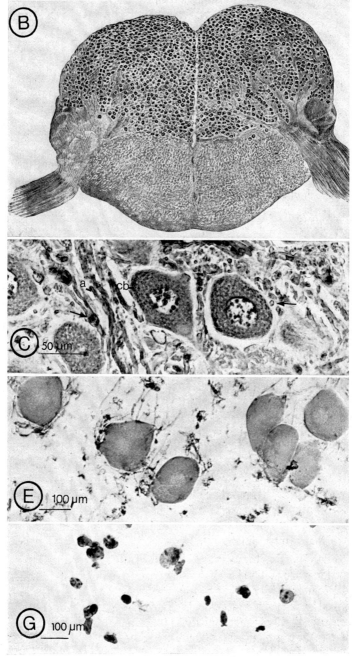

Fig. 1 B, C, E, G

work is severely hampered. We have therefore turned our attention [2, 3] to lower forms, in which the concentration of cholinergic neurons is often far higher than it is in mammals.

The Cholinergic Electromotor System of *Torpedo*

Torpedine fish are elasmobranchs related to the rays and sharks which are characterized by the possession, on each side of the flattened head, of large lobes of electric tissue. The tissue consists of vertical stacks of flattened electroplaque cells (electrocytes) close-packed in a honeycomb pattern, each of which receives a copious cholinergic innervation on its under side. When acetylcholine is released from the nerve terminals, it generates a postsynaptic potential analogous to the end-plate potential in muscle [4] (from which the electrocytes are, indeed, embryologically derived); such potentials sum, during synchronous nerve activity, to generate sizeable electrical discharges which are sufficient to stun prey and frighten away predators. The cholinergic nature of the transmission is well established [5] and the organ contains up to 1000 times more nerve elements than mammalian muscle per unit weight.

The neurons supplying the organ (Fig. 1A—D) comprise a remarkable source of cholinergic nerve tissue all parts of which — cell bodies, axons and nerve terminals — are readily accessible for physiological and biochemical experimentation. The cell bodies of the electromotor neurons (Fig. 1B and C) are extremely large (diam. ~ 120 µm) and contain large clear nuclei (diam. ~ 20 µm) with a single nucleolus. They are packed together in the paired electric lobes which lie on the brain stem just behind the cerebellum and are readily recognized by their yellow color. These cells have few dendrites. They are fired by the command nucleus in the subjacent brain stem by an input which is exclusively axodendritic; there appear to be no recurrent collaterals, interneurons or axosomatic nerve terminals.

The electromotor neurons have axons (Fig. 1A) which run in four large nerve trunks bilaterally between the gill arches to the electric organ, where they ramify profusely. Practically the entire ventral surface of the electrocyte is covered by terminals (Fig. 1D). These are similar in morphology to terminals elsewhere except that their vesicles are larger (~ 90 nm).

The Optic Ganglia of *Loligo*

The cephalopods have the most highly developed nervous system of any invertebrate and show a capacity for learning, visual and tactile pattern recognition and sophisticated behavior superior to many vertebrates [6, 7]. Their nervous systems, especially the optic lobes which receive the primary input from the large and well developed eyes, have long been recognized as being among the richest in acetylcholine of any nervous tissue and, indeed, the first unequivocal identification of acetylcholine as a constituent of nervous tissue was made using octopus brain [8]. The optic ganglia of squid (*Loligo pealei* and *L. forbesi*), for example, weigh over 1 g and contain up to 2000 nmoles of acetylcholine/g of tissue — over 100 times the level found in guinea pig cortex.

Other nervous systems with high acetylcholine levels are those of arthropods, especially insects and lobstes. However, we have found *Loligo*, especially, to be the best for biochemical studies: arthropod tissue is present in much smaller amounts in each specimen so that more specimens must be dissected; owing to the hard chitinous carapace dissection is difficult, and the ganglia (especially in the lobster) are often invested with tough connective tissue.

Results with *Torpedo*

Cell Bodies and Nuclei

The abundance of large-sized and uniform cholinergic cell bodies in the electric lobe of *Torpedo* provides a unique opportunity to isolate such cell bodies in quantity, using the techniques of tissue fractionation which have been applied recently with varying degrees of success to the separation of neuronal and glial cells from mammalian brain [9—12]. In recent work with L. FIORE, we have succeeded in obtaining a remarkably pure preparation of cell bodies of electromotor neurons (Fig. 1 E) by submitting the electric lobe tissue to hand homogenization in 1.8 M sucrose in a small glass Potter-Elvehjem mortar with a loosely fitting Teflon pestle (difference in diameters, 3%) or to chopping followed by suspension in 1.8 M sucrose and dispersion by gentle pressure through nylon bolting: the dispersion is layered onto 2.0 M sucrose containing 1.0 mM-$MgCl_2$ and is covered by a layer of 1.0 M sucrose; after

45 min at $100000\,g$ the almost pure preparation of cell bodies is recovered between the 1.0 and 1.8 M sucrose interface, while axonal fragments float to the top of the tube and small nuclei of glial origin are sedimented (compare Fig. 1 C and G). The yield of cell bodies is 10—20%; fragments of disrupted cells are recovered at the 1.8—2.0 M sucrose interface.

Such cell preparations appear to be much more homogeneous, better preserved and freer from contamination than cell body preparations from mammalian brain, and of course have the advantage of being derived from neurons of only one type. We are currently working on the fine structure of these cells, the compartmentation of the components of the cholinergic system within them, the isolation of their constituent organelles and their metabolism.

The nuclei of the cholinergic electromotor neurons, through clearly visible in the isolated cell bodies (Fig. 1 E), appear to be very labile and very few survive the various methods of cell disruption tried up to now. The nuclear fraction so far isolated (Fig. 1 G) consists almost exclusively of nuclei of the types seen in abundance in the tracts between the electromotor cells. Among these are very small nuclei with a dense nucleoplasm, possibly derived from microglia or endothelial cells and others of larger diameter, a pale nucleoplasm and scattered chromatin, possibly from oligodendrocytes or astrocytes.

Synaptic Components

Isolation of Synaptic Vesicles. Owing to its high collagen content, electric tissue is difficult to homogenize and the nerve terminals do not pinch off in any appreciable numbers to form synaptosomes. Under certain conditions of liquid shear, the non-innervated faces of the electrocytes appear to be shorn away from the innervated faces [2] and the former can be concentrated in a low-speed fraction [2] which is rich in Na^+, K^+-stimulated ATPase.

A more effective way of comminuting the tissue is to render it brittle by freezing it in liquid nitrogen or Freon 12 and then crush it to a coarse powder. This has the effect of breaking open the nerve terminals and permitting the extraction of the terminal cytoplasm including the synaptic vesicles [14]. The extract may be further fractionated by density gradient centrifuging; if this is done in a zonal rotor [15], milligram quantities of almost pure synaptic vesicles may be separated (Fig. 1 F). Two other fractions obtained at the same time contain soluble cytoplasmic components and fragments of post-synaptic membrane, respectively (Fig. 2).

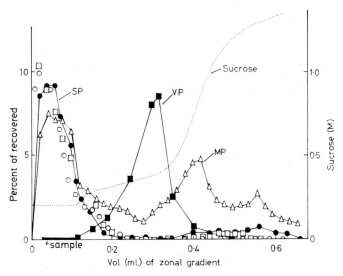

Fig. 2. Separation, in a zonal rotor, of a cytoplasmic extract from the electric organ of *Torpedo*, into fractions containing soluble cytoplasmic protein (●) (SP), synaptic vesicles (VP) and membrane fragments (MP) [16]. The vesicles are identified by their characteristic density, acetylcholine (■) and ATP (Fig. 4) content and morphological appearance (Fig. 1 F); the membrane fragments include pinched-off post-synaptic infoldings identified by their acetylcholinesterase content (△). Note the presence of the soluble cytoplasmic marker, lactate dehydrogenase (○) and the enzyme synthesizing acetylcholine, choline -*O*- acetyltransferase (□) exclusively in SP

Composition of Synaptic Vesicles. Our work on the protein ATP and acetylcholine content of *Torpedo* electric organ synaptic vesicles and the effect of stimulation on the composition and yield of the vesicles [16—19] has been recently reviewed [20—28], so will only be briefly described here.

The vesicle fraction (Figs. 1 F, 2), on dialysis and freeze drying, yields two main protein peaks when submitted to gel filtration on Sephadex G-200; the first of these, passing through in the void volume of the column, consists of vesicle membranes, is rich in lipids and contains three relatively high molecular weight protein components (Fig. 3); the second, rich in non-lipid phosphorus, consists of a single main protein component of mol. wt. about 10000 which comprises 30—40% of the total vesicle protein (Fig. 3,

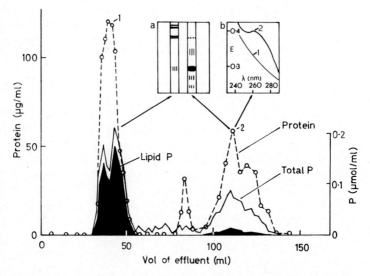

Fig. 3. Separation of synaptic vesicle proteins on Sephadex G-200. The freeze-dried retentate from fraction VP dialysed against distilled water for 60—70 hrs was suspended in 0.2 M KCl, 10 mM-Tris-HCl, pH = 7.4 and eluted with the same buffer. Note the emergence of two protein peaks: the first, in the void volume, contains chloroform-methanol soluble (*i.e.* lipid) phosphorus (black profile), three fairly high molecular weight components in disc-gel electrophoresis (insert a) and a non-specific type of absorption spectrum (insert b); the second, with a mol. wt. of about 10000, is seen to have (insert a) one main low molecular weight component on disc-gel electrophoresis, has a nucleotide-like absorption spectrum (insert b) and has most of its phosphorus (continuous line) in non-lipid form

Table 1). This soluble protein is apparently derived from the core of the vesicle, since it is not released unless the vesicle membrane is disrupted. It is acidic in character (p$I \sim 3$) and somewhat resembles chromogranin A in amino acid composition. Most of the non-lipid phosphorus associated with the core protein ("vesiculin") has been tentatively identified as nucleotide (AMP) phosphorus;

Table 1. Yield and composition of vesiculin preparations

Species of *Torpedo*	Vesiculin			Composition of vesiculin nucleotide:		
	(% of total protein)	(μg/g of tissue)	$\varepsilon_{260} \times 10^5$	Nucleotide mol/mol	Phosphate mol/mol	Phosphate molar ratio
T. nobiliana (5)	42 ± 12	7.2 ± 1.3	1.42 ± 0.13	8.2 ± 0.7	19.9 ± 5.7	2.78 ± 1.0
T. marmorata (4)	43 ± 7	12.1 ± 2.7	1.28 ± 0.50	7.5 ± 3.2	—	—

Values in cols 4–7 assume a molecular weight for vesiculin of 10^4 daltons, that the protein moiety has an ε_{260} of 1.2×10^4 and the putative nucleotide an ε_{260} of 1.54×10^4.

the native vesicle contains considerable amounts of bound ATP (Fig. 4) which presumably breaks down during the isolation of vesiculin.

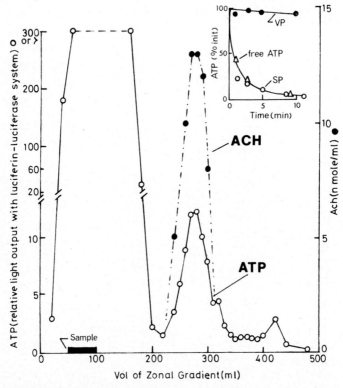

Fig. 4. Similar experiment to Fig. 2, showing presence of ATP as well as acetylcholine (ACh) in vesicle peak. Insert: vesicular ATP (VP) is resistant to the action of an apyrase-myokinase mixture, whereas the ATP present in the soluble protein (SP) peak is hydrolysed at the same rate as an equivalent amount of free ATP

The lipid composition of electric organ vesicles is very similar (Table 2, results of R. R. BAKER) to that of mammalian cortical synaptic vesicles. Noteworthy is the relatively low cholesterol: phospholipid molar ratio, also characteristic of other internal membranes including microsomes, and the negligible lysolecithin content

Table 2. The lipid composition of various storage granules

Organelle	Synaptic vesicles				Chromaffin granules	Storage granules
Tissue	Electric organ	Cortex	Cortex	Brain	Adrenal medulla	Platelets
Species	*Torpedo*	Guinea pig	Guinea pig	Rat	Ox	Rabbit
Reference			[53]	[54]	[55]	[56]
Phospholipid (% of total lipid):						
Lysolecithin	nil	1.2 ± 0.7	ND	1.5	16.8	nil
Phosphatidylcholine	42.8 ± 2.0	38.1 ± 1.1	41.3	42.2	26.0	33.8
Phosphatidylethanolamine	27.4 ± 1.0	29.6 ± 2.0	29.9	36.3	36.1	31.9
Phosphatidylinositol	6.6 ± 0.2	5.8 ± 1.0	5.0	2.9 }	9.2	2.5 }
Phosphatidylserine	12.4 ± 2.0	15.8 ± 1.5	11.1	11.8		11.9
Phosphatidic acid	1.7 ± 1.0	1.2 ± 0.6	1.8	1.8	nil	nil
Sphingomyelin	9.1 ± 2.0	7.8 ± 0.8	11.2	4.9	10.9	17.1
Other	nil	0.6 ± 0.3	0.3	ND	0.6	nil
Cholesterol:phospholipid (molar ratio)	0.45	0.53	0.45	ND	0.56	0.42
Ganglioside (nmol/g of tissue)	0.08	ND	2.0	ND	ND	ND

Unless otherwise stated, figures were obtained by R. R. BAKER and are mean values of 3 experiments $\pm$ S. D. (guinea pig cortex) or of 2 experiments $\pm$ range (electric organ). ND = not determined.

which is in contrast to what has been observed with the membrane of the chromaffin granule (Table 2, Column 6). It now seems clear that the high ($\sim 17\%$) lysolecithin content of chromaffin granule membranes is not generally true of storage granule membranes, and theories of exocytosis based on the presence of lysolecithin in such membranes may thus have to be abandoned.

On stimulation [18], there is a progressive fall in both vesicle numbers and size as indicated by measurements made on electron micrographs of whole tissue; at the same time the external membrane increases in area, with the result that infoldings appear in it and terminal profiles appear smaller and more numerous. These changes are consistent with the loss, by exocytosis, of about 50—70% of the total vesicle population; even on prolonged stimulation, complete depletion of vesicles is not attained. When vesicle fractions are prepared from the stimulated tissue, the reduction in yield (as measured by vesicle protein) exactly parallels the loss estimated from the electron micrographs. However, the remaining vesicles have a lower acetylcholine: ATP ratio than vesicles from unstimulated tissue [17, 18, 29]. The heterogeneity of the vesicle population in unstimulated organs is further shown by significant variations in the acetylcholine: ATP ratio across the vesicle peak in the zonal density gradient [17, 29].

On recovery, vesicle numbers and size rapidly return to normal, but transmitter and ATP content return much more slowly [19]. During this intermediate stage of recovery, the organ is abnormally fatiguable on stimulation, suggesting that a reduced stock of normal vesicles is able to maintain transmitter release at its normal level for a much shorter time. During recovery the acetylcholine: ATP ratio also increases to even higher values than the average seen in unstimulated organs. The significance of these changes in ATP ratio is not entirely clear but points to the presence in unstimulated, and — even more clearly — in terminals recovering from stimulation, of a population of acetylcholine-rich vesicles which is depleted by stimulation and which may comprise vesicles recently arrived at the terminal.

Depletion of vesicle numbers by exocytosis and acetylcholine content on stimulation have also been observed in muscle [30—32], but here the recovery phase is much more rapid and depletion therefore harder to demonstrate.

Components of the Post-Synaptic Membrane. A discussion of the biochemical applications of the cholinergic electromotor system of *Torpedo* would be incomplete without mentioning that the post-synaptic electrocyte membrane is extremely rich in acetylcholine-activated ionophores which constitute the pharmacological receptors for acetylcholine. As will be brought out more fully in another contribution to this symposium (M. RAFTERY, p. 541), several groups [33—38] have succeeded in isolating a protein from the electric organ with a high affinity for drugs or toxins with cholinergic or cholinolytic properties. The specificity of the drug-protein interaction parallels that of the pharmacological receptor and the protein could constitute or be part of the receptor. So far attempts to reconstruct the acetylcholine-induced ionic permeability changes using the "receptor" protein and an artificial membrane have not been successful, and it may well be that the protein is a recognition site rather than the entire system. The relationship of this protein to a proteolipid which *is* claimed to confer acetylcholine-induced ionophoretic properties on artificial membranes [39] is not clear at present.

Axonal Flow

Axonal flow of the characteristic components of the cholinergic neuron, acetylcholine, choline - *O* - acetyltransferase and acetylcholineesterase, is a well-established property of mammalian peripheral cholinergic neurons [40, 41]. The electromotor nerve trunks, owing to their large size and relative accessibility, are almost ideal for axonal flow studies. We and others [42, 43] have investigated the accumulation of vesicle protein, acetylcholine and other components above and below ligatures placed round the nerves.

Electromotor vesicle membrane proteins are antigenic [44, 45]; antibodies to them can be used in the method of indirect immuno-histofluorescence to locate the presence of cholinergic synaptic vesicles in tissues. In this way an accumulation of vesicle protein has been observed to occur above a ligature [42, 43]. Acetylcholine also accumulates (Fig. 5) both above and to some extent below a ligature; the latter may indicate a small amount of reversed flow but could also be accounted for by leakage of acetylcholine from the region of accumulation above the ligature.

Since both vesicle protein and acetylcholine accumulate above a ligature, it may seem reasonable to assume that acetylcholine is travelling down the axon in vesicular form. However, this is by no

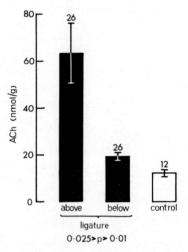

Fig. 5. Accumulation of acetylcholine (ACh) above a ligature. The vertical bars are the S.E.M.'s of the mean values indicated by the blocks; the figures above the blocks give the number of experiments meaned

means proven and attempts to isolate vesicles by homogenizing nerves led to the recovery of the transmitter in a fraction too dense to be synaptic vesicles of the type isolated from the terminals [43].

Results with *Loligo*

Isolation and Properties of Synaptosomes

Synaptosomes may be isolated in good yield and purity from the optic ganglia of *Loligo* utilizing the procedure shown in Fig. 6. When incubated in sea-water (a suitable saline medium for cephalopod tissues), these synaptosomes have a high O_2 uptake which is not greatly increased by the addition of substrates such as glucose unless the synaptosomes have been previously stored. Under metabolizing conditions, they take up choline [46], noradrenaline [47] and 5-hydroxytryptamine [48] by carrier-mediated processes.

Whereas the rates of uptake of noradrenaline and 5-hydroxytryptamine and the levels of these substances in the tissue are comparable to those of mammalian synaptosomes and brain tissue respectively, the uptake of choline is nearly 100 times greater, reflect-

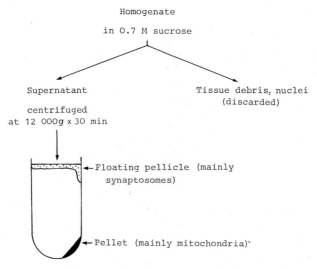

Fig. 6. Preparation of synaptosomes from optic ganglia of *Loligo*

ing the much higher acetylcholine content of squid ganglia and the much greater cholinergic representation. Furthermore, the kinetics of the uptake reveal the presence of a high-affinity uptake system easily overlooked in mammalian preparations [46]. This has a K_m of about 2 µM, about two orders of magnitude less than that of the low-affinity system.

Significance of the High Affinity Choline Carrier

Recent studies by M. J. DOWDALL and K. WÄCHTLER of my Department have indicated a remarkably good correlation between the concentration of the high-affinity choline uptake system and that of acetylcholine both between species and, within a species, in different brain regions (Fig. 7). Such a correlation has also been noted for mammalian brain [49], and degeneration of cholinergic tracts induced by section has been shown to cause the disappearance of the high-affinity carrier system along with choline acetyltransferase [49].

Other evidence that the high-affinity uptake system is a specific component of cholinergic nerve terminals comes from the obser-

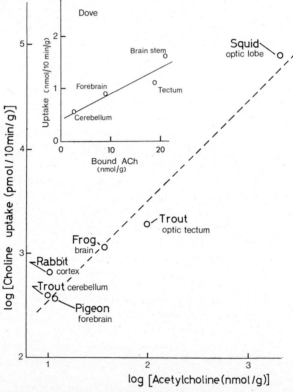

Fig. 7. Correlation diagram showing correlation between magnitude of high affinity choline uptake and acetylcholine content of nervous systems of representatives of various phyla. Insert: correlation for various parts of the brain of one species *(Streptopelia roseogrisea)*. Choline uptake was measured in synaptosome preparations at 23—26° using [*N-Me-³H*] choline and the Millipore filtration technique described by Dowdall and Simon [46]. The incubation media were physiological Ringer solutions buffered to pH 7.2 with 10 mM Tris-HCl. In order to minimize choline uptake due to the low affinity transport system, the uptake was measured at a low (1 μM) choline concentration

vation [50, 51] that both acetylcholine synthesis by intact synaptosomes and the high-affinity uptake system are Na^+-dependent and saturated by concentrations of choline above about 10 μM, while neither is true of the low-affinity system.

We believe that it is through the high-affinity carrier that acetylcholine synthesis is regulated. Choline acetyltransferase, the enzyme synthesizing acetylcholine, is located in the cytoplasm. This is true for *Torpedo* electromotor nerve terminals (Fig. 2) and for synaptosomes generally [52].

Conclusions

Cholinergic neurons are distinguished from other neurons in being able to synthesize three components — or rather categories of components — not found in other neurons. One of these is the enzyme choline -O- acetyltransferase which synthesizes acetylcholine from choline and acetylcoenzyme A. This enzyme (in some species at least two isoenzymes can be distinguished) is a soluble cytoplasmic constituent. It is synthesized in the cell body and moves down the axon by axonal flow until it reaches the nerve terminal where it accumulates in the terminal cytoplasm. The second characteristic group of components is the group of proteins that make up the synaptic vesicles of cholinergic nerve terminals: in *Torpedo*, three main membrane proteins and one main core protein. The vesicles, too, appear to be made in the cell body and to migrate down the axon. The third component is a membrane carrier with a very high affinity for choline — the K_m is about 1 μM, in contrast to a low affinity carrier with a K_m of about two orders of magnitude higher which is found in most cells including kidney and red blood cells. The carrier may well be the site at which acetylcholine synthesis is regulated.

As yet we do not know the site of synthesis of this carrier, how widely diffused in the cholinergic neuron it is, or how it gets to the terminal. The carrier is needed to salvage the choline liberated when acetylcholine is released into the synaptic cleft and is inactivated by being hydrolysed by the large amount of acetylcholinesterase found there.

By contrast, although there is evidence that many central cholinergic cells also manufacture acetylcholinesterase, the distribution of this enzyme is not a reliable guide to cholinergic function. Many instances are known of the occurrence of acetylcholinesterase in the absence of cholinergic neurons. It seems likely that the synthesis of this enzyme — and the acetylcholine receptor — is performed by *cholinoceptive* rather than *cholinergic* cells.

References

1. Smith, A. D.: Biochem. Soc. Symp. **36**, 103—131 (1972).
2. Sheridan, M. N., Whittaker, V. P., Israël, M.: Z. Zellforsch. Mikroskop. Anat. **74**, 291—307 (1966).
3. Dowdall, M. J., Whittaker, V. P.: J. Neurochem. **20**, 921—935 (1972).
4. Grundfest, H.: Progr. Biophys. Molec. Biol. **7**, 1—85 (1957).
5. Feldberg, W., Fessard, A.: J. Physiol. (Lond.) **101**, 200—216 (1942).
6. Young, J. Z.: A model of the brain. Oxford: Clarendon Press 1964.
7. Cousteau, J.-Y., Diolé, P.: Octopus and squid: the soft intelligence. London: Cassell 1973.
8. Bacq, Z. M., Mazza, F. P.: Arch. intern. Physiol. **42**, 43—46 (1935).
9. Rose, S. P. R.: Biochem. J. **102**, 33—43 (1967).
10. Blomstrand, C., Hamberger, A.: J. Neurochem. **16**, 1401—1407 (1970).
11. Johnson, D. E., Sellinger, P. A.: J. Neurochem. **18**, 1445—1460 (1971).
12. Norton, W. E., Poduslo, S. E.: Science **167**, 1144—1146 (1970).
13. Fritsch, G.: Die elektrischen Fische. Leipzig: von Veit 1890.
14. Soifer, D., Whittaker, V. P.: Biochem. J. **128**, 845—846 (1972).
15. Whittaker, V. P., Dowdall, M. J., Dowe, G. H. C., Facino, R. M., Scotto, J.: Brain Res. **75**, 115—131 (1974).
16. Whittaker, V. P., Essman, W. B., Dowe, G. H. C.: Biochem. J. **128**, 833—846 (1972).
17. Dowdall, M. J., Boyne, A. F., Whittaker, V. P.: Biochem. J. **140**, 1—12 (1974).
18. Zimmermann, H., Whittaker, V. P.: J. Neurochem. **22**, 435—451 (1974).
19. Zimmermann, H., Whittaker, V. P.: J. Neurochem. **22**, 1109—1114 (1974).
20. Whittaker, V. P.: Ann. N. Y. Acad. Sci. **186**, 21—32 (1971).
21. Whittaker, V. P.: In: Nahas, G. G., Salamagne, J. C., Viars, P., Vourc'h, G. (Eds.): Le système cholinergique en anesthésiologie et en reanimation, pp. 45—60. Paris: Librairie Arnette 1972.
22. Whittaker, V. P., Dowdall, M. J., Boyne, A. F.: Biochem. Soc. Symp. **36**, 49—68 (1972).
23. Whittaker, V. P., Dowdall, M. J.: In: Fardeau, M., Israël, M., Manaranche, R. (Eds.): La transmission cholinergique de l'excitation, pp. 101—117. Paris: Editions Inserm 1973.
24. Whittaker, V. P.: In: Schneider, D. J. (Ed.): Proteins of the nervous system, pp. 155—169. New York: Raven Press 1973.
25. Whittaker, V. P., Zimmermann, H., Dowdall, M. J.: J. neural Trans. Suppl. XII (1974) (in press).

26. WHITTAKER, V.P., ZIMMERMANN, H.: In: BENNETT, M.V.L. (Ed.): Synaptic transmission and neuronal interaction, pp. 217—238. New York: Raven Press 1974.
27. WHITTAKER, V.P.: Naturwissenschaften 60, 281—289 (1973).
28. WHITTAKER, V.P.: Advanc. Cytopharmacol. 2, 311—317 (1974).
29. DOWDALL, M.J., ZIMMERMANN, H.: Brain Res. 71, 160—166 (1974).
30. KORNELIUSSEN, H.: Z. Zellforsch. mikroskop. Anat. 130, 28—57 (1972).
31. CECCARELLI, B., HURLBUT, W.P., MAURO, A.: J. Cell Biol. 54, 30—38 (1972).
32. CECCARELLI, B., HURLBUT, W.P., MAURO, A.: J. Cell Biol. 57, 499—524 (1973).
33. KARLSSON, E., HEILBRONN, E., WIDLUND, L.: FEBS Letters 28, 107 (1972).
34. CHANGEUX, J.-P.: In: NAHAS, G.-G., SALAMAGNE, J.-C., VIARS, P., VOURC'H, G. (Eds.): Le système cholinergique en anesthésiologie et en réanimation, pp. 99—112. Paris: Librairie Arnette 1972.
35. SCHMIDT, J., RAFTERY, M.A.: Biochem. Biophys. Res. Commun. 49, 572 (1972).
36. KLETT, R.P., FULPIUS, B., COOPER, D., SMITH, M., REICH, E., LOURIVAL, D.P.: J. biol. Chem. 248, 6841—6853 (1973).
37. MILEDI, R., MOLINOFF, P., POTTER, L.T.: Nature (Lond.) 229, 554 (1971).
38. ELDEFRAWI, M.E., ELDEFRAWI, A.T., SEIFERT, S., O'BRIEN, R.D.: Arch. Biochem. Biophys. 150, 210—218 (1972).
39. DE ROBERTIS, E.: Science 171, 963—971 (1971).
40. KÁSA, P., MANN, P.S., KARSCU, S., TÓTH, L., JORDAN, S.: J. Neurochem. 21, 431—436 (1973).
41. SAUNDERS, N.R., DZIEGIELEWSKA, K., HÄGGENDAL, C.J., DAHLSTRÖM, A.B.: J. Neurobiol. 4, 95—103 (1973).
42. ULMAR, G., WHITTAKER, V.P.: Brain Res. 71, 155—159 (1974).
43. HEILBRONN, E., PETTERSON, H.: Acta physiol. scand. 88, 590 (1973).
44. ULMAR, G., WHITTAKER, V.P.: J. Neurochem. 22, 452—455 (1974).
45. WIDLUND, L., KARLSSON, K.A., WINTER, A., HEILBRONN, E.: J. Neurochem. 22, 451—456 (1974).
46. DOWDALL, M.J., SIMON, E.J.: J. Neurochem. 21, 969—982 (1973).
47. POLLARD, H.B., BOHR, V.A., DOWDALL, M.J., WHITTAKER, V.P.: Biol. Bull. Woods Hole 145, 449—450 (1973).
48. FELDMAN, J.L., DOWDALL, M.J.: Biol. Bull. Woods Hole 145, 432—433 (1973).
49. YAMAMURA, H.I., SNYDER, S.H.: Science 178, 626—628 (1972).
50. HAGA, T.: J. Neurochem. 18, 781—798 (1971).
51. HAGA, T., NODA, H.: Biochim. Biophys. Acta 291, 564—575 (1973).
52. FONNUM, F.: Biochem. J. 103, 262—270 (1967).
53. EICHBERG, J., WHITTAKER, V.P., DAWSON, R.M.C.: Biochem. J. 92, 91—100 (1964).
54. BRECKENRIDGE, W.C., MORGAN, I.G., ZANETTA, J.P., VONCENDON, G.: Biochim. biophys. Acta (Amst.) 320, 681—688 (1973).

55. BLASCHKO, H., FIREMARK, H., SMITH, A. D., WINKLER, H.: Biochem. J.
    104, 545—549 (1967).
56. DA PRADA, M., PLETSCHER, A., TRANZER, J. P.: Biochem. J. **127**, 681—
    683 (1972).

Discussion

B. W. AGRANOFF (Ann Arbor, Mich.): I would like to make a comment
about the results of Dr. WHITTAKER. One of the problems for biochemists
that are not equipped with electron microscopes is to find a good marker for
the synaptic vesicles. Of course, if a protein antibody could be found which
is specific — this would certainly be extremely useful. One of the things that
we have used is non-exchangeable acetylcholine in the case of cholinergic
synaptic vesicles because, apparently, the acetylcholine within the vesicles
does not exchange with the cytoplasmic pool, and so I am wondering whether
in regard to the high and low affinity system you would care to say something
about their respective representation in the exchangeable and non-exchangeable pools of acetylcholine?

V. P. WHITTAKER: There is good evidence [HAGA, T., NODA, H.: Bichim.
biophys. Acta (Amst.) **291**, 564—575 (1973); YAMAMURA, H. I., SNYDER,
S. H.: J. Neurochem. **21**, 1355 (1973)] that choline taken up by the high-
affinity system is mostly converted into acetylcholine; that taken up by the
low affinity system probably finds its way mainly into phosphorylcholine.
The subsequent distribution of the acetylcholine between the two main pools
of acetylcholine — the cytoplasmic and the vesicular — depends on the conditions under which the terminals are labeled. In general we can say that
both the cytoplasmic and vesicular pools are labeled *in vivo* [BARKER, L. A.,
DOWDALL, M. J., WHITTAKER, V. P.: Biochem. J. **130**, 1063—1080 (1972)]
but only the cytoplasmic pool is appreciably labeled *in vitro* (*i.e.* using,
synaptosome preparations) [MARCHBANKS, R. M.: Biochem. Pharmacol. **18**
1763—1766 (1969)]. I am afraid I do not know what the relationship between
your "exchangeable" and "non-exchangeable" pools and the "cytoplasmic"
and "vesicular" pools may be: this will probably depend on the techniques
used.

An Experimental Model for Exocytosis of Chromaffin Granules

Stephen Jon Morris

Abteilung für Neurochemie, Max-Planck-Institut für biophysikalische Chemie, D-3400 Göttingen, Postfach 968, Federal Republic of Germany

With 7 Figures

One of the more intriguing aspects of the biochemistry and biophysics of synaptic transmission which is being investigated in V. P. Whittaker's laboratory concerns the mechanism whereby the neurotransmitter, which is stored in the synaptic vesicle storage granules, is released into the synaptic cleft — the space between the pre- and post-synaptic cells. The model for which the most evidence has been accumulated is exocytosis [1—3]. In this model (Fig. 1), the membrane of the storage granule fuses with the pre-synaptic membrane. A connection between the interior of the storage granule and the exterior of the cell is established, and the granule contents are emptied into the synaptic cleft. I would like to comment upon an *in vitro* system which may help to elucidate the processes involved in the membrane fusion which is required by the model [4, 5].

Chromaffin granules, the catecholamine and ATP containing storage vesicles from the adrenal medulla were isolated from fresh bovine adrenal glands essentially by the method of Phillips [6]. Figure 2 is an electronmicrograph of such a preparation. The granules average 3000 Å in diameter and typically appear as a membrane bound space containing a very densely staining cytoplasm. Under certain conditions, if one raises the Ca^{2+} concentration to 5 mM, the granules aggregate (Fig. 3). Along the area of contact, the membranes break up and direct connections between the interiors of the two granules are established (Fig. 4). In some cases this double membrane disappears entirely. The core mate-

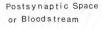

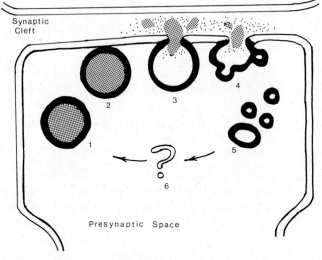

Fig. 1. Exocytosis proceeds as follows: Storage granule (1) fuses with the pre-synaptic membrane (2) establishing a direct connection between the interior of the granule and the exterior of the cell allowing the granule contents to escape into the synaptic cleft (3). The granule membrane is released from the pre-synaptic membrane (4) perhaps at the same time spontaneously vesiculating into smaller hollow pinocytotic spheres (5). The membrane components may be recycled (6)

rials never mix together, however. They are always separated by an electron lucent stripe.

One can reverse this apparent fusion by adding EDTA to the system (Fig. 5). When all the added Ca^{2+} is chelated, one sees only single intact chromaffin granules and a great increase in the number of granule ghosts, which suggests that the granules have the ability to separate and seal up again, although many lyse open and release their contents.

Purified membrane ghosts may be prepared from whole chromaffin granules by cycles of hypotonic lysis in hypotonic media, sedimentation and resuspension in hypertonic media [6]. These appear in electronmicroscopy as hollow spheres (Fig. 6). Addition of Ca^{2+} to the resuspended ghosts fuse them into extremely com-

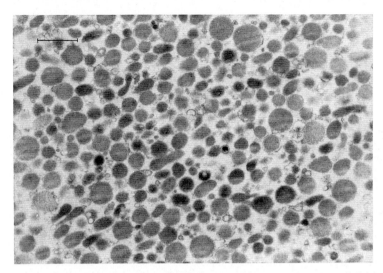

Fig. 2. Electronmicrograph of chromaffin granules prepared as described in Ref. [4]. The black bar is 1 μm

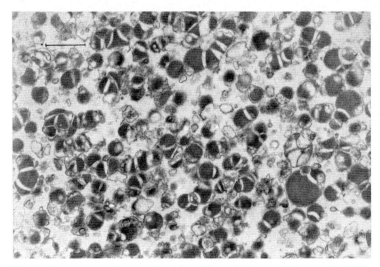

Fig. 3. The same granules after 45 min incubation with 5 mM CaCl₂. Black bar = 1 μm

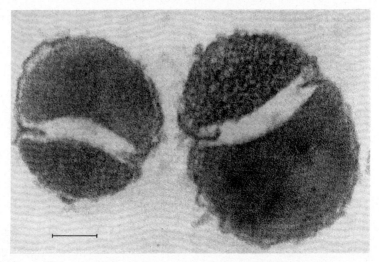

Fig. 4. Higher magnification of Ca^{2+}-treated granules showing apparent lack of dividing membranes. Black bar = 1000 Å

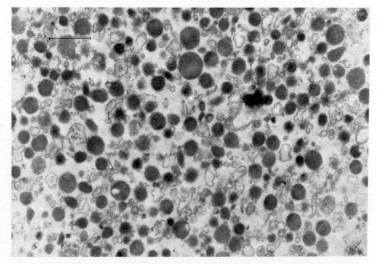

Fig. 5. The granules after 30 min incubation with Ca^{2+} followed by 15 min incubation with 10 mM EDTA. The fusion is apparently reversed. Black bar = 1 μm

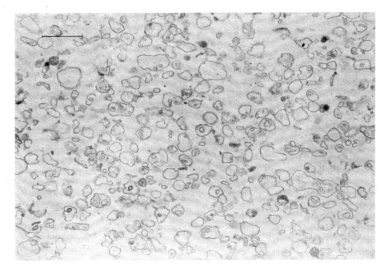

Fig. 6. Granule ghosts prepared as described in Ref. [5]. Black bar = 1 μm

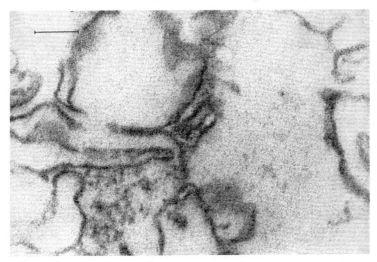

Fig. 7. Granule ghosts after addition of Ca^{2+}. Black bar = 1000 Å

plex arrays (Fig. 7). Again the partitioning double membranes show many breaks. The lysis procedure removes at least 99% of the soluble protein and catecholamine originally contained in the whole granule, which suggests that very little if any energy is required for the fusion to take place.

References

1. DOUGLAS, W. W., NAGASAWA, J., SCHULZ, R.: Mem. Soc. Endocr. **19**, 353—378 (1969).
2. HEUSER, J., REESE, T. S.: J. Cell Biol. **57**, 315 (1973).
3. SMITH, A. D., WINKLER, H.: In: BLASCHKO, H., MUSCHOLL, E. (Eds.): Handbook experimental pharmacology Vol. 33, pp. 538—617. Berlin-Heidelberg-New York: Springer 1972 (review).
4. EDWARDS, W., PHILLIPS, J. H., MORRIS, S. J.: Biochim. biophys. Acta (Amst.) **356**, 164—173 (1974).
5. MORRIS, S. J., EDWARDS, W., PHILLIPS, H. J.: FEBS Letters **44**, 217—223 (1974).
6. PHILLIPS, J. H.: Biochem. J. **136**, 579—587 (1973).

Discussion

E. NEUMANN (Göttingen): I would like to ask what is the time scale on which exocytosis proceeds? Is it minutes, and how does it fit into a model of the cholinergic system?

S. MORRIS: The time scale for the electronmicrograph experiments is 45 min. I can watch the aggregation of the granules by light scattering, but again this proceeds in the order of minutes. If one notes that the time scale for synaptic transmission is in the order of one millisecond for a cholinergic neuromuscular junction, my *in vitro* system seems to be running about 10^4 too slow. However, with better probes, perhaps NMR or the rapid reading light scattering machine which we are developing, we can uncover faster kinetics.

Characterization of an Acetylcholine Receptor[1]

M. A. Raftery, J. Bode, R. Vandlen, Y. Chao, J. Deutsch,
J. R. Duguid, K. Reed, and T. Moody

Church Laboratory of Chemical Biology, Division of Chemistry and Chemical Engineering, California Institute of Technology, Pasadena, CA 91109, USA

With 14 Figures

Introduction

This communication describes recent studies of an acetylcholine receptor from the electric ray *Torpedo californica*. For characterization of neurotransmitter receptors at the biochemical and biophysical levels, it is necessary to obtain at least milligram quantities of the molecules involved. *Torpedo* electroplax constitute an excellent source for these receptors. To understand molecular mechanisms involved in postsynaptic depolarization due to interaction of neurotransmitter with its receptor, studies can and should be conducted at several physical levels, *viz.* cellular, membrane, isolated molecule and reconstituted systems. Most of the work for the study of acetylcholine receptors at the cellular level has been done on vertebrate neuromuscular junctions or on *Electrophorus electricus* electroplax. *Torpedo* electroplax are not so well suited for such studies since the individual cells are basically too thin for the insertion of microelectrodes. Studies on this system can, however, be conducted at the membrane level, on isolated receptor molecules and on reconstituted systems. In this communication we describe studies at two of these levels, the membrane level and isolated receptor molecules. Several important questions can be answered by reconstitution, and this has now been achieved (Michaelson and Raftery, in press, 1974).

---

[1] Contribution No. 4936 from the Church Laboratory of Chemical Biology, California Institute of Technology, Pasadena, CA 91109 USA. Supported by U.S. Public Health Service Grants NS 10294 and GM 06965.

One of the important recent advances that has allowed studies such as those described here to be conducted was the discovery of irreversible effects of certain snake venom neurotoxins on acetylcholine mediated neuromuscular depolarization (Lee and Chang, 1966; Lee et al., 1967). One of the most commonly used of such neurotoxins is α-bungarotoxin (α-Bgt), which can be monoiodinated with ^{125}I to yield a fully active toxin which can be used as a simple assay system for nicotinic acetylcholine receptors (Schmidt and Raftery, 1973).

Membrane Fractionation

Following homogenization, the crude membrane preparation obtained can be fractionated on a sucrose gradient in a zonal rotor to give the pattern shown in Fig. 1. Two fractions of interest are

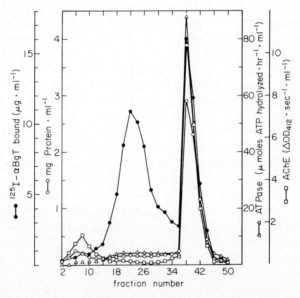

Fig. 1. Fractionation of AcChE- and AcChR-rich membrane fragments from *Torpedo californica* electroplax. 500 gm original electroplax were used and membranes prepared according to Duguid and Raftery (1973). A sucrose gradient (25—55%) was utilized in a Beckman Ti-15 zonal rotor at 30000 rpm for 12 hrs, following which fractions of 20 ml were collected and analyzed by protein content, AcChE activity and ^{125}I-α-Bgt binding as shown. Fractions 4—8 were pooled (AcChE-rich) as were fractions 16—28 (AcChR-rich)

obtained. At the top of the gradient particles which are rich in acetylcholine esterase (AcChE) activity and which contain no ^{125}I-α-Bgt binding ability are obtained, while in the middle of the gradient a fraction very rich in ^{125}I-α-Bgt binding ability is obtained. The heaviest fraction, which will not be discussed here, contains acetylcholine esterase activity, α-Bgt binding ability and ATPase activity. The acetylcholine receptor (AcChR) rich fraction contains from 25—40% of its total protein as AcChR molecules. It is clear from this fractionation procedure that AcChE and AcChR molecules are not associated with the same membrane particles. Studies of the AcChE-rich and AcChR-rich membrane particles by electron microscopy yield some interesting results, as shown in Fig. 2. Negative staining of the AcChR-rich particles reveals closed structures at least 80% of which show masses of particles in the membrane which are approximately 80 Å in diameter and contain a central pit as shown in Fig. 2A. Figure 2B shows these same structures at higher magnification. These results are similar to those previously demonstrated by NICKEL and POTTER (1973) and by CARTAUD et al. (1973) and the consensus seems to be that these structures represent AcChR oligomers embedded in the membrane. In contrast, the AcChE-rich particles can be shown by similar techniques to be quite different. First of all, Fig. 2C shows a thin section of the AcChE-rich particles stained for esterase activity (KARNOFSKY and ROOT, 1964), and it is clear that most of the vesicular structures contain this activity. In Fig. 2D the esterase-rich fragments, using negative staining procedures, seem quite different from the receptor-rich particles. The most obvious difference is the observation of a halo of particles surrounding each fragment. These particles are presumed to be esterase molecules which are somehow stuck into the membrane. It is tempting to conclude that the esterase molecules are attached to these membrane structures by the 150 Å tail-like structure which has been observed recently (RIEGER et al., 1973; DUDAI et al., 1973) by electron microscopy. Such association could be hydrophobic or more likely electrostatic, since the native enzyme can be readily extracted by high ionic strength buffers. The obvious conclusions which can be drawn from these results are: (1) the esterase and receptor molecules are separate entities and, (2) the receptor and esterase molecules are not embedded in, nor associated with, the same mem-

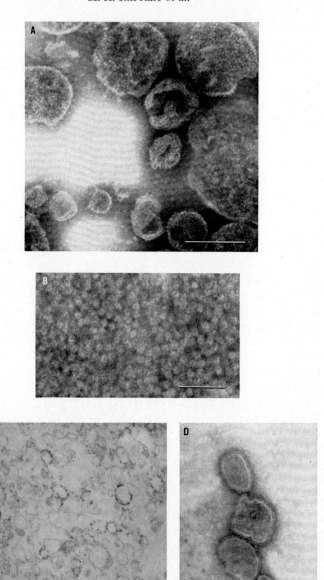

Fig. 2 (Legend see p. 545)

brane. This leaves the possibility that the esterase is associated with an entirely different membrane structure than is the receptor, or that the receptor and esterase molecules are perhaps associated with different regions of the same membrane in the synaptic cleft; that is to say that they are localized in different regions of this cleft. The other striking feature about the receptor-rich particles is that although they appear to be covered with the receptor structures, these structures are not organized in any obvious pattern, *i.e.*, no hexagonal array of these particles has been observed in any of our preparations. It is still possible that clusters of these receptor oligomers exist in the membrane, but there is no obvious lattice extending throughout the membrane.

Isolation and Purification of Acetylcholine Receptor

Unfractionated fragments are generally used for receptor purification. Treatment with 2% Triton X-100 for 15—30 min at 4° C allows quantitative extraction of ^{125}I-α-Bgt binding material from the membranes. Centrifugation of this preparation for 1 hr at $100\,000 \times$ g yields a solution of acetylcholine receptor which is two-fold purified from the crude membrane fraction. Affinity chromatography of this extract on a sepharose column containing the ligand

$$-NH-(CH_2)_5-CONH-(CH_2)_3-\overset{\oplus}{N}(CH_3)_3X^{\ominus}$$ yields a highly purified

preparation as shown in Fig. 3, in which a clear separation of most of the protein from the AcChR and from AcChE can be achieved (SCHMIDT and RAFTERY, 1972, 1973 a). Table 1 summarizes this one-step purification procedure. The most important points are that approximately 100 mg of highly purified receptor can be obtained, representing a 49% yield, from 1 kg of original electroplax tissue, with a specific activity of 10 nmoles of ^{125}I-α-Bgt bound per mg of receptor protein. Some further fractionation can be achieved by

---

Fig. 2 A—D. Electron microscopy of AcChE- and AcChR-rich membrane fragments. (A) Negative staining (uranyl acetate or phosphotungstate) of AcChR-rich fragments; the bar portrays a dimension of 0.5 μ. (B) Same as (A) at higher magnification; the bar portrays a dimension of 500 Å. (C) Thin sectioning of AcChE-rich fragments (stained by the KARNOFSKY and ROOT method), the bar portrays a dimension of 0.5 μ. (D) Negative staining of AcChE-rich fragments (uranyl acetate or phosphotungstate); the bar portrays a dimension of 500 Å

passage of this material through a second affinity column in which the ligand attached to the column is

$$-NH-(CH_2)_2NHCO-(CH_2)_2CONH-(CH_2)_6NHCO-$$
$$(CH_2)_5CONH-\langle\!\!\!\!\!\!\!\!\!\bigcirc\!\!\!\!\!\!\!\!\!\rangle\overset{\oplus}{-}N(CH_3)_3X^{\ominus}.$$

This refractionated material binds one mole of ^{125}I-α-Bgt to 100 000 Daltons of receptor protein and has one of the highest specific

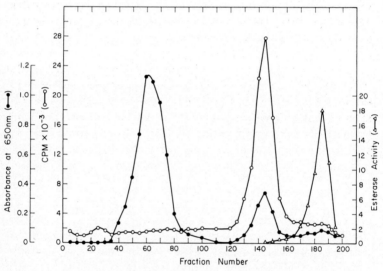

Fig. 3. Purification of AcChR by affinity chromatography according to Schmidt and Raftery (1973a)

Table 1. Purification table-AcChR

	Protein (mgs)	Activity (nmoles)	Specific activity (nmoles/mg)	Purifi- cation	Recovery (%)
Homogenate	18600	1950	0.11	—	100
Membrane suspension	3250	1950	0.60	5.7	100
Triton extract	1350	1950	1.45	13.7	100
Affinity pool	95	950	10	91	49

activities of any receptor preparation reported to date. Although various other procedures have been applied, no further increase in specific activity has been obtained. Fig. 4 shows the results of electrophoresis carried out on this preparation. In non-denaturing gel electrophoresis containing 0.1% sodium cholate the material migrates as essentially one band of high molecular weight, whereas in denaturing gel electrophoresis containing 1% SDS one major polypeptide component of molecular weight approximately 40000 is seen and, in addition, another component of 50000 molecular weight is always present. A minor band at about 65000 molecular weight also seems to be always present. Thus the best receptor preparations do not appear to be composed of a single polypeptide unit.

The molecular properties of the isolated purified receptor can be summarized as follows: By gel filtration the receptor appears to have a Stokes radius corresponding to a molecular weight of approximately 500000, while in sucrose density gradients containing 0.1% Triton X-100 the S value obtained under equilibrium condi-

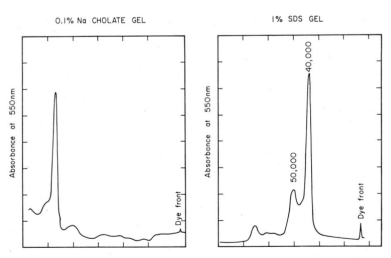

Fig. 4. Left: Gel electrophoresis in 4% gels under non-denaturing conditions at pH = 7.4. The dye front is at a distance of 12—14 cm from the origin. Right: Gel electrophoresis under denaturing conditions according to FAIR-BANKS et al. (1971). The dye front is at a distance of 11.4 cm from the origin

tions corresponds to 9.7 S. The isoelectric point of the isolated receptor is close to 5 and it appears to be a glycoprotein containing N-acetyl-D-glucosamine, mannose and galactose.

Ligand Binding Properties of Acetylcholine Receptor

1. Toxin Sites and Ligand Sites.

The number of α-Bgt binding sites appears to be the same in the membrane bound and Triton X-100 solubilized states, since all of the binding sites can be extracted with detergent. However, in the case of AcChR from *Torpedo californica* electroplax the relationship between toxin binding sites and cholinergic ligand binding sites is not a 1:1 phenomenon. With purified receptor cholinergic ligands appear to bind to half of the toxin binding sites in most cases. This has been shown for acetylcholine, decamethonium and d-tubocurarine (MOODY et al., 1973). In addition, the fluorescent dye *bis*(3-aminopyridinium-)1,10-decane (DAP) has also been shown to bind to half as many sites as does α-Bgt (MARTINEZ-CARRION and RAFTERY, 1973). This effect is shown even more clearly in Fig. 5 where the release of DAP, estimated by

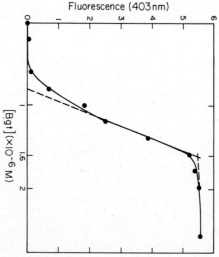

Fig. 5. Release of DAP free into solution from its complex with purified AcChR as a function of added α-Bgt, monitored by the increase in fluorescence (arbitrary units). Initial conditions were such that 96% of DAP binding sites were occupied

increase in fluorescence due to the free dye, is monitored as a function of added α-Bgt. It can be seen that initial additions of the toxin released very little dye but that after 1 equivalent of toxin had been added (in terms of moles of bound DAP), release of further dye was facile. The interpretation of this experiment is that the DAP sites are saturated and the initial added toxin goes preferentially to toxin binding sites not occupied by DAP. Following saturation of these other sites with toxin, the DAP binding sites are occupied with toxin with liberation of the DAP. Extrapolation to the x-axis shows that the DAP sites constitute almost exactly half of the total toxin binding sites (Bode and Raftery, 1974, unpublished). It is possible that DAP would bind more weakly to the other toxin binding sites, but this experiment is very difficult to do using fluorescence techniques. These differences in toxin binding sites and ligand binding sites can be interpreted in a number of ways. The simplest assumption is that toxin binding sites and ligand sites overlap on the receptor molecule. If this is the case, the half-of-the-sites phenomenon could be explained by ligand induced negative cooperativity in binding (Conway and Koshland, 1968) or by pre-existent nonequivalence in binding sites (MacQuarrie and Bernhard, 1971) in the receptor molecule. It is difficult at the present time to distinguish between these alternatives, although the fact that the dissociation constant for DAP changes so little whether the toxin sites unoccupied by DAP are occupied by toxin might argue in favor of a pre-existent nonequivalence model. However, it is also possible that toxin binding sites and ligand binding sites do not overlap but that the competition between these two types of ligand can be explained by conformational processes occurring in the receptor molecule as a function of added toxin or ligand.

2. **Ligand Dissociation Constants.** Dissociation constants can be measured directly on purified membrane fragments or on purified-AcChR by equilibrium dialysis or by centrifugation methods. In addition, two other methods have been used in our laboratory to measure inhibition constants for the same ligands. The first of these involves reduction of the initial rate of ^{125}I-α-Bgt association with receptor in the presence of added ligand (Moody et al., 1973; Schmidt and Raftery, 1974; Deutsch and Raftery, 1974). The second method depends on competition between added ligands and the fluorescent cholinergic analogue DAP (Martinez-Carrion and

Table 2. I_{50} values for AcChR, purified and membrane-bound

	Purified AcChR 5 mM *tris*	AcChR membranes 20 mM NaCl-5 mM *tris*	Ratio
Acetylcholine	2.5×10^{-6}	6×10^{-9}	420
Carbamylcholine	4.5×10^{-5}	4×10^{-8}	1100
Nicotine	8×10^{-5}	1×10^{-7}	800
Phenytrimethyl-ammonium	8×10^{-5}	2×10^{-7}	400
Choline	1.3×10^{-3}	1×10^{-5}	160
Decamethonium	2×10^{-6}	1×10^{-8}	140
Hexamethonium	2×10^{-6}	5×10^{-7}	4.0
d-Tubocurarine	1×10^{-7}	3×10^{-8}	3.3
Gallamine	2×10^{-7}	8×10^{-8}	2.5
DAP	1×10^{-6}	4×10^{-8}	25

RAFTERY, 1973). The four methods have been found to yield numbers for dissociation constants and inhibition constants which agree very closely. Table 2 summarizes some of the pertinent results obtained by inhibition of the initial rate of ^{125}I-α-Bgt association with purified receptor and purified membrane fragments. Inhibition constants vary over three orders of magnitude. The most significant difference observed is in the binding of agonists, acetylcholine, carbamylcholine, nicotine, and decamethonium, where all of these bind considerably more tightly to the receptor in its native membrane environment than they do to the purified material. On the other hand the antagonists, hexamethonium and *d*-tubocurarine display no significant difference in their affinities for the receptor in the purified and membrane-bound states. Effects opposite to these, *i.e.*, agonists binding more strongly to purified receptor than to membrane bound receptor have been observed by MEUNIER and CHANGEUX (1973) in *Electrophorus* electroplax AcChR and these authors have suggested the release of a membrane constraint, yielding a relaxed receptor, as the origin of such effects. It is evident from the data presented in Table 2 that the change undergone by the receptor upon solubilization appears to be restricted to a rather precise region, as discussed in a later section of this communication. The change is localized at the acetylcholine binding subsite and it is not possible yet to say whether quaternary structural changes in the acetylcholine receptor oligomer accompany these tertiary structural changes that are observed. In addition, it is also possible that surface charges, especially negative charges of the membrane particles, exert some effect upon the binding constants for the positively charged ligands that are being studied. The structural change in the receptor is likely to be a very subtle one as evidenced by the greater than 1 order of magnitude difference observed in the ratios for acetylcholine and carbamylcholine (Table 2).

3. Cooperativity in Ligand Binding. Direct determination of dissociation constants for acetylcholine binding to purified receptor or to receptor-rich membrane fragments can be achieved by equilibrium dialysis and centrifugation procedures. Figure 6 shows a Hill plot for the binding of ^{3}H-acetylcholine to purified receptor, and it is apparent that no cooperativity in ligand binding is observed in the concentration ranges studied. Recent results (LEE and RAFTERY unpublished) have demonstrated that at very high acetylcholine concentrations additional binding of the ligand is observed so that the total number of acetylcholine binding sites, both strong and weak, equal the number of toxin binding sites. This result can be

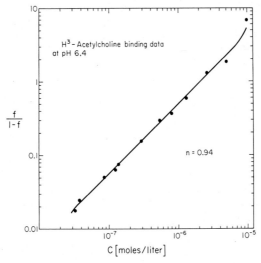

Fig. 6. Hill plot of ^{3}H-acetylcholine binding to purified AcChR from equilibrium dialysis binding data (MOODY et al., 1973)

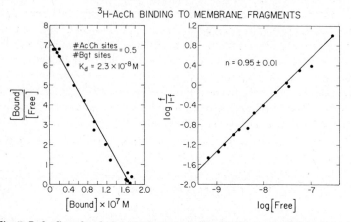

Fig. 7. Left: Scatchard plot of ³H-acetylcholine binding to AcChR-rich membrane fragments showing the values obtained for the dissociation constant and the ratio of acetylcholine to α-Bgt binding sites. Right: Hill plot of the same data

interpreted either as ligand induced negative cooperativity, as preexistent asymmetry of binding sites in the receptor oligomer, or as two classes of acetylcholine binding sites differing in their affinities. These latter results are similar to those observed by ELDEFRAWI (1974) demonstrating negative cooperativity in the binding of acetylcholine to purified acetylcholine receptor from the related species *Torpedo marmorata*.

The binding of acetylcholine to receptor-rich membrane fragments has also been studied, and again we observe no cooperativity for the high affinity acetylcholine binding sites. Figure 7 shows these results and again a Hill coefficient very close to 1 is observed. The significance of these binding studies, both to purified and to membrane-bound acetylcholine receptor, is that the lack of cooperativity in acetylcholine binding is at variance with the previously demonstrated slight positive cooperativity in response, *i.e.*, conductance changes (CHANGEUX and PODLESKY, 1968).

It is not necessary, however, to have positively cooperative ligand binding in order to obtain a positively cooperative response, since the conductance change can occur one or more steps following the initial binding event. This notion has recently been put in quantitative form (LEVITZKI, 1974).

At this point it is pertinent to point out that real differences may exist between AcChR preparations from different sources. While we observe high affinity ligand binding sites equal only to half of the α-Bgt binding sites in the receptor preparations from *Torpedo californica*, MEUNIER and CHANGEUX (1974) observe equal numbers of such sites in membrane preparations from the electroplax from *Torpedo marmorata*, and furthermore they have observed slight positive cooperativity in the binding of acetylcholine to these preparations. Additionally, the acetylcholine receptor from *Electrophorus electricus* appears to behave in the opposite manner to the *Torpedo californica* acetylcholine receptor in comparing dissociation constants for agonists in the membrane-bound and purified states (MEUNIER and CHANGEUX, 1973).

4. Binding of Inorganic Cations to Acetylcholine Receptor. The initial observation that purified AcChR was capable of binding monovalent and divalent cations was made by observing the effects of various cations on the apparent binding constant for the fluorescent cholinergic analogue DAP (MARTINEZ-CARRION and RAFTERY, 1973). Table 3 summarizes the results of these studies for several mono- and divalent cations. In addition to having an effect on the apparent binding constants of various cholinergic ligands, cations also compete with α-Bgt binding sites. Figure 8 demonstrates the effect of millimolar concentrations (1—20) of sodium chloride on the initial rate of ^{125}I-α-Bgt association with purified AcChR. In Table 4 such effects on the rate constant for toxin receptor complex formation are shown. Similar results have also been obtained with receptor-

Table 3. Affinities of various cations to purified *Torpedo* AcCh receptor

Test ions	
NH_4^+, *Tris*, H^+, Na^+, K^+, Li^+, Rb^+, Cs^+	$5.8—6.5 \times 10^{-3}$
Mg^{2+}	2.9×10^{-4}
Ca^{2+}, Sr^{2+}, Ba^{2+}	$1.6—1.9 \times 10^{-4}$
lauryl-, butyryl-, propionyl-, or acetylcholine	$1.0—2.6 \times 10^{-6}$
carbamylcholine	4.5×10^{-5}
butyryl-, propionyl-, or acetyl-thiocholine	$1.2—1.6 \times 10^{-4}$
choline	1.3×10^{-3}
phenyltrimethylammonium	8.0×10^{-5}
tetraethyl or tetramethylammonium	$6.5—9.0 \times 10^{-4}$

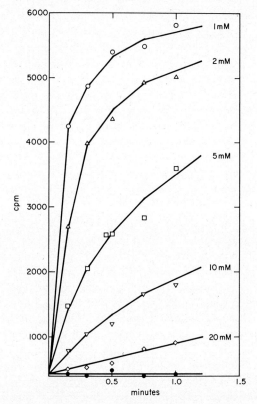

Fig. 8. Rate of ^{125}I-α-Bgt receptor complex formation [cpm bound to DEAE filter discs by the method of SCHMIDT and RAFTERY (1973)] as a function of time in the presence of the indicated mM concentrations of NaCl

Table 4. The toxin binding rate constant as a function of sodium chloride concentration

Expt.	NaCl (m M)	K_1 (M^{-1} sec^{-1})
A		$\gg 3.5 \times 10^6$
B	20	1.5×10^6
C	100	1.8×10^5
D	500	2.5×10^4

rich membrane fragments. Such studies can readily be extended to the effects of high and low salt on the apparent inhibition constants for cholinergic ligand inhibition of ^{125}I-α-Bgt complex formation with receptor-rich membrane fragments. Results of such studies are shown in Table 5. The important point that can be made from such

Table 5. Effects of ionic strength on ligand binding

	20 mM NaCl-5 mM *Tris*	Ringer	Ratio
Acetylcholine	6×10^{-9}	7×10^{-9}	1
Carbamylcholine	4×10^{-8}	1×10^{-7}	3
Nicotine	1×10^{-7}	3×10^{-7}	3
Phenyltrimethylammonium	2×10^{-5}	2×10^{-7}	1
Choline	1×10^{-5}	3×10^{-5}	3
Decamethonium	1×10^{-8}	4×10^{-7}	30
Hexamethonium	5×10^{-7}	6×10^{-5}	120
d-Tubocurarine	3×10^{-8}	9×10^{-7}	30
Gallamine	8×10^{-8}	8×10^{-6}	100
DAP	4×10^{-8}	2×10^{-6}	50

studies is that whereas cation concentration has a dramatic effect on the apparent inhibition constants for doubly charged compounds such as *d*-tubocurarine or bis-quaternary compounds such as hexamethonium and decamethonium, it has a minimal effect on the apparent constants for the agonists acetylcholine, carbamylcholine and nicotine as well as on choline, which are all mono-quaternary compounds. Results which agree with these studies have been obtained from equilibrium dialysis measurements on purified receptor (MOODY and RAFTERY, unpublished). These results are demonstrated in Fig. 9 and they show that sodium cation competes directly with the binding of *d*-tubocurarine to the receptor in a simple competitive fashion. However, sodium chloride has literally no effect on the binding of acetylcholine. The obvious conclusion from these various studies is that cations bind to a specific locus on the receptor molecule, but that this is not the acetylcholine binding site but another anionic site elsewhere in the molecule and that compounds such as decamethonium and hexamethonium obviously also bind to this site. This cation binding site then appears to be a

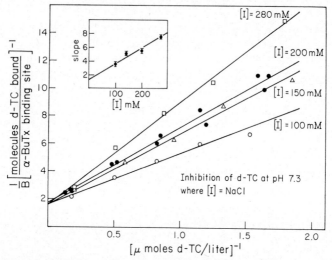

Fig. 9. Double-reciprocal plot of the competition between sodium chloride
and *d*-tubocurarine binding to purified AcChR

peripheral site at some distance from the specific acetylcholine
binding site.

5. Binding Subsites on the Acetylcholine Receptor. Further
understanding of the relationships between the specific acetylcholine binding site and the peripheral cation binding site was obtained by investigation of the competition for these sites between
the cholinergic analogue DAP and various mono- and bis-quaternary
analogues. DAP can be displaced completely from the AcChR into
solution by addition of α-Bgt, and such displacement is readily
monitored since DAP fluoresces when free in solution and is completely quenched when bound to the receptor molecule. Figure 10
demonstrates that hexamethonium can completely displace DAP
with the value for half displacement coinciding with the previously
determined inhibition constant for hexamethonium (MOODY et al.,
1973). On the other hand, carbamylcholine even at very high concentrations is not capable of completely displacing DAP from the
receptor. This prompted the notion that carbamylcholine might
bind to the specific cholinergic binding site but that the DAP
molecule was still bound to the receptor *via* the other end of the

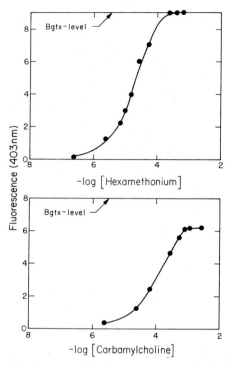

Fig. 10. Displacement of DAP from its complex with purified AcChR as a function of added hexamethonium or carbamylcholine. Bgt-level refers to the relative amount of DAP released by addition of saturating amounts of α-Bgt

DAP molecule. In other words, both carbamylcholine and DAP could be bound at the same time. Similar results were obtained with acetylcholine. It was possible to show directly (BODE and RAFTERY, unpublished) that acetylcholine and DAP could simultaneously bind to the purified acetylcholine receptor with generation of some fluorescence, while the DAP molecule was still associated with the receptor. This was achieved by monitoring the increase in fluorescence in a solution of receptor and DAP caused by addition of various increments of acetylcholine. This increase in fluorescence in the whole solution was compared to the increase in the supernatant following centrifugation of the same solution, at $100\,000\ g$ for 5 hrs so that all DAP associated with the AcChR was pelleted. As shown in Fig. 11, the increase in fluorescence of the whole sample was not observed in the supernatant, thus showing that acetylcholine was displacing only 1/2 of the DAP chromophore from its specific bind-

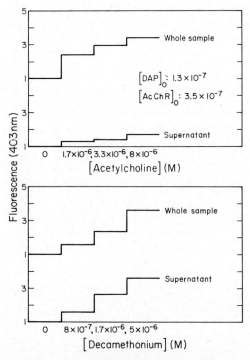

Fig. 11. Increase in fluorescence due to displacement of DAP from its complex with purified AcChR by decamethonium and acetylcholine before and after centrifugation

ing sites but that the DAP molecule still remained associated with the receptor. In Fig. 12 a similar experiment is also shown with decamethonium. In this case it is obvious that decamethonium released the DAP molecule free into solution.

As shown in Fig. 12, decamethonium can smoothly displace all bound DAP from the AcChR with the half point of such displacement agreeing with the known dissociation constant for decamethonium (Moody et al., 1973). A similar experiment with d-tubocurarine yielded a slightly different and interesting result, as also shown in Fig. 12. Half of the total fluorescence was released by addition of d-tubocurarine, and the midpoint for such displacement

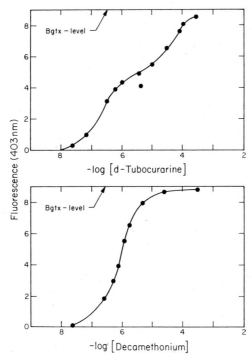

Fig. 12. Increase in fluorescence due to displacement of DAP by α-Bgt or by increasing concentrations of decamethonium or d-tubocurarine

of half of the bound DAP agreed with the known dissociation constant for d-tubocurarine (Moody et al., 1973). However, it was necessary to add d-tubocurarine in concentrations 2 orders of magnitude higher to completely displace DAP. This result can be interpreted to mean that d-tubocurarine, similar to carbamylcholine and acetylcholine, displaces only 1/2 of the DAP molecule from its receptor-bound state and that both molecules can apparently bind simultaneously to the receptor.

6. Chemical Modification of Anionic Sites on the Acetylcholine Receptor. It is reasonable to expect that mono- and bis-quaternary ligands, as well as inorganic cations, bind to negatively charged sites on the receptor molecule. Furthermore, it has been shown (Martinez-Carrion and Raftery, 1973; Schmidt and Raftery, 1974) that DAP and α-Bgt association with the receptor is pH dependent. The amino side chains most likely to be involved in such anionic sites are the carboxylates of aspartic or glutamic acids. The most attractive reagents for modification of such groups are trialkyloxonium salts (Parsons and Raftery, 1970) due to

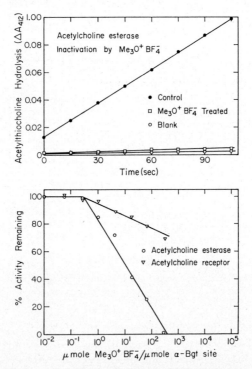

Fig. 13. Modification of AcChE and AcChR with trimethyloxonium fluoroborate. Top: Inactivation of AcChE with respect to hydrolysis of acetylthiocholine, monitored using DTNB to detect thiol production. Bottom: Relative potencies of varying concentrations of trimethyloxonium fluoroborate towards inactivation of AcChE and AcChR (AcChR "activity" measured by binding of ^{3}H-decamethonium)

(1) their ability to modify carboxyls under neutral conditions and, (2) the fact that they are positively charged, thus resembling cations or cholinergic analogues. Trimethyloxonium fluoroborate has recently been used (RAWN and LIENHARD, 1974) to inactivate acetylcholine esterase. In Fig. 13 it is shown that the acetylcholine esterase from *Torpedo californica* can be readily inactivated with trimethyloxonium fluoroborate and a comparison is made between this facile inactivation of enzymatic activity, using acetylthiocholine as a substrate, and the inactivation of the *Torpedo californica* receptor with regard to binding of decamethonium. Such studies (CHAO and RAFTERY, unpublished) have shown that the number of

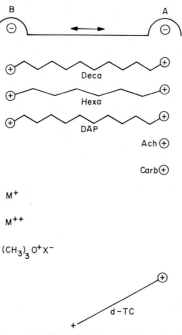

Fig. 14. Schematic view of AcChR binding subsites, showing bisquaternary compounds binding to both sites, monoquaternary compounds binding to subsite *A*, inorganic cations binding to subsite *B* and preferential modification of subsite *B* by trimethyloxonium fluoroborate. This scheme also portrays the binding of *d*-tubocurarine to subsite *A* but not subsite *B*

decamethonium sites are reduced upon treatment of the receptor with trimethyloxonium fluoroborate without affecting the decamethonium binding constant for the residual sites. DAP binding to such esterified AcChR's is completely abolished, while on the other hand acetylcholine binding is unaffected. The simplest interpretation of these results is that the specific acetylcholine anionic binding site is unaffected by reaction with trimethyloxonium fluoroborate, whereas the cation binding site appears to be chemically modified.

7. Summary of Acetylcholine Receptor Binding Subsite Properties. Figure 14 summarizes the results obtained to date for the binding of mono- and bis-quaternary cholinergic analogues and of inorganic cations to the AcChR from *Torpedo californica*. These results indicate that there are two distinct binding subsites for bis-quaternary compounds such as decamethonium, hexamethonium and the fluorescent decamethonium analogue DAP. Acetylcholine and carbamylcholine as well as nicotine bind to subsite "*A*", the specific cholinergic binding subsite, whereas monovalent and divalent cations bind to subsite "*B*", which is also occupied by the bis-quaternary compounds. Additionally, although both sites are probably anionic, the positively charged alkylating agent trimethyloxonium fluoroborate appears to react only with subsite "*B*". It is likely that there is some communication between subsites "*A*" and "*B*", probably of a conformational nature, through the protein structure, since the binding of cations to site "*B*" has some small but measurable effect on the binding of acetylcholine to subsite "*A*".

References

CARTAUD, J., BENEDETTI, E. L., COHEN, J., MEUNIER, J.-C., CHANGEUX, J.-P.: FEBS Letters **33**, 109 (1973).

CHANGEUX, J.-P., PODLESKY, T. R.: Proc. nat. Acad. Sci. (Wash.) **59**, 944 (1968).

CONWAY, A., KOSHLAND, JR., D. E.: Biochemistry **7**, 4011 (1968).

DEUTSCH, J., RAFTERY, M. A.: Biochemistry (1974) (in press).

DUDAI, Y., HERZBERG, M., SILMAN, I.: Proc. nat. Acad. Sci. (Wash.) **70**, 247 (1973).

DUGUID, J. R., RAFTERY, M. A.: Biochemistry **12**, 3593 (1973).

ELDEFRAWI, M. E., ELDEFRAWI, A. T.: Biochem. Pharm. Res. Commun. (1974) (in press).

FAIRBANKS, G., STECK, T., WALLACH, D.: Biochemistry **10**, 2606 (1971).

KARNOFSKY, M., ROOT, L.: J. Histochem. Cytochrome **12**, 219 (1964).

LEE,C.Y., CHANG,C.C.: Mem. Inst. Butantan. Simp. Internac. **33**, 555 (1966).
LEE,C.Y., TSEUNG,L.F., CHIU,T.H.: Nature (Lond.) **215**, 1177 (1967).
LEVITZKI,A.: J. theor. Biol. **44**, 367 (1974).
MACQUARRIE,R.A., BERNHARD,S.: Biochemistry **10**, 2456 (1971).
MARTINEZ-CARRION,M., RAFTERY,M.A.: Biochem. Biophys. Res. Commun.
    55, 1156 (1973).
MEUNIER,J.-C., CHANGEUX,J.-P.: FEBS Letters **32**, 143 (1973).
MICHAELSON,D., RAFTERY,M.A.: Proc. nat. Acad. Sci. (Wash. (1974) (in press).)
MOODY,T., SCHMIDT,J., RAFTERY,M.A.: Biochem. Biophys. Res. Commun.
    53, 761 (1973).
NICKEL,A., POTTER,L.T.: Brain Res. **57**, 508 (1973).
PARSONS,S.M., RAFTERY,M.A.: Biochem. Biophys. Res. Commun. **41**, 45
    (1970).
RAWN,J.D., LIENHARD,G.: Biochem. Biophys. Res. Commun. **56**, 654 (1974).
RIEGER,F., BONS,S., MASSOULIE,T., CARTAUD,J.: Eur. J. Biochem. **34**, 539
    (1973).
SCHMIDT,J., RAFTERY,M.A.: Biochem. Biophys. Res. Commun. **49**, 572
    (1972).
SCHMIDT,J., RAFTERY,M.A.: Anal. Bioch. **52**, 349 (1973).
SCHMIDT,J., RAFTERY,M.A.: J. Neurochem. (1974) (in press).

Discussion

B. W. AGRANOFF (Ann Arbor): I would like to ask you about early
reports that the ratio of choline esterase to receptor (in your system) would
perhaps be one to one. Is there anything to that at the present time?

M. A. RAFTERY: We have not done anything that I would regard as really
quantitative; so I don't know the exact stoichiometry.

E. GROSS (Bethesda): Triethyloxonium tetrafluoroborate abolishes the
choline esterase activity. Is the enzyme potentially a transesterase — could
the carboxyl group which you modify on your protein replace the acetyl
group of acetyl choline? Could you alkylate some other groups?

M. A. RAFTERY: The enzyme has not been shown to be a transesterase
although presumably the reaction it catalyses is reversible. The oxonium
salts we use are specific for esterification of carboxyls at low or neutral pH,
and it is also very rapid. To date we have not conducted experiments to
determine whether the abolition of enzymatic activity is an effect on K_H or
on catalytic steps. Our guess is that it is an effect on binding due to modification of an anionic binding site.

D. E. KOSHLAND JR. (Berkeley): Aren't you a little surprised that the
decamethonium binding is completely wiped out by the alkylation with
oxonium salt?

M. A. RAFTERY: Decamethonium binding is affected as follows: The
number of binding sites is reduced without effect on the dissociation constant

to the remaining sites. DAP binding can be abolished at high oxonium salt concentration. This can be rationalized if we say that the modification occurs at subsite B (since it has no effect on acetyl choline binding, and since modification is reduced in high ionic strength buffers) and that DAP interacts most strongly with this site and perhaps also by means of its methylene groups. In summary, DAP and decamethonium binding appears to be governed mostly by subsite B where the modification preferentially occurs and the number of residual intact sites determines the effect observed.

B. HAMPRECHT (München): You showed the differences in the binding constants for the ligand between the isolated receptor and the receptor on the membrane. What happens to the binding constants of the isolated receptor when lipid from the membranes is added?

M. A. RAFTERY: We are now attempting to find out. We know that such reconstructed materials translocate cations in the presence of cholinergic agonists but we do not as yet know the ligand concentration dependence of this effect.

V. P. WHITTAKER (Göttingen): You use in your last step of purification an affinity column with a choline residue on a hydrophobic rest. Did you leave out once the choline and used only the hydrophobic coated Sepharose?

M. A. RAFTERY: We did not do that but we have been able to show that boiled receptor solutions, which no longer bind α-bungarotoxin, give the same protein profile on the column as do solutions of viable receptor. It is therefore possible that the chromatography but may be due to other types of interaction which luckily give us the preparation we want in a highly purified state.

Biochemistry of Serotonin and Synaptic Membranes in Neurotransmission

W. WESEMANN

Physiologisch-Chemisches Institut der Universität, D-3550 Marburg/Lahn, Deutschhausstraße 1—2, Federal Republic of Germany

With 13 Figures

1. Distribution of Serotonin

According to PAGE [1] "Serotonin made its debut to science in 1868, when it was noted that defibrinated blood caused vasoconstriction" [2], but it was not until 1948 that the vasoconstrictive substance could be identified as 5-hydroxytryptamine (Fig. 1)

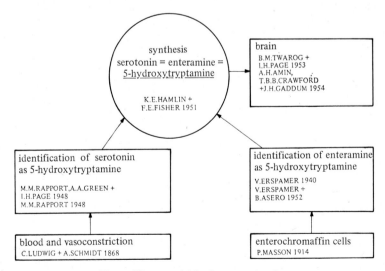

Fig. 1. History of 5-hydroxytryptamine

[3, 4]. The most important localization of 5-HT[1] in mammals is the enterochromaffin cell system of the gastrointestinal tract, where it was discovered by Masson in 1914 [5] because of its chromaffin and argentaffin reactions. This substance was called enteramine. However, identity of enteramine with serotonin [6, 7] and the meanwhile synthesized 5-hydroxytryptamine [8] was established in 1952. The occurrence of 5-HT in brain was only revealed in 1953 during a routine assay of its distribution in different tissues [9, 10]. From thereon research progressed very rapidly in this field.

In contrast to the short scientific history a phylogenetic review must go back to the metazoa, perhaps even to the protozoa. Table 1 lists the 5-HT content in the nervous system of only a few species. Comparison of the 5-HT values of invertebrates and vertebrates neither favours the general assumption that cerebralization and topographic accumulation of 5-HT in brain parallel each other, nor

Table 1. The 5-HT content of nervous tissue in different species

Species	Tissue	5-HT content (μg/g wet tissue)	Ref.
Invertebrates			
Insecta: *Locusta migratoria*	ganglia	<0.2	[11]
Vermes: *Hirudo medicinalis*	nerve cords	6.9	[12, 13]
Mollusca: *Helix pomatia*	ganglia	2—3	[14]
Vertebrates			
Amphia : *Bufo americanus*	brain	9.1	[15, 16]
Bufo marinus	brain	1.5	[15, 16]
Reptilia : *Alligator missis-sipiensis*	diencephalon	0.46—1.56	[17]
Aves : Pigeon	brain	0.7	[15, 16]
Mammalia: Mouse	brain	0.85—1.0	[18]
Rhesus monkey	brain	0.43—0.53	[19]

[1] Abbreviations: 5-HT = 5-hydroxytryptamine (serotonin); 5-HTP = 5-hydroxytryptophan; 5-HIA = 5-hydroxyindole acetaldehyde; 5-HIAA = 5-hydroxyindole acetic acid; 5-HT-ol = 5-hydroxytryptophol; NeuNAc = N-acetylneuraminic acid; MAO = monoamine oxidase; NAcT = N-acetyltransferase; HIOMT = 5-hydroxyindole-*O*-methyltransferase; AANMT = aromatic alkylamine N-methyltransferase; 5-HTP-decarboxylase = aromatic L-amino acid carboxy-lyase, AChE = acetylcholine esterase, ChAc = choline acetylase.

does it prove the contrary. Moreover, it is questionable whether *e. g.* amphibians and mammals can be compared directly with regard to the 5-HT levels since even in one species, *e. g.* the human, 5-HT may take part in such different functions as neurotransmission, hormonal action on the pineal, and control of mood. Contrasting with amphibians in mammals, only the pineal gland can convert serotonin to its N-acetyl-5-methoxy derivative melatonin. Both, conversion and release of melatonin, are controlled by a neuronal signal generated in the retina. The function of the mammalian pineal as a neuroendocrine transducer is quite different from the amphibian organ which is part of a photoreceptor [20].

2. The Serotonin Molecule

Before discussing 5-HT-receptor interactions it is useful to have a look at the 5-HT molecule, since it reveals that the three hetero-atoms may be essential for binding and biological activity (Fig. 2).

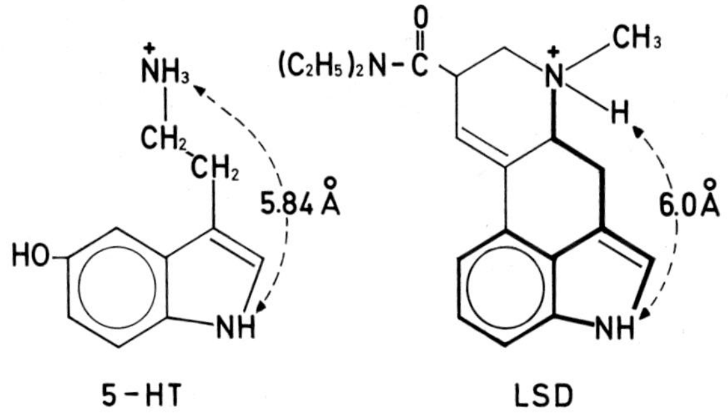

Fig. 2. Structure of 5-hydroxytryptamine and LSD

KIER [21] showed that according to molecular orbital calculations the all-*trans* conformation is the only preferred one. This renders a two-receptor concept for serotonin unlikely. The almost identical inter-nitrogen distance of 5-HT and LSD and the close structural relationship make it conceivable that the prominent antagonist LSD blocks 5-HT receptor sites.

3. Serotonin as Neurotransmitter

When we focus our interest on the possible function of 5-HT as neurotransmitter it must satisfy — like any other transmitter substance in question — a number of criteria. To mention only a few:

1. The brain must contain the possible transmitter substance, the enzymes necessary for its synthesis and the appropiate transport system (availability, synthesis, transport).

2. The substance must be stored in the presynaptic bouton (storage).

3. Presynaptic stimulation must release the substance in question from the terminals into the synaptic cleft (release).

4. The substance must react with specific binding sites of the subsynaptic membrane (transmitter-receptor interaction).

5. The reaction obtained after application of the substance to the presynaptic cell must resemble the synaptic action (functional equivalence of stimulation and transmitter action).

6. The substance must be removed from the subsynaptic binding sites by transport and/or degradation (inactivation).

3.1. Availability, Synthesis, and Transport of Serotonin

Serotonin is found in various amounts in the different areas of the central nervous system (CNS) and is especially concentrated in the older parts of the brain. Rather high concentrations are present in the *bulbus olfactorius*, the *diencephalon*, particularly in the *hypophysis*, and in the *mesencephalon* (Table 2). The fine architecture of the serotonergic neuronal system as revealed by means of histochemical fluorescence techniques, [22,23] shows that from the serotonergic cell bodies in the *raphe* nuclei and in the *formatio reticularis* of the *mesencephalon*, axons are ascending mainly in the medial forebrain bundle terminating *e.g.* in the *neocortex*, the limbic forebrain, and the *hypothalamus*. From the serotonin containing cell bodies in the caudal *raphe* nuclei, axons descend the spinal cord and terminate in segments where motoneurons innervating the limbs are located [24].

Since 5-HT transport to the CNS is hindered either by the blood-brain barrier or by an ineffective transport mechanism [25],

Table 2. 5-HT distribution in different areas of rat brain

Brain area	5-HT (10^{-9} mol/mg protein)
Hypophysis	0.165
Bulbus olfactorius	0.093
Medulla oblongata	0.072
Pons	0.070
Diencephalon	0.065
Mesencephalon	0.065
Nucleus caudatus	0.043
Cortex	0.035
Cerebellum	0.032

the main portion of brain 5-HT is synthesized from tryptophan or 5-hydroxytryptophan [5-HTP] within the brain (Fig. 3). The hydroxylation of tryptophan to 5-HTP by the pteridine requiring enzyme tryptophan-5-hydroxylase [Tryp-OH-ase] is the rate-limiting step in 5-HT biosynthesis. The activity of soluble tryptophan-5-hydroxylase is high in areas rich in 5-HT containing neuronal cell bodies — medulla, ventral midbrain, pons — while it is low in areas that have many serotonergic nerve endings such as corpus striatum [26]. The distribution of the activity of 5-HTP-decarboxylase corresponds in most brain regions to the 5-HT concentration. About 50% of brain 5-HT is removed from brain as 5-hydroxyindole acetic acid [HIAA] ,which is obtained after subsequent oxidation of 5-HT to 5-hydroxyindole acetaldehyde [5-HIA] by the rather unspecific monoamine oxidase [MAO] and to 5-HIAA by an aldehyde dehydrogenase. Only a minor portion of 5-HIA is reduced to 5-hydroxytryptophol [5-HT-ol] by an alcohol dehydrogenase. The diurnal fluctuations of the pineal enzymes N-acetyltransferase [NAcT] and hydroxyindole O-methyltransferase [HIOMT] which convert 5-HT via N-acetyl-5-hydroxytryptamine to N-acetyl-5-methoxytryptamine (melatonin) represent the function of the mammalian pineal as "biological clock". — The extrasynaptosomal localization of aromatic alkylamine N-methyltransferase [AANMT] and its relatively high activities found in nerve ending regions suggest that N-methylation might play a role, though not a predominant one, in the inactivation of released 5-HT [26].

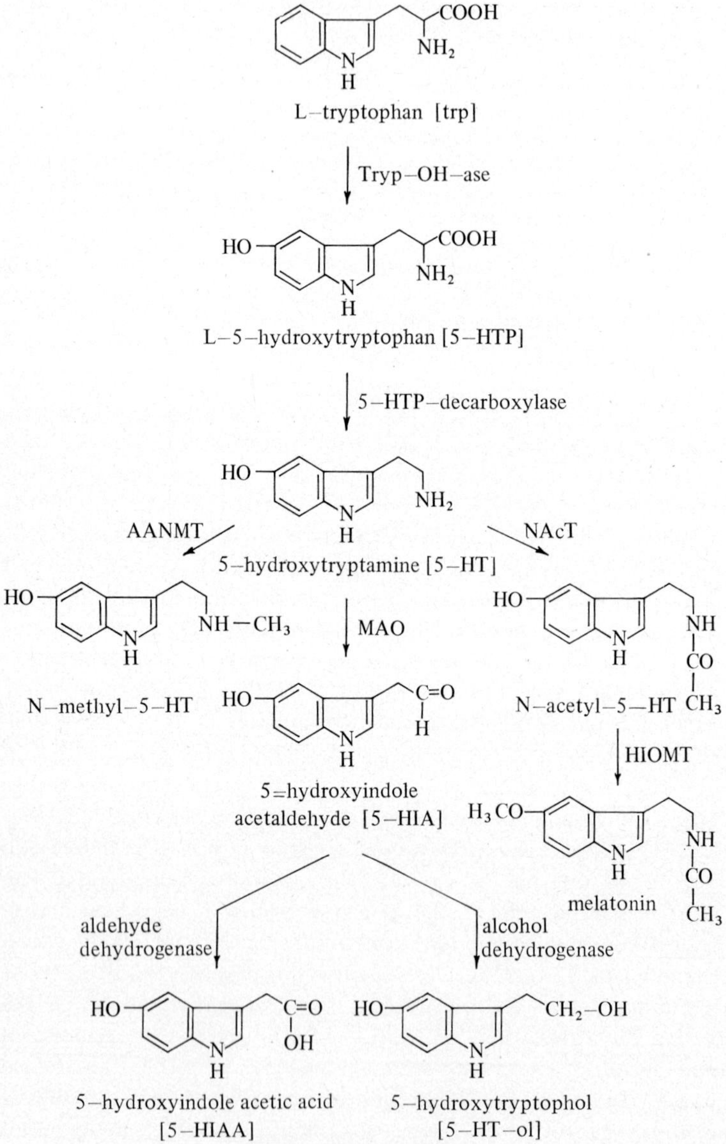

Fig. 3. 5-HT metabolism

Experimental evidence suggests that a least in some brain areas a great portion of the 5-HT is synthesized in the perikaryon and transported via axoplasmic flow to the nerve terminals. Thus only the 5-HT content in the telencephalon is decreased by 78% after medial tegmental lesion [27]; transection of the spinal cord lowers the 5-HT concentration as well as the activity of 5-HTP-decarboxylase and Tryp-OH-ase caudal to the lesion [24]. The axoplasmic transport of 5-HT may be mediated by a carrier molecule, since TAMIR and HUANG [28] detected a soluble protein with high binding affinity for 5-HT in the cytosol of synaptosomes; K_D of the 5-HT-protein complex: 10^{-8} mol/l.

In addition to the availability of 5-HT which is secured by transport and synthesis, a functional interrelationship between 5-HT turnover and electrical activity can also be demonstrated.

Table 3. Interrelationship of 5-HT turnover and electrical activity in raphe nuclei

Stimulus	5-HT content	HIAA synthesis	Firing rate	Ref.
Electrical	↓	↑	—	[29]
LSD	↑	↓	↓	[30—33]
MAO inhibitors	↑	↓	↓	[22, 34]
L-trp	↑	↑	↓	[35, 36]
D-trp	—	—	—	[35]
Imipramine	↑	↓	↓	[35, 37, 38]

Electrical stimulation of the *raphe* nuclei increases the 5-HT turnover, as indicated by a decrease of the 5-HT concentration and an enhancement in 5-HIAA synthesis (Table 3). Substances like LSD, L-tryptophan, Imipramine, and MAO inhibitors raise the 5-HT level and concomitantly reduce the firing rate.

3.2. Storage

The possible transmitter 5-HT which has been synthesized in the perikaryon and which has been transported by means of a carrier mechanism must be stored in compartments of the presynaptic terminal not accessible to the degradation by MAO (Fig. 4). There is accumulating evidence that 5-HT is stored in at least two separate pools [39]: (a) synaptic vesicles can operate as one storage site, (b) the second, the cytoplasmic pool may be identical with carrier bound 5-HT or with low affinity binding sites of 5-HT.

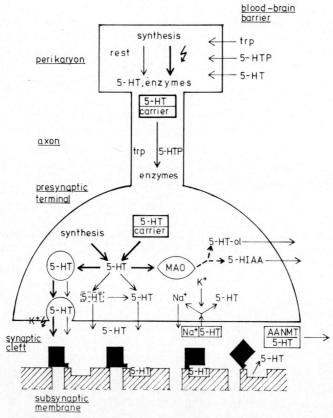

Fig. 4. Metabolism, transport and storage of the putative transmitter 5-HT in the neuronal system

Synaptic vesicles with a 5-HT content of 0,18 nmol/mg protein can be isolated from the 0.2/0.3 M sucrose layer after density gradient centrifugation of ruptured nerve endings (Table 4). These vesicles contain the highest 5-HT concentration of all brain fractions tested so far. After incubation with radioactively labeled

5-HT, the vesicles can accumulate up to 0.85 nmol 5-HT/mg protein [40]. In order to find out whether gangliosides are involved in 5-HT binding, a neuraminic acid analysis was carried out. Though

Table 4

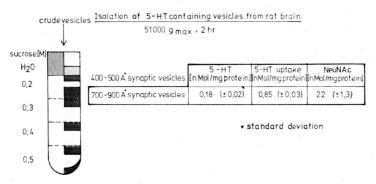

		5-HT [nMol/mg protein]	5-HT uptake [nMol/mg protein]	NeuNAc [nMol/mg protein]
	400–500 Å synaptic vesicles			
	700–900 Å synaptic vesicles	0,18 (±0,02)	0,85 (±0,03)	22 (±1,3)

* standard deviation

22 nmol NeuNAc/mg protein were found in the vesicle fraction, gangliosides could not be detected. Electron micrographs show that the fraction is rich in large and granular vesicles which have in the size-distribution curve a maximum at 735 Å with two shoulders at 600 and 890 Å, indicating three main particle sizes. According to the summation curve, only 3% of the vesicles fall in the range of 300—500 Å characteristic for acetylcholine containing vesicles.

Though part of the 5-HT is metabolized in the terminal by MAO, a significant part is present in the synaptic vesicles and probably in the cytoplasmic pool in a metabolically inert form. This is in accordance with the second postulate that the transmitter in question must be stored in the nerve terminal.

3.3. Release

According to the third criterion, the putative transmitter must be released from the nerve ending into the synaptic cleft on presynaptic stimulation (Fig. 4). Though a decrease of brain 5-HT was measured after stimulation of the *raphe* nuclei [39] and 5-HT was released from brain slices after depolarization of the membranes [29, 41, 42], direct evidence for the validity of this stringent criterion is still missing. In order to study 5-HT metabolism in a more defined system the influence of depolarization on 5-HT release was followed in isolated nerve endings.

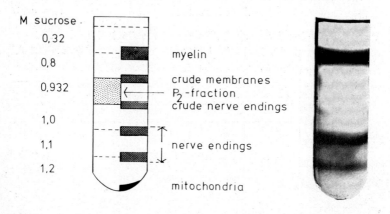

Sucrose density gradient for the isolation of nerve endings at 120000 × g_{max}, 1 hr

Fig. 5. Isolation of nerve endings from rat brain

3.3.1. Isolation of Nerve Endings.

Nerve terminals were isolated either according to BRADFORD (gradient type 3; [43]) or by a procedure developed in our laboratory (Fig. 5). The P_2 fraction (WHITTAKER et al. [44]) was separated by concomitant flotation of myelin and sedimentation of nerve endings and mitochondria in a discontinuous sucrose gradient [45]. Two fractions with nerve endings were obtained. The purity of the fractions was checked by electronmicroscopy, disc electrophoresis, 5-HT content and enzyme analysis. Small nerve endings were enriched in the 1.0/1.1 M sucrose layer, while in the 1.1/1.2 M sucrose fraction mainly bigger nerve endings contaminated with mitochondria were found (Fig. 6a, and b). Impurities resulting from aggregated myelin could be observed neither on the electron micrographs nor after disc electrophoresis. The two very intense amido black positive bands which are present after disc electrophoresis of the myelin fraction are

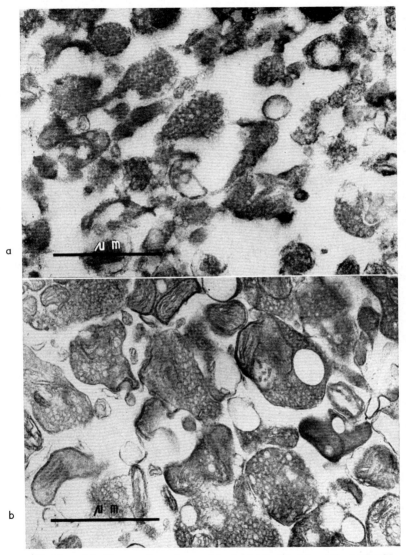

Fig. 6a and b. Nerve endings from rat brain. (a) Isolated from the 1.0/1.1 M sucrose layer. (b) Isolated from the 1.1/1.2 M sucrose layer

absent in the two nerve ending fractions (Fig. 7). As judged by determination especially of 5-HT-decarboxylase activity and 5-HT content (Fig. 8), serotonergic nerve terminals were not significantly concentrated in the 1.0/1.1 M sucrose layer. Therefore, usually the two nerve ending fractions were combined.

3.3.2. Depolarization of Nerve Endings and Serotonin Release.

After incorporation of radioactively labeled 5-HT into isolated nerve endings (see 3.6. Inactivation), the nerve ending membranes were depolarized by incubation in Krebs-phosphate buffer with increasing K^+ concentrations. Compared with the controls contain-

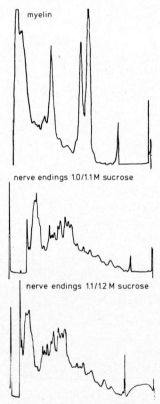

Fig. 7. Densitonetric records after disc electrophoresis of myelin and nerve endings isolated from rat brain, stain: amido black

ing 5 mM K^+, in the presence of 30 mM K^+ the release of radio-actively labeled material, presumably 5-HT and 5-HIAA, is increased by 30%. Addition of Na^+ in the same concentration range does not result in release of significant amounts of radioactivity.

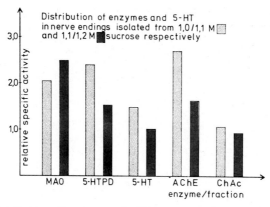

Fig. 8. Distribution of enzymes and 5-HT in nerve endings isolated from rat brain

Encouraged by the fundamental work of MCILWAIN and BRAD-FORD on cerebral excitability [43, 46], we started to measure 5-HT release after electrical stimulation of isolated nerve endings. By means of a stimulation device specially constructed we are able to measure both, electrically triggered release reaction and O_2-consumption (Table 5). After preincubation with radioactively labeled 5-HT followed by a stimulation period of 10 min, about 55% of the total radioactivity incorporated is released as compared with about 25% in the non-stimulated control. The respiration results measured with the Clark electrode — about 66 μmol O_2/100 mg protein/hr during rest and about 97 μM O_2/100 mg protein/hr during stimulation — are in accordance with data obtained by Warburg measurements using brain slices [46], respectively synaptosomal beds and synaptosomal suspensions [47]. The 5-HT release was measured in the presence of the MAO inhibitor Marsilid. Further work has to clarify possible changes in 5-HT metabolism during in vitro stimulation when no MAO inhibitor is present. The two findings, however, (1) that stimulation of the raphe nuclei in situ decreases brain 5-HT and (2) that K^+ and electrical induced depolarization liberates 5-HT from the nerve terminals strongly suggest that *in vivo* 5-HT is also released into the synaptic cleft on presynaptic stimulation.

Table 5

treatment	5-HT-^{3}H		respiration
	total [dpm/mg protein]	% released in medium	μMol O_2/ 100 mg protein / hr
control	368 211	25	66
stimulation	358 959	55	97

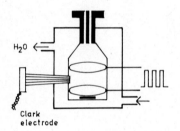

H₂O ←

Clark electrode

After incorporation of ^{3}H - 5-HT, 2×10^{-7} M, nerve endings were incubated with or without stimulation in Krebs - phosphate medium, 6×10^{-3}M Marsilid, for 10' at 37° C.

3.4. Transmitter-Receptor Interaction

In the synaptic cleft the putative transmitter must react with the acceptor molecules of the subsynaptic membranes which become de- or hyperpolarized (Fig. 4). To test the validity of this assumption, nerve ending membranes were isolated by gradient centrifugation according to conventional procedures [40, 44, 48] and analysed for possible binding sites (Table 6). The 5-HT content of the two membrane fractions 40 and 51 pmol 5-HT/mg protein respectively, is second in height from all brain fractions analysed. Binding experiments with radioactively labeled 5-HT show that there is a high affinity binding of 5-HT towards the membrane structures with a rather small dissociation constant, $K_D = 7 \times 10^{-6}$ mol/l [49].

In the last years we have been engaged in studies [49] about the mode of action of the antiviral and antiparkinson compound 1-adamantanamine which interferes with 5-HT distribution in brain, liver, and thrombocytes. Therefore we investigated the action of 1-adamantanamine and its 3,5-dimethylderivative, D 145, on these isolated nerve ending membranes. The modified Dixon plot (Fig. 9) indicates that the 5-HT binding to the membranes is non-competitively inhibited by these two compounds, which are of

Table 6

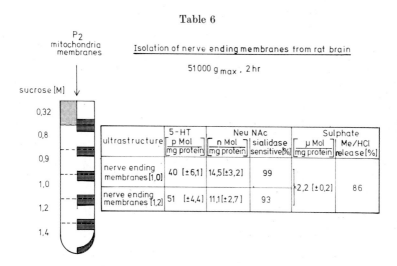

ultrastructure	5-HT [p Mol / mg protein]	Neu NAc [n Mol / mg protein]	sialidase sensitive [%]	Sulphate [μ Mol / mg protein]	Me/HCl release [%]
nerve ending membranes [1,0]	40 [±6,1]	14,5[±3,2]	99	2,2 [±0,2]	86
nerve ending membranes [1,2]	51 [±4,4]	11,1[±2,7]	93		

interest for the treatment of central disorders as well as for studies on neurotransmission. Contrary to reserpine which inhibits the uptake of 5-HT into the vesicles and which can induce Parkinsonism, 1-adamantanamine inhibits both, the uptake of 5-HT into the vesicles and the binding to the nerve ending membranes. Thus, although both substances interfere with the uptake, it is of special interest that adamantanamine, which in addition also inhibits the binding of 5-HT to the membranes, has an antiparkinson effect.

As compared with other neuronal membranes, nerve ending membranes contain a carbohydrate-rich cell coat [50—52]. Sialoglycolipids and sialoglycoproteins appear to be of significance for synaptic transmission, since it was shown that these substances restore the electrical excitability of inactivated brain tissue [46] and possess binding capacity towards cations such as Na^+, K^+, and Ca^{++} [53, 54] and towards transmitter molecules [55]. Sulfated acid mucopolysaccharides are enriched in subcellular fractions of nerve endings where they can regulate activities of enzymes such as tyrosine hydroxylase [56—58]. From the total neuraminic acid, NeuNAc, content of 14.5 and 11.1 nmol/mg protein, respectively, ca. 90—100% can be split off from the membranes by treatment with neuraminidase (Table 6). The rather high sulfate content of

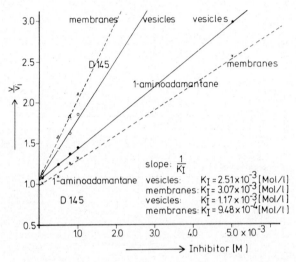

Fig. 9. Inhibition of the 5-HT incorporation into synaptic vesicles and nerve ending membranes by 1-aminoadamantane and D 145 [49]

2.2 μmol/mg protein can be removed almost completely by transesterification with methanol [14].

The specific labeling of the sulfate and NeuNAc-containing structures was attained on the electron microscopical level by treatment with colloidal iron hydroxide (CIH) [59]. At pH = 1.7, CIH was precipitated as electron dense granules with a uniform size of 6—7 nm marking the reaction sites with sulfate and the carboxy group of NeuNAc (Fig. 10a and b). After incubation with neuraminidase which removes NeuNAc, the reactivity of the membranes with CIH is reduced (Fig. 10e and f), since CIH now only reacts with the sulfate groups. When freshly prepared membranes are incubated with methanol/HCl, the reactivity towards CIH is practically lost since the sulfate groups are removed by transesterification and the carboxyl groups of NeuNAc become blocked by

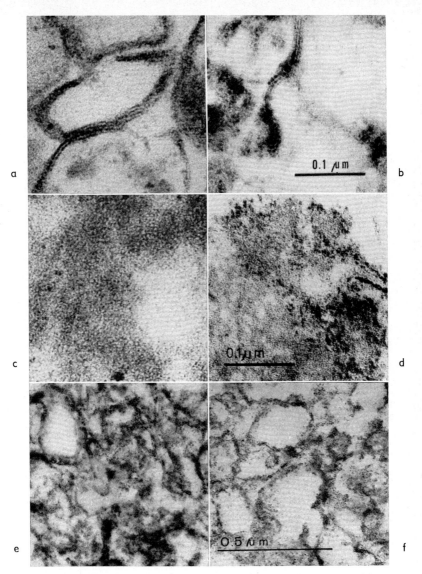

Fig. 10a—f. Electron micrographs of nerve ending membranes isolated from rat brain [59]. (a) Untreated. (b) Treated with colloidal iron hydroxide. (c) Treated with colloidal iron hydroxide after esterification with methanol/ HCl. (d) Treated with colloidal iron hydroxide after esterification and saponification. (e) Treated with colloidal iron hydroxide. (f) Treated with colloidal iron hydroxide preceded by incubation with neuraminidase

esterification (Fig. 10c). After subsequent saponification, the methylester of NeuNAc is hydrolysed and the reactivity towards ClH partly restored. The iron deposits label the acid-resistant neuraminic acid residues of the membrane structure (Fig. 10d). These results confirm that sulfate esters and NeuNAc-containing substances are located at the membranes of the nerve terminals.

Since previous studies in our laboratory on rat stomach fundus have suggested a correlation between 5-HT-induced contraction of smooth muscle and NeuNAc metabolism [60], in the present experiments we analysed the question as to whether 5-HT is also bound to neuraminic acid containing membranes of nerve endings. The relative distribution of NeuNAc and 5-HT in butanol/H_2O extracts of nerve ending membranes which had been preincubated with 5-HT-3-^{14}C indicate that about 50% of the total 5-HT and 25% of the NeuNAc are recovered in the butanol phase, though this phase contains only 7% of the total protein (Table 7). The

Table 7. Relative distribution of protein, N-acetyl-neuraminic acid, and exogenous 5-HT-3-^{14}C in butanol/H_2O extracts of nerve ending membranes

Substance	Distribution % (relative specific concentration)		
	Butanol	H_2O	ppt.
Protein	7%	4%	87%
5-HT-3-^{14}C	49% (7.0)	4% (1.0)	45% (0.5)
NeuNAc	24% (3.2)	4% (0.8)	71% (0.8)

specific concentrations related to protein show that NeuNAc (r.sp.c. 3.2) and 5-HT (r.sp.c. 7.0) are enriched in the butanol phase. Since more 5-HT can be recovered from the butanol phase than can be attributed to unbound 5-HT, the enrichment in the butanol phase could mean that partition is mediated by a NeuNAc containing carrier or acceptor substance which might be identical with the 5-HT binding proteolipid described by FISZER and DEROBERTIS [61].

In our attempts to get further information about the nature of the subsynaptic 5-HT receptor, we recently succeeded in preparing an affinity resin by coupling N-6-(aminohexyl)-tryptamines to

CNBr-activated Sepharose 4 B (Fig.11). The tryptamine derivatives were obtained by subsequent condensation of the corresponding indole derivatives with oxalyl chloride and ε-aminocaproamide and reduction with $LiAlH_4$. The 6-aminohexyl-group was used as

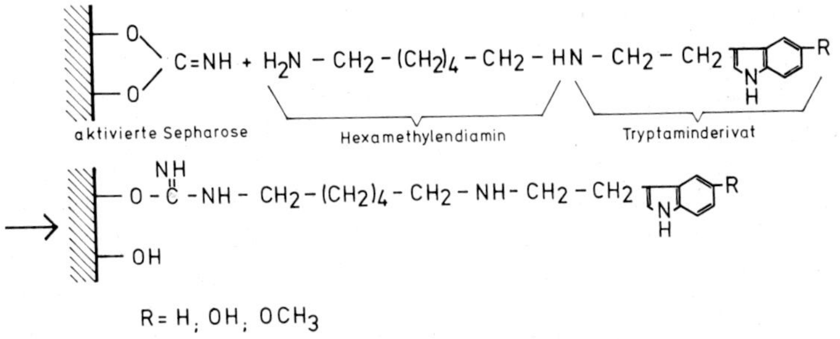

Fig. 11. Synthesis of affinity resin for the chromatography of 5-HT acceptor substance [62]

spacer to link covalently the primary amino group of tryptamine to agarose. A SDS extract from nerve ending membranes was resolved on this affinity resin into two fractions, as compared with only one fraction by the use of unsubstituted Sepharose 4 B (Fig. 12). No obvious differences in the elution pattern were found using indole, 5-methoxy or 5-hydroxyindole derivatives as ligand. Though a clear-cut separation of the two protein fractions was obtained, a satisfying purification of the 5-HT acceptor substance in the second fraction could not be expected since acid substances of the extract will also adhere to the secondary amino groups of the resin and will be found in the same fraction. However, by means of preceding chromatography of a Tween 80 membrane extract on Sepharose 2B part of the unspecific proteins was removed in one fraction, while a second fraction contained a substance with a binding constant towards 5-HT of about 2.5×10^5 l/mol. Rechromatography of this fraction on the affinity column and affinity elution with tryptamine resulted in a ca. 1000 fold enrichment of this substance as compared with the membrane proteins. These first few experiments must be followed by large scale preparation and purification in order to obtain data about the chemical nature and the binding characteristics of the acceptor molecule.

Since we are concerned in our studies with the 5-HT receptor of the subsynaptic membrane, it should also be mentioned that there might exist different types of 5-HT binding with various functions

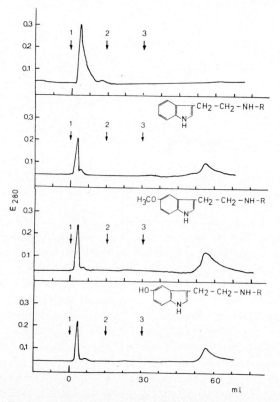

Fig. 12. Affinity chromatography of an SDS extract from nerve ending membranes on Sepharose and on affinity resins with indole-, 5-methoxy-, and 5-hydroxyindole derivatives as ligands [62]

within the neuronal system (Table 8). (1) The 5-HT binding protein described by TAMIR and HUANG [28] is perhaps identical with the carrier which transports the 5-HT molecule from the perikaryon via axon to the synaptic terminal. (2) The synaptic vesicles and the cytoplasmic 5-HT pool in the presynaptic bouton may be regarded

Table 8. Function and localization of possible 5-HT acceptor molecules within the neuronal system

Function	Morphological structure
Transport [carrier]	Perikaryon Axoplasma Presynaptic bouton

Storage	Presynaptic bouton:
	    synaptic vesicles
	    cytoplasmic storage

Release [binding site]	Presynaptic membrane
Retrieval [carrier]	Presynaptic membrane
De- or hyperpolarization ["receptor"]	Subsynaptic membrane

as binding sites. The lipid composition of the vesicles has been investigated by the groups of WHITTAKER and GOMEZ [63, 64]. (3) Since the mechanism of the release reaction has not yet been elucidated, it is uncertain whether there exist binding sites at the presynaptic membrane to which the transmitter molecules are transitorily bound. It is also possible that the transmitter molecules are directly released from the vesicles into the synaptic cleft. (4) A carrier mechanism driven by a cation gradient might operate in order to remove 5-HT from the synaptic cleft. (5) The interaction of 5-HT with the acceptor molecule in the subsynaptic membrane, the "actual receptor", triggers the de- or hyperpolarization of the membrane. The listing of possible binding substances does not mean that further binding sites might not exist or that we really know all these acceptors.

In this context the work of CARNEGIE et al. [65, 66] and SMYTHIES et al. [67] should be mentioned, who isolated a basic protein, the "encephalotogenic" factor from brain. The authors define this protein as a "possible molecular form of a serotonin receptor" [67] or a "possible neuroreceptor" [65] because it interacts with 5-HT. Since this protein is predominantly located in the myelin fraction, it is unlikely that it is specifically involved in the neurotransmitter action at the synaptic celft.

3.5. Functional Equivalence of Stimulation and Transmitter Action

Mainly physiological and pharmacological experiments contributed to the postulate that application of 5-HT to the postsynaptic cell must cause the same reaction as the synaptic action.

Table 9. Response of firing rate in central neurons to 5-HT application

CNS region		Animal	Response	Ref.
Cerebellum:	Purkinje cell	cat	depression	[68—71]
Brain stem:	*pont. raphe*	rat	depression/activation	[72]
Spinal cord:	motor neuron	cat	activation	[24]
	flexor reflex	cat	depression	[24]
Cortex:	*cort. pyriform.*	rat	activation	[73]

Table 9 gives a few examples that 5-HT can stimulate or depress the neuronal action. The inhibitory and stimulating action of 5-HT on the firing of the *pont. raphe* indicates that defined anatomical areas and functional entities can be different in regard to 5-HT action. The response of the Purkinje cells, the *pont. raphe*, the spinal cord and the *cortex pyriform.* to 5-HT application demonstrates the equivalence of stimulation and transmitter action.

3.6. Inactivation

Serotonin can only be classified as neurotransmitter, provided that after the release into the synaptic cleft and the binding to the receptor sites of the synaptic membranes it will be inactivated either by enzymatic degradation or by removal. Previous inactivation is necessary so that the membrane can react with new transmitter molecules in response to new stimuli. Though extra-synaptosomal alkylamine N-methyltransferase was found to convert 5-HT to its biologically inactive mono-methyl derivative [26], the main inactivation mechanism appears to be the retrieval into the nerve endings. The active uptake of 5-HT into isolated nerve endings is time and concentration dependent (Fig. 13). After incubation with a 1 μM solution of 5-HT up to 50 p moles were incorporated per mg protein within 10 min. Adding the MAO inhibitor Marsilid to the incubation medium, the uptake decreases to about 1/10, indicating a high turnover of 5-HT to 5-HIAA. Our results obtained with isolated nerve endings correspond well with studies on brain slices [38, 41] and with the experimental finding that the 5-HT uptake into nerve endings of rat forebrain is reduced after midbrain *raphe* lesion [74—76].

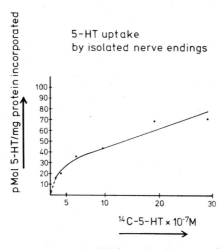

Fig. 13. Retrieval of 5-HT by isolated nerve endings

4. Summary and Conclusion

Experimental evidence is accumulating for the transmitter function of 5-HT. It satisfies some stringent criteria of a neurotransmitter: 5-HT is synthesized, transported and stored in the neuronal system. On stimulation it is released from the nerve terminal into the synaptic cleft where it reacts with acceptor molecules of the subsynaptic membranes, inducing activation or depression of neuronal firing depending on the morphological and functional entity. After the reaction with the subsynaptic membrane, 5-HT is inactivated predominantly by retrieval into the presynaptic bouton. Before 5-HT can be classified definitely as neurotransmitter, the following 3 points should be clarified: (1) The interrelationship of 5-HT mediated transmission with a possible role of cyclic AMP has to be investigated, especially in regard to a possible differentiation between neurotransmitter and neurohormone function. (2) It should be investigated how 5-HT can mediate both, the activation and the depression of neuronal firing patterns. (3) The purification of the subsynaptic receptor molecule and its structural and chemical analysis should be performed. — Further work must be concerned with the biosynthesis of the receptor molecules and its possible dependency on stimulation and drug action.

Acknowledgment

The author is gratefully indebted to Dr. R. Marx, Marburg, and Professor W. Vogell, Konstanz, for carrying out the electron microscopy and co-operating in the histochemical experiments. I wish to express my gratitude to Dr. H. F. Bradford, London, for stimulating and encouraging discussions on the electrical stimulation of isolated nerve endings. I would also like to thank Drs. A. M. Assink, G. Dette, U. Haacke, D. Lathia, and J.-D. Schollmeyer of the University of Marburg, and Dr. F. Seela, at present Max-Planck-Institut f. Exp. Medizin, Göttingen, for their collaboration. This work was supported by grants from the Deutsche Forschungsgemeinschaft.

References

1. Page, I. H., McCubbin, J. W.: Circulation **14**, 161 (1956).
2. Ludwig, C., Schmidt, A.: Arb. physiol. Anstalt (Leipzig) **3**, 12, 1 (1868).
3. Rapport, M. M., Green, A. A., Page, I. H.: J. biol. Chem. **176**, 1243 (1948).
4. Rapport, M. M.: J. biol. Chem. **180**, 961 (1948).
5. Masson, P.: C. R. Acad. Sci. (Paris) **158**, 59 (1914).
6. Erspamer, V.: Arch. exp. Path. Pharmak. **196**, 343 (1940).
7. Erspamer, V., Asero, B.: Nature (Lond.) **169**, 800 (1952).
8. Hamlin, K. E., Fischer, F. E.: J. Amer. chem. Soc. **73**, 5007 (1951).
9. Twarog, B. M., Page, I. H.: Amer. J. Physiol. **175**, 175 (1953).
10. Amin, A. H., Crawford, T. B. B., Gaddum, J. H.: J. Physiol. (Lond.) **126**, 596 (1954).
11. Erspamer, V.: In: Eichler, O., Farah, A. (Eds.): Handbook of exptl., pharmacol, Vol. XIX, p. 162. Berlin-Heidelberg-New York: Springer 1966.
12. Welsh, J. H., Moorhead, M.: Science **129**, 1491 (1959).
13. Welsh, J. H., Moorhead, M.: J. Neurochem. **6**, 146 (1960).
14. Meng, K.: Naturwissenschaften **45**, 470 (1958).
15. Bogdanski, D. F., Bonomi, L., Brodie, B. B.: Life Sci. **1**, 80 (1963).
16. Brodie, B. B., Bogdanski, D. F., Bonomi, L.: In: Richter, D. (Ed.): Comparative neurochemistry, p. 367. Oxford: Pergamon Press 1964.
17. Welsh, J. H.: In: Richter, D. (Ed.): Comparative neurochemistry, p. 355. Oxford: Pergamon Press 1964.
18. Pletscher A.: Helv. physiol. Acta **14**, C 76 (1956).
19. Weissman, A., Finger, K. F.: Biochem. Pharmacol. **11**, 871 (1962).

20. WURTMAN, R. J.: In: LAJTHA, A. (Ed.): Handbook of neurochemistry, Vol. IV, p. 451. New York-London: Planum Press 1970.
21. KIER, L. B.: J. Pharm. Sci. 57, 1188 (1968).
22. DAHLSTRÖM, A., FUXE, K.: Acta physiol. scand, 62, Suppl. 232, 1 (1964).
23. FUXE, K.: Acta physiol. scand. 64, Suppl. 247, 41 (1965).
24. ANDERSON, E. G.: Fed. Proc. 31, 107 (1972).
25. NEAME, K. D.: In: LAJTHA, A. (Ed.): Handbook of neurochemistry, Vol. IV, p. 329. New York-London: Plenum Press 1970.
26. MANDELL, A. J., KNAPP, S., HSU, L. L.: Life Sci. 14, 1 (1974).
27. HELLER, A.: Fed. Proc. 31, 81 (1972).
28. TAMIR, H., HUANG, Y. L.: Life Sci. 14, 83 (1974).
29. AGHAJANIAN, G. K., ROSECRANS, J. A., SHEARD, M. H.: Science 156, 402 (1967).
30. AGHAJANIAN, G. K., FREEDMANN, D. X.: In: EFRON, D. H. (Ed.): Psychopharmacology: a review of progress, p. 1185. Washington: US. Govt.-Printing Office 1968.
31. ANDÉN, N. E., CORRODI, H., FUXE, K., HÖKFELT, T.: Br. J. Pharmacol. 34, 1 (1968).
32. FREEDMAN, D. X.: J. Pharmacol. exp. Ther. 134, 160 (1961).
33. ROSECRANS, J. A., LOVELL, R. A., FREEDMAN, D. X.: Biochem. Pharmacol. 16, 2011 (1967).
34. AGHAJANIAN, G. K., GRAHAM, A. W., SHEARD, M. H.: Science 169, 1100 (1970).
35. AGHAJANIAN, G. K.: Fed. Proc. 31, 91 (1972).
36. AGHAJANIAN, G. K., ASHER, I. M.: Science 172, 1159 (1971).
37. CARLSSON, A.: J. Pharm. Pharmacol. 22, 729 (1970).
38. SHASKAN, E. G., SNYDER, S. H.: J. Pharmacol. expt. Ther. 175, 404 (1970).
39. SHIELDS, P. J., ECCLESTON, D.: J. Neurochem. 20, 881 (1973).
40. WESEMANN, W.: FEBS Letters 3, 80 (1969).
41. CHASE, T. N., KATZ, R. L., KOPIN, I. J.: J. Neurochem. 16, 607 (1969).
42. ANDÉN, N.-E., CARLSSON, A., HILLARP, N.-A., MAGNUSSON, T.: Life Sci. 3, 473 (1964).
43. BRADFORD, H. F.: In: FRIED, R. (Ed.): Methods of neurochemistry, Vol. 3, p. 155. New York: Marcel Dekker 1972.
44. WHITTAKER, V. P., MICHAELSON, I. A., KIRKLAND, R. J.: Biochem. J. 90, 293 (1964).
45. WESEMANN, W., SCHOLLMEYER, J., LATHIA, D.: Proceed. 9th Inter. Congress of Biochemistry, p. 444. Stockholm 1973.
46. MCILWAIN, H.: Chemical exploration of the brain. Amsterdam-London-New York: Elsevier Publish. Comp. 1963.
47. DEBELLEROCHE, J. S., BRADFORD, H. F.: J. Neurochem. 19, 585 (1972).
48. DEROBERTIS, E., ALBERICI, M., DELORES, ARNAIZ, G. R., AZCURRA, J. M.: Life Sci. 5, 577 (1966).
49. WESEMANN, W., FELLEHNER, H., SCHOLLMEYER, J.: Proceed. Special Meeting FEBS, p. 150. Dublin 1972.
50. RAMBOURG, A., LEBLOND, C. P.: J. Cell Biol. 32, 27 (1967).
51. BONDAREFF, W.: Anat. Rec. 157, 527 (1967).

52. BONDAREFF, W.: Z. Zellforsch. mikr. Anat. **81**, 366 (1967).
53. DERRY, D. M., WOLFE, L. S.: Science **158**, 1450 (1967).
54. SPENCE, M. W., WOLFE, L. S.: J. Neurochem. **14**, 585 (1967).
55. WESEMANN, W., HENKEL, R., MARX, R.: Biochem. Pharmac. **20**, 1961 (1971).
56. KUCZENSKI, R., MANDELL, A. J.: J. biol. Chem. **247**, 3114 (1972).
57. KUCZENSKI, R.: J. biol. Chem. **248**, 5074 (1973).
58. KUCZENSKI, R.: Life Sci. **13**, 247 (1973).
59. MARX, R., GRAF, E., WESEMANN, W.: J. Cell Sci. **13**, 237 (1973).
60. WESEMANN, W., ZILLIKEN, F.: Hoppe-Seylers Z. physiol. Chem. **349**, 823 (1968).
61. FISZER, S., DEROBERTIS, E.: J. Neurochem. **16**, 1201 (1969).
62. SEELA, F., WESEMANN, W.: Z. Naturforsch. **29 C**, 248 (1974).
63. EICHBERG, J., WHITTAKER, V. P., DAWSON, R. M. C.: Biochem. J. **92**, 91 (1964).
64. SEMINARIO, L. M., HREN, N., GOMEZ, C. J.: J. Neurochem. **11**, 197 (1964).
65. CARNEGIE, P. R.: Nature (Lond.) **229**, 25 (1971).
66. FIELD, E. J., CASPARY, E. A., CARNEGIE, P. R.: Nature (Lond.) **233**, 284 (1971).
67. SMYTHIES, J. R., BENINGTON, F., MORIN, R. D.: Experientia (Basel) **28**, 23 (1972).
68. BLOOM, F. E., HOFFER, B. J., SIGGINS, G. R., BARKER, J. L., NICOLL, R. A.: Fed. Proc. **31**, 97 (1972).
69. KAWAMURA, H., PROVINI, L.: Brain Res. **24**, 293 (1970).
70. KRNJEVIC, K., PHILLIS, J. W.: J. Physiol. (Lond.) **166**, 296 (1963).
71. PHILLIS, J. W.: The pharmacology of synapses. New York: Pergamon Press 1970.
72. COUCH, J. R.: Brain Res. **19**, 137 (1970).
73. ROBERTS, M. H. T., STRAUGHAN, D. W.: J. Physiol. (Lond.) **193**, 269 (1967).
74. KUHAR, M. J., AGHAJANIAN, G. K., ROTH, R. H.: Brain Res. **44**, 165 (1972).
75. KUHAR, M. J., ROTH, R. H., AGHAJANIAN, G. K.: J. Pharmacol. exp. Therap. **181**, 36 (1972).
76. KUHAR, M. J.: Life Sci. **13**, 1623 (1973).

Discussion

B. HAMPRECHT (München): Dr. WESEMANN, did you perform experiments on the active uptake of serotonin into the vesicles you isolated?

W. WESEMANN: We did not perform detailed studies on the active uptake. However, the serotonin uptake into isolated synaptic vesicles is decreased at 4° C as compared with the incorporation at 37° C. Moreover, the uptake is time dependent and reveals two plateaux corresponding to 0.44 and 0.85 nmoles 5-HT incorporated per mg vesicle protein.

E. MEHL (München): What is the binding capacity in nmoles per mg of protein of your purified fractions?

W. WESEMANN: At this moment I do not know the exact figure for the binding capacity expressed in nmoles per mg protein. But the binding capacity of our purified fraction will be in this order of magnitude, since already the fraction applied to the affinity column binds almost 10^{-10} moles 5-HT/mg protein. The binding constant of this fraction towards 5-HT is about 2.5×10^5 l/mole. We have indications for a second, even higher binding constant. But, as I pointed out in my lecture, first we have to perform large scale preparations before we can extend the Scatchard plot to the low concentration range. The occurrence of two binding sites — first mentioned by MARCHBANKS, R.M. J. Neurochem. **13**, 1481 (1966) — could mean that the retrieval of 5-HT is mediated by two different uptake processes as suggested by the two slopes in Fig. 13. — In contrast to Dr. MEHL who eluted the protein fractions from the LSD affinity column with a SDS containing buffer, we use SDS only to compare the resolution power of our affinity resins with Sepharose 4B. All other experiments — measurements of the binding capacity as well as chromatography — were performed with Tween 80 extracts of the membranes, since SDS may interfere with the reconstitution of membrane proteins and thus with binding phenomena. The affinity elution was achieved with tryptamine without SDS or a salt gradient. The specific eluted fractions resulted in an enrichment of protein by factor 1000 as compared with membrane proteins, and 100000 with regard to total proteins.

Purification of Serotonin- and LSD-binding Proteins from Synaptic Membranes

E. MEHL and L. WEBER

*Max-Planck-Institut für Psychiatrie, Neurochemische Abteilung,
D-8000 München, Federal Republic of Germany*

With 1 Figure

We have been working on the isolation of serotonin-binding proteins from pig brain using affinity chromatography [1, 2]. In contrast to the approach with tryptamine derivatives of the preceding paper, the affinity gels were prepared with the LSD-analogue D-lysergic acid diaminohexane amide, a serotonin antagonist of high affinity, and the elution was of increasing specificity using D,L-tryptophan, serotonin, 1-methyl-D-lysergic acid butanolamide and finally D-LSD. According to LSD-binding data with crude membranes, a purification higher than 100000-fold would be necessary. To differentiate between synaptic and extra-synaptic origin of binding proteins, detergent extracts of two types of subcellular fractions were subfractionated in parallel on two affinity columns, and the dialysed fractions were compared for their ^{3}H serotonin binding capacity. The binding profiles of total particulate fraction (Fig. 1A) and external synaptosomal membranes (Fig. 1B) have four binding protein peaks in common, indicating extra-synaptic origin. The most specifically eluted binding protein (Fig. 1 B, indicated by arrow) is the most concentrated one in synaptic membranes, as would be postulated for a receptor. Upon radio-iodination and sodium dodecylsulfate (SDS) gel electrophoresis of this fraction, the apparent molecular weights of the five protein zones can be given a mono-, di-, and hexamer of a 35000 dalton unit and as mono- and dimer of a 40000 dalton unit. After preparative affinity chromatography of extracts from the total particulate fraction of 200 g cortex on 20 ml-affinity gels, the LSD-eluted fraction was characterized further. LSD-binding data indicated dissociation constants of about 10 nM and 1 μM, and optimal binding at pH = 6.5. These figures resemble very closely those obtained with

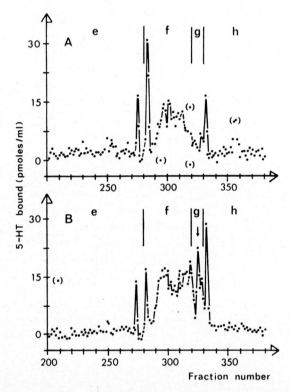

Fig. 1A and B. Profiles of ³H serotonin-binding capacity of 2.7 ml-fractions after affinity chromatography of extracts from total particulate fraction (A) and external synaptosomal membranes (B). Proteins were extracted with 0.1% SDS in 50 mM sodium phosphate, pH = 7.4 (2.5 mg membrane protein/ml). The extracts and the eluents were pumped at a rate of 5 ml/hr onto 2 ml-columns. The eluents (a to h) contained standard buffer (150 mM NaCl, 50 mM *Tris*-HCl, pH = 7.4, 0.1% SDS, 0.02% NaN₃) plus various additions: 0.6 M NaCl (*b*, 100 ml), 2.0 M urea (*c*, 100 ml) 5 mM D, L-tryptophan (*d*, 220 ml), a linear gradient of serotonin, 0.1-30 mM (*e*), 1 mM 1-methyl-D lysergic acid butanolamide (*f*), 0.7 mM D-LSD (*g*), 2.0 M urea, pH = 10 (*h*). After exhaustive dialysis, binding capacity was assayed in 400 μl-ultrafiltration cells in presence of 20 nM ³H serotonin and 0.012% SDS native, unextracted synaptic membranes [3]. So far tested, the binding is rather specific (Table 1).

Thus, the purified high affinity LSD- and serotonin-binding protein fulfils some of the limited criteria [3] applicable for receptor identification.

Table 1. Specificity of binding

Substance (50 nM)	Binding capacity (nmoles/mg protein)
D-LSD	1.27
Serotonin	0.5
Tyramine	0.06
Dopamine	<0.006
D, L-Norepinephrine	<0.006
Histamine	<0.03
Acetylcholine	<0.03

References

1. MEHL, E., WEBER, L.: Abstr. 4th Int. Meeting Int. Soc. Neurochem., No. 111. Tokyo 1973.
2. MEHL, E., WEBER, L.: Advances in biochemical psychopharmacology. In: COSTA, E., SANDLER, M. (Eds.): Serotonin, Vol. 11. New York: Raven Press 1974, p. 105—108.
3. FARROW, J. T., VAN VUNAKIS, H.: Biochem. Pharmacol. **22**, 1103—1113 (1973).

Biochemistry of Learning Processes

Biochemical Concomitants of the Storage of Behavioral Information

BERNARD W. AGRANOFF

Neuroscience Laboratory and Department of Biological Chemistry, The University of Michigan Ann Arbor, MJ 48101 USA

With 1 Figure

Introduction

The topic of the 25th Mosbach Colloquium testifies to the significant recent interest, as well as progress, in understanding sensory mechanisms. While it is logical to think of sensory reception as the beginning of a coding process and to therefore next consider the storage of encoded information, it is appropriate to first address ourselves to the vast conceptual gap between receptor interactions and the subsequent processing steps in the nervous system. In the recent studies on *E. coli* chemotaxis [1, 2], we see the beginning of a complete story, albeit at an elementary level — of how a sensory input is used to elicit a response of biological significance to the organism. In a higher animal, sensory information is first transduced into nerve impulses which are centrally processed and in some way associated with temporally related events. This paper will describe biochemical attempts, particularly over the past 10 years in our laboratory as well as those of others, to understand *when*, in relation to the learning process memory storage occurs, *where*, if at all, memory storage functions are localized in the vertebrate brain and *what* kinds of molecular events appear to mediate the process.

Two problems immediately present themselves. The first concerns the quantification of learning and memory. In behavioral experiments, we establish whether or not an animal responds in a predicted fashion. The gross behavior observed is the summation of a great number of factors, and it is not immediately apparent which of many behavioral measures is most useful [3]. For example, the latency or time interval between presentation of a stimulus and the response is often used. Alternatively, one can record the number of errors made in acquiring a predetermined performance criterion, or the rate of repetitive responding in a given time period. Computations can be based on absolute or relative scores, in which a measure of performance in a retraining session is compared with that seen on initial training. No one behavioral measure or method of computation would appear *a priori* to be more representative than another of the underlying biological processes, yet depending upon which variable is used, quite different conclusions can be drawn [4]. Genetic differences among individual animals can account for some of the variability seen in behavioral studies [5—7], but even genetically similar or identical animals such as clones [8] will learn a given task in somewhat different ways, depending on their previous life experience and the details of presentation of each training trial. Because of the high degree of inherent variability in behavioral experiments, psychologists tend to use learning paradigms and scoring systens that give the greatest degree of reliability, arrived upon on an empirical basis, and to rely heavily on experimental design, including appropriate control groups to validate their experiments. For these reasons, comparison of experiments between laboratories is often difficult. The most useful behavioral findings have resulted from continued efforts within a single laboratory using the same experimental system.

In studies on memory, we must infer from the measured performance of experimental subjects conclusions regarding the associative strength of a newly learned behavior. When we intervene experimentally to cause a reduction in subsequent performance, great caution must be taken in the interpretation of the results. Before we can conclude that we have disrupted memory, we must consider the alternative explanation that (1) lingering effects of the putative disruptive agent may still be effective at the time of retraining. If an injected drug produces disorientation or confusion, it may be blocking the retrieval of encoded memory. If we wait for the effect to wear off, we should ultimately see recovery of the learned behavior; (2) aversive (unpleasant) stimulus effects of a drug or physical agent might serve as a punishment, so that when it is given following training it will discourage the subject from subsequent performance of the learned behavior. Other aspects of these problems will be discussed in relation to specific experiments.

A second major problem category for the biochemist is that he has no idea how much of a biochemical change to expect when an animals' behavior is permanently altered as a result of experience. Considering the enormous capacity of the brain, implicit from the diversity of possible behavioral responses, it would seem that the amount of expected change in the total isotopic labeling of brain RNA or protein associated with learning a single novel task should be quite small. This then casts considerable doubt on whether such gross studies as biochemical concomitants of behavior in whole brain [9] are worth pursuing. Even when we examine a specific brain area known by various considerations to participate in the learning of a new task [10], we must still bear in mind that many other behaviors are very likely mediated by brain cells in the same region.

Why then should a biochemist be encouraged to believe that he can learn something significant about higher brain function ? It is based largely on the belief that since behavioral memory is long-lasting, its formation should be mediated by a process of covalent bond formation or destruction [11]. The alternative mechanism of feedback loops such as reverberating electrical circuits seems highly unlikely, since production of electrical silence in the brain by spreading depression [12] or hypothermia [13] does not destroy the subsequent ability of an animal to perform learned behavior. The hypothesis that permanent chemical changes in the brain result from experience is consistent with a "connectionist" neuronal model of the brain. Whether the putative brain changes involve activation of preexisting pathways, formation of new synaptic connections or, alternatively, the inactivation or destruction of existing ones is, of course, of great importance to biochemical strategies for the study of memory formation.

Structural and Physiological Considerations

On inspection, it is immediately apparent that the brain is enormously more complicated than any other organ. The high degree of differentiation is also evidenced by an unusually large amount of unique sequence RNA in the brain relative to other organs [14]. Of particular interest is the report that human brain RNA is more diverse than human embryonic brain or adult mouse brain, and that a significantly higher level of unique sequence RNA was found in the left cerebral hemisphere than in the right [15]. Brain diversity is also evidenced by the precision of connectivity of neurons. This can be demonstrated in a number of ways. SPERRY showed some years ago [16] that the cut optic nerve in the goldfish will regenerate itself in such a way that each retinal ganglion cell finds its way back to the appropriate region of the optic tectum, even if the distal end of the nerve has been rotated 180° following the cut. This point-to-point specification recapitulates events which must occur during development, and suggests the existence of a cellular chemical coding process. In a sense, the brain may represent a better model for studying cell recognition than do simpler biological systems. Interesting preliminary results suggest that cells from different retinal regions in the developing chick reaggregate with specific tectal cells [17]. While it is not possible, even with precise stereotactic electrodes, to map the location of a given neuron in the brain, this can be done in selected simple systems. The abdominal ganglion of *Aplysia* has been mapped and neuro-transmitters identified in a number of specified neurons, giving further evidence of the high degree of order in nerves and nerve networks that is genetically specified [18]. By means of recording electrophysiological responses, we have learned that neurons have rather characteristic repertoires of firing patterns. Some fire constantly at a high rate while some are restricted to a low rate, and still others fire intermittently or variably [19]. As a result of sensory stimulation, some neurons can be shown to be "on" and others "off" units. In many instances, there is a relationship between the type of neuron and its neurotransmitter. For example, γ-amino-butyric acid is generally an inhibitory transmitter [20]. Before an electrical impulse is transmitted to the next neuron in a polysynaptic pathway it must first be converted to a chemical signal and cause the release of neurotransmitter which is "tasted" by the post-synaptic membrane, leading to depolarization and further impulse conduction. DALE's principle that each neuron has only one neuro-transmitter [21] has held up through the years, and if exceptions are found they will probably serve only to prove the rule.

Since neurotransmitter synthesis is ultimately regulated at the nucleus, we must first remember that neurons differ from other cells in their sizes and shapes — the presynaptic terminals of a neuron in a large animal might be a meter away from its cell body. Enzymes of neurotransmitter synthesis can be shown to migrate towards the presynaptic region together with other neuronal proteins by the process of axonal flow [22]. While this flow is proximo-distal (centrifugal), there is evidence for the presence of disto-proximal flow as well, that is, in a direction from the synaptic region to the nucleus [23]. The latter may be the means whereby the signal to make more transmitter synthetic enzyme following presynaptic neurotransmitter depletion reaches the nucleus and the polysomal synthetic apparatus. When labeled amino acids are injected, they are taken up by neurons but are not transported axonally. However, if they are incorporated into proteins that migrate *via* axonal flow, a radioactive proximo-distal flow can be observed. This technique cannot be used to observe reverse flow, since little or no protein appears to be synthesized in the presynaptic region. We can observe proximo-distal axonal flow in the fish visual system by injecting labeled amino acid precursor into the eye, and at a later time measuring the appearance of radioactivity in the brain [24]. Fish have completely crossed optic nerves and each tectum receives only contralateral fibres. When labeled leucine is used as precursor, a considerable amount of radioactive amino acid escapes from the eye, enters the circulation, and subsequently labels protein both the contralateral and ipsilateral optic tectum locally. By subtracting the radioactivity on the ipsilateral side from that of the contralateral side, one can calculate the amount of protein which is transported axonally. Using this method, it has been established that there are two rates of axonal flow [24]. In the fish, there is a rapid rate of about 70 mm/day at 20°. In homoiotherms, the rapid rate is about 400 mm a day. The slow rate is approximately 0.5 mm/day. In an attempt to develop a radioautographic method for axonal flow, we tested the relative efficacy of labeling of transported proteins compared to local labeling with a number of precursors. We found that ^{3}H-proline was an excellent precursor of transported protein in the fish visual system and produced only a minimal amount of systemic labeling [25]. It is thus particularly well-suited for the study of neuronal pathways. By injecting into the region of a cell body and waiting an appropriate amount of time, radioautograms can be made that will identify the presynaptic terminals [26]. While there is no direct evidence of changes in bulk flow as a result of stimulation, specific components can be inferred to change from assays for specific enzyme activities [27] or from postsynaptic electrophysiological changes [28].

In sharp contrast to the various lines of evidence indicating a precise relationship of neurons to one another, is the important observation that the firing pattern of nerve networks are probabilistic in nature [29]. When a stereotypic muscle movement such as the walking of an insect is studied in regard to the discharge sequence of identified neurons involved in the movement, it is found that the discharges of individual nerves are not as precise as the resultant muscular movement. It follows that the explanation of behavioral patterns in terms of oligosynaptic circuits such as reflex arcs is over-simplistic. We must invoke the participation of nerve networks. The idea that each neuron has a distinct chemical specifier may or may not prove to be true, but there is no reason to expect that a given behavior will be mediated by a single protein. As discussed below, such a finding would certainly transcend all we presently know about the nervous system.

Plasticity in the Nervous System

There are no striking anatomical, physiological or biochemical alterations of a lasting nature that have yet been reliably demonstrated as a result of the learning of a new behavior. It is also generally accepted that neurons do not replicate following early development, while glia do [30]. Numerous experiments purporting to show some environmental effects on brain structure have previously been reported. Perhaps the most extensive study was that of Krech and coworkers [31], who compared the brains of groups of rats maintained for several weeks under drastically different environmental conditions. One group was kept under conditions of deprivation — isolated, quiet and dimmed lights. The second group was kept in an enriched environment — several animals per cage, many bright objects and opportunity for exploration of their surroundings. Although relatively minor biochemical changes were observed, there was a marked thickening of the occipital cortex. More recently, electron microscopic findings have resulted in the claim of increased size of synaptic regions and increased numbers of dendritic spines and branching in cortical neurons [32—34]. Such changes may not be permanent, but correlated with the period of stimulation.

The question then remains as to what chemical events in the brain occur as a result of experiences that permanently alter subsequent behavior. It is convenient to describe three biochemical approaches:

1. Biochemical concomitants of behavior.
2. Specific enhancement of memory by various biological or pharmacological means.
3. Behavioral effect of substances known to block specific molecular processes.

Biochemical Concomitants of Behavior

This approach is exemplified by the work of GLASSMAN et al. [35]. Mice were trained to jump up on a shelf to avoid a punishing shock upon the presentation of a light-buzzer signal. Just before training, an animal was anesthetized and injected intracerebally with ^{3}H- or ^{14}C-labeled uridine. The mouse was decapitated a few minutes after training and its brain was combined with that of a resting mouse or yoked control (an animal receiving the same amount of light-buzzer and shock, but not having the opportunity to jump up on the shelf), given the second isotope. At the end of the incorporation period, brains of pairs of animals, such as from a yoked control and trained mouse were combined. The intention of such double-labeled experiments was to detect the possible existence of a minor component of labeled RNA that could be correlated with the training experience. The double-labeled technique is ideal for the detection of the proverbial "needle in the haystack". The result was, however, that the investigators found a haystack full of needles: differences were found throughout the RNA fractions. They observed a general increase in RNA labeling not only among molecular weight species, but in RNA from different subcellular fractions. The increase, however, was seen only in brain and not in other organs. The ^{14}C/^{3}H concentrations in the acid-soluble fraction was measured, and corrections for precursor pool size were made. This calculation was probably inadequate for a number of reasons. The specific activity of the UTP pool was not measured and, further, it is not in any event possible to measure with certainty the relevant pool that was precursor to the incremental labeled RNA. Since it is unlikely that the learning of a new behavior would involve such a large change in RNA labeling in relation to the information specific process, we conclude that (a) the observed RNA labeling may be more closely related to some more global pheno- menon or epiphenomenon of the learning process, such as stress, and not to an information-specific process or (b) it is possible that the changes seen reflect altered precursor pool sizes rather than increas- ed RNA synthesis. When goldfish are injected with labeled orotic acid, radioactivity is ultimately found in both uridine and cytidine moieties of the brain RNA [36]. As a result of training in a shuttle- box, the ratio of U/C is increased. This was shown to be a result of the stress associated with learning and could, further, be attributed to precursor pool size [37]. Hence, in this instance, both arguments (a) and (b) apply. A further reason that the increase in RNA label- ing seen in the mouse experiment is not likely to reflect net increase in RNA synthesis is that in the cited studies, there has not been reported a concomitant increase in protein labeling. Since mes- senger, transfer and ribosomal RNA subserve protein synthesis, one might have anticipated a comparable or even greater effect on protein labeling under the conditions that stimulate RNA labeling.

BATESON et al. [38] have studied uracil incorporation into brain RNA in the newborn chick in relation to an imprinting paradigm. In this case, one measures the chick's preference to follow an object to which it was exposed shortly after hatching. The imprinting process is effective only during a critical period shortly following hatching, and the imprinted preference remains with the animal. Increased labeling of RNA during the imprinting session was found in the anterior part of the forebrain. While the results are subject to the same criticism raised concerning the mouse studies, these and other reported localizations of such effects may be extremely useful findings [39, 40]. Even though all of these reports may reflect changes in precursor pool sizes rather than RNA synthesis, they might indicate specific brain regions that mediate some part of the learning process. Nucleotide pools may well be affected by changes in regional metabolism and/or cerebral blood flow. Such hypotheses can be examined in the whole animal by techniques developed by SOKOLOFF. A radioautographic technique for studying changes in regional cerebral blood flow involves the use of labeled inert substances such as Antipyrine, whose diffusion into the brain is limited by cerebral blood flow. By injecting such substances and killing animals before there is complete equilibration between blood and brain, cerebral blood flow can be measured. By this technique, SOKOLOFF has been able to show increased blood flow in the optic radiation following visual stimulation in the cat [41]. More recently, by means of labeled deoxyglucose, he has been able to estimate the rate of regional glucose utilization. Deoxyglucose is phosphorylated at a rate which reflects that of glucose, but the resulting 2-deoxyglucose 6-phosphate remains in the brain for considerable periods of time [42]. These radioautographic techniques have not yet been applied to behavioral paradigms, but the above RNA experiments suggest that this might well prove profitable.

Enhancement of Memory

Loss of the ability to form new permanent memory is a characteristic of the ageing brain, and there are numerous anecdotal as well as documented scientific reports of agents which have been claimed to improve memory. Various central nervous system excitants in small amounts, such as strychnine and picrotoxin have been used [43]. The beneficial effects of agents reported to stimulate brain RNA synthesis or hydrolysates of RNA itself have been described [44], but in general there is no evidence to indicate that any of these agents are useful. There has been considerable interest and controversy regarding the claim that extracts from brains of trained animals can be injected into naive recipients who then perform the learned task — so-called memory transfer experiments [45]. Many questions have been raised regarding the reproducibility of the observed phenomena and the nature of synthetic peptides purported to mediate the effect [46]. As stated previously, behavioral experiments are generally not as easily reproduced from laboratory to laboratory as biochemical ones, and many of the memory-transfer reports have come from investigators who have had no previous background in behavioral research. Other questions are based on whether the injected substances lead to production of the claimed behavior, *i.e.*, memory of a stimulus-specific nature. Many substances cause nonspecific activation or depression and can alter the behavior of an animal in a way that could be interpreted as evidence of learned behavior. The question of stimulus specificity thus becomes crucial. In the end, such experiments will be judged by sustained efforts by laboratories in which well-described paradigms are developed and which can be reliably reproduced in other laboratories, and in which the injected material can be shown to produce stimulus-specific effects and, ultimately, demonstrable biochemical effects. The demonstration of transfer of memory would, at face value, transcend our present knowledge, not only of neurobiology but of all biological sciences. We know sufficiently little about how the brain functions at the molecular level that we cannot simply discount such hypotheses. Since the experimental findings themselves appear to be in question, I can only at this point add my own prejudices, which I am confident I have already done.

Behavioral Effects of Substances Known to Block Specific Molecular Processes

This approach deals with use of substances of known structure and mode of action that block at specific metabolic sites, and the correlation of their actions with observed behavioral effects.

For the past 10 years, our laboratory has used antimetabolites that block macromolecular synthesis in the goldfish brain. We selected the common goldfish, *Carassius auratus*, because of its availability and our impression that it was the simplest animal we could train predictably and easily. Its brain resides in a roomy cranial cavity that is easily accessible to injection of various drugs by syringe [47]. By means of a labeling pulse of radioactive amino acids or nucleosides given at various times following intracranial injection of the inhibitors, we established the degree of block of total protein or RNA synthesis in the brain [48]. Our first behavioral observation was that fish swam about normally and showed usual fear responses and feeding behavior under conditions of greatly reduced RNA or protein synthesis — 90 or more percent inhibition. We could then ask the question, what effect do these agents have on learning and memory ? For our behavioral assay, we taught fish to swim over a barrier upon a light signal to avoid a punishing electrical shock (Fig. 1). Fish were trained to swim back and forth, hence the name "shuttle-box" for the training apparatus. In the earlier studies referred to here, fish received 30 training trials and their responses were automatically recorded by means of photocells on either sides of the barrier (shuttle-boxes were ultimately interfaced with a computer that measured the individual responses in 10 shuttle-boxes simultaneously). Each training trial lasted one minute and began with a 20-sec period in which a light signal was present on the side of the apparatus containing the fish. This was followed by another 20-sec period in which the light remained on, but an intermittent punishing shock was administered through the

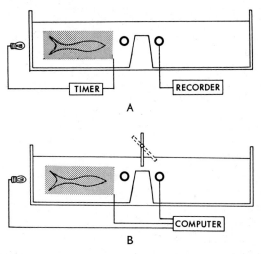

Fig. 1 A and B. Shuttle-boxes used for study of learning and memory in the goldfish (from AGRANOFF, Ref. [48]). (A) Automated shuttle-box used in initial studies on memory. Twenty seconds after onset of light on the side of the apparatus in which the fish was located an intermittent electrical shock was administered, causing the fish to escape to the dark, unshocked side. Light and shock remained in the starting compartment until the 40th second of the trial. After 20 sec of darkness, the second trial began with onset of light on the previously dark side. Fish eventually learned to swim over the barrier during the first 20 sec, avoiding shock. Fish position was established by photodetectors. (B) A more recent shuttle-box in which the fish must also deflect a clear plastic gate to cross the barrier. This results in lower initial scores and discourages spontaneous crossing. Light and shock are terminated when the fish crosses the barrier. Latencies to avoid and escape are recorded on paper or magnetic tape. Signal lights and electrodes are shown on only one side

water. This was followed by 20 sec of no-shock and with the signal
lights off. Untrained fish did not ordinarily cross the barrier during
the first 20 sec. Without prior training, they escaped to the dark
side of the apparatus after a few shocks had been administered.
This was the unconditioned escape response. What we were trying
to teach the fish was to go over the barrier during the first 20 sec,
with the light alone — in other words, to learn that the onset of
light indicated that a shock would be given which could be avoided
only by swimming over the barrier. On the average, untrained
(naive) fish demonstrated an avoidance response twice during the
first 10 trials, about four times during a subsequent block of
10 trials and six times during the last 10 trials, that is, trials 21—30.
The increasing probability of avoidance indicated that fish were
learning the task. We found that if we presented the first 20 trials
in a single session, returned fish to their individual storage tank
for 3—7 days, and then gave them the third set of 10 trials, their
avoidance scores were still about what we would have seen had
they received their final 10 trials in the first session — the 60%
responding rate (about six avoidance responses in 10 trials). Since
such a score distinguished the trained fish from untrained ones, we
had evidence of memory of the training for a several day period.
The 20-trial training session and the 10-trial retraining session
given several days later furnished us with an estimate of both
learning and memory. To reduce individual variability and to compensate for seasonal variation in fish performance, we utilized a
regression equation [50]. This means that we estimated, on the basis
of a large number of control experiments and on weekly control
groups, how a given fish should do for trial 21—30 from analysis of
his first 20 trials. Fish that did well on the first 20 trials did better
on the last 10 trials than those who did poorly on the first 20 trials.
For each fish we have then a predicted score for trials 21—30 which
we compare with the achieved score. The greater the difference
between these two scores, the greater the computed memory
deficit.

Studies with Puromycin

Table 1 shows the result of an experiment in which puromycin
was injected intracranially. Three groups of fish are represented.
The first is the control group, given 20 trials on Day 1 and then

Table 1. Effect of puromycin and puromycin moieties injected after training on memory (From AGRANOFF et al., Ref. [48])

No.	Trials Day 1 1—10	11—20	Treatment	Trials Day 4 21—30 A	21—30 P	Retention score (A—P)
73	2.3	3.4	Uninjected	5.3	5.3	0
36	2.5	3.8	Puromycin dihydro- chloride 170 µg, immediate	2.7	5.4	—2.7
35	2.5	4.6	Puromycin dihydro- chloride 170 µg, 60 min delay	5.5	5.6	—0.1
23	2.0	3.2	Puromycin amino- nucleoside 90 µg, immediate	5.1	5.0	+0.1
81	2.5	3.5	O-Methyltyrosine hydro- chloride, 70 µg, immediate	5.2	5.4	—0.2

returned to storage tanks for three days. On Day 4 they were given their last 10 training trials. They had complete memory of the training, as evidenced by the agreement of their predicted and achieved scores. A second group of fish were trained similarly but was given puromycin intracranially just after trial 20. They appeared to have no memory of their training as evidenced by a low Day 4 score, significantly lower than the one predicted for them. Was this a memory deficit or was it an indication of residual damage of the drug injection? For example, if the antibiotic caused blindness, animals would be expected to do poorly on retraining. Lingering effects of the injection were completely ruled out by the third experimental group, given the puromycin injection an hour after trial 20 on Day 1. On Day 4 this group had no performance deficit on retraining. Puromycin could thus block memory only if given shortly after training. This experiment in the fish demonstrated the production of a retrograde amnesia — an apparent loss of memory after the initial experience, and indicated the "fixation" or consolidation of memory. This is analogous to the amnesia seen in man after a blow to the head or from similar trauma. For example, following an automobile accident, memories of events immediately preceding the accident are lost. In man and animals alike, electroconvulsive shock also produces a retrograde amnesia [51]. The difference between the physical, traumatic or electroshock amnesia and the presently described antibiotic-mediated one is that in the case of the antibiotic treatment, the experimental subjects do not lose consciousness. This experiment put to rest the idea that early memory could be disrupted only by some sort of electrical storm that destroyed reverberating circuits. It also prompted our next experiment, to inject the antibiotic before training. When we inject-ed fish intracranially with puromycin prior to training [48], we found that they learned at the same rate as uninjected fish, even though their brains were not making very much protein. On retrain-ing these same animals three days later, they had as low a per-formance level as that seen in the animals that were injected immediately after training. The agent produced an anterograde amnesia in this instance. These experiments show that the sort of memory that is associated with learning itself, what we call "short-term memory", does not require normal ongoing protein synthesis in the brain. The formation of long-term or permanent memory, however, does.

These experiments did not distinguish between a block of formation of a permanent form of memory and the formation of a faulty, rapidly decaying memory. In either event, once memory had become "fixed", puromycin had no effect.

Animals trained and injected with puromycin just before retrain-ing showed normal retention scores. Puromycin-treated animals can retrieve old memories, they can also form new ones, but cannot store them for long periods of time. They are thus somewhat similar to humans with memory disorders, seen in old age and as a sequela of acute alcoholism and malnutrition, the Wernicke-Korsakoff syndrome [52]. In the fish, the lesion is temporary. They recover after the blocker wears off and can again learn and store memories normally.

When a fish is injected with puromycin, amnesia is not pro-duced instantly, as might be predicted from the pre-trial injection experiment. Animals given 20 training trials, injected with puro-mycin and retrained immediately show usual scores for trials 21—30, about six avoidance responses. If we take groups of animals, each given 20 trials and injected immediately with puromycin, then retrained at various intervals after injection, we find that short-term memory does not disappear instantaneously but decays over a period of three days [53]. It seems then that puromycin does not destroy memory but prevents formation of a long-term form, or perhaps produces an increasing interference leading to the irretrievability of memory [50].

The Environmental Trigger

In the course of these experiments, we observed a striking phenomenon. The fixation process (that is, the growing insusceptibility to puromycin) following training did not begin unless the animals were removed from the training apparatus and placed into their storage tanks. If fish remained in the apparatus for 1—3 hrs after trial 20, puromycin injection would produce the amnestic response on Day 4, even though injection was no longer effective if given after immediate return to the home tanks [53]. We interpret this interaction of the environment with the ongoing memory process to mean that a signal elicited by termination of the training session is required before the experimental animal can make permanent memory of shock-avoidance learning.

Other Blocking Agents

Table 2 summarizes a number of studies in the goldfish. It can be seen that several inhibitors of protein and RNA synthesis block memory, while an analog of puromycin and a DNA inhibitor do not. It should also be noted that none of the agents used produced a measurable effect on acquisition. We have noted no significant differences in pre-training or post-training injections, or short-term decay effects of the various effective RNA and protein blockers. It appears that the acquisition of a new behavior does not require normally ongoing macromolecular synthesis, while the formation of permanent memory does. Protein inhibitors appear to block labeling of DNA from thymidine, as has been observed previously in other systems [63]. However, the fact that arabinosyl cytosine has no effect on memory suggests that the former agents are blocking memory *via* inhibition of protein synthesis.

BARONDES [64] found that puromycin was an amnestic agent in the mouse, as was originally shown by FLEXNER [65]. The former authors postulated at one time that puromycin exerted its amnestic effect by producing abnormal electrical activity in the brain. They

Table 2. Summary of actions of various agents on macromolecular labeling
and on behavior in goldfish

	^{3}H-Thymidine uptake	^{3}H-Uridine uptake	^{3}H-Leucine uptake	Seizures	Memory	Ref.
Puromycin (170 µg)	B	O	B	P	B	[48, 54]
Puromycin aminonucleoside (92 µg)	—	M	O	P	O	[48, 54]
O-Methyl tyrosine (70 µg)	—	O	O	O	O	[48, 54]
Puromycin (170 µg) plus Acetoxycycloheximide (0.2 µg)	—	—	B	P	B	[48, 54, 55]
Acetoxycycloheximide (0.2 µg)	B	O	B	O	B	[48, 54]
Actinomycin D (2.0 µg)	—	B	M	O	B	[56, 57]
Camptothecin (25 µg)	—	B	M	—	B	[57]
Arabinosyl cytosine (100 µg)	B	O	O	—	O	[58]
5-Bromotubercidin (50 µg)	—	B	O	—	B	[59]
5-Fluorouridine (50 µg)	—	B	O	—	O	[59]
KCl (600 µg)	—	—	M	X	B	[60, 61]
electroconvulsive shock	—	—	M	X	B	[62]

B = block; O = no effect; M = moderate or slight effect; X = produces
seizure; P = potentiates pentylenetetrazol seizure.

showed that while puromycin did not produce frank convulsions,
it potentiated the convulsant action of pentylenetetrazol (PTZ).
Animals primed with puromycin would convulse with subthreshold
doses of PTZ [66]. We obtained a similar result in the fish. We
found, however, that puromycin aminonucleoside, an analog of
puromycin [54] that did not block protein synthesis, also potentiated PTZ-induced seizures, and had no effect on memory formation [48]. We thus dissociated the possible convulsive action of the
drug from its effect on memory. Furthermore, cycloheximide and
acetoxycycloheximide were both shown to be amnestic agents but
not to potentiate seizures. These glutarimide derivatives were subsequently shown to be effective amnestic agents in the mouse [67].

This was further evidence that the blockers did not exert their effects on memory as convulsants. Actinomycin D, an RNA blocker, has been shown to be an effective amnestic agent [56]. It is quite toxic and, therefore, not an ideal agent for behavioral studies. More recent studies in our laboratory with camptothecin [57], 5-bromotubercidin and 5-fluorouridine indicate that normally ongoing RNA synthesis may also be required for normal brain function. While uridine incorporation RNA was blocked by both the bromotubercidin and fluorouridine, the latter had no effect on memory. This result is consistent with the proposal that memory formation is dependent upon messenger RNA, since bromotubercidin blocks both messenger and ribosomal RNA synthesis, but 5-fluorouridine blocks only ribosomal RNA synthesis [68]. Additional support for this thesis comes from recent studies in mice indicating that α-amanitin [69] blocks memory formation. The action of puromycin, of the glutarimide antibiotics and of actinomycin D have been confirmed in the mouse [70] and, more recently, in the chick [71]. While it still remains unclear whether these agents are producing effects on memory by their purported blocking actions on macromolecular synthesis, the production of amnesia in at least three diverse species using somewhat different experimental paradigms speaks for a relative high degree of consistency for the thesis that memory formation is somehow RNA and protein-dependent.

The Effect of Temperature

Since the fish is poikilothermic, it is well-suited for studying the temperature-dependence of memory formation. By measuring changes in the rate of development of susceptibility of memory to electroconvulsive shock or to puromycin, we have been able to show that (1) lowering the temperature 10° C after training extends the period of susceptibility of memory to disruptive agents, (2) increasing temperature 10° C immediately following training decreases the period of susceptibility of memory to consolidation, and (3) cooling fish for 24 hrs following training results in a profound decrease in protein synthesis, but does not produce a selective block of memory [72]. Apparently, the metabolic machinery must be functioning in the face of a decrease in macromolecular synthesis in order for memory to be disrupted.

Interaction of Parameters of the Learning Paradigm and Blocking Agents

One way to explore the nature of the action of the antibiotics in blocking memory is to explore the variety of behavioral tasks whose retention can be blocked. For example, it has been suggested that in the shuttle-box experiments, puromycin blocks only a "conditioned fear" component [73]. We explored this possibility by taking advantage of an old observation — that when fish are alerted or threatened, there is a slowing of the heart rate and that this response could be conditioned by presenting to the fish a light signal followed by an unavoidable electrical shock [74]. The conditioned response was the appearance of cardiac deceleration on presentation of light alone. By giving fish 10 such trials and measuring their heart rate by means of implanted electrodes, we studied both learning and memory of this conditioned emotional response [75]. On retesting three days after the 10 training trials, fish were given 10 extinction trials. This means they were presented with light alone until they no longer showed the conditioned response (slowing of the heart rate). We could not block memory of the response by injection of puromycin immediately following training. We reasoned that perhaps in this case memory was being consolidated during training instead of afterwards, so we repeated the experiment, but gave puromycin before training. Fish showed normal acquisition scores and again had good memory of the training [76]. We then attempted the same training paradigm giving fish only five training trials with the hope that this "weaker" learning would now be susceptible to the antibiotic, but it was not. We found that electroconvulsive shock was also ineffective in blocking this memory. It appears then that the cardiac conditioned response in the goldfish is not susceptible to the usual disruptive agents. It also appeared that in this instance, the agent was not blocking fear-conditioning. Further evidence that the antibiotics do not selectively block fear-conditioning comes from a number of studies including some in mice, in which various protein inhibitors have been shown to block memory of passive avoidance [77], appetitive tasks and a number of discrimination paradigms [78]. In mice, the number of training trials and stimulus strength appear to play an important role in the measured performance seen on retraining. For example, in an aversive training situation in which mice receive foot shock, increasing the intensity of the shock can lead to some retention even when protein inhibitors have been given [79, 80]. Also, increasing the number of training trials can in some instances lead to retention [78]. Since there is an interaction between the amount and intensity of the training stimuli and the inhibition of protein synthesis, it appears then that there is a kind of "neuronal watershed" effect following the training, in which the neural signals that survive are strengthened and those that are weakened are lost [50]. If this strengthening process is occurring in the synaptic region, and if protein and RNA blockers inhibit this step, then perhaps we can explain the resistance of the conditioned emotional response to puromycin on the basis that it involves a smaller synaptic network than does the operant task. The loss of a fixed fractional efficacy at each synapse in an oligosynaptic circuit would not result in the same degree of loss of signal that the same fractional loss would produce in a longer chain [75].

A number of experiments have been performed to investigate the possibility that the antibiotics are producing an effect which can be explained purely on a behavioral basis, that is, that some aspect of the injection of the drugs produces an aversive or punishing effect on the animal, and thus he will not perform the learned task. This would appear to be quite unlikely in the fish, since even when the puromycin is administered a day before training, we find an effect on memory tested several days later. It is not likely that a fish would associate punishment with an injection given a day before training, and not the same dose given a few hours afterwards. Furthermore, we find that fish that are anesthetized immediately following training, given puromycin and then allowed to remain anesthetized for four hours, still show the amnestic effect, while the anesthetic alone has no effect on memory [50].

Mice that appear to be amnestic for a learned task as a result of antibiotic treatment can in some cases be shown to have partial memory if given a behavioral reminder [81]. In other words, they are not completely amnestic. Such experiments have been interpreted to mean that antibiotics do not produce an effect on memory, but on retrieval. A more precise interpretation of such results is that the memory that is lost is not complete, but sufficient to prevent demonstration of the learned task. So amnesia has after all been produced but is not complete, and we should therefore be cautious in the use of the term. It is hard to ask the animal what part of the task he remembers. We all know that for us, recall is more difficult than recognition.

Other Agents that Block Memory

In the fish, both electroconvulsive shock and KCl convulsions can produce a profound amnesia along a temporal gradient, somewhat like that seen with the antibiotics. These agents were initially believed to destroy the short-term form of memory, while the antibiotics affected the long-term form. This distinction is not straightforward, since KCl can produce an amnestic effect following training far after the antibiotics are no longer effective [61]. Furthermore, if electroconvulsive shock is given *before* training and fish are allowed to recover, they show poor memory several days later, just as was observed with the antibiotics [82]. Fish given electroconvulsive shock immediately following training and retested a few hours later have been shown to have a short-term memory decay, as was demonstrated with the antibiotics. Protein synthesis is decreased following electroconvulsive shock [83] but only to a minor degree, and if a small dose of puromycin is given to mimic this degree of inhibition, there is no memory loss. The convulsants therefore share some of the properties of the antibiotics on memory, but appear to act *via* a different mechanism.

A block of memory can be produced in the rat by intracerebral injections of diisopropylfluorophosphate, an anticholinesterase, and it has been proposed that the antibiotics might exert their amnestic effect *via* some cholinergic mechanism [84]. Similarly, diethyl dithiocarbamate, a dopamine β-hydroxylase inhibitor, has also shown to be an effective amnestic agent [85], and it has been proposed that puromycin action can be reversed by drugs that compete for adrenergic receptor sites in the mouse [86].

Route of Injection

An important consideration in all of these experiments is the route of injection of the drug. When drugs are injected intracerebrally, it is often very difficult to tell whether they are acting locally or have penetrated the entire brain. In early studies,

FLEXNER indicated that fresh memories could be blocked by temporal injections of puromycin, and that by means of three bilateral injections older memories could be disrupted as well [65]. It has subsequently been shown that the needle track itself can have some disruptive effects [87]. This problem has been dealt with in a number of ways. In the fish, the needle does not penetrate the brain and because of the fishes' primitive meninges, the antibiotic can penetrate the entire brain from the cranial fluid. In mammalian brain the injection must be intracerebral and bilaterally administered, usually into an anesthetized animal. In the mouse, subcutaneous injection of a sufficient quantity of cycloheximide or anisomycin produces a protein block in the brain [79]. By this route, however, protein synthesis is also blocked throughout the body, and the peripheral effects can complicate interpretation of results. Localized injections to establish precisely where in the brain the various agents are acting have not been exploited. We have found local intracerebral injection difficult in the fish because of the small size of the brain and the lack of good streotactic landmarks. We have, however, demonstrated localized reversible lesions in monkey brain by means of implanted cannulae and radioautography [88].

Discussion and Conclusions

On the basis of ablation experiments, LASHLEY concluded many years ago [89] that the conditioned response could not be localized within the brain. It is high time to reinvestigate this challenge with the more sophisticated tools now in hand. Since many antibiotics produce a reversible block of macromolecular synthesis in the brain, the same animal can be used many times in behavioral experiments. Both from the standpoint of antibiotic injection and measurement of concomitants of macromolecular synthesis and cellular metabolism, regional brain studies deserve more emphasis.

Of various biochemical approaches to the difficult problem of memory formation and storage, probably the most consistent and thoroughly explored approach thus far has been the use of blocking agents in whole animals. The thesis is presented on the basis of our work and that of others, that long-term memory formation requires normally ongoing RNA and protein synthesis during a critical period of time following the actual learning experience. Even in the presence of a drastic reduction in these macromolecular processes, there is little or no measurable effect on acquisition of a new behavior. This finding is perhaps as significant as is the profound effect demonstrable on long-term storage. We have discussed the possibility that macromolecular synthesis in specific synapses are involved in the new learned behavior or, alternatively, that some non-information containing step which "fixes" nascent memories accounts for the action of the blocking agents. The former possibility is supported by the relatively high susceptibility of memory of what appear to be more complex tasks to the blocking agents, and by evidence that stimulus strength and amount of training can override the protein block. The alternative hypothesis that the agents block a generalized fixation signal or process is supported by the fact that consolidation does not start until after training, and by the demonstration of an environmental effect on its onset. Perhaps the agents are effective in both ways. In any event, the evidence points to the participation of the cell nucleus at some distance from the synapse. The amount of time necessary for intracellular chemical communication will depend on axonal flow rates and the dimensions of the cells mediating the behavioral change. It is of interest that colchicine, an agent known to bind microtubular protein and thus block axonal transport, has recently been reported to block memory in the goldfish [90]. Further consideration must also be given to non-neuronal elements. While glia are often depicted as supporting cells, their role in higher brain function is unknown. They have been shown to contain neurotransmitter-related enzymes [91].

That macromolecular synthesis is involved in memory formation remains an hypothesis. Proof can come only from studies which, in the absence of inhibitors, demonstrate molecular alterations in the brain as a result of behavioral experience — if not for specific memories, for what goes on in the brain at a time when new memories are being formed.

References

1. ADLER, J.: This book, p. 107ff.
2. KOSHLAND, D.: This book, p. 133ff.
3. KIMBLE, G. A.: In: HILGARD, E., MARQUIS, D. (Eds.): Conditioning and learning, 2nd ed. New York: Appleton-Century-Crofts 1961.

4. FLOOD, J.F., BENNETT, E.L., ROSENZWEIG, M.R., ORME, A.E.: Physiol. Behav. **9**, 589 (1972).
5. WAHLSTEN, D.: Behav. Biol. **7**, 143 (1972).
6. VAN ABEELEN, J., DAEMS, J., DOUMA, G.: Physiol. Behav. **10**, 751 (1973).
7. FLOOD, J.F., ROSENZWEIG, M.R., BENNETT, E.L., ORME, A.E.: Behav. Biol. **10**, 147 (1974).
8. REIGE, W.H., CHERKIN, A.: Nature (Lond.) New Biol. **240**, 28—29 (1972).
9. GLASSMAN, E.: Ann. Rev. Biochem. **38**, 605 (1969).
10. YANIGAHARA, T., HYDEN, H.: Exp. Neurol. **31**, 151 (1971).
11. AGRANOFF, B.W.: In: QUARTON, G.C., MELNECHUK, T., SCHMITT, F.O. (Eds.): The neurosciences: A study program. New York: The Rockefeller University Press 1967.
12. BURES, J., BURESOVA, O.: J. Comp. Physiol. Psychol. **53**, 558 (1960).
13. RANSMEIER, R.E., GERARD, R.W.: Amer. J. Physiol. **179**, 663 (1954).
14. BROWN, I.R., CHURCH, R.B.: Biochem. Biophys. Res. Commun. **42**, 850 (1971).
15. GROUSE, L., OMENN, G.A., McCARTHY, B.J.: J. Neurochem. **20**, 1063 (1972).
16. SPERRY, R.N.: Proc. nat. Acad. Sci. (Wash.) **50**, 703 (1963).
17. BARBERA, A.J., MARCHASE, R.B., ROTH, S.: Proc. nat. Acad. Sci. (Wash.) **70**, 2482 (1973).
18. KANDEL, E.R., SPENCER, W.A.: Physiol. Rev. **48**, 65 (1968).
19. EVARTS, E.V.: In: QUARTON, G.C., MELNECHUK, T., SCHMITT, F.O. (Eds.): The neurosciences: A study program. New York: The Rockefeller University Press 1967.
20. ECCLES, J.C.: The physiology of synapses. New York: Academic Press, Inc. 1964.
21. DALE, H.H.: Proc. roy. Soc. Med. **28**, 319 (1935).
22. LASEK, R.J.: Int. Rev. Neurobiol. **13**, 289 (1970).
23. LAVAIL, J.H., LAVAIL, M.M.: Science **176**, 1416 (1972).
24. McEWEN, B.S., GRAFSTEIN, B.: J. Cell Biol. **38**, 494 (1968).
25. ELAM, J.S., AGRANOFF, B.W.: J. Neurochem. **18**, 375 (1971).
26. NEALE, J.H., NEALE, E.A., AGRANOFF, B.W.: Science **176**, 407 (1972).
27. COYLE, J.T., WOOTEN, G.F.: Brain Res. **44**, 701 (1972).
28. CUENOD, M., BOESCH, J., MARKO, P.: Int. J. Neurosci. **4**, 77 (1972).
29. BRAZIER, M.A.B., WALTER, D.O., SCHNEIDER, D. (Eds.): Neural modelling, brain information service research report No. J. Los Angeles: Univ. of California 1973.
30. DAVISON, A.N., DOBBING, J.: In: Applied neurochemistry. Philadelphia: F. A. Davis, Co. 1968.
31. DIAMOND, M.C., KRECH, D., ROSENZWEIG, M.R.: J. Comp. Neurol. **123**, 111 (1964).
32. VOLKMAR, F.R., GREENOUGH, W.T.: Science **176**, 1445 (1972).
33. SCHAPIRO, S., VUKOVICH, K.R.: Science **167**, 292 (1970).
34. ROSENZWEIG, M.R., BENNETT, E.L., DIAMOND, M.C.: J. Comp. Physiol. Psychol. **82**, 175 (1973).

35. ADAIR, L. B., WILSON, J. E., GLASSMAN, E.: Proc. nat. Acad. Sci. (Wash.) **61**, 606 (1968).
36. SHASHOUA, V. E.: Proc. nat. Acad. Sci. (Wash) **65**, 215 (1968).
37. BASKIN, F., MASIARZ, F. R., AGRANOFF, B. W.: Brain Res. **39**, 151 (1972).
38. BATESON, P. P. G., HORN, G., ROSE, S. P. R.: Brain Res. **39**, 449 (1972).
39. MACKINNON, P. C. B., SIMPSON, K. A., MACLENNON, C.: J. Anat. **104**, 351 (1969).
40. BOWMAN, R. E., STROBEL, D. A.: J. Comp. Physiol. Psychol. **67**, 448 (1969).
41. SOKOLOFF, L.: In: KETY, S. S., ELKES, J. (Eds.): The regional chemistry, physiology, and pharmacology of the nervous system. Oxford: Pergamon Press 1961.
42. SOKOLOFF, L., REIVICH, M., PATLAK, C. S., PETTIGREW, K. D., DES ROSIERS, M.: Trans. Amer. Soc. Neurochem. **5**, 85 (1974).
43. McGAUGH, J. L.: In: Psychopharmacology: a review of progress 1957—1967. USPHS Publication No. 1836 (1968).
44. PLOTNIKOFF, N.: Science **151**, 703 (1966).
45. UNGAR, G., DESIDERIO, D. M., PARR, W.: Nature (Lond.) New Biol. **238**, 198 (1972).
46. STEWART, W. W.: Nature **238**, 202 (1972).
47. AGRANOFF, B. W., KLINGER, P. D.: Science **146**, 952 (1964).
48. AGRANOFF, B. W., DAVIS, R. E., BRINK, J. J.: Brain Res. **1**, 303 (1966).
49. AGRANOFF, B. W.: In: McGAUGH, J. L. (Ed.): The chemistry of mood, motivation, and memory. New York: Plenum Press 1972.
50. AGRANOFF, B. W.: In: HONIG, W. K., JAMES, P. H. R. (Eds.): New York: Academic Press 1961.
51. MILNER, P.: In: Physiological psychology. New York: Holt, Rinehart, Winston 1970.
52. VICTOR, M., ADAMS, R. D., COLLINS, G. H.: The Wernicke-Korsakoff syndrome. Philadelphia: F. A. Davis, Co. 1971.
53. DAVIS, R. E., AGRANOFF, B. W.: Proc. nat. Acad. Sci. (Wash.) **55**, 555 (1966).
54. AGRANOFF, B. W.: In: LAJTHA, A. (Ed.): Protein metabolism of the nervous system. New York: Plenum Press 1970.
55. LIM, R., BRINK, J. J., AGRANOFF, B. W.: J. Neurochem. **17**, 1637 (1970).
56. AGRANOFF, B. W., DAVIS, R. E., CASOLA, L., LIM, R.: Science **158**, 1600 (1967).
57. NEALE, J. H., KLINGER, P. D., AGRANOFF, B. W.: Science **179**, 1243 (1973).
58. CASOLA, L., LIM, R., DAVIS, R. E., AGRANOFF, B. W.: Proc. (Wash.) nat. Acad. Sci. **60**, 1389 (1968).
59. AGRANOFF, B. W.: Unpublished.
60. AGRANOFF, B. W.: In: BYRNE, W. L. (Ed.): Molecular approaches to memory and learning. New York: Academic Press 1970.
61. DAVIS, R. E., KLINGER, P. D.: Physiol. Behav. **4**, 269 (1969).
62. DAVIS, R. E., BRIGHT, P. I., AGRANOFF, B. W.: J. Comp. Physiol. Psychol. **60**, 162 (1965).
63. VERBIN, R. S., FARBER, E.: J. Cell Biol. **30**, 13 (1966).

64. BARONDES, S. H., COHEN, H. D.: Science **151**, 595 (1966).
65. FLEXNER, J. B., FLEXNER, L. B., STELLAR, E.: Science **141**, 57 (1963).
66. COHEN, H. D., ERVIN, F., BARONDES, S. H.: Science **154**, 1557 (1966).
67. BARONDES, S. H., COHEN, H. D.: Brain Res. **4**, 44 (1967).
68. BRDAR, B., RIFKIN, D. B., REICH, E.: J. biol. Chem. 2397 (1973).
69. THUT, P. D., HRUSKA, R. E., KELTER, A., MIZNE, J., LINDELL, T. J.: Psychopharmacologia (Berl.) **30**, 355 (1973).
70. SQUIRE, L. R., BARONDES, S. H.: Nature (Lond.) **225**, 649 (1970).
71. MARK, R. F., WATTS, M. E.: Proc. roy. Soc. (Lond.) B **178**, 439 (1971).
72. NEALE, J. H., KLINGER, P. D., AGRANOFF, B. W.: Behav. Biol. **9**, 267 (1973).
73. POTTS, A., BITTERMAN, M. E.: Science **158**, 1594 (1967).
74. OTIS, L. S., CERF, J. A., THOMAS, G. J.: Science **126**, 263 (1957).
75. SCHOEL, W. M., AGRANOFF, B. W.: Behav. Biol. **7**, 553 (1972).
76. SCHOEL, W. M., AGRANOFF, B. W.: In preparation.
77. GELLER, A., ROBUSTELLI, F., JARVIK, M. E.: Psychopharmacologia (Berl.) **21**, 309 (1971).
78. BARONDES, S. H.: Int. Rev. Neurobiol. **12**, 177 (1970).
79. FLOOD, J. F., BENNETT, E. L., ROSENZWEIG, M. R., ORME, A. E.: Physiol. Behav. **10**, 555 (1973).
80. QUARTERMAIN, D., McEWEN, B. S.: Nature (Lond.) **228**, 677 (1970).
81. QUARTERMAIN, D., McEWEN, B. S., AZMITIA, E. C.: Science **169**, 683 (1970).
82. SPRINGER, A. D., SCHOEL, W. M., KLINGER, P. D., AGRANOFF, B. W.: Behav. Biol. (in press).
83. DUNN, A. J.: Brain Res. **35**, 254 (1971).
84. DEUTSCH, J. A., HAMBURG, M. D., DAHL, H.: Science **151**, 221 (1966).
85. RANDT, C. T., QUARTERMAIN, D., GOLDSTEIN, M., ANAGNOSTE, B.: Science **172**, 498 (1971).
86. ROBERTS, R. B., FLEXNER, J. B., FLEXNER, L. B.: Proc. nat. Acad. Sci. (Wash.) **66**, 310 (1970).
87. BOHDANECKA, M., BOHDANECKY, Z., JARVIK, M. E.: Science **157**, 334 (1967).
88. EICHENBAUM, H., BUTTER, C. M., AGRANOFF, B. W.: Brain Res. **61**, 438 (1973).
89. LASHLEY, K. S.: Brain mechanisms and intelligence: a quantitative study of injuries to the brain. Chicago: University of Chicago Press 1929.
90. CRONLY-DILLON: J. Physiol. (Lond.) **234**, 104 p. (1973).
91. SCHRIER, B. K., THOMPSON, E. J.: J. biol. Chem. **249**, 1769 (1974).

Discussion

H. GRISEBACH (Freiburg): I do not know whether it was your intention — but you did not mention the popular scotophobin experiment. Could you comment on scotophobin and on the experiments on different choline esterase levels in trained and untrained rats by E. BENNETT in Berkeley?

B. W. AGRANOFF: I did not go into the so-called memory-transfer on purpose, because I think we are going to hear something about it. And I guess that some of you know that I am — let us say — an agnostic, and it would take a miracle to convert me. But I retain the privileges of conversion and last rites. — In relation to the work of BENNETT — that is an approach that is described in my written paper (Ref. [31]) — the idea is, if we make the assumption that whatever change is going on is going to be quite small — why not flood an animal's experience over a long time period and then analyze for the difference ? In this case, there are two groups of animals — environmentally deprived or enriched — and after some period of time, the authors examined the brains. They first thought that there was a difference in cholinesterase, but it turned out to be primarily anatomical, a thickening of the sensory cortex. They subsequently reported (Ref. [34]) increased size of synapses by electron microscopy, something of the order of 10% between the experimental and the controls. One of the interesting aspects of this is that, apparently, the cortical thickening is not permanent. If the animals are removed from the two environments and retained in a common environment for some period of time, the change either disappears or is greatly attenuated.

D. NACHMANSOHN (New York): I am quite familiar with these experiments on cholinesterase, as you can imagine. I think we have something to comment on this. I know the statements about increased cholinesterase after learning. They report that after learning there is a statistically significant increase of 2% of cholinesterase in the brain. Now, I would like to say that it is impossible with available methods to measure 100% differences. And I think that answers the question.

B. W. AGRANOFF: I should mention one approach using a blocking agent. DEUTSCH in San Diego (Ref. [81]) has injected DFP into rats and claimed to block memory and, under different conditions, to actually improve memory, depending on the state of the animal's learning. That is just another approach.

D. E. KOSHLAND, JR. (Berkeley,CA.): What about positive responses ? — Are there any compounds that improve them — such as, say, glutamate ?

B. W. AGRANOFF: The question then was: What could improve memory ? — thus far, very little! — There is a large history of substances that have been claimed to be effective, including strychnine and picrotoxin (in small amounts!) — but to my knowledge, there is not yet an agent about which one could say that it definitely improved memory storage.

H. STIEVE (Jülich): Can you say something about the forgetting of the conditioned response of the ECG as compared to the forgetting of the trained response ?

B. W. AGRANOFF: That is quite difficult. In the case of the conditioned response, we measured extinction. In the training test that I described first, there is no difference between a training trial and a testing trial. If an animal does not avoid, it is then trained again. In the case of the cardiac conditioning we use only extinction training. That is, the animals receive light alone until the effect disappears. But if you are asking in general: does one have better memory of visceral type conditioning as compared to instrumental— I don't think so!

H. STIEVE: Could it be possible that in your experiments learning occurs at one place which cannot be reached by erasing drugs, and therefore you can only erase the trained behavioral response and not the conditioned response of the ECG ?

B. W. AGRANOFF: Yes, that is quite possible. I would say that my current interpretation would not be different from what you have just said.

B. HAMPRECHT (München): You were testing the effect of your drugs on avoidance responses — what is the effect of the drugs on rewarding responses ?

B. W. AGRANOFF: There is no effect on the escape response, of course. If there were, that would be pretty good evidence that the drug was doing something other than blocking memory. But there is no effect at all on the performance. But if you mean, for example, an appetitive response in which the animal receives food, a positive reward of some sort ? — No, we have not done that, but it has been reported to be successful in mice with appetitive responses.

Besseres Lernen und Behalten in Schwerem Wasser bei Fischen

E. Lehr[1]

*Max-Planck-Institut für Hirnforschung, Arbeitsgruppe Neurochemie,
D-6000 Frankfurt/M.-Niederrad, Bundesrepublik Deutschland*

M. Wenzel

Pharmazeutisches Institut der Freien Universität Berlin, D-1000 Berlin

G. Werner

*Max-Planck-Institut für Hirnforschung, Arbeitsgruppe Neurochemie,
D-6000 Frankfurt/M.-Niederrad, Bundesrepublik Deutschland*

With 2 Figures

Wenn Fische in Wasser mit 12,5% bzw. 25% D_2O-Gehalt leben, erlernen sie eine Farblicht-Unterscheidungsaufgabe schneller [1], und eine, gleichgültig ob in H_2O oder H_2O/D_2O-Gemisch, erlernte Aufgabe behalten sie länger ([1, 2]; vgl. Abb. 1).

Die Ergebnisse stehen in Einklang mit der Erfahrung, daß durch die Einwirkung des Schweren Wassers physiologische Prozesse verlangsamt und morphologische Strukturen gefestigt werden (vgl. [2—5]). Eine derartige Stabilisierung könnte Gedächtnisstrukturen unmittelbar betreffen, z. B. durch gefestigte Konformation denkbarer „Informationsmoleküle" nach Austausch von Wasserstoff gegen Deuterium. Sie könnte aber auch indirekt bewirkt werden, da durch D_2O die Aktivität von Enzymen gesenkt wird [3], wodurch auch solche enzymatisch-katabolische Vorgänge gebremst werden sollten, die zu Gedächtnisverminderung führen. Möglicherweise wirken beide Prozesse zusammen. Der schnellere Lernerfolg bei D_2O-Einwirkung in unseren Versuchen ließe sich ebenfalls mit verzögertem Vergessen erklären, indem der Informationsverlust zwischen den einzelnen Lernakten vermindert werden könnte. Da-

---

[1] Neue Anschrift: Abteilung Pharmaforschung-Biologie, C. H. Boehringer Sohn, D-6507, Ingelheim, Bundesrepublik Deutschland.

gegen dürfte die stabilisierende Wirkung von D_2O nicht ausreichen, die Codierung beim Lernvorgang zu verhindern, weil dann
erschwertes Lernen die Folge sein sollte.

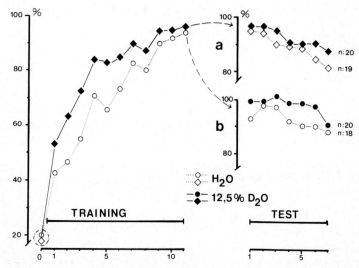

Abb. 1. Lernen und Vergessen bei Fischen *(Scardinius erythrophthalmus)* mit
und ohne Einfluß von Schwerem Wasser. Abszisse: Versuchstage mit je
10 Wahl-Darbietungen pro Fisch. Ordinate: % dressurgemäße Richtigwahlen

Die Abfrage der Lernaufgabe bei zwei Fischgruppen, die abwechselnd immer 24 Std lang von H_2O in ein H_2O/D_2O-Gemisch
und umgekehrt eingesetzt wurden, zeigte: Unter dem Einfluß von
D_2O wählten die Tiere langsamer (Abb. 2, unten). Zugleich wurde
hierbei (abgesehen vom ersten Versuchstag) das Erlernte in D_2O
weniger zuverlässig wiedergegeben (Abb. 2 oben).

Dieser Effekt war bereits 2 Std nach dem Auswechseln von
H_2O gegen H_2O/D_2O-Gemisch erkennbar, wie durch auffälliges
Überkreuzen der Kurven unmittelbar nach jedem Umsetzen deutlich wird.

Beide Versuchsreihen machen wahrscheinlich, daß die D_2O-
Wirkung keinesfalls auf einem verbesserten Wiedergeben des
Erlernten beruht. Im Gegenteil, unter D_2O-Einfluß verhielten sich

die Fische auffallend träger und zeigten sich unsicherer, dressurgemäß zu wählen. Da die beiden Fischgruppen identisch dressiert worden waren, läßt sich unseres Erachtens das verbesserte Behalten einer erlernten Aufgabe bei Einwirkung von D_2O nur durch eine stabilisierte Informationsspeicherung interpretieren.

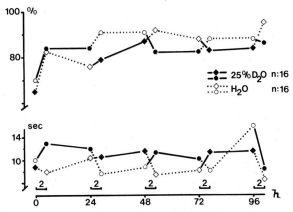

Abb. 2. Wahlsicherheit (oben) und Aktivität (unten) bei Fischen *(Scardinius erythrophthalmus)* abwechselnd unter Einfluß von Schwerem Wasser. Obere Ordinate: % dressurgemäße Richtigwahlen. Untere Ordinate: Zeit bis zur Wahlentscheidung in sec. Abszisse: Versuchsablauf in Stunden; pro Meßpunkt 5 Wahldarbietungen pro Fisch

Literatur

1. LEHR, E., WENZEL, M., WERNER, G.: Besseres Lernen in Schwerem Wasser bei Fischen. Naturwissenschaften **61**, 399—401 (1974).
2. LEHR, E., WENZEL, M., WERNER, G.: Einfluß von Schwerem Wasser auf das Gedächtnis von Fischen. Naturwissenschaften **57**, 521—524 (1970).
3. THOMSON, J. F.: Biological effects of deuterium. London-Oxford-New York-Paris: McMillan 1963.
4. WENZEL, M., STÖHR, W.: Schutzeffekt von D_2O gegen die Hyperthermieschädigung von Ascites-Tumorzellen. Hoppe-Seylers Z. physiol. Chem. **351**, 737—740 (1970).
5. HAESER, P. E., LEHR, E., WERNER, G.: Verminderter Sauerstoff-Verbrauch bei Fischen in Schwerem Wasser. Naturwissenschaften **59**, 123 (1972).

Versuche zur chemischen Übertragbarkeit erworbener Informationen

G. F. DOMAGK

Physiologisch-Chemisches Institut der Georg-August-Universität Göttingen,
D-3400 Göttingen, Humboldtallee 7, Bundesrepublik Deutschland

With 7 Figures

In dem vorangegangenen Vortrag wurde klargestellt, daß die Gedächtnisspeicherung mit chemischen Veränderungen im Gehirn einhergeht. Zahlreiche Arbeitsgruppen haben Beweise für eine lernabhängige Biosynthese von Proteinen bzw. Ribonucleinsäuren erbracht. Experimente zur Stützung der Hypothese, daß diese Makromoleküle informationsspezifisch aufgebaut sind, wurden erstmals 1962 von McCONNELL [J. Neuropsychiat. **3**, Suppl. 1, 42 (1962)] angeführt, als es ihm gelang, durch Extrakte aus trainierten Planarien von diesen Spendern erworbene Informationen durch Injektionen oder durch Kannibalismus auf naive Plattwürmer zu übertragen. Aus verschiedenen hier nicht zu diskutierenden Gründen haben die Planarienexperimente zum „Memory-Transfer" einer heftigen Kritik unterlegen. Wenige Jahre später wurden dann aber auch Versuche zur chemischen Übertragung erworbener Informationen bei höheren Tieren publiziert. Generell werden hierbei Tiere durch Training auf ein für sie ungewöhnliches Verhalten trainiert, wobei Bestrafung durch Elektroschock oder Futterbelohnungen lernverstärkend wirken. Aus so vorbereiteten Spendertieren werden dann Gehirnextrakte bereitet, deren Injektion bei vorgetesteten Empfängertieren eine Verhaltensänderung bewirkt, obwohl bei den nachfolgenden Testen der Extraktempfänger die Bestrafung durch Elektroschock bzw. die Belohnung durch Futter nicht mehr erfolgt.

Die weitestgehenden Schlußfolgerungen aus derartigen Transfer-Versuchen zog G. UNGAR in Houston, Texas, der u. a. bei Ratten durch Elektroschocks eine quantitav meßbare Dunkelfurcht erzeugt hatte. Hirnextrakte aus so vorbehandelten Spendern bewirken bei den Empfängertieren eine verkürzte Aufenthaltszeit im Dunkeln. Aus den vereinten Gehiren von 4000 derartig vorbehandelten Spendertieren gelang es Ungar und seinen Mitarbeitern, 300 µg eines Pentadecapeptids anzureichern, das in ng-Mengen i.p. gespritzt, bei Mäusen eine Dunkelfurcht verursachte. Nach der Strukturaufklärung der Verbindung gelang in Houston auch eine synthetische Herstellung des hochwirksamen Peptids, dem Ungar den Namen *Scotophobin* gab. Wir selbst haben vor einigen Jahren Versuche mit synthetischem Scotophobin durchgeführt. Spritzt man Fischen, wie z. B. den sehr lichtscheuen Schleien, intercranial ng-Mengen des Peptids ein, so verbringen die Tiere in einem Hell-Dunkel-Wahlapparat beträchtliche Anteile der Versuchszeit im beleuchteten Teil des Aquariums. Der niederländische Pharmakologe DeWied [In: H. P. Zippel (Ed.): Memory and Transfer of Information, p. 380. New York-London: Plenum Press 1973] hat unter Scotophobin eine vom Hell-Dunkel-Verhalten unabhängige Extinktionsverzögerung, also eine Gedächtnisverbesserung, bemerkt.

Da die Publikation des Scotophobin-Versuchs [Ungar u. Mitarb.: Nature **238**, 198 (1972)] einer heftigen Kritik ausgesetzt war [Stewart: Nature **238**, 202 (1972)], hat mein Mitarbeiter Penschuck derartige Experimente in Göttingen durchgeführt (Dissertation, Mediz. Fakultät Göttingen; in Vorbereitung). Wir verwendeten dabei einen etwas veränderten Apparat in Gestalt eines Y-Labyrinths, bei dem das Tier nach Öffnen des Startbox die Möglichkeit zum Betreten eines Dunkelraums oder des beleuchteten Labyrinthschenkels hat (Abb. 1). Es wurde gefunden, daß unter diesen Bedingungen fast alle untrainierten Ratten eine Dunkelpräferenz zeigen. Das ,,Training", bestehend aus mehreren 5 sec dauernden Fußschocks, die an 5 aufeinanderfolgenden Tagen während des Aufenthalts der Tiere in der Dunkelkammer gegeben wurden, bewirkt bei den Tieren eine starke Furcht vor dem Betreten des Dunkelraums. So vorbehandelten Tieren wurde das Gehirn entnommen, sofort eingefroren, sodann homogenisiert und hochtourig zentrifugiert. Der dabei erhaltene Überstand wurde als ,,Gehirnextrakt" bezeichnet; Kontrolltiere erhielten einen ebenso bereiteten Extrakt, der aus dem Gehirn naiver Ratten bereitet worden war. Die besten Transfer-Ergebnisse wurden erhalten,

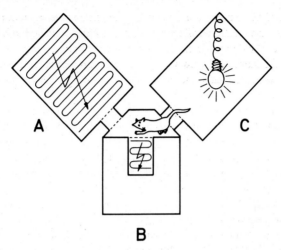

Abb. 1. Apparat zum Ausbilden und Messen der Dunkelfurcht von Ratten

wenn eine 0,2-Gehirnäquivalenten entsprechende Extraktmenge an, bezüglich ihres Hell-Dunkelverhaltens vorgetestete Ratten, i.p. injiziert wurde. Wie Abb. 2 zeigt, wurde bei den Empfängern „trainierter Hirnextrakte" eine signifikante, etwa 1 Woche anhal-

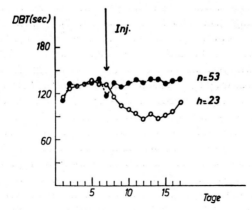

Abb. 2. Bei Ratten durch i.p. Injektion von Gehirnextrakt (0,2 Hirn-äquivalente) hervorgerufene Dunkelfurcht. ● Empfänger von Kontroll-extrakten; ○ Empfänger von „trainiertem Extrakt"

tende Verminderung der Dunkelpräferenz gefunden, während die Empfänger von Kontrollextrakten im allgemeinen keine Veränderung ihres Verhaltens zeigten. Ungewöhnlich ist die Dosis-Wirkungs-Abhängigkeit, die in Abb. 3 aufgezeichnet ist: Die beste

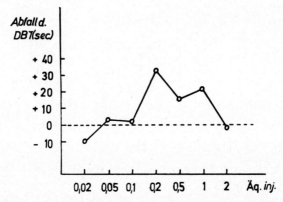

Abb. 3. Dosisabhängigkeit der übertragenen Dunkelfurcht. Abszisse: i.p. verabfolgte Hirnäquivalente. Ordinate: Verkürzung des Aufenthalts im Dunkeln (DBT) bei Versuchsdauer von 180 sec

Wirkung der Extrakte war zu beobachten, wenn 0,2 — 1 Gehirnäquivalente i.p. verabfolgt wurden. Eine solche ungewöhnliche Dosisabhängigkeit hat Rosenblatt [Proc. nat. Acad. Sci. (Wash.) **64**, 661 (1969)] auch bei andersartigen Transfer-Versuchen beschrieben. Da die Wirksamkeit der Gehirnextrakte nach kurzfristiger Inkubation mit Pronase aufgehoben ist, kann man annehmen, daß es sich bei diesen wirksamen Extrakten, wie bei dem Ungarschen Scotophobin, um eine Polypeptid handelt (Abb. 4).

1969—1971 hat der Amerikaner Levan [Experientia (Basel) **26**, 648 (1970)] in mehreren Arbeiten die Transferierbarkeit einer Röntgenstrahl-induzierten Geschmacksaversion beschrieben. Die Unterdrückung einer angeborenen Geschmackspräferenz durch eine einmalige Röntgenbestrahlung war erstmalig von Garcia [Science **122**, 157 (1955)] beobachtet worden. Gibt man einer Maus nach 20stündiger Durstperiode für 30 min das spontan bevorzugte Saccharin zu trinken, unmittelbar gefolgt von einer Bestrahlung mit 400 r, so rühren die Tiere in der Folgezeit wochenlang nicht mehr das Saccharin an, sondern trinken Wasser (Abb. 5). Durch Verwendung von sowohl Saccharin wie Äthanol gegenüber Wasser bevorzugenden C 57 Bl-Mäusen konn-

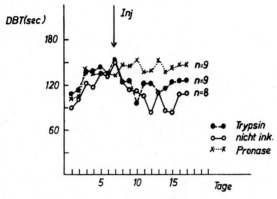

Abb. 4. Inaktivierung der Dunkelfurcht-induzierenden Hirnextrakte durch Inkubation mit Pronase

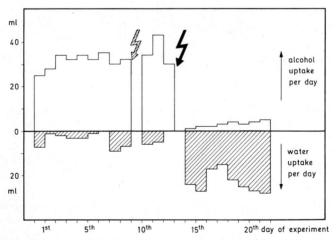

Abb. 5.   Röntgenstrahlbedingte Aversion gegen Trinken von Alkohol. 10 Mäuse wurden zusammen am 9. und 13. Versuchstag auf Durst gesetzt. 30 min vor der nachfolgenden Bestrahlung wurde 10% Äthanol, aber kein Wasser gegeben. ⚡ Scheinbestrahlung ⚡ Gabe von 450 r

ten wir zeigen, daß die Röntgen-bedingte Umstellung reiz-
spezifisch erfolgt: nur der unmittelbar von der Bestrahlung
gegebene Geschmacksreiz wird in der Folgezeit abgelehnt, andere
Präferenzen bleiben bestehen (Abb. 6).

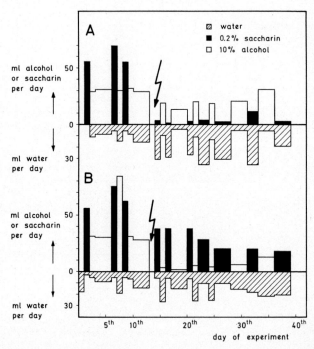

Abb. 6. Spezifität der Röntgen-induzierten Geschmacksaversion. 2 Mäuse-
gruppen (je 10 Tiere) erhielten alternierend Wasser und Saccharin bzw. Wasser und 10% Äthanol geboten. Trinkpause am 13. Tag. Nach 24 Std Durst
erhielt Gruppe A für 30 min nur Saccharin, Gruppe B nur Äthanol. Beide
Tiergruppen erhielten dann 450 r und an den Folgetagen wieder alternierend
Wasser/Saccharin bzw. Wasser/Äthanol

Zu unseren diesbezüglichen Transferversuchen haben wir bei
Saccharin trinkenden NMRI/HAN-Mäusen eine Saccharin-Aversion
durch s.c. Injektion von 50 μg Apomorphin erzeugt. 24 Std nach
der dadurch bedingten Umstellung der Geschmackspräferenzen
(es wird jetzt Wasser statt Saccharin getrunken) wurden den
Spender- und Kontrolltieren die Gehirne entnommen. Sofort

schloß sich dann folgender Arbeitsgang an: Homogenisieren, Zentrifugieren, Dialysieren und Gefriertrocknen. Das lyophilisierte Dialysat, also niedermolekulare Hirnbestandteile, wurde in die Gehirnventrikel vorgetesteter Empfängertiere injiziert. Abbildung 7 zeigt

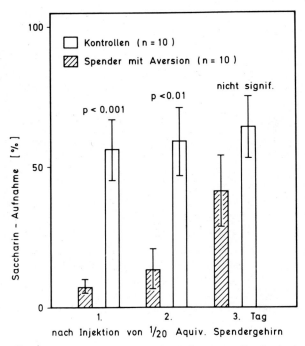

Abb. 7. Übertragung einer Apomorphin-induzierten Saccharin-Aversion durch intraventrikuläre Injektion von Gehirnextrakten

einen sehr gut gelungenen, von Frau Dr. Kübler durchgeführten Versuch, bei dem die Empfängertiere von „Sacchararin-Aversions-Extrakt" 2 Tage lang eine signifikante Saccharinaversion zeigten, während die Empfänger von Kontrollgehirn-Extrakten weiterhin Saccharin tranken.

Zwei in der Folgezeit durchgeführte Versuche mit größeren Tierzahlen hatten ein eindeutig negatives Ergebnis: hier hatten auch alle Empfänger von „Kontrollgehirnextrakt" ihre Saccharin-Präferenz aufgegeben. Inzwischen sind uns die Bedingungen, unter denen der Effekt reproduzierbar ist, bekannt; möglicherweise handelt es sich nicht um den Transfer einer „erlernten" Geschmacksaversion. Wenn man die von AGRANOFF erwähnte Abhängigkeit des Lernverhaltens von der Jahreszeit oder die von ROSENBLATT beschriebene Abhängigkeit des Transfer-Erfolgs von der Menge der injizierten Extraktmenge vor Augen hat, so wird die Schwierigkeit derartiger Versuche erkennbar.

Da manchmal der Vorwurf erhoben wird, Transfer-Effekte seien fast immer nur bei Vermeidens-Reaktionen beschrieben worden, so versuchen wir seit einiger Zeit, ein operantes Verhalten zu übertragen. Diese, von meinem Mitarbeiter LAUFENBERG (Dissertation, Mediz. Fak., Göttingen; in Vorbereitung) angestellten, Versuche an Mäusen, die bei Ertönen eines Summerzeichens den Futtertrog verlassen und in die andere Käfighälfte überwechseln müssen, um einen Fußschock zu vermeiden, sind ganz ermutigend. Zur Publikation fehlen aber bislang noch die wichtigsten Kontrollversuche mit Normalgehirnen.

Hin und wieder wird die Frage gestellt, ob es rein von der substantiellen Kapazität her denn möglich sei, daß man die im Laufe eines Lebens gesammelten Erfahrungen in Form chemischer Verbindungen mit sich trage. Wenn wir vereinfachend rechnen, daß ein Mensch 100 Jahre alt werde und daß jedes Jahr 1000 Tage habe, so ergibt das eine Lebensspanne von 10^5 Tagen. Würde unser „Normalmensch" nun an jedem seiner Tage 100 im Langzeitgedächtnis zu fixierende Eindrücke sammeln, so benötigte er dafür 10^7 „Gedächtnismoleküle". Würden diese Substanzen in Gestalt von mittelkettigen Peptiden (ca. 10 Aminosäuren, somit Molekulargewicht etwa 1000) vorliegen, so käme man, wenn von jeder dieser Substanzen 1 Nanomol gespeichert wäre, auf eine Peptidmenge von 10 g, eine Größenordnung also, die durchaus diskutiert werden kann. Nach der derzeit im wesentlichen von UNGAR vertretenen Hypothese sollen diese Peptide lernabhängig die funktionelle Zusammenschaltung zahlreicher Nervenzellen des Gehirns bewirken.

Discussion

E. GROSS (Bethesda, Md.): If scotophobin transfers learned dark avoidance — as you say it does — how does it do it? What is the mode of action in the animal to which you administer the peptide? Is there a concept for the sequence of events following the injection of scotophobin?

G. F. DOMAGK: No — there is not, so far. The only thing which is known is that even by i.p. injection the scotophobin reaches the brain. There has been one experiment in which synthetic scotophobin was labeled with radioactive iodine. But there is no explanation so far as to whether it acts on the synapse or what is the mechanism of action of these "memory molecules".

B. W. AGRANOFF (Ann Arbor, Mich.): This remark is directed not at you, but at the area of memory transfer in general. It is a case where fewer experiments would be more impressive than more. That is to say, I find it puzzling to see a number of positive experiments, none of which have been pursued biochemically. This leads me to suspect that the actual experimental findings are insufficiently robust for use as a test system, hence the continued search. Why do you not exploit any one of the systems you have presented?

G. F. DOMAGK: I think that is right. We ourselves did not want to embark upon the scotophobin story after it has been elaborated by UNGAR, and it does not seem worthwhile to extract another scotophobin peptide. But we are still screening for procedures, and as soon as we have one which gives reliable and reproducible results, we will continue on this and hope to make it also work in the hands of other researchers.

Epilogue

L. Jaenicke

Institut für Biochemie der Universität Köln, 5 Köln 1, An der Bottmühle 2,
Federal Republic of Germany

When I first proposed the theme of this symposium, it was with the throught in mind that we biochemists cannot too often be reminded of the origins of our craft, and I therefore welcomed the opportunity of once again blending biochemistry with physiology. Biochemists and biophysicists have tended to drift away from biology and physiology, and this has resulted in a biased, almost sterile *l'art pour l'art* attitude against the "old-fashioned" approach that embraced whole areas of the natural sciences. This deplorable situation is also reflected by physiologists, who often assume a truculent, if not hostile stance when biochemists try to invade their ivory towers with molecular explanations of physiological phenomena. Obviously, the long-term effects of such reductionist behavior are regrettable and harmful for all life sciences.

I had hoped to enjoy the passive role of listener and hear first-hand, detailed accounts of research in a field that is not my own, but that has captivated my attenion and imagination for many years. However, things turned out differently. I was charged with the honorable but nevertheless nerve-wracking task of organizing this, the 25th Mosbacher Colloquium. As it was a Jubilee-Symposium, I thought it appropriate to "celebrate the feasts as they fall". I was able to compose the program contained in this book thanks to the largesse of the Directing Board of the Gesellschaft für Biologische Chemie, thanks to private and public Maecenates, thanks, too, to my colleagues — in alphabetic order — Drs. R. Jaenicke, K.-E. Kaissling, H. Stieve, and U. Thurm, for their kind advice and helpful piloting when my heavily loaded ship threatened to run aground. Last but not least, my thanks go out to all the speakers and guests for their cooperation, without which the whole event would not have been possible.

In order to achieve continuity, I asked some of the speakers to deliver broad and introductory accounts of the state of their research fields, while more detailed accounts were requested from other speakers. I sought to admix a good deal of membrane and sensory physiology into a basically biochemical symposium, and hoped so to encourage the presentation of fruitful, well-founded models and speculations bridging the gap between "jump and juice". Still, it is beyond my competence to weigh, evaluate and summarize the work presented during this Mosbach Colloquium on the *Biochemistry of Sensory Functions*. We have heard of the development of our knowledge on the structure and function of visual energy transformation and of exciting recent trends in research on chemoreception and chemotaxis. We have been given an experimental basis for new and stimulating thoughts on the transformation of sensory inputs into energy stimuli and their biophysical integration into a "searching" hypothesis, the heuristic value of which will, I hope, become evident in the near future. Finally, we were given a timely warning to be critical about unduly simplistic explanations in such a complex filed as the biochemistry of the senses, and reminded not to neglect checks and controls. I thank all the speakers, who cooperated with my request to be temperate and timely and not to be led astray by their enthusiasm for their own exciting work, but to fit it into the general frame of the perception, transmission, transformation and storage of signals from without and within. This has made this year's Mosbach Colloquium — following its five-and-twenty years' tradition — more than just a punctual affair, but a refresher course and a stimulating review of one of the most interesting lines of research in the borderline field that stretches between biochemistry, biophysics, and pharmacology — to coin a polysyllable, the field of molecular biodynamics.

A colloquium is a forum of discussion. Therefore, thanks are due to the discussants, who helped to clarify and to round up some topics with their questions and remarks; thanks are also due to the speakers, who sometimes answered and commented in a hilarious *extempore* manner, thus providing the informal atmosphere that is required for a fruitful dialogue.

A symposium is a hospitable meeting, and this it was in the traditional surroundings of the town of Mosbach, thanks to the hospitality of its citizens.

Finally I have to thank Professor E. AUHAGEN for his saintly patience, the secretaries of the Gesellschaft für Biologische Chemie, Mmes. J. LAHMANN, U. LAUENSTEIN, and E. MERTENS for their unfailing coordinative efforts and, last but certainly not least, my coworkers, Dr. G. BÄHR, Miss U. KLEIN, Messrs. J. N. HOWELL, J.-C. JÉSIOR, F.-J. MARNER, and K. SEFERIADES for helping with the behind-the-scences drudgery and providing the electronic know-how.

With the help of all involved, this book provides a black-and-white reminder to those who attended the 25th Mosbach Colloquium and should give its prospective readers sufficient information of more than ephemeral interest — if only to give a benchmark for evaluating the progress, which, let us hope, will not fail to come, in the biochemistry of sensory functions.

Springer-Verlag Berlin Heidelberg New York

Biochemistry and Physiology of Visual Pigments

Symposium Held at Institut für Tierpsychologie,
Ruhr-Universität Bochum / W.Germany,
August 27–30, 1972
For the Organizing Committee
Edited by Helmut Langer
With 202 figures. XIII, 366 pages. 1973
Cloth DM 38,–; US $15.50
ISBN 3-540-06204-1

Contents: Pigment Structure and Chemical Properties. Photolysis and Intermediates of the Pigments.
Regeneration of the Pigments. Excitation and Adaptation of Photoreceptor Cells. Ionic Aspects of Excitation and Regeneration. Enzymology and Molecular
Architecture of the Light Sensitive Membrane.

Information Processing in the Visual Systems of Arthropods

Symposium Held at the Department of Zoology,
University of Zurich, March 6–9, 1972
Edited by R. Wehner
With 263 figures. XI, 334 pages. 1972
DM 40,–; US $16.40
ISBN 3-540-06020-0

Contents: Anatomy of the Visual System. Optics of
the Compound Eye. Biochemistry of Visual Pigments.
Intensity – Dependent Reactions. Wavelength –
Dependent Reactions. Pattern Recognition. Visual
Control of Orientation Patterns. Storage of Visual
Information. Methods of Quantifying Behavioral Data.

Prices are subject to change without notice

Handbook
of Sensory Physiology
Outline

Distribution rights for India:
UBS, New Delhi

For further information
please ask for special leaflets

Springer-Verlag
Berlin
Heidelberg
New York